Fourth Edition

EXERCISE PHYSIOLOGY

LABORATORY MANUAL

Gene M. Adams

California State University
Fullerton

McGraw Hill

Boston   Burr Ridge, IL   Dubuque, IA   Madison, WI   New York   San Francisco   St. Louis
Bangkok   Bogotá   Caracas   Kuala Lumpur   Lisbon   London   Madrid   Mexico City
Milan   Montreal   New Delhi   Santiago   Seoul   Singapore   Sydney   Taipei   Toronto

McGraw-Hill Higher Education

A Division of The **McGraw-Hill** Companies

EXERCISE PHYSIOLOGY LABORATORY MANUAL, FOURTH EDITION

Published by McGraw-Hill, a business unit of The McGraw-Hill Companies, Inc., 1221 Avenue of the Americas, New York, NY 10020. Copyright © 2002, 1998, 1994, 1991 by The McGraw-Hill Companies, Inc. All rights reserved. No part of this publication may be reproduced or distributed in any form or by any means, or stored in a database or retrieval system, without the prior written consent of The McGraw-Hill Companies, Inc., including, but not limited to, in any network or other electronic storage or transmission, or broadcast for distance learning.

Some ancillaries, including electronic and print components, may not be available to customers outside the United States.

 This book is printed on recycled, acid-free paper containing 10% postconsumer waste.

2 3 4 5 6 7 8 9 0 QPD/QPD 0 9 8 7 6 5 4 3 2

ISBN 0–07–232903–3

Vice president and editor-in-chief: *Thalia Dorwick*
Publisher: *Jane Karpacz*
Executive editor: *Vicki Malinee*
Developmental editor: *Carlotta Seely*
Senior marketing manager: *Pamela S. Cooper*
Project manager: *Richard H. Hecker*
Production supervisor: *Sherry L. Kane*
Designer: *K. Wayne Harms*
Cover/interior designer: *Rokusek Design*
Cover image: *Robert Llewellyn/SuperStock*
Senior supplement producer: *Tammy Juran*
Media technology producer: *Judi David*
Compositor: *Shepherd, Inc.*
Typeface: *10/12 Times*
Printer: *Quebecor World Dubuque, IA*

Library of Congress Cataloging-in-Publication Data

Adams, Gene M.
    Exercise physiology laboratory manual / Gene M. Adams. — 4th ed.
        p.   cm.
    Includes bibliographical references and index.
    ISBN 0–07–232903–3
    1. Exercise—Physiological aspects—Laboratory manuals. I. Title.

QP301 .A244   2002
612'.044—dc21   2001044673
                                                 CIP

The Internet addresses listed in the text were accurate at the time of publication. The inclusion of a website does not indicate an endorsement by the authors or McGraw-Hill, and McGraw-Hill does not guarantee the accuracy of the information presented at these sites.

www.mhhe.com

CONTENTS

PREFACE

The fourth edition of *Exercise Physiology Laboratory Manual* is faithful to its original objective of familiarizing students with many of the basic laboratory procedures and tests in exercise physiology. It is designed to complement the typical exercise physiology lecture course. No single manual can be an exhaustive survey of all laboratory tests or experiments in this field.

The field and laboratory experiences are designed to reinforce the basic principles learned in the lecture course and to teach the fundamental principles and skills of measurement and evaluation in the field of exercise physiology. Although computerized and automated methods facilitate testing, particularly calculations, they often do not provide an optimal understanding of testing principles. Too often, the underlying concepts are lost when all that is required is pressing a "magic button" on an instrument.

Organization

My goal has been to make this manual as generic as possible, so that it is applicable to most exercise physiology laboratories. The framework is flexible enough for instructors to substitute their own tests and equipment, while assuring that laboratory procedures follow the basic principles of testing. Each chapter may stand alone to accommodate flexible scheduling of laboratory sessions.

Part 1, Orientation to Measurement in Exercise Physiology, contains the first three chapters. Chapter 1 (Terminology) begins with the terms that are important for understanding and measuring exercise, such as those related to *fitness, mass, force, work, velocity, power,* and *energy.* It continues with a discussion of meteorological terms, such as *temperature* and *relative humidity.* In addition, the chapter presents some common statistical terms used in exercise physiology, such as *variable, relationship, norms,* and *standards.* Chapter 1 also summarizes the types of tests often associated with fitness and exercise. These are categorized into three types: field, field/laboratory, and laboratory tests. Chapter 2 (Scientific Units of Measure) begins with a discussion of the latest recommendations for the International System of measurement. This logically leads to a comparison of the American and metric systems. The units of these two systems dealing with length, mass, volume, and other concepts presented in the first chapter are discussed with respect to their conversions and precision. Chapter 3 (Collection of Basic Data) includes a discussion of basic data, such as name, date, and gender that are usually required for data collection in all laboratory tests. Measurements of body weight and height introduce students gradually to the scientific approach.

The initial chapters present field and laboratory tests for strength (Part 2) and anaerobic fitness (Part 3). The middle chapters present aerobic fitness tests (Part 4), including cardiovascular (Part 5) and pulmonary (Part 6) tests. Part 7 (Range of Motion) discusses flexibility of the lower trunk. Part 8 (Body Composition) contains chapters on body mass index, girth, skinfolds, and hydrostatic weighing.

New or Expanded Topics

Chapter 1: Terminology
- Biochemical pathways
- Revised fitness vs. time continuum to agree with latest research
- All new figures for fitness continuum

Chapter 2: Scientific Units of Measure
- Latest International System recommendations for units of measure
- International System's spelling and abbreviations
- Barometric pressure

Chapter 3: Collection of Basic Data
- Distinction among mass, force, and weight
- Procedures for measuring stature and body mass
- Improved form for recording stature and body mass

Chapter 4: Dynamic Strength
- Effect of rebounding (bouncing) weight during repetitions
- Distinction between vertical displacement and distance
- Procedures for testing Direct 1 RM

Chapter 5: Static Strength
- Procedures for adjusting grip size and number of trials
- Accuracy of grip strength testing
- Calibration of grip dynamometers
- New figure: posture and Lafayette dynamometer

Chapter 6: Isokinetic Strength
- Peak torque
- Fiber typing
- Eccentric testing and significance
- Leg strength vs. injury incidence
- Accuracy of isokinetic testing with various machines

Chapter 7: "Horizontal Power"—Sprinting
- Physiological rationale of sprint
- Effect of sprint-training
- Accuracy of sprint tests
- Biomechanics of sprinting
- New figure: run velocity vs. time curve

Chapter 8: Vertical Power—Jumping
- Bases of countermovement jumping
- Electronic measure of vertical power
- Summary of procedures (steps)
- Absolute vs. relative power

Chapter 9: Anaerobic Cycling
- Accuracy of Wingate Cycle Test
- Easy-to-follow calculations of power and work
- New figures: graph of metabolic contributions; weight cycle ergometer; graphic relationship between power and time

Chapter 10: Anaerobic Stepping
- Physiological rationale
- Accuracy of test results

Philosophical Approach

My philosophical approach to learning laboratory procedures is consistent with the following quote.

> A learner does not act without thinking and feeling, or think without acting and feeling, or feel without acting or thinking.[a]

This means that teachers encourage students to be *active* during the laboratory session and to *feel* what it is like to be tested and to administer tests. Then teachers encourage students to *think* about their actions and feelings, so students can truly *know* the topic.

Acknowledgments

This manual is a fruitful combination of the "knowing" given to me by my former teachers, role models, colleagues, and students. My first teacher, the late Dr. Larry Morehouse, introduced me to exercise physiology and contributed to the framework for building my future knowledge in this field. My second teacher, Dr. Herbert deVries, contributed to my technical and research skills, while enhancing my knowledge and encouraging my involvement in the profession. My role model, Dr. Fred Kasch, showed me how to apply what I knew to the general public and to students. These three men contributed to my admiration for all pioneers of exercise physiology and to my excitement about exercise physiology. I am grateful to my colleagues from all parts of the country, such as Dr. William Beam, Dr. Ronald Deitrick, Dr. James Hodgdon, and Dr. Robert Ruhling, who contributed their encouragement and ideas. Thanks go to these professionals who reviewed this manual: Cheryl J. Cohen, Western Illinois University; Sheri Colberg, Old Dominion University; Patricia Pierce, Slippery Rock University; Robert O. Ruhling, George Mason University; Robert D. Weathers, Seattle Pacific University; Loretta Quinnan Wilson, Tulane University; Frank B. Wyatt, Wichita State University.

A big thank-you goes to my wife, Janet, the illustrator for this book, and to my son, Mannie, and my daughter, Shawn, who served as my wife's models. Finally, thanks and appreciation go to all my students for their enthusiasm, which continues to inspire me.

---

[a]Barrow, H. M., & McGee, R. (1971). *A practical approach to measurement in physical education* (p. 145). Philadelphia: Lea & Febiger.

ORIENTATION TO MEASUREMENT IN EXERCISE PHYSIOLOGY

Persons who are tested in an exercise physiology laboratory are usually there for more than one reason. They may wish to evaluate[2]

- Their functional capacity, whether it is for athletics, recreation, occupation, or routine daily tasks
- The safety of their exercise and work roles
- The effects of any interventions, such as diet, exercise, and medications
- Their future (prognosis) status with respect to morbidity and mortality

The laboratory investigators, clinicians, and technicians are there to serve the needs of the participants, but they also gather research that may lead to better understanding of exercise, which they or others can use to develop more effective health and fitness programs. Also, the laboratory personnel are hopeful that the testing will increase the motivation of their clients or participants.

The students in an exercise physiology laboratory class are usually there to enhance their understanding of the content presented in the exercise physiology lecture class. Students typically like to apply their learning to their personal lives. Fortunately, a laboratory experience that complements the classroom topics can be an effective motivational method. Students may be doubly motivated if these laboratory experiences include both their acute effects of exercise and their fitness evaluations.

Students of exercise science can be assured of the importance of an education in exercise science laboratories by knowing that the field's professional organizations also affirm their importance. For example, the Exercise Science Council of the National Association for Sport and Physical Education (NASPE) states that students of exercise science are expected to "demonstrate the use of (1) health and fitness field and laboratory instruments, (2) techniques, [and] (3) procedures . . . ."[22] The council asserts that, in conjunction with this basic standard, students should be able to "evaluate and interpret exercise testing results." The logical first step in acquiring such abilities for the exercise physiology student is to master the scientific language, or terminology, of physiological testing.

The beginning student of exercise physiology is introduced to many new terms and often is exposed to unfamiliar measuring units. If these are not mastered early, the performance tests administered in a laboratory course of exercise physiology will have little meaning. It would be similar to studying a new subject written or taught in a foreign language. Former editors of the highly respected journal *Medicine and Science in Sports and Exercise* emphasized the importance of standardizing terminology and measuring units in the field of exercise physiology.[14,33,52,53] The terms and units presented in *Exercise Physiology Laboratory Manual* are faithful to these editors' recommendations.

Familiarization with the terms and units of exercise science helps students administer appropriate tests, record the results, and interpret the results. Similarly, the collection of data reinforces this learning. Collecting basic data and measuring the environmental conditions are the best places to start in learning the principles of data collection. Students are already familiar with most of the terms that define basic data, such as *name, date, time, gender, age, height (stature), and weight (mass).* The recording of basic data and environmental conditions is a part of every variable's data collection form in this manual. Thus, I have placed it in Chapter 3 as the first data collection experience in the manual.

TERMINOLOGY

Many of the terms used to orient the beginning student in a course of exercise physiology laboratory may be organized into the following seven categories: (1) fitness, (2) measurement, (3) meteorological, (4) statistical, (5) calibration, (6) types of tests, and (7) research abstract terms.

Fitness Terms

Familiarization with fitness terms is essential for understanding the measurement of physical performance. Performance is often related to a person's fitness. One simple definition of physical fitness is "the ability to carry out physical activities satisfactorily."[27] Because the term *satisfactorily* has many interpretations, it behooves kinesiologists to describe fitness more precisely in order to make the appropriate fitness measure. One perspective is to view fitness as having various components. Some of the health-related components of fitness can be placed into time-continuum models.

Health-Related Fitness

Fitness and health are not the same. For example, the exercise recommendation of the American College of Sports Medicine (ACSM) and the American Heart Association for improving cardiovascular *fitness* (cardiorespiratory endurance)[49] has a higher minimum intensity of exercise than their recommendation for improving cardiovascular *health*[10,24,48] or longevity.[45] Regardless of the differences between fitness and health, five traditional fitness components (Table 1.1) are often classified as health-related fitness components:[2]

- Strength
- Muscular endurance or muscle endurance
- Cardiorespiratory endurance or cardiovascular endurance
- Flexibility
- Body composition or morphological fitness

These supposedly independent fitness components are directed not only at exercise performance but also at diseases (e.g., cardiovascular) or functional disabilities (e.g., obesity, musculoskeletal pain) associated with hypokinetic (low activity) lifestyles. Table 1.1 gives examples of traditional health-related fitness components that are frequently measured outside the exercise physiology laboratory (field test) and inside the laboratory ("lab" test).

Fitness-Time Continuums

Models using time continuums enhance our understanding of fitness terms. A time continuum means that fitness components can be categorized across a continuous time line from zero seconds to infinity. I present two models of continuums—one that emphasizes the three health-related fitness components of strength, muscular endurance, and cardiorespiratory endurance; and one that emphasizes the bioenergetic pathways of strength-power, power-endurance, mixed endurance, and cardiorespiratory endurance. Both continuums use time measured in units of seconds (s), minutes (min), or hours (h). The continuums base each fitness component upon a performer's time for sustaining a maximal effort at an optimal pace. Thus, the continuum relies upon the performers to make their best effort over the given time zone of the continuum. A runner, swimmer, or cyclist, for example, would be expected to travel as far as possible for any given time within the allotted time zone for each fitness category.

Time Continuum for Health-Related Fitness

Table 1.1 and Figure 1.1 show that the general fitness-versus-time relationship is faithful to most tests that measure strength, muscular endurance, and cardiorespiratory endurance. For example, it usually takes about 5 s or less for a person to perform most strength tests, such as a maximal lift of one repetition (1 RM)[42] or a maximal static force[40] or isokinetic force.[1] It may take up to 15 s to perform most power tests (a combination of strength and speed), such as short sprints, repetitive jumps, or repetitive heavy lifts. It usually takes no more than 2 min for a young adult to perform most traditional muscular endurance tests, such as sit-ups, pushups, or a run of four hundred meters (m). It usually takes 2 min or more to perform most cardiorespiratory endurance tests.

Although *muscular endurance* has been the popular term for short, sustained efforts and the term *cardiorespiratory endurance* has been popular for longer efforts, we should recognize that cardiorespiratory endurance also requires the endurance of the muscular system. Although I prefer the term *power endurance* instead of *muscular endurance,* I will use the term occasionally due to its overwhelming popularity. The two other traditional health-related components of fitness—flexibility and body composition—cannot be categorized meaningfully

Table 1.1 Traditional Health-Related Fitness Components and Examples of Their Measurement in Field Testing and Laboratory Testing

Health-Related Fitness Components	Measurement Examples	
	Field Testing	**Laboratory Testing**
Strength	Maximal lift (e.g., 1 RM Test)	Peak torque (e.g., isokinetic dynamometry)
Muscular endurance (or muscle endurance)	Timed repetitions (e.g., sit-ups)	Mean power (e.g., Wingate cycle ergometry)
Cardiorespiratory endurance (or cardiovascular endurance)	Timed distance (e.g., 1.5-mile run)	Maximal oxygen consumption (e.g., graded exercise test)
Flexibility	Linear range of motion (e.g., sit-and-reach)	Degrees range of motion (e.g., Leighton flexometry)
Body composition (or morphological fitness)	Height-weight relationship (e.g., body mass index)	Lean-fat relationship (e.g., hydrostatic weighing)

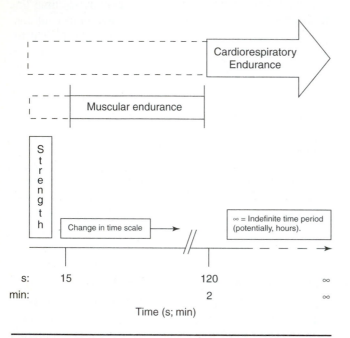

Figure 1.1 Three of the traditional health-related fitness components are related to approximate time zones. Strength contributes to activities requiring maximal forces and power lasting for several seconds (s). Muscular endurance often describes the type of fitness for activities that can be continued longer than about 15 s but usually not longer than 2 min. Cardiorespiratory endurance often describes fitness for activities that can be continued longer than 2 min.

into this health-related time continuum of fitness. Perhaps body composition is an expected *by-product* of a person's participation in the activities that relate to the time-designated fitness components.

Bioenergetic-Time Continuum of Fitness

One problem with relating three of the traditional health-related fitness components—strength, muscular endurance, and cardiorespiratory endurance—to the time zones in Figure 1.1 is that significant fitness differences exist within each designated time zone. Hence, more specific terminology may be applied to a fitness-time continuum by subdi-

viding the time zones based on physiological factors, especially bioenergetic (metabolic) factors. Thus, identifying more specific fitness components leads to more valid testing and training procedures (Table 1.2, Figure 1.2, Figure 1.3).

The bioenergetic-time continuum approximates the classification of exercise or fitness based on the various analyses of world-record running events[30,51,59,61,62,64] and reports of the associated predominant bioenergetic systems.[12,13,21,25,36,37,44,50,59,60,62,65,70] Mathematical models of running records contribute surprisingly consistent data, which help validate the bioenergetic-time continuum of fitness.[69] The continuum's four major fitness components based on bioenergetic pathways are

- Strength/power
- Power-endurance
- Mixed endurance
- Cardiorespiratory endurance (Aerobic fitness)

The aerobic fitness component is further divided into short aerobic and long aerobic components, whereby the latter considers nutritional and hydration factors.

From the bioenergetic point of view, exercise and fitness may be categorized based upon the predominant metabolic pathways for producing adenosine triphosphate (ATP) (Table 1.2). The anaerobic pathway is a high-power system producing ATP at high rates, but it is a low-capacity system producing ATP in relatively small amounts. The aerobic pathway, which traditionally is viewed as responsible for cardiorespiratory endurance, is just the opposite of the anaerobic pathway; it is a low-power but high-capacity system.

Again, it is important to remember that the time ranges for the bioenergetic-time continuum are based upon maximal efforts at optimal paces. As an example of a submaximal effort, if performers slowly walked for 30 s they would begin by using predominantly the phosphagenic pathway for a few seconds. However, by the end of the 30 s walking period, they would have used the oxidative pathway to produce most of the ATP, and not by using the phosphagen and glycolytic pathways of anaerobic metabolism. Thus, the oxidative pathway would be the predominant pathway for this low-intensity submaximal effort despite the short

Table 1.2 Subdivisions of the Bioenergetic-Time Continuum of Fitness Based on the Predominant Bioenergetic Pathways for the Production of Adenosine Triphosphate (ATP)

Fitness Category	Bioenergetic Pathway	Time Period
	Anaerobic	≈ 1 s – ≈ 60 s
Strength/power (power includes speed)	Phosphagenic	≤ 15 s
Power-endurance (sustaining power and speed)		
	Phosphagenic and glycolytic	≈ 15 s – ≈ 60 s
	Ph ≈ Gly	≈ 15 s – ≈ 30 s
	Glycolytic > Ph	≈ 30 s – ≈ 60 s
		≈ 0.5 min – ≈ 1 min
Mixed endurance (muscle and cardiorespiratory endurance)	**Anaerobic and aerobic** Glycolytic and oxidative	≈ 60 s – ≈ 120 s ≈ 1 min – ≈ 2 min
Cardiorespiratory endurance[a]	**Aerobic**	≥ 120 s (≥ 2 min)
Short-aerobic	Oxidative (mitochondrial respiration[b])	≈ 2 min – ≈ 60 min
Long-aerobic	Oxidative + euhydration[c] + proper nutrition	≥ 60 min[d]

Note: The symbol ≈ means "approximately." [a]In all but the elite aerobic athlete, the term *cardiorespiratory endurance* reflects muscle mitochondrial respiration as a single limiting factor more than it reflects the respiratory system (e.g., ventilation). [b]The term *mitochondrial respiration* is technically more accurate because anaerobic glycolysis contributes some ATP during "aerobic" exercise.[56] [c]The term *euhydration* means "normal balance of fluid." [d]The time criterion for the hydration factor of long-aerobic fitness varies with the environmental temperature and relative humidity.

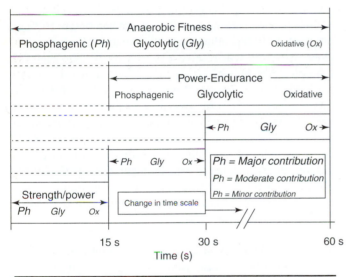

Figure 1.2 The bioenergetic-time continuum of anaerobic fitness relates strength/power and power-endurance to time and the bioenergetic pathways for producing ATP. For strength/power fitness (≤ 15 s) the phosphagenic (*Ph;* largest italics) is the major ATP producer, with the glycolytic (*Gly;* moderate italics) pathway making a moderate contribution and the oxidative (*Ox;* smallest italics) pathway making a minor contribution. From about the 15th s to the 30th s of power-endurance fitness, the phosphagenic and glycolytic make moderate contributions, whereas the oxidative pathway makes a minor contribution. From about the 30th s to the 60th s of power-endurance activities, the glycolytic pathway is the major contributor, with the oxidative pathway making a moderate contribution and the phosphagenic pathway making a minor contribution.

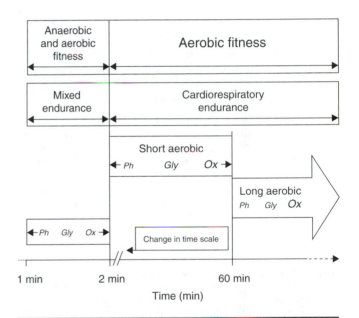

Figure 1.3 The bioenergetic-time continuum of mixed anaerobic/aerobic fitness and of aerobic fitness relates mixed endurance and cardiorespiratory endurance to time and the bioenergetic pathways for producing ATP. For anaerobic/aerobic fitness (1 min to 2 min), the glycolytic (*Gly;* moderate italics) and oxidative (*Ox;* moderate italics) pathways are the major ATP producers, with the phosphagenic (*Ph;* smallest italics) pathway making a minor contribution. From about the 2nd min to the 60th min of short-aerobic cardiorespiratory endurance, the phosphagenic makes a minor contribution and the glycolytic makes a moderate contribution, whereas the oxidative pathway makes a major contribution. Beyond the 60th min, the oxidative pathway remains the major ATP contributor, whereas the glycolytic and phosphagenic pathways are minor contributors. Hydration and nutrition are also major considerations for long-aerobic fitness.

duration of 30 s. Conversely, if a person sprints all-out for 30 s, then the sprinter relies mainly on the phosphagenic and glycolytic systems as predominant producers of the total ATP. A basic tenet of the continuum is that performers must pace themselves optimally. Thus, they must not run the first several seconds as fast as possible, or jog the first several seconds, but run at an optimal speed throughout the performance. The goal is to cover the longest distance within a given time period.

The bioenergetic pathways are metabolic paths that are responsible for providing the energy substance adenosine triphosphate (ATP) for muscle action. As noted in Table 1.2 and Figures 1.2 and 1.3, the two major metabolic pathways—aerobic and anaerobic—produce this useable ATP chemical energy, so that the muscles can transfer it to mechanical energy (movement). The broad categories of anaerobic metabolism and aerobic metabolism have been determined routinely by direct measurement of oxygen consumption combined with the estimation of either accumulated oxygen deficit[38,62] (a relatively new laboratory method) or oxygen debt (an older laboratory method). The subdivisions of anaerobic metabolism—phosphagenic and glycolytic—have been harder to decipher and require technical procedures beyond the scope of this text. For example, directly measured phosphagen stores require a detailed biopsy analysis of a muscle sample[12] or a radioactive isotope of phosphorus combined with magnetic resonance spectroscopy.[25] Until the newer research methodologies provide more data, it is somewhat presumptuous to assign specific time zones to the continuum's anaerobic fitness components. Nevertheless, I present a model for a bioenergetic continuum with approximate designations that might enhance our general understanding of exercise and fitness. I have modified the fitness time zones presented in former editions of the laboratory manual due to some of the more recent studies[12,59,61,62,69] showing a greater contribution of the aerobic pathway than that which was traditionally accepted.

Anaerobic Pathway The anaerobic pathway is the predominant producer of ATP for movements requiring strength and power in addition to activities related to power-endurance. The **phosphagenic** predominates for **strength and power** movements requiring immediate maximal efforts of several seconds (e.g., ≤ 15 s).[13] The force of these movements also depends upon the muscle mass and neuromuscular recruitment.

The **phosphagenic** and **glycolytic pathways** contribute substantially to sustaining **power-endurance** activities that last from approximately 15 s to 30 s. Long sprinters, for example, who have improved their power-endurance fitness will be able to sustain faster running speeds for distances ranging between 150 m and 250 m. Power-endurance actions receive most of their energy from two bioenergetic pathways: (1) fast phosphagenic resynthesis of ATP by combining two adenosine diphosphate molecules[13,56] and by splitting phosphocreatine and (2) glycolytic synthesis of ATP from carbohydrates. The closer the exercise duration

comes to 30 s, or the farther from 15 s, the greater becomes the contribution from the glycolytic pathway.

The glycolytic pathway dominates for activities longer than about 30 s to those shorter than approximately 60 s. The nonoxidative system causes performers of these events to accumulate high lactate values due to rapid glycolysis. Although the phosphagenic pathway is not a dominant pathway of the production of ATP for maximally paced activities slightly longer than 30 s, it does contribute a meaningful amount of ATP. The oxidative pathway contributes a meaningful amount of ATP for maximal-effort activities closer to 60 s, but it is not the dominant pathway. However, the glycolytic pathway consistently dominates in its contribution of ATP for this 30 s to 60 s time period.

Mixture of Anaerobic and Aerobic Pathways **Mixed-endurance fitness** is the term for optimally sustained movements lasting between approximately 60 s (1 min) and 120 s (2 min). It relies on substantial contributions from both the aerobic and anaerobic pathways. The ATP contributions of each pathway oscillate above and below 50 % of the total ATP depending upon the duration. Performances closer to 1 min will receive a greater (> 50 %) anaerobic (phosphagenic plus glycolytic) contribution than those all-out performances nearing 2 min, when > 50 % of the contribution comes from the oxidative pathway.[59,62] A typical event for this pathway is the 800 m run in elite runners. As with the predominant glycolytic pathway, the maximal-effort activities of mixed-endurance fitness also cause high lactate values, attesting to the significant contribution of the glycolytic pathway. But, as the *mixed* term implies, successful performance is equally dependent upon the contribution from the aerobic pathway.

Aerobic Pathway **Cardiorespiratory endurance** is dependent upon the aerobic pathway,[a] which is an oxidative pathway that predominates in optimally paced exercise of duration longer than 2 min. It may be divided into two major portions—one, called short-aerobic fitness, from about 2 min to 60 min and another, called long-aerobic fitness, for prolonged efforts greater than 60 min. Long-aerobic tasks still depend on the oxidative pathway but require more consideration of nutritional and hydration factors for successful performance than do the short-aerobic tasks.[5] However, the need for fluids occurs earlier than 60 min when exercising in hot and humid environments.

Summary of Bioenergetic-time Continuum Many of the performance tests presented in this manual may be categorized according to the bioenergetic-time continuum—that is, the predominant metabolic pathway being evaluated by the test (Table 1.3). Flexibility and body composition tests

---

[a]Technically, part of the "aerobic" pathway's production of ATP is from glycolysis, which is nonoxidative.[56]

Table 1.3 Performance Tests Presented in This Laboratory Manual Categorized According to the Predominant Bioenergetic Fitness Category

Strength (≤ 5 s) (Phosphagenic)	Anaerobic (≤ 60 s)		Anaerobic and Aerobic (60 s–120 s)	Short Aerobic (2 min–60 min)
	Power (≤ 15 s) (Phosphagenic)	Power-Endurance (15 s–60 s) (Phosphagenic-Glycolytic)	Mixed Endurance (Oxidative-Glycolytic)	Cardiorespiratory Endurance (Oxidative)
Dynamic free-weights: Direct 1 RM	Sprints: 40 yd, 50 yd, 60 yd; Indirect 1 RM	Wingate cycle: Mean anaerobic power	Slow treadmill run (most men and some women)	1.0-mile (9 min) run; 1.5-mile (12 min) run
Static dynamometry: Handgrip	Vertical jump; Wingate cycle: Peak anaerobic power	Fast treadmill run (some men, some women)	Anaerobic step	Aerobic step; Åstrand cycle
Isokinetic: Leg extension/flexion:	Fast treadmill run (most women students, some men students)	Slow treadmill run (most women and some men)		Maximal oxygen consumption; Exercise electrocardiogram; Exercise blood pressure; Exercise respiration

Traditional Health-Related Tests Not a Part of a Fitness-Time Continuum

Flexibility: Sit-and-reach

Body composition (Morphological fitness): Stature-weight indexes; girth; skinfolds; hydrodensitometry

are referred to as noncontinuum types of traditional health-related fitness tests.

Measurement Terms

When kinesiologists measure fitness or exercise performance, they usually use such terms as *mass, force, work, velocity, speed, power,* and *energy*. See Appendixes B, C, and D for more examples of measurement terms and their conversions.

Mass (M)

Mass is a basic physical quantity that is defined as the quantity of matter in an object. Under normal acceleration of gravity, mass is equivalent to weight. The base unit of measure for mass or weight is the kilogram (kg).

Force (F)

Force is a term derived from the product of mass and acceleration. It is defined as that which changes or tends to change the state of rest or motion in matter.[4] Thus, muscular activity generates force. Mass and force are two basic quantities that are similar under certain circumstances. For example, there are times when you will use your body weight (mass) as a measure of force in order to calculate your work load or work rate. A person applying a maximal force to a resistance or load, whether it is against gravity or a lever, is displaying the fitness component of strength. Most muscular activity, however, uses submaximal forces.

The intensities of forces applied during exercise are associated with three of the traditional fitness components. In other words, each component can be associated with an estimated range for the percentage of a maximal contraction. Strength, for example, is a health-related fitness component that requires forces at or very near 100 % of maximal. The forces necessary to perform activities associated with muscle endurance have a large range and are less than those required for strength. Based on the relationship between the number of maximal repetitions and one maximal repetition when weight lifting (see Chapter 4) and the approximate amount of time it would take to perform such repetitions, muscular endurance actions may be estimated to require about 40 % to 80 % maximal force. The forces necessary to perform the number of lifts inherent to cardiorespiratory endurance are usually less than 40 % maximal contraction.[16] This model should illustrate how forces can be related to fitness components for some activities—in this case, weight lifting.

Work (w)

Work is derived from the product of two basic quantities—force and length (distance, displacement). Often, work is thought of as the force applied upward *against* gravity for a given displacement (d) or distance (D). This may be classified as positive work ($^+$w), or concentric exercise (Eq. 1.1). For example, the work or exercise performed while ascending steps or running on an up-sloped treadmill is calculated as positive work. Positive work also occurs when exercising on a cycle ergometer. For example, the pendulum-type Monark® cycle ergometer shows clearly the vertical force by the lift of the weight pendulum on the ergometer, in addition to the dial indicator at the top-front panel of the ergometer. When the force is combined with the distance traveled—as measured by an odometer or calculated from the revolutions per minute—then work can be calculated.

$$^+w = F \times D \qquad \text{Eq. 1.1}$$

The work calculated for step tests should consider the negative work ($-$w) or eccentric component. Eccentric exercise represents the muscle action when descending the step. For step-test purposes, negative work is considered to be about one-third of the positive work[2,43] and can be calculated two ways (Eq. 1.2a, 1.2b).

$$\text{Multiplication: } -w = 0.33 \times {^+w} \qquad \text{Eq. 1.2a}$$

$$\text{Division: } -w = {^+w} \div 3 \qquad \text{Eq. 1.2b}$$

The combined components of positive work and negative work constitute total work (w). This combination can be presented either as an addition equation (Eq. 1.3a) or a multiplication equation (Eq. 1.3b). The horizontal component of stepping work, consisting of the back and forth movements, usually is considered when calculating the total energy cost in terms of oxygen consumption.

$$\text{Addition: } w = {^+w} + {^-w} \qquad \text{Eq. 1.3a}$$

$$\text{Multiplication: } w = 1.33 \times {^+w} \qquad \text{Eq. 1.3b}$$

Velocity (v) and Speed

Velocity is the quotient of *displacement* divided by time (d/t), where displacement represents the straight-line distance between your starting point and your ending point (Eq. 1.4a, 1.4b). The layperson often uses the term *velocity* when talking about speed, but, mechanically speaking, speed and velocity are different.[28] **Speed** is the quotient of *distance* divided by time (D/t), where the distance represents the actual length covered (Eq. 1.5). Displacement and distance first appear to be the same thing, but displacement represents how far away the body was at the end of the event from the beginning of the event; it is basically what we commonly call "the distance that the crow flies." For example, batters who hit inside-the-park home runs end up where they started—at home plate. Their displacement was zero; therefore, their average velocity was zero meters per second (m/s; m·s^{-1}). Obviously, they had to run fast. Thus, the more meaningful description uses their *average* speeds (pace) calculated by dividing the distance they covered (minimum of 360 ft or 110 m) by their times.

$$\text{Average } v = d / t \qquad \text{Eq. 1.4a}$$

$$\text{Average } v = d \div t \qquad \text{Eq. 1.4b}$$

$$\text{Average speed} = D / t \qquad \text{Eq. 1.5}$$

The fitness components can be related either to average speed or to maximal velocity based on world-record times for various running events. The reference points for maximal velocity and maximal average speed are often based on the 100 m event, in which runners achieve maximal velocity within 4 s to 6 s, or between 30 m and 50 m[20,68] and might maintain this up to the 11th s.[68] A former world-record holder in the 100 m run reached a maximal velocity of 12.1 m·s^{-1} (27.0 mph) at the 40 m mark, but the average speed over the entire 100 m was slightly less than 10.2 m·s^{-1} (22.8 mph). The average speeds for the other running events, and their associated bioenergetic fitness components are depicted in Figure 1.4 as a percentage of the maximal pace (average speed) for the world record (as of the year 2000) 100 m and 200 m runs. Interestingly, a static muscle action exhibits zero velocity and zero speed because there is no visible movement, thus zero displacement and zero distance.

Power (P)

Power is the term for the *rate* of work. It is the mathematical product of force and velocity.[67] Power can be expressed five ways (Eq. 1.6a, 1.6b, 1.6c, 1.6d, 1.6e). In Chapter 4 we will use any one of these to calculate our power after having indirectly measured our strength.

$$P = w / t^b \qquad \text{Eq. 1.6a}$$

$$P = w \cdot t^{-1} \qquad \text{Eq. 1.6b}$$

$$P = F \times v \qquad \text{Eq. 1.6c}$$

$$P = F \times (d \cdot t^{-1}) \qquad \text{Eq. 1.6d}$$

$$P = F \times (d / t) \qquad \text{Eq. 1.6e}$$

Notice that the format in two of the formulas (Eq. 1.6b, 1.6d) multiplies by the negative power exponent (e.g., $^{-1}$). This is the recommended reporting style of the International System of Nomenclature[62] used by most scientific journals.

Power is also a term often used when referring to the rate of transforming metabolic energy to physical performance,[34] such as aerobic power and anaerobic power. However, instead of viewing these metabolic terms as power terms, as would a physicist, the exercise physiologist would probably view them as energy terms.

Energy (E)

Energy is a term describing the amount of metabolic energy released due to the combination of visible mechanical work and the heat of the body itself. It may be calculated from the total amount of work produced and the known or estimated efficiency of the exerciser. The metabolic oxygen cost during exercise on a cycle ergometer is estimated from the power level plus the oxygen cost of free-wheel (unloaded) cycling and resting metabolism.[35]

Meteorological Terms

Meteorology is the study of weather or the environmental conditions. The primary meteorological variables most likely to affect physiological responses in a laboratory are temperature, relative humidity, and barometric pressure. Each variable's lower and upper criteria of neutral—normal physiological effect—may differ depending upon the type of laboratory test. For example, higher laboratory temperatures are allowable for testing a person at rest than for testing a person at exercise. The acclimatization and fitness of the person are two other factors that may affect the neutral zone of each meteorological variable.

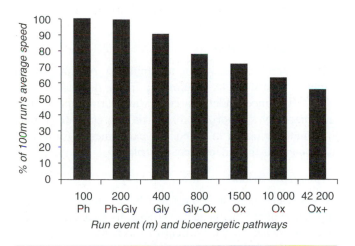

Temperature (*T*)^c

High air temperatures in the laboratory affect physiological responses at rest and exercise. For example, heart rate increases at exercise by approximately one beat per minute

Figure 1.4 The average speeds for various running events and their associated bioenergetic fitness components are depicted as a percentage of the maximal pace (average speed) for the men's world-record times (as of 2000) of the 100 m and 200 m runs. The pace of running decreases from the 100 % reference speed of the 100 m run and the 200 m run to the marathon's low of 55 % of the reference speed. (Ph = phosphagenic; Gly = glycolytic; Ox = oxidative; Ox+ = oxidative + hydration + nutrition).

^{b}The abbreviation for the basic quantity of time is an italicized *t*. The *t* can be written with a slanted stem when writing it by hand.
^{c}Temperature's abbreviation *T* is italicized because it is a basic quantity.[63]

for every degree Celsius (C) over twenty-four degrees (24 °C = 75.2 °F).[46] Americans are familiar with the Fahrenheit (F) scale, but the two most common scales for scientists are the Celsius scale and the scale using kelvin (K) units.[d] Usually, the Fahrenheit scale is not printed in scientific research journals, although sometimes it is presented in parentheses after the Celsius degree.

Fahrenheit (F)

Gabriel Fahrenheit chose the number 32 to designate the melting point of ice. He assigned the number 96 to the temperature of human blood. Although this range of temperatures accommodates most of Earth's weather situations, it is not as convenient for calculations as the Celsius and kelvin scales. Thus, the Système International d'Unités (SI)[62] does not recommend its use as a measurement scale.

Celsius (C)

Celsius was formerly called the centigrade scale, but now the appropriate term is Celsius.[6] Anders Celsius, a Swedish mathematician, arbitrarily chose to make the freezing and boiling points of water 0 °C and 100 °C, respectively.

Kelvin (K)

The basic thermal unit for the International System (SI) is the kelvin, named after 19th-century physicist William Kelvin. It has an absolute zero, meaning that the coldest possible temperature truly is zero kelvin (0 K), meaning there is no *minus* or *below zero* temperature for this scale. A temperature of 0 °C or 32 °F is a temperature of 273.16 K.

Relative Humidity (RH)

High relative humidity exacerbates the effect that temperature has on heart rate. Instead of heart rate increasing by only one beat per minute (1 b/min) for every degree Celsius over 24 °C, high humidity can double, triple, or quadruple that rate (2 b/min to 4 b/min for each degree Celsius > 24 °C).[46] Humidity, or air saturation, is a meteorological term indicating the relative amount of water in the air. If the RH is 100 %, then the air contains the most amount of water it can possibly hold at that air temperature. Air can hold more water at higher temperatures than it can at lower temperatures. Typically, relative humidity at exercise is not apt to affect exercise if between 20 % RH and 60 % RH.[e] Relative humidity percentages below or above this neutral range are often referred to as *arid* or *humid,* respectively.

---

[d]Although Dr. Kelvin originated the kelvin unit, the *k* is not capitalized because it is an approved SI base unit. However, the abbreviated symbol *K* is capitalized (uppercase).

[e]The SI style requires a space between the percent symbol (%) and the number (% = 0.01).[63]

Barometric Pressure (P_B)

The term *barometric pressure* refers to the air pressure of the environment. Altitudes can be estimated from air pressures, and weather patterns can be dictated by changes in air pressures. Normal exercise responses occur at barometric pressures common near sea level. However, aerobic power is usually less at the barometric pressures associated with altitudes above 1500 m (4920 ft).[15] Barometric pressures are used to correct respiratory ventilation volumes and metabolic volumes.

Statistical Terms

The term *statistics* can have more than one meaning.[39] In a broad sense, it includes the method of organizing, describing, and analyzing quantitative (numerical) data, in addition to predicting outcomes or probabilities. The combined term *basic statistics* is sometimes used to describe group data with such statistics as the mean (average, *M*) and standard deviation *(SD).*

Some of the statistical terms commonly used in an exercise physiology laboratory are (a) **variables,** (b) **relationships,** and (c) **norms/standards.**

Variables

A variable is a characteristic. The characteristics, or variables, mentioned in this manual usually have quantitative values that vary among the members of a sample or population. Some of the measured variables discussed in this manual are strength, run/walk time, oxygen consumption, heart rate, blood pressure, and percent body fat. A variable is either independent or dependent.

Independent Variable

An independent variable is manipulated, or changed, in order to determine its relationship to the dependent variable.[66] The independent variable's measuring unit is usually placed on the horizontal (X) axis of a graph (e.g., time in minutes or power in watts). The experimenter (or technician) controls the independent variable.[32]

Dependent Variable

A dependent variable is measured before and/or after manipulation of the independent variable. Its measuring unit is usually placed on the vertical (Y) axis of a graph (e.g., heart rate in b/min).

Relationships

Certain visual relationships may be observed when one variable is plotted on a graph with another variable. When the graphic line (best fit) is straight and ascending, it is called a positive linear relationship (see Chapter 12's Figure 12.1). Thus, an increase in one variable causes—or is associated with—a proportional increase in the other variable. When the plotted points on the graph form a descending straight line, it is called a linear negative (inverse) relationship. In this case, an increase in one variable causes—or is associated with—a proportional decrease in the other variable. Many graphic relationships are positive or negative curvilinear. Chapter 4 contains a graph (Figure 4.1) that depicts a linear negative line and a negative curvilinear line to describe the relationship between the percent of a maximal lift and the number of repetitions possible. Chapter 5's Figure 5.1 depicts the positive curvilinear relationship between time and a maximal static muscle action.[40]

Certain relationships allow the **prediction** of one variable by knowing the value of another variable. Many relationship terms use the unit of measure called the **correlation coefficient** to express the extent of the relationship. The correlation coefficient may describe the accuracy of a test, such as its **reliability, validity,** and **objectivity.**

Prediction

The relationship between one variable and one or more other variables allows transformation into an equation to estimate one of the variables. The line of best fit of the graphic plot of one variable to another is termed a **regression line;** when it is transformed into an equation, it is called a **regression equation.** Sometimes regression equations are presented in the form of a **nomogram.** A nomogram is a series of two or more vertical or diagonal lines by which to predict one variable from one or more other variables without having to perform any calculations. For example, Figure 8.3 in Chapter 8 enables a person to find the vertical power of a jumper by placing a straight edge across the left and right vertical lines for the jumper's distance and the jumper's body mass (weight), respectively. The jumper's vertical power is where the straight edge intersects the middle vertical line.

The statistical term that describes the predictive error of a regression equation is the **standard error of estimate (SEE).** This is a type of standard deviation around the predicted scores from the regression line. For example, if the predicted lean body mass is 40 kg, and the *SEE* is 5 kg, then 68 % of the scores will be between 35 kg and 45 kg. Thus, the standard error of the estimate indicates the amount of error to be expected in a predictive score.[8] For example, one researcher[19] suggests an acceptable *SEE* criterion of less than 15 % for aerobic fitness predictions.

Reliability

Reliability is an estimate of the reproducibility or consistency of a test. Reliabilities of tests should be based on a sample of at least 30[41], or 30 to 60 participants. A reliable test generates high intraclass correlation coefficients (*R*) and high interclass correlation coefficients (*r*) when data from repeated trials of that test are compared. Based on input from other investigators,[11,29,38,54,58] I have summarized the correlation coefficient criteria that may be used to

Table 1.4 **Some Criteria for Qualifying Test-Retest Reliability Correlations**

Category	Correlation Criteria
High	≥ .9
Good	.80–.89
Fair	.70–.79
Poor	< .70

Note: The correlation coefficient is a decimal number that does not require the zero preceding it. This is because there are no correlation numbers less than −1.0 or greater than 1.0.

qualitatively categorize reliability ranging from poor to high (Table 1.4). The criterion for an acceptable correlation may vary with the opinions of various investigators; a recommended minimum test-retest correlation can be as low as .70[52,58] or, more stringently, as high as .85.[29] A perfect correlation is +1.0 or −1.0, but this would occur rarely. The intraclass correlation coefficient is a better estimate of reliability because it permits more than two scores, and is more sensitive to measurement errors.[8]

The reliability of a test may be affected by the experimental and biological error (variability). Experimental variability is due to lab procedures, instrumentation, and environment; thus, it represents the technical error in a test. Biological variability or error is due to the natural periodicity (hourly, daily, weekly) or inherent biological fluctuations of the human participant.[31] Although a test may exhibit acceptable reliability coefficients, the stable reliability can be affected by a participant's learning or familiarity with a test. If this occurs, usually the second or subsequent trials improve, compared with the initial trial. A one-way analysis of variance (ANOVA), which is beyond the scope of this text, is a good statistical method to calculate *R*, thus checking the stable reliability of test scores.[54]

Objectivity

Although similar to reliability, objectivity is distinct in that it represents the ability of a test to give similar results when administered by different administrators. It is sometimes referred to as *inter-observer reliability.*

Validity

Criterion validity is a measure of the test's ability to measure what it claims to measure. A test with high validity has a good correlation *(r)* with the criterion measure (actual or true). For example, run-walk distances or times are often judged for validity by their correlation with scores on maximal oxygen consumption tests. The guidelines for qualifying meaningful criterion validity coefficients need not be as high as for those guidelines that qualify reliability coefficients, which are listed in Table 1.4. For example, correlation coefficients ≥ .70 are sometimes deemed "moderately high." Two other types of validity are content validity and construct (discriminant) validity. Content validity relies on expert opinion or past research, and construct validity indicates the test's ability to discriminate among groups.[54] Most validity coefficients described in this text are based on criterion validity.

Norms and Standards

Norms and standards enhance the interpretation of test scores. Although the two terms are often used interchangeably, they are different.

Norms

Norms are values that relate a person's score to those of the general population. Some authorities[7] suggest that the minimum number of participants to establish norms be set at 100 for each category. If the population sample number is less than 100, or if the samples within a population (e.g., specific age groups) are less than 100, it is probably more appropriate to refer to the data as *comparative scores,* rather than norms. The derived percentiles *(%ile)* or standard deviations[f] *(SD)* developed from norms are often described in accordance with such descriptive categories as poor, below average, average, above average, and excellent (Figure 1.5). For example, if a person is categorized as excellent in a certain fitness component on the Canadian Standardization Test, then that person ranks better than 80 % of the population.[23] Table 1.5 shows three categorization scales based on percentiles.[23,26,55]

Standards

Standard is a term often used synonymously with *norms.* However, more appropriately it is used to connote a desirable or recommended value or score.[3] The term *criterion-referenced standards (CRS)* is a professionally popular term.[18] It has an advantage over normative standards for fitness tests because CRS indicate the levels necessary for good health, regardless of the level of physical fitness of the reference group.[9,17,47,57] The CRS for fitness tests may be based upon professional expertise and scientific research, in addition to normative data.[17] Thus, CRS are standards that represent recommended levels of performance. Because the CRS are absolute standards, they do not consider the number of persons who meet the standard. For example, a normative standard such as the mean or the 50th *%ile* may not meet the desirable level of performance. The CRS levels allow easy recognition of the adequacy or inadequacy of a person on that particular fitness/health variable. Also, as long as a person meets the CRS criterion, he or she has the same merit as someone who scores extremely high on the variable.

Because the criterion standards are based partially on human judgment, and because of testing errors or participant motivation, the cutoff scores may cause false merit or false nonmerit. Also, the merit levels usually do not indicate fitness levels at which a person may need to be successful in recreational or competitive sports; they are concerned mainly with health-related fitness.

Thus, norms describe a person's position within a population, whereas *standards* describe the criteria suggested for appropriate health-related fitness of a population. The American Alliance for Health, Physical Education, Recreation and Dance (AAHPERD) Health-Related Test is a test battery that provides both norms and standards.

Calibration Terms

The term **calibration** refers to the process of verifying the accuracy of the measuring instruments in order to enhance the reliability, validity, and objectivity of testing. Often, an

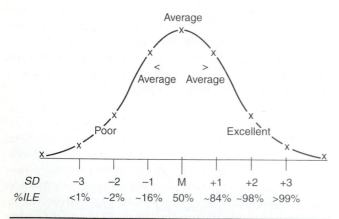

Figure 1.5 A typical normal curve and possible placement of qualitative categories (Canadian Standardization Test) based on a chosen multiple of the standard deviation and percentiles.

SD	−3	−2	−1	M	+1	+2	+3
%ILE	<1%	~2%	~16%	50%	~84%	~98%	>99%

| Table 1.5 | Descriptive Categories Based on Percentiles |
| | |

	Percentiles	Categories
Canadian Standardization Test[23]	81–100	Excellent
	61– 80	Above average
	41– 60	Average
	21– 40	Below average
	1– 20	Poor
Institute for Aerobics Research,[a]YMCA[26]	90–100	Well above average
	70– 89	Above average
	50– 69	Average
	30– 49	Below average
	10– 29	Well below average
Functional Fitness Test[55]	76–100	Above average
	25– 75	Average
	1– 24	Below average

Based on [23]Fitness and Amateur Sport Canada. (1987). *Canadian Standardized Test of Fitness (CSTF) operations manual* (3d ed.). Ottawa, Canada: Author. [a]Institute for Aerobics Research, Dallas, TX. [26]Golding, L. A., Myers, C. R., & Sinning, W. E. (Eds.). (1989). *Y's way to physical fitness.* Champaign, IL: Human Kinetics. [55]Rikli, R. E., & Jones, C. J. (1999). Functional fitness normative scores for community-residing older adults, ages 60–94. *Journal of Aging and Physical Activity, 7,* 162–181.

[f]Notice that all statistical abbreviations are placed in italics; underlining is acceptable if italics are not available. The symbol *%ile* is my abbreviation.

instrument is calibrated at three or more points along its measurement scale. These points usually include the lowest point (e.g., zero), an approximate midpoint, and the highest point. For example, a platform scale for measuring body mass may be calibrated at the zero point (0 kg), at the approximate midpoint (70 kg) and at the high point (136 kg). The **zero** point usually can be adjusted on most scientific weighing scales. The **midpoint** and **high-point** calibrations use "certified" weights. Certified weights are those measured on a highly accurate scale at an official weighing center. Weights can unofficially be certified in an exercise physiology laboratory with accurate, previously calibrated scales. Midpoint and high-point adjustments cannot be made on many instruments. Thus, the experimenter may develop a correction factor based upon any discrepancy between the observed and known values at the high points and midpoints, or the experimenter may adjust the zero to minimize or eliminate the discrepancy at the most critical interval of the particular measurement.

Types of Tests

Nearly two-thirds of the 30 or more tests described in this manual are tests that require measurements during exercise or recovery conditions, not resting conditions. The value of performance testing of humans is analogous to that of testing a car; the best way to test the performance of the car is not solely by examining it as it sits there but by examining it as it motors along the highway. Similarly, the best way to evaluate human performance is to measure the human during exercise. The next-best way is to measure the human during recovery from exercise. The various tests used to measure physical performance may be based upon their predominant use on the field, in the laboratory, or both. Thus, the tests described in this manual are designated as one of three types: (a) **field**, (b) **field/lab**, or (c) **laboratory.**

Field Tests

Field tests are common in physical education/kinesiology. Exercise physiologists need to be familiar with field tests because they often measure or estimate variables (e.g., physical fitness components) that are discussed in a course of exercise physiology. Field tests in physical education were developed at the turn of the 20th century in order to test large groups of persons as accurately and economically as possible outside of a laboratory setting. Unless extrinsic variables (e.g., weather, terrain, motivational) are strictly controlled, field tests are not as appreciated in research as are the more controlled laboratory tests. However, this does not mean that field tests cannot be as valid as some laboratory tests. In addition to their use in physical education classes, field tests are popular as screening and maintenance tests for military and safety/emergency personnel (e.g., firefighters, lifeguards, police, and rangers) and for college or professional sports recruiters. Some familiar

field tests are sit-ups, pushups, and pull-ups. Two *aerobic* field tests described in this manual are the 1.5-Mile Run Test and the AAHPERD 1.0-Mile Run Test.

Field/Lab Tests

Field/lab tests may be administered under either field or laboratory conditions. This usually means that minimal equipment is required but that the test should be performed under conditions that approximate those in the laboratory setting. In other words, slightly more stringent controls are placed on field/lab tests, compared with those placed on field tests. An example of a field/lab test is the Aerobic Step Test. It can be administered in the laboratory using a small step platform to test one person at a time. Also, a longer step bench or stadium bleacher may be used outside the laboratory facility, along with the accessory equipment, such as metronome and stopwatch, to accommodate the simultaneous testing of a large group of participants. Thus, a field/lab test uses essentially the same equipment whether it is administered in the laboratory or outside the laboratory (in the "field").

Laboratory Tests

Laboratory tests often require more sophisticated, expensive, and/or bulky equipment than the field or field/lab tests. In addition, more rigid controls are placed upon some of the extraneous variables, such as weather and motivation. These controls are made not only during the test but also prior to the test. For example, a participant[g] undergoing a true lab test should not be influenced by such factors as a heavy meal or a cup of coffee. Due to the more stringent controls and greater complexities in laboratory tests, technicians must be more knowledgeable and skilled in testing procedures and interpretation of testing. Laboratory tests do not lend themselves well to testing more than one person simultaneously and, therefore, require more time per participant. In general, compared with field tests, laboratory tests offset their less practical characteristics by virtue of their more precise and accurate characteristics.

Table 1.6 provides a summary of the tests described in this manual under the headings *Field Tests, Field/Lab Tests,* and *Laboratory Tests.* Some of these may be placed in two or all three categories depending upon the sophistication applied by the investigator or technician. For example, densitometry (hydrostatic weighing) can be performed in a swimming pool and without any measurement of residual volume. It can also be measured in the pool but this time calculated using the prior measurement of residual

---

[g]I prefer the more benign terms such as *participant, performer,* and *person* over the traditional term *subject,* which is appropriate for animals. *Participant* also appears to be the favored term by the *Publication Manual of the American Psychological Association* (pp. 13–14).[6]

volume. Finally, it can be measured in the laboratory underwater tank at appropriate water temperature with accurate scales and using the residual volume measured in the water. Thus, depending upon the sophistication selected, it can be classified as a field test, a field/lab test, or a laboratory test.

Research Abstract Terms

The parts of a research article in scientific journals have traditional terms or headings. The abstract of an article briefly covers the same sections but is much shorter than the full-length journal article and acts as a summary of the study. Research articles often range in length from about three to six pages in many scientific journals and may even exceed 100 pages in special journal supplements, master's theses, and doctoral dissertations. However, these articles may be reduced to merely 150 to 500 words in an abstract. For example, one journal in the field, *Research Quarterly for Exercise and Sport,* presently averages about 200 words per abstract, whereas another, *Medicine and Science in Sports and Exercise,* averages about 325 words. Also, when researchers submit abstracts for presentation at conventions, they often are given special forms with an outlined "box" (about 13 cm × 13 cm; 5 in. × 5 in.) by which to limit the length of their abstract (see Box 1.1 and Form 3.3 in Chapter 3). There is abundant use of abbreviations in abstracts in order to squeeze as many words as possible into this box. The writer must address the following sections of the abstract:

1. Introduction (may include a one-sentence or two-sentence summary of the review of literature)
2. Purpose (sometimes combined with the introduction)
3. Method
4. Results and discussion (sometimes these are separate sections)
5. Conclusion

An abstract of a research study is usually placed at the front of the written article. However, if it does not appear at the beginning, it may be presented as a summary at the end of the article.

Abstract Introduction

An abstract should first catch the reader's attention by stating the *importance* or *significance* of the study. Perhaps the study settles some controversial issue or benefits a particular group, such as educators, coaches, or scientists. Sometimes a brief historical perspective is included. The statement of the importance/significance is usually no longer than one or two sentences.

Abstract Purpose

The purpose of the study concerns the problem that the study is trying to solve. It may be presented in research question form, such as "What is the aerobic fitness level of the students in our exercise physiology lab class?" It also may be stated definitively, such as "The purpose of this study was to

Table 1.6	Categorization of Tests According to Field, Field/Lab, and Laboratory Test	
Field Tests	**Field/Lab Tests**	**Laboratory Tests**
Free-Weight Strength	Handgrip Dynamometry	Isokinetic Leg Strength
Sprints	Vertical Jump	Maximal Oxygen Consumption
40 yd	Anaerobic Step	Treadmill Anaerobic Power
50 yd	Wingate Cycle	Exercise Electrocardiogram
60 yd	Rockport Walk	Vital Capacity
1.5 Mile Run	Aerobic Step	Forced Expiratory Volume
12 min Run	Aerobic Cycle	Lung Volumes
AAHPERD Run	Blood Pressure	Maximal Voluntary Ventilation
Stature-Weight	Sit-Reach Flexibility	Exercise Ventilation
Body Mass Index	Girth	Exercise Tidal Volume and Frequency
	Skinfolds	Densitometry (Underwater Weighing)

BOX 1.1 Title of Abstract

Name(s) of investigator(s):
Institution(s) or affiliation(s) of investigator(s): City, state, and e-mail address, if available, of primary (first-listed) author
Introduction: Importance, significance, and possibly a brief review of the topic
Purpose: Statement of the problem or research question or goal or specific objectives; hypotheses and their rationale
Methods: Description of participants, informed consent statement, instrumentation (apparatus), procedures, experimental design and statistical methods
Results: Summary of major findings, statistical values in text, tables, or figures
Discussion: Explanations (rationale) and implications of the findings; interpretation; confounding variables; confirmation or refutation of prior studies; future studies; some journals delete this heading and put its contents in the results section
Conclusion: The conclusion is usually so brief that it can be included in the discussion section; it is a final statement related to the purpose; it is the answer to the research question

Note: Sometimes the names and affiliations of the investigators are not included within the box when submitting abstracts for blind review. The subheadings per se (e.g., "Methods") printed here usually are not included in the abstract box for convention presentation but are often included in the journal's full article (e.g., *Medicine and Science in Sports and Exercise*).

determine the level of fitness in the exercise physiology lab class." Sometimes there is more than one purpose to a study, or one of the purposes is secondary to another.

The purpose may include the hypothesis of the investigators. This is a statement regarding the expected outcome. For instance, the investigators might feel that physical educators have higher fitness levels than that of the average person. A **physiological rationale,** which provides the basis for the study or for the type of test chosen to solve the problem, may be included. Thus, statements regarding the physiology, validity, and reliability of a test may be included here.

Abstract Methods

The description of the methods for solving the research problem follows the purpose section. Often, this portion of the abstract is overdone; three or four statements should be sufficient for most method sections of an abstract, unless the investigators are concerned with a research problem dealing with the type of methodology per se.

The methods portion of an abstract often includes the following: (1) description of participants; (2) general description of the instrumentation, procedures, and calculations; and (3) experimental design, statistical method, and sampling procedure.

Abstract Results and Discussion

The results usually summarize and evaluate the group data from a tabular form to a statistical form. Thus, the results include such statistical data as the means, standard deviations (sometimes the range), and statistically significant differences.

The discussion includes the investigators' interpretation of the results. These may be best applied if norms and standards exist for the particular testing method of the study. The discussion should include a physiological rationale (a reason) or justified speculations for the results and

Table 1.7 **Summary of Terms for Fitness, Measurement, Meteorology, Statistics, Calibration, Types of Tests, and the Scientific Abstract**

Term	Description
Fitness	Ability to carry out physical activities satisfactorily
Health-related continuum	Strength, muscular endurance, cardiorespiratory endurance
Noncontinuum health-related	Flexibility, body composition
Bioenergetic-related continuum	Strength/power (phosphagenic); power-endurance (phosphagenic-glycolytic; glycolytic); mixed endurance (glycolytic-oxidative); cardiorespiratory endurance (oxidative; aerobic)
Measurement	Measure of the quantity or quality of anything
Force (F)	Changes or tends to change the state of rest or motion of matter
Work (w)	Product of force and distance
Velocity (v)	Displacement divided by time
Speed	Distance divided by time
Power (P)	Rate of work
Energy (E)	Visible mechanical work plus body heat
Meteorology	Study of weather or environmental conditions
Temperature (T)	Degree of hotness or coldness of anything measured by three temperature units—degrees Fahrenheit, degrees Celsius, and kelvin
Relative humidity (RH)	Amount of water in the air relative (%) to the most water air could hold at that temperature
Barometric pressure (P_B)	Environmental (atmospheric) air pressure
Statistics	Method of organizing, describing, and analyzing data
Independent variable (X axis)	Characteristic that the investigator controls
Dependent variable (Y axis)	Characteristic that changes due to the change in the independent variable
Visual relationships	Linear and curvilinear graphics, which can be positive, negative, or both
Predictive relationships	One variable can be predicted (estimated) from knowing another variable by using a regression equation.
Norms	Allow for the interpretation of data by observing the mean, standard deviation, and percentiles
Criterion-reference standard	Established by expert opinion
Calibration	Assures the accuracy of the measuring instruments
Zero point	Lowest point in the range of a measuring instrument
Midpoint	Within the measuring instrument's middle part of the range
High point	Peak in the range of the measuring instrument
Types of Tests	
Field	Convenient, simple, and inexpensive tests for large groups outside the laboratory
Field/lab	A more controlled field test or a less controlled laboratory test
Laboratory	Usually restricted to testing no more than a few controlled persons simultaneously in an environmentally controlled laboratory that has relatively expensive equipment and skilled technicians
Scientific Abstract	Brief summary of the research, which includes introduction/purpose, method, results, discussion, and conclusion

may include any confounding variables affecting the results. It may mention whether the findings confirm or refute previous research. Also, the findings may have raised questions that may be answered by further research.

Abstract Conclusion

The conclusion should be very succinct, simply answering the research question that was proposed in the purpose section of the abstract. It should be as obviously presented as the purpose. Thus, it sometimes begins as follows: "The investigators concluded . . ." or "The data suggest . . . ." It is often the last sentence of the abstract. The abstracts of some journals (e.g., *Medicine and Science in Sports and Exercise*) use boldface type for the four or five distinct section headings. Thus, the conclusion and the other sections are obvious to the reader.

Summary of Terminology

Many of the basic terms and units used in exercise physiology are summarized in Table 1.7. As with learning any new language, the beginner should practice using these terms and units, so that they become a natural part of the exercise physiology vocabulary. The student activities listed in Box 1.2 should help students familiarize themselves with the terms used in this text.

References

1. Abernethy, P. J., & Jurimae, J. (1996). Cross-sectional and longitudinal uses of isoinertial, isometric, and isokinetic dynamometry. *Medicine and Science in Sports and Exercise, 28,* 1180–1187.
2. American College of Sports Medicine (ACSM). (2000). *ACSM's guidelines for graded exercise testing and prescription.* Philadelphia: Lippincott Williams & Wilkins.
3. American College of Sports Medicine (ACSM). (1988). ACSM opinion statement on physical fitness in children and youth. *Medicine and Science in Sports and Exercise 20,* 422–423.
4. American College of Sports Medicine (ACSM). (1999). Information for authors. *Medicine and Science in Sports and Exercise, 31*(1), i–v.
5. American College of Sports Medicine, American Dietetic Association, & Dietitians of Canada. (2000). Nutrition and athletic performance. *Medicine and Science in Sports and Exercise, 32,* 2130–2145.
6. American Psychological Association. (1994). *Publication manual of the American Psychological Association.* Washington, DC: Author.
7. Barrow, H. M., & McGee, R. (1971). *A practical approach to measurement in physical education.* Philadelphia: Lea and Febiger.
8. Baumgartner, T. A., & Jackson, A. S. (1987). *Measurement for evaluation in physical education and exercise science.* Dubuque, IA: Wm. C. Brown.
9. Blair, S. N., Falls, H. B., & Pate, R. R. (1983). A new physical fitness test. *The Physician and Sportsmedicine 11,* 87–91.
10. Blair, S., & Morrow, M. S. (1997). Surgeon general's report on physical fitness: The inside story. *ACSM's Health & Fitness Journal, 1*(1), 14–18.
11. Blesh, T. E. (1974). *Measurement for evaluation in physical education.* New York: Ronald Press.
12. Bogdanis, G. C., Nevill, M. E., Boobis, L. H., & Lakomy, H. K. A. (1996). Contribution of phosphocreatine and aerobic metabolism to energy supply during repeated sprint exercise. *Journal of Applied Physiology, 80,* 876–884.
13. Brooks, G. A., Fahey, T. D., White, T. P., & Baldwin, K. M. (2000). *Exercise physiology: Human bioenergetics and its application* (pp. 26–27). Mountain View, CA: Mayfield.
14. Buskirk, E. R. (1987). Implementation of the use of SI units. *Medicine and Science in Sports and Exercise, 19*(6), 545.
15. Buskirk, E. R. (1969). Decrease in physical work capacity at high altitude. In A. H. Hegnauer (Ed.), *Biomedicine of high terrestrial elevations* (pp. 204–222). Natick, MA: U.S. Army Research Institute of Environmental Medicine.
16. Chilakos, A. (1974, December). Cardiovascular endurance training through weight training. *The Physical Educator,* 179–180.
17. Corbin, C. B., & Pangrazi, R. P. (1992). Are American children and youth fit? *Research Quarterly for Exercise and Sport, 63,* 96–106.
18. Cureton, K. J., & Warren, G. L. (1990). Criterion-referenced standards for youth health-related fitness tests: A tutorial. *Research Quarterly for Exercise and Sport, 61*(1), 7–19.

19. Davies, C. T. M. (1968). Limitations to the prediction of maximum oxygen intake from cardiac frequency measurements. *Journal of Applied Physiology, 24,* 700–706.

20. Dintiman, G. B. (1984). *How to run faster.* New York: Leisure Press.

21. Edington, D. W., & Edgerton, V. R. (1976). *The biology of physical activity.* Boston: Houghton Mifflin.

22. Exercise Science Council of NASPE. (1995, September/October). Basic standards for the programs preparing students for careers in exercise science. *UPDATE* (NASPE Suppl), 2.

23. Fitness and Amateur Sport Canada. (1987). *Canadian Standardized Test of Fitness (CSTF) operations manual* (3rd ed.). Ottawa, Canada: Author.

24. Fletcher, G. F., Balady, G., Blair, S. N., Blumenthal, J., Caspersen, C., Chaitman, B., Epstein, S., Froelicher, E. S., Froelicher, V. F., Pina, I. L., & Pollock, M. L. (1996). Statement of exercise: Benefits and recommendations for physical activity programs for all Americans. A statement for health professionals by the Committee on Exercise and Cardiac Rehabilitation of the Council on Clinical Cardiology, American Heart Association. *Circulation, 94,* 857–862.

25. Foss, M. L., & Keteyian, S. J. (1998). *Fox's physiological basis for exercise and sport.* Boston: McGraw-Hill.

26. Golding, L. A., Myers, C. R., & Sinning, W. E. (Eds.). (1989). *Y's way to physical fitness.* Champaign, IL: Human Kinetics.

27. Gutin, B., Manos, T., & Strong, W. (1992). Defining health and fitness: First step toward establishing children's fitness standards. *Research Quarterly for Exercise and Sport, 63,* 128–132.

28. Hay, J. G., & Reid, J. G. (1982). *The anatomical and mechanical bases of human motion.* Englewood Cliffs, NJ: Prentice-Hall.

29. Johnson, B. L., & Nelson, J. K. (1974). *Practical measurements for evaluation in physical education.* Minneapolis: Burgess.

30. Jokl, P., & Jokl, E. (1977). Running and swimming world records. *Journal of Sports Medicine and Physical Fitness, 17*(2), 213–229.

31. Katch, V. L., Sady, S. S., & Freedson, P. (1982). Biological variability in maximum aerobic power. *Medicine and Science in Sports and Exercise, 14*(1), 21–25.

32. Kirk, R. E. (1968). *Experimental design: Procedures for the behavioral sciences.* Belmont, CA: Brooks/Cole.

33. Knuttgen, H. G. (1995). Force, work, and power in athletic training. *Sports Science Exchange, 57*(4), 1–6.

34. Komi, P. V., & Knuttgen, H. G. (1994). Sport science and modern training. In J. D. Halloran, P. V. Komi, H.G. Knuttgen, P. DeKnop, P. Oja, & F. Roskam (Eds.), *Sport science studies* (pp. 44–62). Germany: Verlag Karl Hofmann Schondorf.

35. Lang, P. B., Latin, R. W., Berg, K. E., & Mellon, M. B. (1992). The accuracy of the ACSM cycle ergometry equation. *Medicine and Science in Sports and Exercise, 24* (2), 272–276.

36. McArdle, W. D., Katch, F. I., & Katch, V. L. (1996). *Exercise physiology: Energy, nutrition, and human performance.* Baltimore: Williams & Wilkins.

37. McGilvery, R. W. (1975). *Biochemical concepts.* Philadelphia: W. B. Saunders.

38. Medbø, J. I., Mohn, A. C., Tabata, I., Bahr, R., Vaage, O., & Sejersted, O. (1988). Anaerobic capacity determined by maximal accumulated O_2 deficit. *Journal of Applied Physiology, 64,* 50–60.

39. Minium, E. W. (1970). *Statistical reasoning in psychology and education.* New York: John Wiley and Sons.

40. Morris, A. F., Clarke, D. H., & Dainis, A. (1983). Time to maximal voluntary isometric contraction (MVC) for five different muscle groups in college adults. *Research Quarterly for Exercise and Sport, 54,* 163–168.

41. Morrow, J. R., & Jackson, A. W. (1993). How "significant" is your reliability? *Research Quarterly for Exercise and Science, 64,* 352–355.

42. Murray, J. A., & Karpovich, P. V. (1956). *Weight training in athletics.* Englewood Cliffs, NJ: Prentice-Hall.

43. Nagle, F. J. (1971). Effects of activity: Metabolic effects. In American College of Sports Medicine, (Ed.), *Encyclopedia of sport sciences and medicine* (pp. 212–15). New York: Macmillan.

44. Newsholme, E. A., Blomstrand, E., & Ekblom, B. (1992). Physical and mental fatigue: Metabolic mechanisms and importance of plasma amino acids. *British Medical Bulletin, 48,* 477–495.

45. Paffenbarger, R. S., Kampert, J. B., Lee, I.-M., Hyde, R. T., Leung, R. W., & Wing, A. L. (1994). Changes in physical activity and other lifeway patterns influencing longevity. *Medicine and Science in Sports and Exercise, 26,* 857–865.

46. Pandolf, K. B., Cafarelli, E., Noble, B. J., & Metz, K. F. (1975). Hyperthermia: Effect on exercise prescription. *Archives of Physical Medicine and Rehabilitation, 56,* 524–526.

47. Pate, R. (1983). *South Carolina physical fitness test manual.* Columbia: South Carolina Association for Health, Physical Education, Recreation and Dance.

48. Pate, R. R., Pratt, M., Blair, S. N., et al. (1995). Physical activity and public health: A recommendation from the Centers for Disease Control and Prevention and the American College of Sports Medicine. *J.A.M.A: The Journal of the American Medical Association, 273,* 402–407.

49. Pollock, M. L., Gaesser, G. A., Butcher, J. D., Despré, J-P., Dishman, R. K., Franklin, B. A., & Garber, C. E. (1998). ACSM position stand on the recommended quantity and quality of exercise for developing and maintaining cardiorespiratory and muscular fitness, and flexibility in healthy adults. *Medicine and Science in Sports and Exercise, 30,* 975–991.

50. Powers, S. K., & Howley, E. T. (2001). *Exercise physiology.* Boston: McGraw-Hill.

51. Purdy, J. G. (1974). Least squares model for the running curve. *Research Quarterly, 45,* 224–238.

52. Rarick, G. L., & Dobbins, D. A. (1975). Basic components in the motor performance of children six to nine years of age. *Medicine and Science in Sports and Exercise, 7,* 105–110.

53. Raven, P. B. (1998). Information for authors. *Medicine and Science in Sports and Exercise, 30*(1); i–iv.

54. Rikli, R. E., & Jones, C. J. (1999). Development and validation of a functional fitness test for community-residing older adults. *Journal of Aging and Physical Activity, 7,* 129–161.

55. Rikli, R. E., & Jones, C. J. (1999). Functional fitness normative scores for community-residing older adults, ages 60–94. *Journal of Aging and Physical Activity, 7,* 162–181.

56. Roberts, R. A., & Roberts, S. O. (1997). *Exercise physiology.* St. Louis: Mosby-Year Book.

57. Safritt, M. J. (1981). *Evaluation in physical education.* Englewood Cliffs, NJ: Prentice Hall.

58. Safritt, M. J. (1990). *Introduction to measurement in physical education and exercise science.* St. Louis: Times Mirror/Mosby.

59. Savaglio, S., & Carbone, V. (2000). Human performance: Scaling in athletic world records. *Nature, 404,* 244.

60. Serresse, O., Lortie, G., Bouchard, C., & Boulay, M. R. (1988). Estimation of the contribution of the various energy systems during maximal work of short duration. *International Journal of Sports Medicine, 9,* 456–460.

61. Sparling, P. B., O'Donnell, E. M., & Snow, T. K. (1998). The gender difference in distance running performance has plateaued: An analysis of world rankings from 1980 to 1996. *Medicine and Science in Sports and Exercise, 30,* 1725–1729.

62. Spencer, M. R., & Gastin, P. B. (2001). Energy system contribution during 200- to 1500-m running in highly trained athletes. *Medicine and Science in Sports and Exercise, 33,* 157–162.

63. Taylor, B. N. (1995). *NIST special publication 811, 1995 edition: Guide for the use of the International System of Units (SI).* Gaithersburg, MD: United States Department of Commerce, National Institute of Standards and Technology.

64. Thibault, G., & Peronnet, R. (1988). Physiological analysis of world running records. *Medicine and Science in Sports and Exercise, 20* (2, Suppl.): Abstract #294, p. S49.

65. Thomson, J. M., & Garvie, K. J. (1981). A laboratory method for determination of anaerobic energy expenditure during sprinting. *Canadian Journal of Applied Sport Science, 6,* 21–26.

66. Van Dalen, D. B. (1973). *Understanding educational research.* San Francisco: McGraw-Hill.

67. Vandewalle, H., Peres, G., & Monod, H. (1987). Standard anaerobic exercise tests. *Sports Medicine, 4,* 268–289.

68. Volkov, N. I., & Lapin, V. I. (1979). Analysis of the velocity curve in sprint running. *Medicine and Science in Sports, 11,* 332–337.

69. Ward-Smith, A. J. (1999). Aerobic and anaerobic energy conversion during high-intensity exercise. *Medicine and Science in Sports and Exercise, 31,* 1855–1860.

70. Wilmore, J. H., & Costill, D. L. (1999). *Physiology of sport and exercise.* Champaign, IL: Human Kinetics.

SCIENTIFIC UNITS OF MEASURE

Measuring units is the term given to describe the type of measure being made. For instance, in the United States we use pounds to describe our weight and feet and inches to describe our height. The units most commonly used in exercise physiology are those that measure variables associated with exercise, physiology, and meteorology. Some of these were introduced in Chapter 1—"Terminology." In accordance with the International System (SI) of nomenclature, numerous variables are described with such measuring units as kilogram, liter, meter, and kelvin. Many variables combine two or more measuring units to form such units as liters per minute and milliliters per kilogram per minute.

The quantification of exercise physiology requires that all variables have well-defined units of measure. Americans are already familiar with such units as inches, feet, and pounds, which they use in their daily lives. However, the single measuring system that is officially approved worldwide by scientists is the International System of Units—abbreviated as "SI" from its French name, "Système International."[3,15,16] SI is based upon the decimal and metric systems, thus simplifying the conversion of one unit to another.[10]

Only three countries in the world—the United States, Burma, and a part of an island of Borneo in Indonesia have not adopted, or are not committed to, the metric system.[9] Therefore, with apologies to Burma and Borneo, we can justify calling the nonmetric system the American system. However, American scientists, including exercise physiologists, have adopted SI metric units of measure. Although U.S. legislation has discouraged the use of the nonmetric system, it is dying much too slowly, according to most American scientists and the general population in the rest of the world. Americans often overlook metric designations on such objects as engine sizes (e.g., cubic centimeters), food containers (e.g., grams), and liquid containers (e.g., liters). Metric markers in America are sometimes found on road mileage/kilometer signs, auto tachometers, and speed-limit signs. Some U.S. buildings display temperature readings in Celsius. Hopefully, as more students become familiar with SI nomenclature—specifically, the metric system—the United States population will adopt, and use routinely, the worldwide metric system.

Recognizing and Reporting SI (Metric) Units

It is important to recognize SI units of measure when you see them and to know how to report them after making measurements. As with learning any language, students must be concerned with spelling, punctuation, and grammar of the SI "language." With respect to **spelling,** the SI guide published by the United States National Institute of Standards and Technology[15] permits American scientists to spell *liter* and *meter* as such, whereas a Briton may spell them as litre and metre, respectively. Although Mr. Kelvin originated the kelvin temperature scale, the *k* is not capitalized when referring to the unit and not to him directly, because the unit "kelvin" is adopted as one of the seven *base* units[a] of the International System of Units.[15] The same rationale applies when spelling out some of the derived units, whose names are those of persons, such as newton, watt, joule, and pascal.[b] When expressing the full name, not the abbreviation, of a two-component unit such as newton meter, use a space between the two words. Do not use a hyphen (e.g., not "newton-meter") and do not link terms absent of a space (e.g., not "newtonmeter").

Obviously, **symbols and abbreviations** of measuring units avoid spelling problems and are convenient and space-efficient. However, abbreviations (e.g., kg) and symbols (e.g., °) of measuring units should be used only when associated with the numeric value.[16] For example, *kilogram* should not be abbreviated as expressed in the present sentence. But it should be used if reporting that a person's body weight (mass) is 60 kg. Abbreviations are not capitalized unless associated with a person's name, such as N, W, C, and K, for Misters Newton, Watt, Celsius, and Kelvin, respectively. Also, scientists in the United States should use the uppercase L when abbreviating the unit for liter. This will avoid any confusion with the numeral one (1). Plural abbreviations are not acceptable in the SI. Thus, 60 kg or 175 cm is not reported as 60 kgs or 175 cms. Abbreviations are followed by a period only for the American abbreviation inches (in.) or at the end of a sentence. A space is also required between the numeral and the unit;[c] thus, the technician records "60 kg," not "60kg," or records "10 %," not "10%."

---

[a]The SI base units are meter (m), kilogram (kg), second (s), ampere (A), kelvin (K), mole (mol), and candela (cd).[15]

[b]Derived units are mixtures of base units or other derived units such as $m \cdot kg \cdot s^{-2}$, J/s, N·m, and N·m².[15]

[c]Expressions such as "sixty degrees per second (60°·s⁻¹)" or "an angle of ninety degrees (90°)" are examples of exceptions to the rule regarding a space between the numeral and the symbol or abbreviation.

When abbreviating a two-component unit, use a centered dot (·) or a space to separate each component.[d] Thus, one may abbreviate "newton meter" as "N·m" or "N m," but not the joined "Nm." Unit abbreviations and unit names are not mixed; thus, one should not use a mixed expression, such as "newton·m" or "N·meter." Similarly, one does not mix numerals and names; thus, "the static force was 500 N," not ". . . 500 newtons," or ". . . five-hundred N." The symbols for the expressions "greater than" and "less than" are ">" and "<," respectively. The symbols for "equal or greater than" and "equal or less than" are "≥" and "≤," respectively.

The recommended style of expressing **per** in combined units, such as liters per minute, is to use the centered dot preceding the unit with its negative exponent. Thus, the unit would appear as $L \cdot min^{-1}$, unless this is impractical for certain computers or typewriters. In that case, one slash (solidus; /) is acceptable (e.g., L/min). However, it is incorrect to use more than one solidus (accent on the first syllable säl) per expression, such as "mL/kg/min." The latter could be expressed with one solidus as $mL/(kg \cdot min)$ or as $mL \cdot kg^{-1} \cdot min^{-1}$. The following provides the mathematical rationale for using the negative exponent in place of the solidus:

$kg / 1 = kg^1 = kg$ to a power of 1 (positive exponent)

reciprocal of $kg / 1 = 1 / kg = kg^{-1}$ (negative exponent)

$mL / kg = mL \times 1 / kg = mL \cdot kg^{-1}$

The SI style also calls for scientists to record some **numbers** differently than what we are used to seeing. The general rule for numerical values with more than four digits is to insert a blank space to separate groups of three digits on either side of the decimal. For example, we are familiar with writing the number 10,500 with a comma, but we need to write it as 10 500 in accordance with SI recommendations (requirements). The one exception to this is when there are only four digits to the left or right of the decimal. For example, it is appropriate to record the number as 1500, or 1 500 for uniformity of numbers in a table, but not as 1,500. One reason for such rules is to avoid confusion where some countries use a comma instead of a decimal point.

Common Units of Measure in Exercise Physiology

The common variables in exercise physiology and their accompanying measuring units to quantify exercise are force, work, velocity, power, and energy. These terms were introduced in Chapter 1. Chapter 2 will include descriptions of their measuring units and their metric interconversions, in addition to American vs. metric conversions. It will also include descriptions of the units for time and meteorological conditions.

Force (F)

The recommended measuring unit for force is newton (N), named after a mid-19th-century scientist. The author of the guide published by the National Institute of Standards and Technology states, "In science and technology, weight is a force, for which the SI unit is the newton; in commerce and everyday use, weight is usually a synonym for mass, for which the SI unit is the kilogram."[15]

Although the kilogram (kg) unit is a weight (mass) unit, laboratories often use it as a measure of the force necessary to (a) lift a weight or one's own body weight, (b) crank a cycle ergometer, and (c) press against a dynamometer (a strength-measuring device that may be squeezed, pressed, or pulled). Many cycle ergometers (e.g., Monark™) in laboratories display kg or kp[e] or N as the force units. Ideally, the kilogram should be replaced by the newton (N) for all force measures (ergometry and dynamometry) in scientific publications, but the popularity of the kilogram and its presence on the dial of the instruments prevent the exclusive use of newtons as force units in this manual.

Work (w)

The unit of measure for work combines the basic physical quantity length (or distance) with the derived quantity force. Thus, the force unit—newton—and the distance unit—meter—combine to produce the work unit—newton meter (N·m). The newton meter is equivalent to another universally approved term, *joule* (J). Although the kilogram meter (kg·m) and newton meter are still common, the preferred expression for work is the joule, because it represents the totality of work rather than its two separate components. In other words, newtons (N) multiplied by meters (m) equals joules (J); thus, one may as well use the product term, joules, rather than its components, newtons and meters. For angular motion, or "rotational force," such as when measuring the strength of leg extensors on an isokinetic machine, the most appropriate term for the "moment of force"[f] is torque, and its unit of measure is newton meter (N·m). In this case, the newton meter is preferred over the unit joule. Thus, torque is the product of the force in newtons multiplied by the distance in meters.

Velocity (v) and Time (t)

Velocity is commonly measured in miles per hour (mph; $mi \cdot h^{-1}$) but should be reported scientifically as kilometers per hour (km/h; $km \cdot h^{-1}$), meters per minute (m/min; $m \cdot min^{-1}$), or meters per second (m/s; $m \cdot s^{-1}$). When the motion is angular, such as actions on an isokinetic machine,

---

[d]The use of the space is a recent interpretation of SI by an author (B. N. Taylor) of publications by the National Institute of Standards and Technology (NIST). Also, he reports that spaces on each side of the centered dot are now optional. (http://physics.nist.gov/cuu/Units/units.html)

[e]The unit kilopond represents the force at normal acceleration of gravity that is dependent upon the global latitude. For example, a person has a greater mass when at the North Pole than at the Equator due to the greater force of gravity at the Pole. The difference between kg·m and kp·m has little practical significance for exercise physiologists.

[f]The "moment of force" is based on the length of the moment arm which is measured from the center of rotation to the point where the external force is applied. (See Chapter 6—"Isokinetic Strength")

the appropriate units of measure are degrees per second (°/s; °·s⁻¹) or radians per second (rad/s; rad·s⁻¹). Although SI accepts the abbreviations of min, h, and d (day) for time units, it states that "if a standarized symbol for the unit is not available, the name of the unit should be written out in full."[15] Thus, it appears that full names should be given for week, month, and year.[3,15] However, it is not unusual to see wk, mo, and yr or y in scientific publications.

Power (P)

Common units of measure for power are (a) watts (W), (b) joules per second ($J \cdot s^{-1}$), (c) kilogram meters per minute ($kg \cdot m \cdot min^{-1}$), (d) newton meters per minute ($N \cdot m \cdot min^{-1}$), and horsepower (hp). Although $kg \cdot m \cdot min^{-1}$ has been a popular term for power by many exercise physiologists, and hp is the popular term for most Americans, neither of these is an acceptable SI power unit. The units kilogram meters per minute and horsepower should be converted to watts (W), the accepted unit of measure for power by the international scientific community. The watt is equal to the force (N) times the distance (m) that the object moves divided by the time (s) spent moving the object. The symbol for watt is the uppercase W, not to be confused with the lowercase w for work. When the unit watt is spelled out in full, it should not begin with a capital letter, despite the fact that the unit was named after Mr. Watt. This rule applies to all units that are proper names (e.g., newton, kelvin, joule, pascal).

Energy (E)

The most popular unit for energy or heat among laypersons is the kilocalorie (kcal). However, the **joule (J)** is the universally approved unit of measure for metabolic energy release and of work (exercise) and heat. The joule was named after scientist James Joule, who proposed the law of the conservation of energy. Notice in Equation 2.1 that all three variables use the joule as the unit of measure.[11]

$$\text{Metabolic Energy Release (J)} = \text{w (J)} + \text{Heat (J)} \qquad \text{Eq. 2.1}$$

The exercise physiologist often measures internal energy in terms of the metabolic consumption of oxygen in **liters per minute** ($L \cdot min^{-1}$) or in relative terms as in milliliters per kilogram body weight ($mL \cdot kg^{-1} \cdot min^{-1}$), or in **metabolic equivalents** (MET). The symbol MET denotes a multiple of the resting oxygen consumption. In absolute terms, resting oxygen consumption approximates $0.25 \ L \cdot min^{-1}$; thus, a MET value of 10 represents an oxygen consumption of $2.5 \ L \cdot min^{-1}$. In relative terms, resting oxygen consumption[1] is approximately $3.5 \ mL \cdot kg^{-1} \cdot min^{-1}$ and caloric expenditure is $1 \ kcal \cdot kg^{-1} \cdot h^{-1}$.

A close relationship exists between the exercise units of work and power and the physiological unit for oxygen consumption. Thus, the steady-state oxygen cost ($\dot{V}O_2$; $mL \cdot min^{-1}$) of cycle ergometry at a person's low or moderate level may be estimated ($SEE = \pm 6 \% \text{ to } \pm 7 \%$) from the known power output during cycle ergometry.[1,5,12] This relationship assumes that the exercise intensity is below the person's lactate threshold,[8] thus low and moderate exercise intensities. I have used Equations 2.2 to 2.4 on many occasions to estimate the oxygen cost (mL/min) at low and moderate power levels. The "300" represents the oxygen cost of sitting on the cycle ergometer without pedaling. A more individualized approach uses the participant's weight (kg) multiplied by 1 MET ($3.5 \ mL \cdot kg^{-1} \cdot min^{-1}$), instead of adding the generic resting metabolism of 300 mL/min.

$$\dot{V}O_2 \text{ (mL / min)} =$$

$$[\text{P (in } N \cdot m \cdot min^{-1}) \times 0.2] + 300 \qquad \text{Eq. 2.2}$$

$$[\text{P (in } kg \cdot m \cdot min^{-1}) \times 2] + 300 \qquad \text{Eq. 2.3}$$

$$[\text{P (in W)} \times 12] + 300 \qquad \text{Eq. 2.4}$$

For example, if a person is cycling long enough to reach steady state (usually $\geq$ 3 min for low to moderate intensities) at a power level of 100 W, then the following calculation would estimate that person's total oxygen cost in milliliters per minute:

$$\dot{V}O_2 \text{ (mL / min)} = (100 \times 12) + 300$$

$$= 1200 + 300$$

$$= 1500 \text{ mL / min} = 1.5 \text{ L / min}$$

Once the oxygen cost is known, it is possible to calculate the caloric and kilojoule (kJ) expenditure simply by multiplying the liters of oxygen consumed by 5 (Eq. 2.5) and 21 (Eq. 2.6), respectively.

$$\text{kilocalorie cost (kcal)} = 5 \times \dot{V}O_2 \text{ (L / min)} \qquad \text{Eq. 2.5}$$

where:

$$1 \text{ L / min} = 5 \text{ kcal}$$

$$\text{kilojoule cost (kJ)} = 21 \times \dot{V}O_2 \text{ (L / min)} \qquad \text{Eq. 2.6}$$

where:

$$1 \text{ L / min} = 21 \text{ kJ}$$

Thus, a layperson would say that the person in the prior example "burned" 7.5 kcal/min based on the product of 5 times 1.5 L/min. The scientist would say that the person's metabolic energy release was 31.5 kJ/min based on the product of 1.5 times 21.

Table 2.1 provides the energy values associated with low to moderate cycling intensities progressing by 25 W intervals. Keep in mind that the table and these equations do not account for the slow component of high-intensity exercise that occurs above the lactate threshold.[8] Hence, they would underestimate slightly the true oxygen cost for high-intensity exercise. What is deemed "high" is determined by the fitness of the exerciser, whereby the higher the fitness, the higher the lactate threshold. The oxygen rates include the 9 % $\dot{V}O_2$ increase due to chain friction inherent in many friction-loaded cycle ergometers.[4]

Table 2.1

Table 2.1 The Energy Cost Measured as Oxygen Consumption ($\dot{V}O_2$; L/min), Joules per minute (J/min), and kiloJoules per minute (kJ/min) at Low-to-Moderate Power Levels (kg·m·min⁻¹; N·m·min⁻¹; W) of Cycle Ergometry[a]

Power			Energy Rate		$\dot{V}O_2$
kg·m·min⁻¹	N·m·min⁻¹	W	J/min	kJ/min	L/min
150	1 500[b]	25	1 500	1.5	0.6
300	3 000	50	3 000	3.0	0.9
450	4 500	75	4 500	4.5	1.2
600	6 000	100	6 000	6.0	1.5
750	7 500	125	7 500	7.5	1.8
900	9 000	150	9 000	9.0	2.1
1050	10 500	175	10 500	10.5	2.4
1200	12 000	200	12 000	12.0	2.8

Note: [a]Based on approximate conversion factors. [b]The four-digit numbers in column two and column four are separated by a space at the third digit to the left of the decimal in order to have a uniform column of numbers. This is an approved SI style.

Also, the steady-state oxygen cost of exercise can be estimated for walking and running, on both a level and sloped terrain.[1,13] Equation 2.7 shows that the total or gross oxygen cost (mL·kg⁻¹·min⁻¹) for walking on a level treadmill is a function of adding resting metabolism to walking metabolism—basically, the same principle as applied to cycling. Thus, walking is equal to 1 MET (3.5 mL·kg⁻¹·min⁻¹) plus one-tenth of the walking speed (m/min).

Estimated Oxygen Cost (ml·kg⁻¹·min⁻¹)

for Walking on Horizontal Treadmill =

$(0.1 \times$ speed in m / min$) + 3.5$ mL·kg⁻¹·min⁻¹   Eq. 2.7

Equation 2.7 is intended for low (50 m/min; 3 km/h; 1.87 mph[g]) to moderate (100 m/min; 6 km/h; 3.73 mph) walking speeds. For example, if a person was walking on a level treadmill at a speed of 60 m/min, then the following calculation would produce the gross oxygen rate:

Horizontal Oxygen Rate (mL·kg⁻¹·min⁻¹)

$= (0.1 \times 60$ m / min$) + 3.5$ mL·kg⁻¹·min⁻¹

$= 6.0 + 3.5$ mL·kg⁻¹·min⁻¹

$= 9.5$ mL·kg⁻¹·min⁻¹

The MET equivalent is calculated by dividing the gross oxygen rate—9.5 mL·kg⁻¹·min⁻¹—by the resting metabolic rate (1 MET)—3.5 mL·kg⁻¹·min⁻¹. Thus, the following calculation provides the MET quantity of 2.7 for the prior example:

MET (ratio of exercise $\dot{V}O_2$ rate to resting $\dot{V}O_2$ rate)

$= 9.5$ mL·kg⁻¹·min⁻¹ $\div 3.5$ mL·kg⁻¹·min⁻¹ $= 2.7$

Table 2.2 shows the conversions for the units presented in this chapter.

Meteorological Units

The primary meteorological concerns of the exercise physiologist are temperature, relative humidity, and barometric pressure. The units presented here for these terms are those accepted by the scientific community or adopted as the SI style.

Temperature (T)[h]

The temperature units are apt to be confused by exercise physiology students because of the three scales available for temperature—Fahrenheit, Celsius, and kelvin. In general, Fahrenheit and Celsius conversions need not be memorized, because most laboratory thermometers have Celsius degrees, which are accepted as SI units.[i] Fahrenheit degrees are not accepted by the International System; therefore, laboratory students do not need to convert the Celsius degrees to Fahrenheit degrees. However, if Celsius thermometers are not available, then the Fahrenheit degrees have to be converted to the Celsius degrees or kelvin. Students are encouraged to make approximate estimates of Celsius degrees from any given Fahrenheit degrees by using certain mnemonics or by memorizing some of the most important Fahrenheit-to-Celsius degrees, such as core temperature, freezing point, and boiling point. Accurate Celsius determinations require mathematical conversions. The decimal conversions (0.56 or 1.8), rather than the fractions (5/9 or 9/5), are more compatible with pocket calculators (Eq. 2.8 and Eq. 2.9). Remember, the first step you make in converting Fahrenheit degrees to Celsius degrees is to subtract 32 from the given Fahrenheit degrees. The last thing you do to convert degrees Celsius to degrees Fahrenheit is to add 32 to the product of 1.8 and degrees Celsius.

---

[g]The units of measure "mph" and "mi·h⁻¹" are not accepted as appropriate SI abbreviations but are used here because of their presence on the speedometers of most U.S.-manufactured treadmills.

[h]The symbol for temperature is an italicized *T*.
[i]Although it is discouraged, the SI style is flexible enough to allow the Fahrenheit degrees (or other American units) to be placed in parentheses after the SI unit for the enhanced understanding of a special audience (e.g., American laypersons).

Measuring Unit	Exact (=) Conversion (Research)	Approximate (≈) Conversion (Classroom)
Force (F)		
N	1 N = 0.1019 kg	1 N ≈ 0.1 kg
kg	1 kg = 9.8066 N	1 kg ≈ 10 N
Work (w)		
kJ	1 kJ = 1000 J	
J; N·m	1 J = 1 N·m = 0.1019 kg·m	1 N·m ≈ 0.1 kg·m
kg·m	1 kg·m = 9.8066 N·m	1 kg·m ≈ 10 N·m
Velocity (v)		
m·min^{-1} (m/min)	1 m·min^{-1} = 0.04 "mi·h^{-1}"	
km·h^{-1} (km/h)	1 km·h^{-1} = 0.6214 "mi·h^{-1}"	1 km·h^{-1} ≈ 0.6 mi·h^{-1}
	= 16.7 m·min^{-1}	
	= 0.28 m·s^{-1}	
"mi·h^{-1} (mph)"[a]	1 "mi·h^{-1}" = 26.8 m·min^{-1}	1 "mi·h^{-1}" ≈ 27 m·min^{-1}
	= 0.447 m·s^{-1}	≈ 0.45 m·s^{-1}
Power (P)		
W	1 W = 6.118 kg·m·min^{-1}	1 W ≈ 6 kg·m·min^{-1}
	= 0.1019 kg·m·s^{-1}	≈ 0.1 kg·m·s^{-1}
J·s^{-1} (J/s); J·min^{-1} (J/min)	= 1 J·s^{-1} = 60 J·min^{-1}	= 1 J·s^{-1} = 60 J·min^{-1}
N·m·s^{-1}; N·m·min^{-1}	= 1 N·m·s^{-1} = 60 N·m·min^{-1}	= 1 N·m·s^{-1} = 60 N·m·min^{-1}
kg·m·min^{-1}	1 kg·m·min^{-1} = 0.1635 W	1 kg·m·min^{-1} ≈ 0.16 W
Energy (E)		
J	1 J = 1 N·m = 0.000239 kcal	
kJ	1 kJ = 1000 J = 0.2389 kcal	1 kJ ≈ 0.24 kcal
kcal[a]	1 kcal = 4186 J = 4.186 kJ	1 kcal ≈ 4200 J ≈ 4.2 kJ
V̇O$_2$	1 L = 5.05 kcal = 21.14 kJ	1 L ≈ 5 kcal ≈ 21 kJ
MET	1 MET = 3.5 mL·kg^{-1}·min^{-1}	
	= 1 kcal·kg^{-1}·h^{-1}	

Note: Spaces are optional alongside the centered dot (half-line dot; middle period). [a]The U.S unit miles (mi) and kilocalorie (kcal) are not approved SI units of measure. For quick reference, place an adhesive tab on the edge of this page.

°F to °C: °C = 0.56 (°F − 32) or

$$= (°F - 32) / 1.8 \qquad \text{Eq. 2.8}$$

°C to °F: °F = (1.8 × °C) + 32   Eq. 2.9

The conversion of Celsius to kelvin is made simply by adding the Celsius degrees to 273.15 K (≈ 273 K)[j] or by subtracting if the temperature is below 0 °C (Eq. 2.10).

$$K = 273.15 + (°C) \qquad \text{Eq. 2.10}$$

For example, the following calculation is made to convert the normal core temperature of 37 °C to kelvin:

$$37 °C = 273 + 37 = 310 K$$

If an environmental Celsius temperature is a minus value, such as −10 °C, then the calculation is

$$-10 °C = 273 + (-10) = 263 K$$

Relative Humidity (RH)

Many laboratories have a hygrometer instrument to measure relative humidity. These instruments simply state the relative humidity in units of percent (e.g., 50 %). No con-

versions are necessary because the percent unit is universal. Ideally, laboratories should have instruments that display directly or indirectly the wet-bulb globe temperature index (WBGT index). This index considers the interaction among relative humidity, air temperature, and radiant temperature.

Barometric Pressure (P$_B$)

Altitudes higher than 1500 m (4920 ft) produce barometric pressures less than 840 hPa (hectopascal; 630 torr; 630 mm Hg). Usually, an exercise physiology laboratory has mercury or aneroid barometers to measure atmospheric (barometric) pressure in units of millimeters of mercury (mm Hg). Home and nautical barometers usually have pressure units in inches of mercury (in. Hg). Many of the weather reports on U.S. television and radio state the air pressure in inches of mercury. SCUBA gauges use units of pressure called atmospheres (atm) and "pounds per square inch" (psi) but these are not acceptable SI units. Although we will see "mm Hg" and "torr" (and occasionally more recently, hPa) in the scientific literature dealing with atmospheric pressure, the 1995 SI recommended unit is pascal (Pa).[15] Because the pascal is small, which produces large, cumbersome numbers such as 101 325 Pa for sea level pressure (760 mm Hg), the most convenient unit for environmental pressures are the hectopascal (hPa) and the kilopascal (kPa). I have only seen the kilopascal unit on tire

---

[j]Kelvin is a basic unit that does not need a degree (°) symbol preceding it. Thus, one can say, "273 K," not "273 °K."

Table 2.3

Table 2.3 Meteorological Units, Conversions, and Mnemonics for Temperature and Barometric Pressure

Temperature (T)	Barometric Pressure (P$_B$)
273 K = 0 °C = 32 °F	760 torr = sea level
–40 °C = – 40 °F	760 torr = 29.92 in. Hg[a]
0 °C = 32 °F (freezing)	760 torr = 1 atmosphere (atm)
10 °C = 50 °F	760 torr = 1013 mbar
16 °C ≈ 61 °F (60.8 exactly)	1 in. Hg = 25.4 mm Hg = 25.4 torr
22 °C ≈ 72 °F (71.6 exactly)	750 torr = 999.75 mbar ≈ 1000 mbar
28 °C ≈ 82 °F (82.4 exactly)	1 torr = 133.3 Pa = 1.333 hPa = 0.133 kPa
37 °C = 98.6 °F (T$_{core}$)	1 kPa = 7.50 torr
40 °C = 104.0 °F	1 hPa = 0.750 torr
100 °C = 212 °F (boiling)	

Note: The symbol ≈ means "approximately." [a]Mnemonic for 29.92: the number is the same when read backwards.

gauges, not laboratory barometers. In accordance with SI style, scientists should convert the observed millimeter of mercury unit into a hectopascal unit, or the temporarily accepted millibar unit of measure.[15] The hectopascal (1 hPa = 100 Pa) has the same numerical value as the millibar (mbar; 1/1000 bar), which is a common unit for meteorologists. The barometric pressure at sea level is commonly given as 760 mm Hg, 760 torr, or 29.92 in. Hg. In hectopascal, kilopascal, and millibar units, sea level is 1013 hPa, 101.3 kPa, and 1013 mbar. Because the pascal unit is unfamiliar to the U.S. population, including many of its scientists, it may be justified (and approved by SI style) to first record the SI unit "hPa" and then to place the U.S. unit immediately following in parentheses. Thus, sea level might be indicated as "1013 hPa (760 mm Hg)." The lowest *natural* occurring barometric pressure at sea level ever recorded was 840 hPa (630 mm Hg). Pressures from this lowest value to 1066 hPa (800 mm Hg) would not be expected to influence exercise performance.[6,14] The lowest barometric pressure I ever observed in my laboratory at an altitude of ≈ 48 m (157 ft) was 993 hPa (745 mm Hg) during a severe El Niño storm in 1998. Table 2.3 gives an assortment of SI unit conversions, along with some temperature mnemonics (memory aids) that may be helpful for quick conversions.

The American College of Sports Medicine permits exceptions to the SI units for physiological and gas pressures.[2] Thus, blood pressure units and lung pressures are reported in millimeters of mercury (mm Hg) in the journal *Medicine and Science in Sports and Exercise.*

Metric Conversions

Metric units are much simpler to use than the traditional units of the American system. The metric system facilitates the transition (or conversion) from weight and length measures to volume measures and vice versa.

The following conversion factors are categorized according to length, force, weight (mass), and volume mea-

sures. The conversions from the metric dimension to the American dimension are helpful for Americans in visualizing the size of the object. However, it is best to visualize in metrics. That is, as you learn the metric system, let the metric value itself be meaningful by visualizing it before making a conversion to the American value. For example, when in the presence of a woman who says that her body weight (body mass) is 60 kg and that she is 160 cm or 1.60 m tall, let her image linger in your thoughts before making the conversion to the American system. Thus, picture her in the metric perspective, and then, if you must, make the conversion where she is revealed as being 5 ft 3 in. tall and her weight is 132 lb.

Fortunately, most instruments in an exercise physiology laboratory are labeled in metric units. Thus, there are not many occasions when students need to convert to metrics. A pocket calculator with basic functions, such as addition, subtraction, multiplication, division, and square root, is adequate for most calculations in this laboratory manual, including those needed for making conversions. Some calculators have automatic functions for metric conversions, but your instructor may not wish you to use these during exams.

Length Measures

Every exercise physiology student is expected to respond quickly and correctly in metric units to the question "What is your body weight (mass) and stature (height)?" Virtually all Americans fail to express common length measures, such as their height, in metric units. Most Americans cannot visualize metric dimensions accurately. For example, the average height for an American woman between the ages of 18 y and 35 y is 163 cm or 1.63 m. However, many can only picture this height after converting it to ≈ 64 in. or 5 ft 4 in. Also, Americans refer to typical sheets of paper as "8 1/2 by 11 in.," not "21.5 cm by 28 cm." Rarely would Americans refer to a mountain location at an altitude of 9900 ft as being located at 3000 m, nor would they relate a 55 mph (or mi·h^{-1}) speed limit to about 90 km/h (km·h^{-1}).

The metric unit of measure for length is the meter (m). Body height, or stature, is often expressed in meters or centimeters. The length of one centimeter is about 40 % the length of one inch. To convert the average height of 69.5 in. for men between the ages of 18 y and 35 y[7] to centimeters, the inches may be divided by the metric conversion factor 0.3937, or multiplied by 2.54 as follows:

$$cm = 69.5 \div 0.3937 = 176.53$$

$$= 176.5 \text{ to closest tenth centimeter}$$

$$cm = 69.0 \times 2.54 = 176.53$$

$$= 176.5 \text{ to closest tenth centimeter}$$

I encourage students to visualize metric dimensions. For example, Figure 2.1 shows the size of a 10 cm or 0.1 m line. Students should practice visualizing 10 cm by noting nearby objects that seem about 10 cm in length.

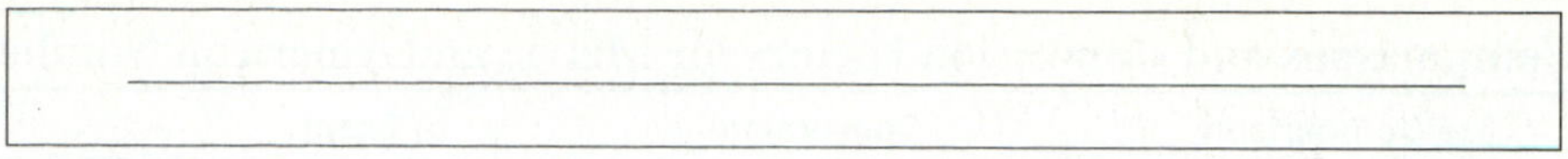

Figure 2.1 Visualization of a 10 cm line (also 100 mm or 0.1 m).

BOX 2.1 | **Length Units**

1 m = 100 cm = 1000 mm = 39.370 in.
    = 3.281 ft (≈ 3.3 ft) = 1.0936 yd
1 cm = 10 mm = 0.01 m = 0.3937 in.
1 mm = 0.001 m (≈ 1/25 in.)
1 km = 1000 m = 0.62137 mi
Mnemonic: 165.1 cm = 65 in.
1 in. = 2.54 cm = 25.4 mm
1 ft = 0.3048 m
1 yd = 0.914 m
1 mi = 1609.35 m = 1.609 km ≈ 1.6 km

BOX 2.2 | **Mass**

1 kg = 1000 g = 2.2046 lb ≈ 2.2 lb
1 g = 1000 mg = 0.0022 lb = 0.0352 oz
1 lb = 0.453 59 kg ≈ 0.45 kg
1 oz = 28.3495 g

BOX 2.3 | **Volume**

1 L = 1000 mL = 1.0567 qt ≈ 1.06 qt
1 qt = 0.9464 L
Avogadro number = 6.02217×10^{23} molecules in a mole (mol) of any substance
1 mol of any gas = 22.414 L at standard temperature and pressure

---

BOX 2.4 | **Interconversion of Units**

1 cm^3 = 1 mL
1000 cm^3 = 1000 mL = 1 L = 1 kg

Common SI metric units

Common SI metric units and the accepted SI symbols are presented for length, weight (mass), and volume in Boxes 2.1–2.4. The metric value of one meter (1 m) presented in Box 2.1 originally represented the fractional distance from the equator to the geographic North Pole—that is, one-tenth millionth (0.1/1 000 000). The SI now defines it as the path traveled by light in vacuum during a time interval of 1/299 792 458 s.[15]

Weight (Mass: M) Measures

In responding to the question "What is your body weight?" exercise physiologists respond using the metric unit called the kilogram. They also describe components of body mass, such as lean body mass and fat mass, using the kilogram unit. And, when they measure underwater body mass to obtain body density and percent fat, they use the gram. Box 2.2 relates the gram to its metric counterparts the kilogram and milligram. Additionally, it points out that the metric kilogram is more than twice as heavy as one pound. A body weight, or body mass, of 144 lb can be converted to the closest kg by dividing the American value by the approximate conversion factor

2.2 or multiplying by the approximate conversion factor 0.45 as follows:

$$kg = 144.0 \div 2.2 = 65$$

or

$$= 144.0 \times 0.45 = 65$$

Force (F) Measures

The SI unit for force, the newton (N), signifies the product of mass (kg) and acceleration (a), which is expressed as $kg \cdot m \cdot s^{-2}$, or $kg \times m/s^2$. A kilogram is approximately (≈) 10 times more forceful than one newton. Thus, 1 kg is equal to 9.806 N, or, approximately, 1 kg is 10 N. Conversely, 1 N is equal to 0.1019 kg, or, approximately, 1 N is 0.1 kg.

Volume (V) Measures

Exercise physiologists use volume measures for such variables as oxygen consumption, lung volumes, sweat loss, fluid replacement, and cardiovascular measures of cardiac output and stroke volume. The basic unit of measure for volume is the liter (L); it is 5.67 % larger than an American system's quart (qt) unit. Box 2.3 presented the metric vs. American conversions, in addition to the descriptions of Avogadro's number and a mole of gas. The latter are helpful in understanding pressure and volume relationships, which are discussed in Chapter 15.

Interaction of Length, Mass, and Volume Units

The metric system facilitates the conversion from mass (weight) and length measures to volume units of measure

Table 2.4 Size Comparisons and Conversion Factors for Metric and American Numbers

Variable	Size Comparison	Conversion	Exact	Approximate (≈)
Length	1 cm < 1 in.	in. to cm	in. ÷ 0.3937	≈ 0.4
			in. × 2.54	same (2.54)
	1 m > 1 ft	ft to m	ft ÷ 3.281	≈ 3.3
			ft × 0.3048	≈ 0.3
	1 m > 1 yd	yd to m	yd ÷ 1.0936	≈ 1.1
			yd × 0.914	≈ 0.9
	1 km < 1 mi	mi to km	mi ÷ 0.621	≈ 0.6
			mi × 1.609	≈ 1.6
Mass	1 g < 1 oz	oz to g	oz ÷ 0.0352	≈ 0.035
			oz × 28.3495	≈ 28
	1 kg > 1 lb	lb to kg	lb ÷ 2.2046	≈ 2.2
			lb × 0.453 59	≈ 0.45
Volume	1 L > 1 qt	qt to L	qt ÷ 1.0567	≈ 1.06
			qt × 0.9464	≈ 0.95

BOX 2.5 Possible Student Activities

- Students list metric items, metric markers, and metric reports that they observe in their daily lives over the next few days.
- Students estimate the metric lengths of various items in the laboratory.
- Using Figure 2.1, each student places the right hand with all digits together, so that the thumb's edge is at the left edge of the 10 cm line. Is the edge of the little finger within 2 cm of the end of the line?
- Students hold and then estimate the mass in kilograms of various items (e.g., lifting weights, beaker with water).
- Students estimate the stature and body mass of other students.
- Each student weighs one of his or her shoes to the closest hundredth of a kilogram on a triple beam scale or a sensitive electronic scale. For example, if a shoe is 316 g, then its mass to the closest hundredth kilogram is 0.32 kg. Record the mass here: ____ g, ____ kg.
- Students compare a "meter stick" with a "yard stick."
- Students solve the problems presented in Box 2.6, then check answers with those in Box 2.7.
- Students are encouraged to bring a digital wrist-stopwatch and a pocket calculator to each laboratory session.

BOX 2.6 Metric Problems

Most of the problems presented here may be solved in more than one way. These different approaches to the same problem may sometimes produce small differences in the answers. Also, differences may be produced due to rounding off of the various conversion factors. These differences are small enough to be of little practical significance in most exercise physiology laboratory classes.

Before starting any calculations, students are encouraged to "guesstimate" the answer. Guessing will prevent making obvious errors, such as placement of the decimal point, and will force metric thinking and visualization.

1. Which of these two lengths is longer—250 yd or 240 m?
2. A ski length of 68.9 in. is how many centimeters?
3. 35 mph = ? km·h^{-1}
4. Most distance racing shoes have a weight less than 10 oz. How many grams is this?
5. 2.5 gal = ? L and ? mL
6. True or False: 12.5 qt is > 13 L
7. Twenty-eight miles per gallon = ? km/L
8. True or False: 82 °F is < 30 °C
9. A barometric pressure equal to 29.92 in. Hg is equal to ? hPa.

---

and vice versa. For example, when a length unit such as a centimeter (cm) is cubed (cm^3), it becomes a volume unit of measure.[k] Thus, 1000 cm^3 is the same as 1000 mL (or 1 L), a volume measure (Box 2.4). Also, one liter of water, a volume unit of measure, is equivalent to one kilogram, a mass unit of measure. It is easier to remember and rationalize that one liter equals one kilogram than to remember and rationalize that one quart equals 2.09 lb.

Converting mass to volume has practical significance to an exercise physiologist who is concerned about a performer's water loss via perspiration under hot conditions. Using a sensitive weight scale, the physiologist can calculate the amount (volume) of water lost during exercise by simply subtracting the person's weight after exercise from the weight before exercise. For example, if a person rapidly lost 1 kg of body mass while exercising in a sauna, it would require 1 L of fluid to restore normal water balance (assuming that fat loss was insignificant).

Summary of Metric Conversions

Some metric units have sizes that are greater than (>) their respective American sizes. For example, one meter is about 10 % longer than one yard (1 m > 1 yd). Contrarily, there are some metric sizes that are less than (<) their respective American sizes, such as the centimeter which is about 40 % the length of an inch (cm < in.).

Table 2.4 presents other examples of these size comparisons and provides the necessary values for converting

---

[k]The abbreviation "cc" for cubic centimeter is not recommended as an International System unit.

References

1. American College of Sports Medicine (ACSM). (2000). *ACSM's guidelines for graded exercise testing and exercise prescription.* Philadelphia: Lippincott Williams & Wilkins.
2. American College of Sports Medicine (ACSM). (1999). Information for authors. *Medicine and Science in Sports and Exercise, 31*(1), i–v.
3. American Psychological Association. (1994). *Publication manual of the American Psychological Association* (p. 105). Washington, DC: Author.
4. Åstrand, P.-O. (1988). *Work tests with the bicycle ergometer.* Varberg, Sweden: Monark Crescent AB.
5. Åstrand, P.-O., & Rodahl, K. (1977). *Textbook of work physiology.* San Francisco: McGraw-Hill.
6. Buskirk, E. R., Kolias, J., Ackers, R. F., Prokop, E. K., & Reategui, E. P. (1967). Maximal performance at altitude and on return from altitude in conditioned runners. *Journal of Applied Physiology, 23,* 259–266.
7. Frisancho, A. R. (1990). *Anthropometric standards for the assessment of growth and nutritional status.* Ann Arbor: University of Michigan Press.
8. Gaesser, G. A., & Poole, D. C. (1996). The slow component of oxygen uptake kinetics in humans. In J. O. Holloszy (Ed.), *Exercise and sport sciences reviews* (pp. 35–70). Baltimore: Williams & Wilkins.
9. Garrett, W. E. (1985). Editor's comment. *National Geographic, 167* (6): 693.
10. Knuttgen, H. G. (1986). Quantifying exercise performance with SI units. *The Physician and Sportsmedicine, 14*(12): 157–161.
11. Knuttgen, H. G. (1995). Force, work, and power in athletic training. *Sports Science Exchange, 57*(4): 1–6.
12. Lang, P. B., Latin, R. W., Berg, K. E., & Mellon, M. B. (1992). The accuracy of the ACSM cycle ergometry equation. *Medicine and Science in Sports and Exercise, 24,* 272–276.
13. Powers, S. K., & Howley, E. T. (2001). *Exercise physiology.* Boston: McGraw-Hill.
14. Squires, R. W., & Buskirk, E. R. (1982). Aerobic capacity during acute exposure to simulated altitude, 914 to 2286 meters. *Medicine and Science in Sports and Exercise, 14,* 36–40.
15. Taylor, B. N. (1995). *NIST Special Publication 811, 1995 Edition: Guide for the use of the International System of Units (SI)* (p. 4). Gaithersburg, MD: United States Department of Commerce, National Institute of Standards and Technology.
16. Young, D. S. (1987). Implementation of SI units for clinical laboratory data. *Annals of Internal Medicine, 106,* 114–129.

American values to metric ones. For example, if the length of a sprint is 50 yd, then by dividing 50 yd by 1.0936 the metric distance is 45.7 m. Rarely is it necessary in exercise physiology to convert metric units to American units, unless the reading or listening audience has not yet learned to visualize the metric values. Even in that exception, the presenter should mention the metric value as an "aside" or in parentheses. The student activities listed in Box 2.5 should assist in the learning of the units in this chapter. Boxes 2.6 and 2.7 show examples of metric problems and solutions.

Nearly all test forms (data collection forms) include basic information about the participants. The information is sometimes referred to as either basic data or vital data, including such items as (1) name, (2) date, (3) time, (4) age, (5) gender, (6) height, and (7) weight. Often, vital data include heart rate and blood pressure; however, these last two variables are omitted in this manual's data forms except in Part 5—"Cardiovascular Testing." Form 3.1, at the end of this chapter, may be used to record *basic data* and, in some cases, to calculate metric conversions for basic data.

Recording Basic Data

The art and technical skills of administering tests include the precise and thorough recording of all basic data. Some of the comments here may appear so obvious that they are unnecessary, but I have witnessed numerous occasions when seemingly obvious items of basic data were omitted, much to the later chagrin of the investigators or the participants.

Names, Date, and Time

Names are always written with the last name first, followed by a comma and then the first name. In potentially publishable research, an identification number (ID#) replaces the name for anonymity and confidentiality purposes. Also, to resolve discrepancies or errors it helps to include the technician's (tester's) initials, especially if technicians have interobserver differences.

The test **date** is presented with the month in numerical form at the beginning of the date. For example, September 4, 2002 would be recorded as 9/4/02 (or 09/04/02). Besides recording these on the data collection form (e.g., Form 3.1), name and date should be recorded on any type of chart paper, such as the electrocardiogram or isokinetic machine's recording paper.

It is important to record test **time** on the data collection form because of the diurnal or circadian variations of certain biological and performance variables.[7,8,9] It is best to repeat tests on the same person as closely as possible to the original time of the test.

Age and Gender

Age is recorded to the closest year (y), except when it may be important to record to the closest tenth year. For exam-

ple, if someone turned 72 y of age four months ago, then the age might be recorded as 72.3 y.

Gender (sex) for a person is abbreviated as M (male) or F (female). For a group of persons over 17 years of age, the recommended group designation is M (men) and W (women).[2] But, as long as there is a single participant under 18 y of age, the group's designation is male or female, not men or women.

Height (Stature) and Body Weight (Mass)

The anthropometric[a] term for height is **stature,** because the latter refers to a human's height, not a tree's height or a building's height.[6] The term **mass,** as noted in Chapter 2, is synonymous with *weight* under normal acceleration of gravity. Obviously, people's weights or masses are measured at normal (Earth's) gravitational force. The body mass and body weight of a person use the same unit of measure—the kilogram (kg). In Chapter 4, we will see that we will use body weight as a force measure to calculate work and power. In that case, we will use the SI unit for force—the newton (N).

The technician records stature to the nearest tenth of a centimeter (0.1 cm; 1 mm) if the height scale (stadiometer; anthropometer) has such graduations (markings). If the platform scale's anthropometer is only in inches and its graduations are ¼ in. or ½ in., then the technician records the inches to the closest ¼ in. or ½ in., respectively. Then the inch value is converted and recorded to the legitimately rounded centimeter or decimal centimeter.

The main considerations in rounding off numbers are conventionality, consistency of the significant digits, and precision of the measurement. The appropriate conventionality guide is that of the International System (SI).[13] SI recommends using the "5 rule" when reducing a certain number of digits to the significant digits. Fortunately, it is the rule with which most Americans are familiar. "If the digits to be discarded begin with a digit less than 5, the digit preceding the 5 is not changed." For example, the number 7.44 changed to a two-digit number would become 7.4; changed to a one-digit number, it would become 7 (but not 7.0). Conversely, if the discarded digit or digits begin with a number greater than 5, then the digit preceding the 5 is in-

---

[a]The term *anthropometric* means "measurement of humans."

creased by 1. For example, 167.66 cm becomes 167.7 cm as a four-digit number and becomes 168 as a three-digit number. If the discarded digit or digits begin with a 5 and are followed by no digit or zeros, then the preceding number remains even, or becomes even if it had been odd. For example, 77.5 kg, or 77.50 kg, become 78 kg as a two-digit number; however, 66.5 kg and 66.50 kg, are rounded to the even number 66 kg as a two-digit number.

The degree of precision sought in a measure or mathematical calculation is dependent upon the purposes of the measurement and the precision of the instrument. For example, in the United States the stature of a person is often stated to the closest ½ in. (1.27 cm) or ¼ in. (≈0.6 cm), depending upon the accuracy of the stadiometer. Thus, when the mean *(M)* height is calculated from the heights of several persons, it should be rounded off either to the closest ½ in. or ¼ in., respectively. If converting the inches to centimeters, both the ½ in. (0.5 in.) and ¼ in. (0.25 in.) values should not be rounded to the closest tenth centimeter because the stadiometer does not justify such precision. The closest 0.5 cm would be a justifiably rounded number for the ¼ in. scale and to the closest centimeter for the ½ in. scale. Rounding off to the closest *tenth* centimeter provides unwarranted and false information. However, if the purpose of the investigators is to detect the change in height in persons from morning to evening, then they should choose a more precise stadiometer (stadio = stature; meter = measurement). By choosing a centimeter scale with graduations in tenths, they can record height to the closest 0.1 cm (1 mm or ≈ 1/25 in.).

Methods of Measuring Height (Stature) and Weight (Body Mass)

I encourage my students to test other students rather than a student testing oneself. Although this can take more time, it mimics typical research procedures and it gives students, referred to as "technicians," or "testers," practice in their personal relationship with a participant. As an example of the latter, technicians should call participants by their names and thank deserving participants for their cooperation and effort.

You may recall from Chapter 1 that one of the major sections of an abstract is the "Method" section. The method sections in this manual usually include two major phases—preparations and procedures. Three items are usually included in the procedures phase—the technician's steps for administering the test, the calculations and conversions, and the recording of the data onto the forms. Box 3.1 discusses the accuracy of stature and weight measures.

Stature (Height) Method

Height—or the more technical term, *stature*—is a variable that is not usually as significant as weight (mass) in most exercise physiology evaluations. However, it is a basic variable that is routinely measured in all laboratories; thus, its accurate and standardized measurement should be given serious attention. Our **purposes** for measuring stature are (1) to familiarize students with standardized stature measurements; (2) to characterize, or describe, the participant; (3) to relate the participant's height to U.S. norms; and (4) to relate the participant's body mass (weight) to stature (height) based on U.S. norms.

Stature may be measured on a physician's scale or platform-beam scale (review Figure 3.1) if the scale's stadiometer has been checked for accuracy. Most U.S. platform scale's stadiometers (or anthropometers) now have both centimeter and inch graduations on the sliding vertical bar. The bar has a hinged lever, which the technician can swing upward to a 90° angle onto the crown of the participant's head.

Inexpensive wall-mounted stadiometers with a horizontal head lever that slides between two stoppable grooves are convenient and accurate (e.g., Seca™; www.seca.com). A stadiometer can be improvised by attaching a metric-graduated tape against a wall. Then any right-angled device can be placed against the crown of a person's head and

---

BOX 3.1 **Accuracy of Stature and Body Mass (Weight) Measures**

Stature

The test-retest reliability of height measurements is very high. My correlation coefficient (*r*) was .998 for 28 men tested about one week to two weeks apart. Others have reported correlation coefficients of 0.89 for within-day trials and day-to-day trials.[3]

Body Mass

Body mass is a very reliable measurement. In two separate studies, my **test-retest correlations** for the participants' body mass were as high as .99 and .995 in 93 and 28 men, respectively. Others have found similarly high (*r* = .99) values.[3] Body mass is often measured on a platform scale that has a balancing beam with two moveable weights and one tare-screw weight (Figure 3.1). The **sensitivity** and graduated marks of these common scales usually is 1/4 lb (0.113 kg; 4 oz). Some types of laboratory scales (Precision Scale™) for measuring body mass are sensitive enough to detect weights to the closest 20 g (0.02 kg; 0.71 oz), about the mass of three U.S. quarters plus a penny. Not even this sensitive scale is sensitive enough to measure the mass of a dime (2.2 g), a penny (2.4 g), or a nickel (5.0 g). However, a triple-beam scale, which is sometimes called a chemistry scale, is sensitive enough to measure the mass of any U.S. coin to a tenth of a gram (0.1 g). The upper limit of a person's body mass on most U.S. platform scales is 159 kg (350 lb).

against the wall. Instead, a mark may be made at the lower edge of the right-angled device, and then the height of that mark can be measured with, ideally, a metal metric tape. It may be convenient to have a short stool, bench, or step-ladder for the technician to stand on to measure tall persons. The following procedures may help to standardize and enhance the accuracy of stature measurements:

Preparation

1. If using the platform-beam scale, check its accuracy by confirming the distance from the platform base to the first graduated measure on the stadiometer.
2. Complete Form 3.1 with the prior basic data information (name, date, time, age, and gender).

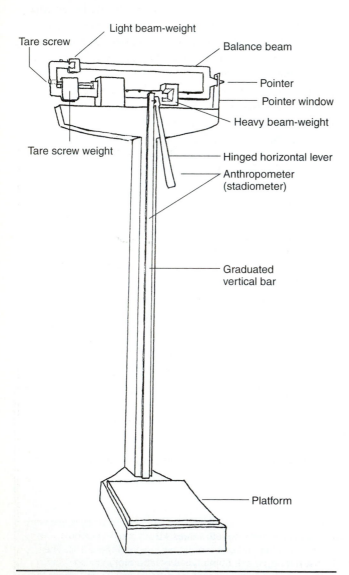

Figure 3.1 The platform scale is an instrument for body weight (mass) and height (stature). The anthropometer (stadiometer) with the sliding vertical bar and hinged horizontal head lever is the portion of the platform scale that measures height.

3. Ask the participant to remove shoes; thin socks may remain. Also, if weight is measured simultaneously, ask the participant to remove as many clothes and jewelry as feasible.

Procedures for Stature (Height) Measurement

1. The participant steps onto the platform scale and then turns, facing away from the balance beam and the stadiometer. The technician, probably standing on a stool, asks the participant to lower the head in order to clear the swing of the hinged lever to a horizontal position. If using a "wall stadiometer," the participant stands facing away from the wall, with heels, scapulae, and buttocks in contact with the wall. Some persons will not be able to maintain a natural stance if the posterior of the head is also touching the wall.[6]
2. The participant stands as tall as possible with heels together and feet evenly balanced at an angle of approximately 60°, using the medial borders (inside) of the feet and the wall as the reference lines.[13] For example, a 90° angle would indicate that the feet were pointed directly forward.
3. As the participant inhales deeply and maintains the designated position, the technician places one edge of the right-angled object against the wall and places the other edge on the top of the participant's head. If using the platform scale's stadiometer, the technician places the stadiometer's hinged lever on top of the participant's head, so that the horizontal lever forms a right angle with the graduated vertical rod.
4. The technician records (Form 3.1) the height to the nearest tenth of a centimeter (0.1 cm) if using a precise stadiometer. However, if the platform scale's stadiometer is only in inches and its graduations are ¼ in. or ⅛ in., then the technician records the inches to the closest ¼ in. or ⅛ in., respectively, onto Form 3.1.
5. The technician converts the inch length to centimeter length and then records it to the legitimately rounded centimeter of 0.5 cm (if ¼ or ⅛ in.) or 1 cm (if ½ in.) onto Form 3.1.
6. Although weather conditions have no known effect on stature, the technician should get into the habit of recording meteorological data onto the data collection form. These data may be recorded before or after the stature measurement.

Body Mass (Weight) Method

Body mass is probably the most measured variable in exercise physiology laboratories. This basic variable is factored into many of the other variables described in this laboratory manual; hence, its importance cannot be overestimated.

Participants can be weighed in the attire that corresponds to the reference source. For example, if the reference source for comparison allowed 0.3 kg (300 g; ≈ ⅔ lb) of clothing, such as underwear, shirt, and shorts, dress, or trousers, then the person may be weighed in such attire. In the exercise physiology laboratory, often the nude, or nearly nude, person is weighed for tests that relate the fitness score to body mass. Nude weight is always preferred for tests of body composition. If a person wears only a disposable paper gown, it may be deemed as nude weight.[6] Although weighing the nude person is ideal, it may be more convenient to weigh the person's clothes prior to weighing that person wearing those clothes. Then the nude weight is simply the weight of the clothes subtracted from the weight of the person wearing those clothes. The exercise-clothed weight should be used for the calculation of work or power when the participants are lifting their own weight, such as in bench stepping, uphill walking, or uphill running. This is because the participants are lifting the weight of the apparel in addition to their own body weight. The following methods are helpful when measuring a participant's body mass:

Preparation by the Technician

1. Calibrate the weighing scale if it has not been calibrated within a month (Box 3.2).[5]

2. Insert the acquired basic data, such as participant's name, date, time, age, gender, and technician's initials, onto Form 3.1.
3. Weigh the person's weigh-in clothing excluding shoes.
4. Record the mass of the weigh-in clothing onto Form 3.1 to the closest ¼ lb if weighed on a nonmetric scale or to the closest 0.02 kg if weighed on a sensitive metric scale.
5. Ask the participant to put on the clothes that were weighed previously and to remove shoes, thick socks, and jewelry.

Procedures for Body Mass (Weight) Measurement

1. The participant, now wearing the weigh-in clothing, stands on and faces the scale. If stature was just measured, then the person simply turns to face the scale while the technician acts as an assistant or spotter (vice versa if stature will be measured after the weight measurement).
2. To avoid disturbing the participant, the technician stands behind the platform scale when reading and adjusting the beam weights. Most platform scales have graduations on both sides.
3. The technician places the heavy beam weight (lower lever) to the estimated graduation mark.

BOX 3.2   Example of Calibration Procedures for the Platform Scale

Zero Calibration

1. Set both moveable beam weights of the scale to the zero positions.
2. Observe the position of the pointer; it should come to rest in midair between the top and bottom of the pointer window.
3. If necessary, balance the pointer in this midair position by using a dime, screwdriver, or strong thumbnail to adjust the tare-screw weight of the platform scale. Turning the tare screw clockwise moves the tare-screw weight toward the screw's head, thus lifting the pointer higher in the pointer window.

High-Point Calibration

1. Set the beam weights to the highest position for which you have calibration weights or to the position of the highest expected body mass of your participants. Typical platform scales cannot read body masses above 159 kg (350 lb). Ideally, if you have 350 lb of certified weights, place them on the scale. But, if you have only 100 kg (220.5 lb to closest 0.1 lb) certified weights, or weights that you have "certified" on a precision scale, then set them on the scale and adjust the beam weights accordingly. For example, set the heavy beam weight to 200 lb and set the light beam weight to 20.5 lb.
2. Observe the position of the pointer. If it is balanced in midposition in the pointer window, then the scale is accurate at body masses near the high-point range.
3. If the pointer is above the balanced point, then adjust the light lever weight, if necessary, to the pointer's midair position.
4. Record any discrepancy between the original set position and the final balanced position.
5. If needed, derive a correction factor for the high-point readings. For example, if 120 kg of "certified" high-point weights showed 121 kg on the scale, then subtract 1 kg from those persons' body weights that were between 110 kg and 130 kg (range chosen arbitrarily).

Midpoint Calibration

1. Estimate the average body mass of the participants.
2. Place "certified" weights on the scale that come close to the estimated participants' average weight. (A Cybex™ machine has certified weights.)
3. Balance the pointer to the midair position. If it is already balanced, then the scale is accurate near the midpoint position of the pound or kilogram scale.
4. If the pointer is not in the midair position, adjust the light beam weight to the balanced position.
5. Record any discrepancy between the original set position and the final midair position.
6. If needed, derive a correction factor for midpoint readings or readjust the tare-screw weight to the pointer's midair position. Unfortunately, this will change the zero point, thus distorting low-range body masses.

4. The technician places the light beam-weight (upper lever) to the graduation mark that causes the pointer to balance in the midair position within the window. If the pointer cannot be balanced with the light beam-weight, then the heavy beam-weight must be readjusted.

5. The technician records the body mass to the closest ¼ lb onto Form 3.1. If the technician weighs the person on a sensitive electronic scale, then the person simply steps on the platform and waits until the technician records the body mass to the closest 0.02 kg (20 g) onto Form 3.1. The rounded off 2.2 (or 2.20) conversion factor for American-to-metric may be used instead of the exact 2.2046 conversion value in order to calculate weight to the closest 0.1 kg.

6. The technician assists the participant off the scale and reminds the person of any jewelry that might have been removed.

7. The technician, using Tables 3.1, 3.2 (Men), or 3.3 (Women), records participant's relationship to U.S. average and percentile onto Form 3.1.

8. The technician, using Table 3.4 and the 85 % criterion, records only the woman participant's optimum weight onto Form 3.1.

9. The technician, using Table 3.4 (Women) or 3.5 (Men), records participant's relationship to U.S. average onto Form 3.1.

10. The technician, using Table 3.6, records "Yes" or "No" onto Form 3.1, depending if the participant was within the acceptable weight range for his or her given age-height group.

11. The technician, using Table 3.7 and the $M \pm 11.0$ kg criterion, records the person's percentile category of "average," "above average," or "below average" onto Form 3.1.

Table 3.1 Two Reports of Average Stature (cm) of Men and Women, Ages 18 y to 34 y

	Food & Nutrition Board[a]	Frisancho[b]
Men	177.8	176.5
Women	162.6	162.9

Sources: [a]Food & Nutrition Board, National Academy of Science—National Research Council. (1980). Recommended dietary allowances (9th ed., revised.) In K. L. Jones, L. W. Shainberg, & C. O. Byer (Eds.), *Dimensions* (5th ed.) San Francisco: Harper & Row. [b]Frisancho, A. R. (1990). *Anthropometric standards for the assessment of growth and nutritional status.* Ann Arbor: University of Michigan Press.

Table 3.2 Average Stature (cm) and Percentiles (%ile) for American Men, Ages 18 y to 75 y

Age (y)	Height (M) (cm)	Percentiles (%ile) 5th	10th	15th	25th	50th	75th	85th	90th	95th
18–24.9	176.6	165.4	167.8	169.5	171.9	176.6	181.2	183.7	185.5	188.6
25–29.9	176.7	165.1	167.8	169.4	172.0	176.6	181.5	184.0	185.7	188.0
30–34.9	176.2	164.8	167.4	169.0	171.5	176.2	180.9	183.3	184.8	187.2
35–39.9	176.1	164.0	166.8	168.8	171.9	176.1	181.0	183.5	185.0	187.7
40–44.9	175.9	165.0	167.2	168.9	171.4	176.0	180.3	182.7	184.2	186.9
45–49.9	175.2	163.8	166.5	168.0	170.6	174.8	180.2	182.9	184.5	186.6
50–54.9	174.6	164.2	166.4	167.8	170.2	174.6	178.8	181.4	183.2	185.3
55–59.9	173.9	163.2	165.0	166.8	169.3	173.8	178.7	181.0	182.3	184.6
60–64.9	173.0	161.9	165.0	166.4	168.7	173.0	177.4	179.8	181.3	183.7
65–69.9	171.5	159.7	162.9	164.5	166.7	171.6	176.3	178.6	180.1	182.5
70–74.9	170.6	159.5	162.0	163.6	165.8	170.7	175.0	177.4	179.4	182.0

Permission from: Frisancho, A. R. (1990). *Anthropometric standards for the assessment of growth and nutritional status.* Ann Arbor: University of Michigan Press.

Table 3.3 Average Stature (cm) and Percentiles (%ile) for American Women, Ages 18 y to 75 y

Age (y)	Height (M) (cm)	Percentiles (%ile) 5th	10th	15th	25th	50th	75th	85th	90th	95th
18–24.9	163.0	152.3	154.8	156.4	158.8	163.1	167.1	169.6	171.0	173.6
25–29.9	162.9	152.6	155.2	153.6	156.6	162.8	167.1	169.5	170.9	173.3
30–34.9	162.6	152.9	155.2	156.4	158.4	162.4	166.8	169.2	171.2	173.1
35–39.9	162.8	152.0	155.0	156.4	158.6	162.7	167.0	169.4	171.0	173.5
40–44.9	162.6	151.6	154.3	156.2	158.1	162.7	166.7	168.8	170.5	173.2
45–49.9	162.0	151.7	154.0	155.4	157.9	162.0	166.3	168.4	169.9	172.2
50–54.9	161.2	151.3	153.8	155.3	156.9	161.1	165.1	167.3	169.2	171.0
55–59.9	160.3	149.8	152.7	154.1	156.7	160.3	164.4	166.6	167.8	170.1
60–64.9	159.6	149.2	151.4	153.0	155.6	160.0	163.7	166.1	167.3	169.8
65–69.9	158.6	148.5	150.7	152.4	154.8	158.8	162.6	164.8	166.2	168.1
70–74.9	157.6	147.2	150.0	151.7	153.7	157.4	161.5	163.8	165.5	167.5

Permission from: Frisancho, A. R. (1990). *Anthropometric standards for the assessment of growth and nutritional status.* Ann Arbor: University of Michigan Press.

Results and Discussion of Stature and Body Mass

The results section of a scientific report or study simply presents the findings in the text, tables, and figures. In the exercise physiology classroom, the results of the measurements are recorded also on the individual data collection form (e.g., Form 3.1) and the group data collection form (e.g., Form 3.2). The group form may use the participant's ID number or initials, instead of the name. The group results often include the mean *(M)*, standard deviation *(SD)*, and range of scores—that is, the lowest (minimum) to the highest (maximum) score.

The discussion section of a scientific report provides the reader with an interpretation of the results or measured values. The interpretation of the individual's stature or body mass and the average of the group can be made by re-ferring to the appropriate tables, which give the values from a much larger—but, ideally, a similar—population.

Stature

An interpretation of body stature may be made by comparing the person's height with that of the same age group and gender. In some cases, the stated values for the age categories may differ from one source to another. For example, the Food and Nutrition[4] source gives a higher average height for men between the ages of 18 y and 34 y, than does the Frisancho[5] source.

Effect of Aging on Stature   The average heights for younger men and women are greater than the average heights when all adult ages are included in the norms. Thus, it is not unusual

---

Table 3.4   **Average Weights[a] of American Women, Ages 18 y to 74 y by Age and Height**

| | | Age Group (y) | | | | | | | | | | | |
| | | 18–24 | | 25–34 | | 35–44 | | 45–54 | | 55–64 | | 65–74 | |
in.	cm	lb	kg	lb	kg	lb	kg	lb	kg	lb	kg	lb	kg
57	144.8	114	51.8	118	53.6	125	56.8	129	58.6	132	60.0	130	59.1
58	147.3	117	53.2	121	55.0	129	58.6	133	60.5	136	61.8	134	60.9
59	149.9	120	54.5	125	56.8	133	60.5	136	61.8	140	63.6	137	62.3
60	152.4	123	55.9	128	58.2	137	62.3	140	63.6	143	65.0	140	63.6
61	154.9	126	57.3	132	60.0	141	64.1	143	65.0	147	66.8	144	65.5
62	157.5	129	58.6	136	61.8	144	65.5	147	66.8	150	68.2	147	66.8
63	160.0	132	60.0	139	63.2	148	67.3	150	68.2	153	69.5	151	68.6
64	162.6	135	61.4	142	64.5	152	69.1	154	70.0	157	71.4	154	70.0
65	165.1	138	62.7	146	66.4	156	70.9	158	71.8	160	72.7	158	71.8
66	167.6	141	64.1	150	68.2	159	72.3	161	73.2	164	74.5	161	73.2
67	170.2	144	65.5	153	69.5	163	74.1	165	75.0	167	75.9	165	75.0
68	172.8	147	66.8	157	71.4	167	75.9	168	76.4	171	77.7	169	76.8

Source: Abraham, S., Johnson, C. L., & Naijar, M. F. (1979). *Weight by height and age for adults 18–74 years.* Publication No. (PHS) 79-1656. Hyattsville, MD: U.S. Department of Health, Education, and Welfare. From the NHANES data.
Note: [a]Includes clothing weight between 0.1 to 0.3 kg without shoes; pound-to-kg conversion uses 2.2.

Table 3.5   **Average Weights[a] of American Men, Ages 18 y to 74 y, by Age and Height**

| | | Age Group (y) | | | | | | | | | | | |
| | | 18–24 | | 25–34 | | 35–44 | | 45–54 | | 55–64 | | 65–74 | |
in.	cm	lb	kg	lb	kg	lb	kg	lb	kg	lb	kg	lb	kg
62	157.5	130	59.1	141	64.1	143	65.0	147	66.8	143	65.0	143	65.0
63	160.0	135	61.4	145	65.9	148	67.3	152	69.1	147	66.8	147	66.8
64	162.6	140	63.6	150	68.2	153	69.5	156	70.9	153	69.5	151	68.6
65	165.1	145	65.9	156	70.9	158	71.8	160	72.7	158	71.8	156	70.9
66	167.6	150	68.2	160	72.7	163	74.1	164	74.5	163	74.1	160	72.7
67	170.2	154	70.0	165	75.0	169	76.8	169	76.8	168	76.4	164	74.5
68	172.8	159	72.3	170	77.3	174	79.1	173	78.6	173	78.6	169	76.8
69	175.3	164	74.5	174	79.1	179	81.4	177	80.5	178	80.9	173	78.6
70	177.8	168	76.4	179	81.4	184	83.6	182	82.7	183	83.2	177	80.5
71	180.3	173	78.6	184	83.6	190	86.4	187	85.0	189	85.9	182	82.7
72	182.9	178	80.9	189	85.9	194	88.2	191	86.8	193	87.7	186	84.5
73	185.4	183	83.2	194	88.2	200	90.9	196	89.1	197	89.5	190	86.4
74	188.0	188	85.5	199	90.5	205	93.2	200	90.9	203	92.3	194	88.2

Source: Abraham, S., Johnson, C. L., & Naijar, M. F. (1979). *Weight by height and age for adults 18–74 years.* Publication No. (PHS) 79-1656. Hyattsville, MD: U.S. Department of Health, Education, and Welfare. From the NHANES data.
Note: [a]Includes clothing weight between 0.1 to 0.3 kg without shoes; pound-to-kg conversion uses 2.2.

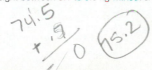

Table 3.6 Acceptable Weights for Men and Women, 19 Years of Age and Older

Height		Weight			
		19 y to 35 y		> 35 y	
in.	cm	lb	kg	lb	kg
60.0	152.4	97–128	44.0–58.1	108–138	49.0–62.6
61.0	154.9	101–132	45.8–59.9	111–143	50.3–64.9
62.0	157.5	104–137	47.2–62.3	115–148	52.2–67.1
63.0	160.0	107–141	48.5–64.0	119–152	69.1–68.9
64.0	162.6	111–146	50.3–66.2	122–157	55.3–71.4
65.0	165.1	114–150	51.8–68.0	126–162	57.3–73.5
66.0	167.6	118–155	53.6–70.3	130–167	59.1–75.8
67.0	170.2	121–160	55.0–72.6	134–172	60.8–78.0
68.0	172.8	125–164	56.8–74.4	138–178	62.7–80.7
69.0	175.3	129–169	58.6–76.6	142–183	64.5–83.0
70.0	177.8	132–174	60.0–78.9	146–188	66.4–85.3
71.0	180.3	136–179	61.8–81.2	151–194	68.6–88.0
72.0	182.9	148–195	67.3–88.5	164–210	74.5–95.3

Source: Joint Dietary Guidelines Advisory Committee of U.S. Departments of Agriculture and Health and Human Services. (1990). *Nutrition and your health: Dietary guidelines for Americans.* Home and Garden Bulletin No. 232: U.S. Department of Agriculture.
Note: Men are in upper-half of range, women in lower-half.

Table 3.7 Percentiles and Expected Distance from the Mean Weight for All Participants[a] and for a Sample Group[b]

Percentile	All Participants[a] (± of the M kg)	Women's Sample Group[b] (kg)
95th	$M + 20.5$	83.7
90th	$M + 16$	79.2
80th (above average)	$M + 11$	74.2
50th (average)	M	63.2
20th (below average)	$M - 11$	52.2
10th	$M - 16$	47.2
5th	$M - 20.5$	42.7

Source: Abraham, S., Johnson, C. L., & Najjar, M. F. (1979). *Weight by height and age for adults 18–74 years.* Publication No. (PHS) 79-1656. Hyattsville, MD: U.S. Department of Health, Education, and Welfare. From the NHANES data.
Note: [a]Any of the average weights in the NHANES tables (3.4 and 3.5). [b]25-year-old to 34-year-old women, 160 cm tall, mean weight 63.2 kg.

for height to decrease starting in the thirties and continuing to decrease throughout older adulthood. Table 3.2, for example, shows the mean heights for men 18 y to 24.9 y as 176.6 cm and from 25 y to 29.9 y as 176.7 cm. But the mean height decreases by 0.5 cm to means of 176.2 cm and 176.1 cm in 30 y to 34.9 y and 35 y to 39.9 y men, respectively.[5] The seventy-year-old men in this cross-sectional study were 6.0 cm shorter ($M = 170.6$ cm) than the youngest age group (176.6 cm). The loss in stature for the women (Table 3.3)[5] was similar to the loss for the men.

Interpretation of Stature Percentiles Average heights (cm) and percentiles (%ile) in men and women ages 18 y to 75 y were presented in Tables 3.2 and 3.3, respectively.[5]

Table 3.3 showed that women's heights between the ages of 18 y and 24.9 y average 163.0 cm and that the 50th %ile is 163.1 cm. The values for the mean and the 50th %ile of any variable, not just stature, are always similar. Determining the percentile from Table 3.3 of a 24-year-old woman who is 171.0 cm tall is simply a matter of finding the row that includes her age group and then moving across the table to the column containing her height. Thus, the woman's percentile is the 90th %ile, meaning that she is taller than 90 % of all women between the ages of 18 y and 24.9 y and is 8.0 cm taller than the average (163. cm) for her age group.

But how would the percentile be determined if the person's height were not on the table? We could accept the percentile column that is closest to the person's height, but we would lose some accuracy. We could be more accurate by using a method called interpolation.[b] Interpolation means that we choose an appropriate percentile according to a height that is between two other percentile columns. For example, if the 24-year-old woman's height is 170.3 cm, then her percentile lies midway between the 85th %ile (169.6 cm) and the 90th %ile (171.0 cm). This places this woman at the 87.5 %ile; by using our "5" rule for rounding off to an even number, she is at the 88th %ile.

Body Mass (Weight)

Body masses, are more meaningful if they are categorized according to height and age. The average American body

---

[b]A method called extrapolation is used for determining the more appropriate percentile for heights that are either higher or lower than any age group's heights. For women ages 18 y to 24.9 y, these would be < 152.3 cm and > 173.6 cm.

masses are listed in Tables 3.4 (women) and 3.5 (men).[1] The weights of these persons between 18 y and 75 y of age included clothing weight up to 0.3 kg, but without shoes.

Effect of Height and Age on Weight   *Men's* weights appear to increase by about 5 lb (2.3 kg) for each inch (2.54 cm) of increased height. For example, the average weight of men between the ages of 18 y and 24.9 y who are 68 in. (172.8 cm) tall is 159 lb (72.3 kg), whereas the average weight of men the same ages who are 69 in. (175.3 cm) tall is 164 lb (74.5 kg). The greatest weight gain in men occurs between the ages of 25 y and 34 y.

Women's weights increase about 3 lb (1.4 kg) for each inch of increased height. Their greatest weight gain occurs between the ages of 35 y and 44 y. It is important to recognize that the weights listed in Tables 3.4 and 3.5 are average weights, not recommended weights.

Interpretation of Weight Percentiles   Table 3.7 provides percentiles that can be used with all age-height categories. A broad designation of "average weights" is assigned to percentiles from the 20th %ile to the 80th %ile. This range represents plus or minus 11 kg ($\pm$ 11 kg) from the 50th %ile or the mean (*M*). For example, if a 25-year-old woman is 160 cm (63 in.) tall and her body mass is 74.4 kg (164 lb), then she is 11.2 kg from her age-height (25 y to 34 y) group's mean weight of 63.2 kg listed in Tables 3.4 and 3.7. This places her slightly above the 80th %ile, thus categorizing her as "above average" body mass. This procedure can be used to categorize body weights for all other age-height groups into "average," "above average," and "below average."

Acceptable and Optimum Body Weights for Women   The body weights listed in Tables 3.4 and 3.5 are average weights, not acceptable body weights and not optimal body weights. The acceptable body weights for men and women listed in Table 3.6 are from the 1990 Joint Dietary Guidelines Advisory Committee.[10] The committee gives quite a large range of acceptable weights for each age-height category. For example, a "big-boned" man between the ages of 19 y and 35 y whose height is 167.6 cm (66.0 in.) can have a body weight from 53.6 kg (118 lb) to 70.3 kg (155 lb) and still be deemed "acceptable."

One group of investigators suggested a method for determining the optimal weights for women.[12] Based on over 100 000 nonsmoking women nurses in the United States who were studied over a 16-year period starting at ages 30 y to 55 y, the study concluded that a direct relationship exists between body weight and risk of death. The investigators suggested that optimum weights for women are 85 % of the U.S. average for women of the same age and stature as those listed in Table 3.4. Using Equation 3.1, the optimum weight may be calculated from the average weight for women of a specific age-height group.

$$\text{Optimum wt for women} \qquad \text{Eq. 3.1}$$
$$= 0.85 \times \text{U.S. ave. for age and ht}$$

For example, a woman between 18 y and 24 y of age who is 165.1 cm (65 in.) tall is in a group with an average weight of 62.7 kg (138 lb) based on Table 3.4. Thus, by using Equation 3.1, the optimum weight in terms of reduced mortality is

$$0.85 \times 62.7 \text{ kg} = 53.3 \text{ kg (117.25 lb)}$$

Although no similar study has derived optimal weights for men based solely on age and height, the body mass index explained in Chapter 23 of this laboratory manual acts similarly as a criterion for reducing mortality risk.

A woman's weight gain after the age of 18 y is an important factor in mortality that should not be overlooked. A weight gain of 9 kg (20 lb) and 18 kg (40 lb) was associated with a 2.5 and 7.0 times greater risk of death from heart disease, respectively, compared with those women maintaining the weights they had had at the age of 18 y.[12]

Figures 3.2 (men) and 3.3 (women) depict percentiles based on the combined first and second National Health and Nutrition Examination Surveys (NHANES).[5] However, the figures comprise all adult ages from 18 y to 74 y, rather than 6-year or 10-year categories for this age group, as in Tables 3.4 and 3.5. The figures also provide five bold and curved lines that categorize weights into "low weight," "below average," "average," "above average," and "heavy weight." For example, if a man between the ages of 18 y and 74 y has a body weight of 78 kg (171.6 lb) and is 175 cm tall, then he would be placed at the 50th %ile.

Data Collection Forms

It might be said that data collection is only as good as the forms onto which you record the data. Forms do not only provide a record of the raw data but can also remind the investigators of the procedural steps to be performed to gather the data. Form 3.1—"Individual Basic Data"—is a good example of both of these characteristics. The data inserted on it are meant for *one* participant, whereas Form 3.2 provides an example of how a form can facilitate data analysis, such as calculating the mean and the range of scores from a *group* of participants. Form 3.3 provides an example of a research abstract and allows you to fill in some of the basic data and results. Form 3.4 provides a template, which may be used to write your own research abstract. It might be helpful to copy this form before writing on it, so that it can be used for future abstracts of test data collected from the later chapters.

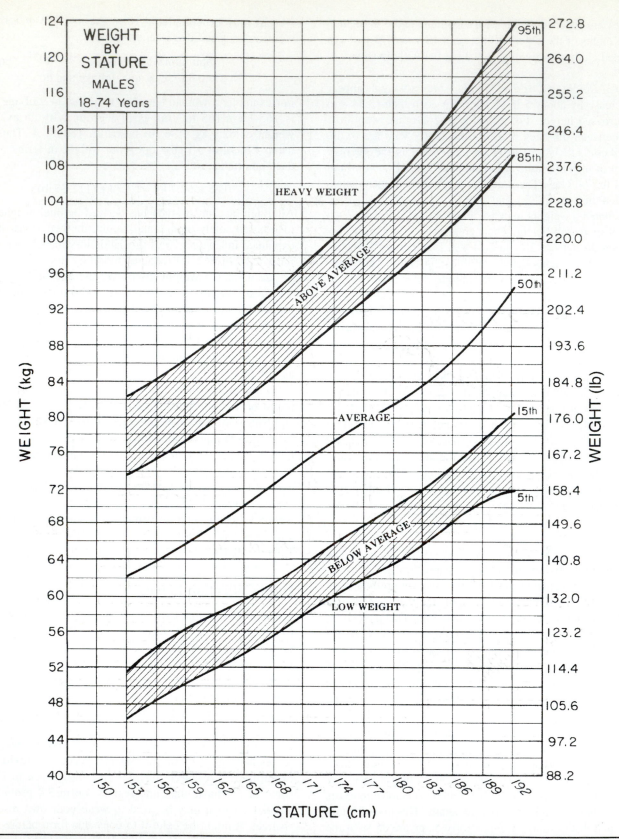

Figure 3.2 Percentiles of weight (kg; lb) based on the stature (cm) of men between the ages of 18 y and 74 y in the NHANES Surveys From: Frisancho, A. R. (1990). *Anthropometric standards for the assessment of growth and nutritional status.* (p. 77). Ann Arbor: University of Michigan Press. The figure allows us to find the percentile of any man between the ages of 18 y and 74 y by using the meeting point of his weight (kg and lb) on the Y axes and his stature (cm) on the X axis. For example, if the man's body weight is 64 kg (140.8 lb) and he is 174 cm tall, then he is in the "below average" category and near the 12th %ile.

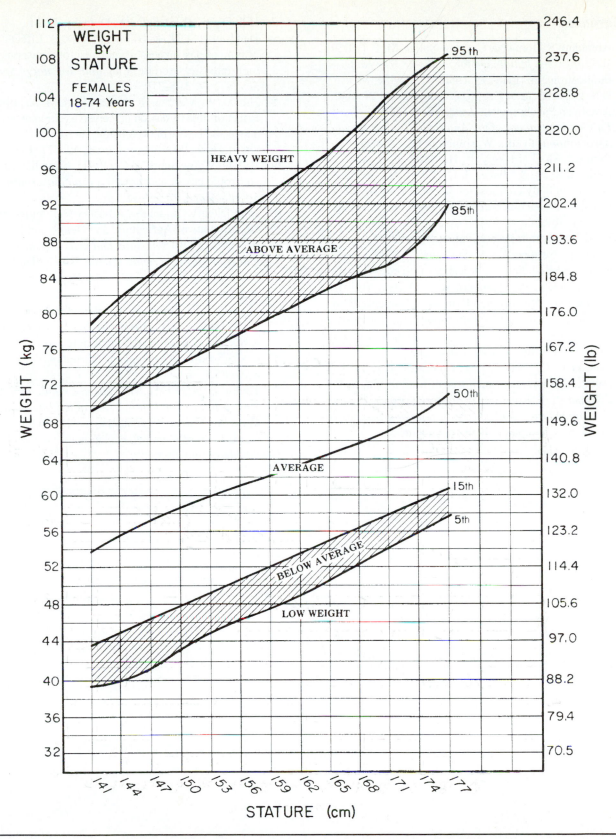

Figure 3.3 Percentiles of weight (kg; lb) based on the stature (cm) of women between the ages of 18 y and 74 y in the NHANES surveys. From Frisancho, A. R. (1990). *Anthropometric standards for the assessment of growth and nutritional status* (p. 80). Ann Arbor: University of Michigan Press. The figure allows us to find the percentile of any woman between the ages of 18 y and 74 y by using the meeting point of her weight (kg and lb) on the Y axes and her stature (cm) on the X axis. For example, if her body weight is 64 kg (140.8 lb) and her geight is 174 cm, then she is in the "average" category and near the 33rd %ile.

References

1. Abraham, S., Johnson, C. L., & Naijar, M. F. (1979). *Weight by height and age for adults 18–74 years.* Publication No. (PHS) 79-1656. Hyattsville, MD: U.S. Department of Health, Education, and Welfare.
2. American Psychological Association. (2001). *Publication manual of the American Psychological Association* (5th ed.). Washington, DC: Author.
3. Bemben, M. G., Massey, B. H., Bemben, D. A., Boileau, R. A., & Misner, J. E. (1995). Age-related patterns in body composition for men aged 20–79 years. *Medicine and Science in Sports and Exercise, 27,* 264–269.
4. Food & Nutrition Board, National Academy of Science—National Research Council. (1980). Recommended dietary allowances (9th ed., revised). In K. L. Jones, L. W. Shainberg, & C. O. Byer. (Eds.), *Dimensions* (5th ed.). San Francisco: Harper & Row.
5. Frisancho, A. R. (1990). *Anthropometric standards for the assessment of growth and nutritional status.* Ann Arbor: University of Michigan Press.
6. Gordon, C. C., Chumlea, W. C., & Roche, A. F. (1988). Stature, recumbent length, and weight. In T. G. Lohman, A. F. Roche, & R. Rartorell (Eds.), *Anthropometric standardization reference manual* (pp. 3–8). Champaign, IL: Human Kinetics.
7. Hill, D. W., Borden, D. O., Darnaby, K. M., Hendricks, D. N., & Hill, C. M. (1992). Effect of time of day on aerobic and anaerobic responses to high-intensity exercise. *Canadian Journal of Sport Science, 17,* 316–319.
8. Hill, D. W., Cureton, K. J., & Collins, M. A. (1989). Effect of time of day on perceived exertion at work rates above and below the ventilatory threshold. *Research Quarterly for Exercise and Sport, 60,* 127–133.
9. Hill, D. W., & Smith, J. C. (1991). Circadian rhythm in anaerobic power and capacity. *Canadian Journal of Sport Science, 16,* 30–32.
10. Joint Dietary Guidelines Advisory Committee of U.S. Departments of Agriculture and Health and Human Services. (1990). *Nutrition and your health: Dietary guidelines for Americans* (Home and Garden Bulletin No. 232). Washington, DC: U.S. Department of Agriculture.
11. Manson, J. E., Willett, W. C., Stampfer, M. J., Colditz, G. A., Hunter, D. J., Hankinson, S. E., Hennekens, C. H., & Speizer, F. E. (1995). Body weight and mortality among women. *New England Journal of Medicine, 333,* 677–685.
12. Taylor, B. N. (1995). *NIST Special Publication 811, 1995 Edition: Guide for the use of the International System of Units (SI).* Gaithersburg, MD: United States Department of Commerce, National Institute of Standards and Technology.

STRENGTH TESTING

The terms used to describe and quantify exercise are dependent upon the type of muscular action.[17,18] The two major types of exercise are dynamic and static. Dynamic exercise consists of muscle actions that are concentric or eccentric, depending on whether the muscles are shortened (concentric) or lengthened (eccentric). During most dynamic exercises, the speed of movement is variable throughout the movement, such as when lifting a barbell. Thus, the load being lifted changes speed, due to biomechanical, physiological, and anatomical factors of the lifter, but the absolute load itself (the mass of the load) does not change. The other type of exercise—static—utilizes a muscular action that is isometric. The muscles do not change their length, except

that caused by the elasticity of the muscle and connective tissues. Another type of muscle action, called isokinetic, may be proposed on the basis of the isokinetic apparatus. These machines alter the resistance of the load, causing the load to move at a constant speed[12] although the muscle movement itself may not always be constant.[18]

Strength may be defined as the maximal force generated at a given velocity of exercise.[19] The velocity of exercise may include muscle actions that cause muscle fibers to lengthen (eccentric), remain the same length (isometric), or shorten (concentric). At zero velocity the exercise is static, whereas all other velocities of exercise include muscle actions that are dynamic. Therefore, the ideal profile of a person's strength would include measurements of that person's forces under all possible velocities. The practical approach, however, would be to measure strength during a movement at variable speed, during muscle action at zero speed, and during movements at designated constant speeds. Chapter 4 focuses on dynamic strength (free weights)—that is, strength during a movement in which the body part is changing its speed of movement.

DYNAMIC STRENGTH

F ield tests of strength have existed since at least the time of the ancient Olympics, when contestants were required to lift a ball of iron in order to qualify for the games. In 1873, Dudley Sargent, M.D., a pioneer in early physical education, initiated strength testing at Harvard University.[8] Currently, many strength trainees measure their dynamic concentric strength in the weight room using free weights and weight machines.

Two popular free-weight exercises that are described as dynamic strength tests in this chapter are the bench press, and the two-arm curl. Depending on the controlled or standardized conditions, the free-weight field tests described here could be classified also as field/lab or, possibly, laboratory tests.[10,34] This chapter includes a description of both direct and indirect (predicted; estimated) measures of dynamic strength for the muscle groups used in performing the two free-weight exercises.

Rationale

One of the most operational (easily applied) definitions for dynamic strength states that it is manifested as a person's *one repetition maximal,* or *1 RM,* for a specific movement.

Direct 1 RM

A direct measure of strength is the maximal weight that a person can lift in the prescribed manner only one time. A brief preview of the traditional 1 RM test would show that it requires a person to exert maximally on a selected weight, chosen as close as possible to the person's expected 1 RM weight. If the person cannot lift it with correct form, then a lower weight is tried after a rest interval; if the person properly lifts the weight twice, then the performer stops. After a rest interval, a small additional weight is added, and the person tries again. This process is repeated until only one repetition is possible.[25] Obtaining the 1 RM value for the first time in a person may be inaccurate and time consuming because of the number of attempts at achieving one, and only one, repetition at a given weight[22] and a lack of standardizing the lifting position or procedures. Direct 1 RM measurements also may be injurious for some persons, especially the elderly[32] and children.[15] The American Academy of Pediatrics[1] and the National Strength and Conditioning Association[30] endorse this sentiment in not recommending 1 RM performances by children.

Indirect 1 RM

Fortunately, the 1 RM value may be approximated by knowing any number of maximal repetitions from two to 20 for any given weight lifted. Thus, the 1 RM may be calculated from equations based upon either a curvilinear (exponential) or a linear relationship between the percent of one repetition maximal (% 1 RM) and less than 20 repetitions maximal (20 # RM).

The indirect 1 RM method is based on a negative **linear relationship** between % 1 RM and the number of RM. The 1 RM can be estimated from measuring the number of RM at intensities between 80 % and 100 % 1 RM,[14,16,20,23] and possibly extended from intensities as low as 60 % RM.[14,27] In general, the percent of a 1 RM load decreases by about 2 % to 2.5 % for each increase in the number of maximal repetitions (Figure 4.1). Thus, the 1 RM load represents 100 % 1 RM that can be lifted only once, whereas a 90 % 1 RM load could be lifted about five times. Equation 4.1 and a sample calculation are presented here.

$$1 \text{ RM (kg or lb)} = \frac{\text{kg or lb at \# RM 2 to 20}}{1.00 - (\# \text{ RM} \times 0.02)} \qquad \text{Eq. 4.1}$$

where:

    1 RM = one repetition maximal; predicted strength

    # RM = number of repetitions possible

    1.00 = 100 % as a decimal

    0.02 = 2 % as a decimal

For example, if a person can lift 100 kg (≈220 lb) only one time, then the 100 kg represents one repetition maximal, or 1 RM or 100 % 1 RM. However, if this person lifts 80 kg 10 times (10 # RM), then the 1 RM of 100 kg is derived without directly measuring it by using Equation 4.1 as follows:

$$1 \text{ RM (kg)} = 80 \text{ kg} / [1.00 - (10 \times 0.02)]$$

$$= 80 \text{ kg} / (1.00 - 0.20)$$

$$= 80 \text{ kg} / 0.80$$

$$= 100 \text{ kg}$$

The reverse is also true; if the 1 RM is known, it is possible to predict the approximate load that can be lifted a given number of times. For example, if a person's 1 RM is 100 kg, it is likely that about 75 % to 80 % of 100 kg

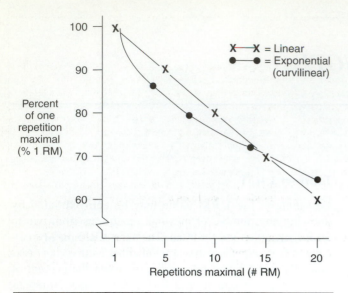

Figure 4.1 The curvilinear and linear relationships between the percent of one repetition maximal (% 1 RM) and the number of repetitions maximal (# RM).

Table 4.1 Primary Muscles for Two-Arm Curl and Bench Press

Two-Arm Curl	Bench Press
Arms	Shoulders
Biceps brachii	Anterior deltoid
Brachioradialis	Coracobrachialis
Brachialis	Chest
	Pectoralis
	Arms
	Triceps brachii

(then 75 kg to 80 kg) could be lifted no more than 9 to 12 times (9 # RM to 12 # RM), or about 10 times.[20]

Bioenergetic Rationale

The biochemical pathway for maximal muscle actions—that is, strength—is the phosphagenic pathway. Even the longest of 1 RM movements is completed in less than 10 s; this includes the time spent holding the weight prior to the movement, raising the weight, holding it in the lifted position, and lowering the weight.[29] Thus, the actual time spent raising the weight is usually less than three seconds. As illustrated in the fitness continuum (Figures 1.2 and 1.3 in Chapter 1), maximal exercise efforts of this duration are placed within the strength fitness category.

Anatomical Rationale

The major muscles that are used to execute the two strength tests described here are presented in Table 4.1. These popular strength-training exercises emphasize the upper body musculature, particularly the arms, shoulders, and chest.[39]

Purpose of the Free-Weight Strength Tests

Strength testing serves purposes related to both health and performance. Persons, especially women, who habitually exert forcefully against resistances may protect themselves from losing some bone density.[2,4] It seems plausible that stronger persons are more likely to provide the necessary forces to prevent the advent of porous bones, associated with osteoporosis. Before embarking on strength-training programs, it is meaningful to evaluate participants in order to prescribe their programs and monitor their progress. For example, a trainee's exercise prescription may include performing two or three sets of maximal repetitions at 80 % of the 1 RM load.

Additionally, the purpose of the Free-Weight Tests as performed in *Exercise Physiology Laboratory Manual* goes beyond the mere measurement of strength. Because of the distinct terminology and measurements in exercise physiology, another purpose of these tests is to familiarize the student with common exercise terms and measurements associated with work and power. Thus, in addition to learning how to administer the strength tests, students will learn how to measure positive (concentric) work, negative (eccentric) work, total work, and mean power.

Method

The method section of a research paper should enable the readers to replicate the researcher's study. This means that the equipment (instruments and materials), procedures, and calculations (analysis) are described in the Method section. Box 4.1 provides a summary of the accuracy of 1 RM testing.

Equipment

Various instruments are available to measure muscle strength. Some of these are (a) free-weights (e.g., barbells), (b) dynamometers, (c) cable tensiometers, (d) load cells (electromechanical devices), and (e) isokinetic devices. The equipment for the dynamic strength and power tests includes the following: (1) weighing scale (e.g., platform scale or electronic scale); (2) bar; (3) assorted free-weights ranging from 1 kg ($\approx$ 2.5 lb; 10 N) to 10 kg ($\approx$ 25 lb; 100 N) each; (4) barbell collars (unless weights are welded onto the bar); (5) stopwatch capable of measuring to a tenth of a second; and (6) a metric tape or stick.[a]

---

[a]Technicians measuring vertical displacement for a *laboratory* test, rather than a field test, might use a linear transducer (e.g., Unimeasure™, Corvalis, OR) accurate to the closest 0.01 cm.[10]

BOX 4.1 Accuracy of 1 RM Testing

Regardless of the accuracy of the equipment and the diligence of the examiner and participant, strength scores in participants will vary due to daily biological variability; this may cause strength scores in an individual to change by 2 % to 12 %.[36] When the 1 RM strength was determined for a two-arm curl performed two days apart on a custom-made weight machine, the test-retest correlation was .98. This correlation may not be as high, however, for two-arm curls performed with free-weights because of less standardization of body position and movement.[35] The test-retest variation of 1 RM and predicted 1 RM ranges from 5 % to 15 %.[3] Thus, if on one day a person's maximal lift is 50 kg, or is predicted to lift 50 kg, then on a subsequent day that person's 1 RM, or predicted 1 RM, may be any value between 47.5 kg and 52.5 kg if at the least variability, and 42.5 kg and 57.5 kg at the most variability. Test-rest reliability is likely to be higher if the average of a few trials is used rather than the highest score of a few trials.[6]

The traditional direct method of measuring dynamic strength is not without its inconsistencies, especially for inexperienced lifters. Because 1 RM strength trials may increase significantly from trial one to trial two, especially in older adults,[33] the second trial of another day should be used[3] as the baseline for strength-training intervention studies. It would be inappropriate to attribute all strength gains to the resistance training program on the basis of strength scores from trial one.

Although the National Football League's (NFL) Test of strength for prospective players is not exactly like the predictive ones described here, it is similar enough to provide some input as to the accuracy of such predictive 1 RM tests. The NFL prescribes an absolute weight of 225 lb (102 kg) to be bench pressed as many times as possible (repetitions maximal; RM). Their valid test ($r = .96$) predicted 1 RM strength in college football players, who required about seven repetitions to fatigue. The prediction appeared to be most accurate for those players who performed 10 RM or less.[6]

When predicting 1 RM from repetitions maximal, some inaccuracy may occur in assuming that there is a 2 % to 2.5 % decrease in any given person's 1 RM mass for each single increase of repetitions maximal. For example, this would assume that 10 RM is approximately 80 % of 1 RM mass. However, one reviewer reported a range from 60 % to 90 % for persons performing 10 repetitions maximal.[28] The initial strength and resistance training experience of the performer can affect the prediction of 1 RM.[5] This negative linear relationship also appears to vary with different muscle groups.[7]

The measurement of power for the bench press, using a 90 % 1 RM method, revealed a test-retest correlation of .97.[3]

BOX 4.2 Safety Checklist for Free-Weight Lifting

1. Be alert for situations that might cause collisions, stumbles, and dropped weights:
   people   weights   mats   benches   overhangs
2. Perform a prior exercise regimen of loosening up (stretching) and warming up (light lifting).
3. Use the hooked-thumb grip, not a thumbless grip.
4. Check adjustable collars for tightness.
5. Use spotters wisely:
   Place the spotter behind the bench-press performer if you use only one spotter.
   Place the spotters at each end of the barbell if you have two spotters.
   Communicate clearly between spotter(s) and performer:
   "Ready"—spotters help remove bar from holders and place into performer's starting position.
   "Done"—performer announces "done" on the last repetition; spotters help return bar to the rack.
6. Protect the back by
   Keeping weights close to the body when handling the weights during loading the bar and lifting.
   Avoiding twists while handling the bar.
   Activating abdominal muscles while lifting.
7. Breathe properly by exhaling out of the mouth during the concentric execution and inhaling upon returning the weight via eccentric action.
8. Children (≤ 16 y) and novice older adults (≥ 60 y) should not compete for 1 RM.
9. Technicians should keep injury records for 3 y to 5 y and
   Provide a brief factual description of how the injury occurred.
   Review the files annually to analyze possible causes of injury.

Weighing scales, used to measure the mass and force components, were discussed in Chapter 3. Most weight rooms have barbells and weights to measure the force component of work and power. A total weight of about 90 kg (198 lb) should accommodate most performers. One bench is needed for one of the two strength exercises described here. Most exercise physiology laboratories have measurement tapes (preferably, metric) and stopwatches to measure the distance and time components of work and power. Although the calculations of work and power may be performed without a calculator, the proper use of a pocket calculator minimizes time and assures accuracy. Students are encouraged to bring their own pocket calculators and wrist stopwatches to every laboratory session.

Safety is a concern for all fitness tests, especially those requiring intense or explosive movements and those leading to exhaustion. Box 4.2 provides a safety checklist for technicians and performers.

Executing the Two-Arm Curl and Bench Press

The accuracy of free-weight strength testing is enhanced if the execution of the lifts is standardized. The prescribed positions of the two-arm curl and bench press are illustrated in Figures 4.2, and 4.3, respectively. These movements should be practiced a few times with only the bar. The technician ensures that the performer executes properly.

Two-Arm Curl

1. The performer stands with the feet parallel and shoulder width apart.
2. With straightened arms hanging down at the sides and with the hands taking a supinated grip (palms facing out, thumbs lateral), the bar is held against the thighs.
3. The performer then raises the bar to the chest by flexing at the elbow joint and without bending the legs and back. (By standing with the back near the wall, it might ensure that the performer does not lean backwards.)
4. After reaching the fully flexed position, the performer returns the bar to the preparatory position.
5. Subsequent repetitions require a stop for ≥ 0.5 s but ≤ 1.0 s at the initial position. Rebounding from each repetition causes an enhancement (8 % to $\approx$ 16 %) of strength due to prior eccentric muscle action.[10] Thus, the technician does not permit rebounding.

Bench Press

1. The performer lies supine on a wide bench with the knees bent and the soles of the feet on the bench. However, if the performer is in jeopardy of toppling from the bench, the feet may be on the floor and straddling the bench as in power-lifting competitions. Some might argue that, by placing the feet on the floor it causes the back to arch, thus risking injury.[9,24]
2. Two technicians, or spotters, at each side of the performer or one spotter behind the performer, place the barbell in the performer's pronated hands (thumbs medial) spaced about shoulder width apart and at chest level.
3. The performer raises the weight to a straightened-arms position directly above the chest.
4. The performer returns the barbell to the preparatory position.
5. The performer stops subsequent repetitions at the initial position for ≥ 0.5 s but ≤ 1.0 s.

Preparation for 1 RM, Work, and Mean Power

As with all of the tests performed in this manual, the first two steps are to record the **basic** and **meteorological data.** Thus, the name, date, time, age, gender, height, weight, environmental temperature, relative humidity, and barometric pressure are recorded on Form 4.1. An additional factor, specific for free-weight testing, might be the recording of

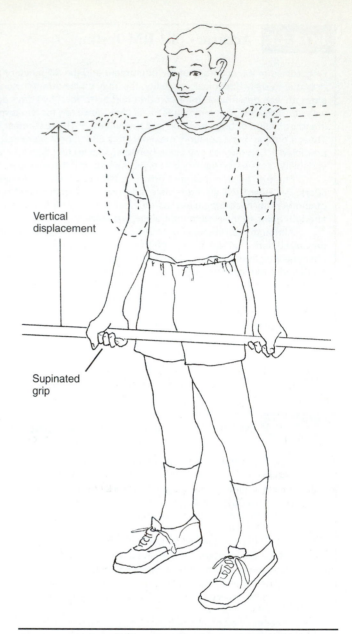

Figure 4.2 The beginning and end positions for the two-arm curl. The arrow denotes the vertical displacement measurement needed for calculating work and power.

the performer's experience in lifting free-weights. The body weight should be as close to the nude weight as possible and measure according to the procedures described in Chapter 3.

Another universal step is to **calibrate** the test equipment. The calibration of the platform scale was described in the calibration Box 3.2 of Chapter 3. Usually, the stopwatch can be assumed to be accurate, but, to be sure, it might be compared with another from a reputable dealer.

It is not unusual for the poundage of commercial weights to be labeled inaccurately. For example, in one instance a sand-filled weight that was marked as 8.8 lb (4.0 kg), really weighed 10.4 lb (4.7 kg). Hence, the

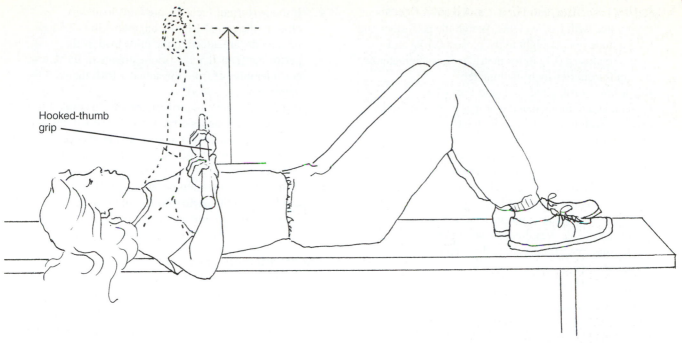

Figure 4.3 The beginning and end positions for the bench press. An alternate bench position places the performer's feet on the floor. The arrow denotes the vertical displacement measurement needed for calculating work and power.

Hooked-thumb grip

weights, barbells, and collars that are to be used for testing should be verified on an accurate scale prior to testing. The actual pound or kilograms should be labeled with an appropriate marking device (e.g., chalk) on the barbells or weights.

In some instances, **mass** is considered equal to the force lifting the mass, such as when lifting a barbell against gravitational forces. The mass (free-weights), which in this case is the **force,** should be weighed on a metric scale to the closest tenth kilogram or be converted to metrics after being weighed on a nonmetric scale. All values are recorded on Form 4.1.

Before the subject performs the maximal repetitions for a given weight, **displacement (d)** measurements must be made for each of the two exercises in order to calculate the work (w = F × d) accomplished. The displacements[b] are measured to the closest centimeter with a metric tape and are recorded on Form 4.1. They can be made with the performer using an imaginary or unloaded bar at two points: the preparatory and endpoints of each movement. The criteria for measuring these lengths were illustrated in Figures 4.2 and 4.3. Suggested weights for the Indirect 1 RM Test and the landmarks for measuring displacements of the two free-weight exercises are presented in Table 4.2.

After making the vertical displacement measures, the performer should be given 5 min to 10 min of **prior exercise,** consisting of loosening-up and warming-up exercises.

---

[b]The term *displacement* represents the straight-line length of the concentric phase of the exercise. The term *distance* includes the curved-line length (the arc) of concentric and eccentric phases of the exercise.

Table 4.2	**Landmarks for Measuring Displacements for the Indirect 1 RM Test**	
Exercise	**Bar Starting Point**	**Bar Endpoint**
Two-Arm Curl	Against thighs	Fully flexed arm-curl position near chest
Bench Press	On chest	Straightened-arms position over head

Note: Use 80 % 1 RM if the approximate 1 RM is known.

Obviously, these exercises should incorporate the muscles to be used in the two strength tests. Thus, the loosening-up exercises should stretch the upper body muscles and tendons. One warm-up set of about eight repetitions should mimic the executions of each lift, but with weights that are about 40 %[37] to 60 %[21] of an estimated one repetition maximal. This can be followed by another set of three repetitions between 50 % and 70 %, of estimated 1 RM or three to five reps at 60 % to 80 %. These preliminary estimates are rather exploratory for first-time performers (novices).

Summary of Preparatory Steps

Technician (Tester/Examiner/Investigator/Researcher)

1. Calibrate the platform scale or electronic scale. (Refer to the calibration Box 3.2 in Chapter 3.)
2. Weigh and mark the barbells and assorted weights. Labeling them in newton (N) units can simplify work and mean power calculations.

3. Record basic data onto Form 4.1. Ask performer about experience with free-weights. Weigh the performer and record nude body weight to the closest 0.1 kg and height to closest 0.1 cm for metric wall stadiometer or 0.5 cm for quarter-inch stadiometer.
4. Record meteorological data onto Form 4.1.
5. Explain and demonstrate the proper execution of the two free-weight lifts using only the bar (see step 3 of performer).
6. Measure and record (Form 4.2) the vertical displacement of one concentric action of the performer's two-arm curl and benchpress (refer to Figures 4.2 and 4.3 and Table 4.2).
7. Load the bar with an appropriate weight for the performer (Table 4.2). Record weight onto Form 4.1.
8. As the final preparatory step, the technician prescribes a prior-exercise regimen (see performer's final step).

Performer (Participant)

1. Provide technician with basic data factors, such as name, age, and experience with free-weights.
2. Provide technician with clothes to be worn during weigh-in or be scantily clothed, so that weight is nearly nude weight.
3. Practice the lifts until performance is satisfactory.
4. Hold the starting and endpoint positions for each lift, so that the technician can record the displacement measurements.
5. As the final preparatory step, the performer loosens up and warms up by following the prior exercise regimen:
   a. Loosen up with 2 min to 3 min of stretching (ballistic and static) the muscle groups for the two lifts.
   b. Warm up with one set of 8 reps at ≈ 40 % to 60 % of estimated 1 RM; rest for 1 min with stretching. Do another set of 3 to 5 reps at ≈ 60 % to 80 % of estimated 1 RM; rest with stretching for 1 min.

Test Procedures for the Direct 1 RM

The direct method is the traditional trial-and-retrial method. The results may be compared with the results of the indirect method. Hence, the comparison can serve as a validation of the indirect method.

The procedures outlined here[21,31,37] combine those described by others. The procedural steps for the traditional direct measurement of 1 RM are as follows:

1. The performer follows the prior exercise regimen as described in step 5 of the performer's preparatory steps. Record loads of ≈ 40 % to 60 % 1 RM and ≈ 60 % to 80 % 1 RM onto Form 4.1.
2. The performer attempts a single lift at a load that is close (95 %) to the perceived 1 RM. Record load onto Form 4.1.
3. Most performers would need a recovery period of 2 min to 10 min.

4. If the performer feels the previous load was close to the actual 1 RM load, then 5 lb (≈2.5 kg) increments are added to the prior load; if the performer feels that the prior estimate of 95 % was considerably off from the actual 1 RM, then > 5 lb increments are added.
5. If the performer can properly execute a single lift, but no more than one repetition, on the second, third, or fourth retrial, then this load should be recorded as the 1 RM on Form 4.1. Allow 2 min to 7 min for recovery between trials.
6. If more than four attempts at the 1 RM value are needed, then the performer should be retested on another day with the advantage of having the knowledge gained from this session's trials.[37]

Test Procedures for the Indirect 1 RM Test and the Mean Power Test

Indirect 1 RM The prediction of 1 RM may be made based on either a linear relationship or a curvilinear relationship between % 1 RM and # RM. The focus of the following is based on the more popular, but not necessarily more accurate, linear relationship. The ultimate step in predicting 1 RM is to determine the performer's maximal number of repetitions for a given weight (force). Repetitions maximal (# RM) is defined as the number of repetitions, without a rest interval, performed until no other properly executed repetition can be completed. In order to comply with the linearity rationale, it is best if the number of maximal repetitions does not exceed 20. If it is apparent that the performer is about to exceed 20 repetitions, then stop the performer and wait for 5 min to 10 min before repeating the exercise at a heavier weight.

Mean Power of # RM Timing the durations of each of the two free-weight lifts is necessary when calculating power because power is the rate of doing work. The timer should start the stopwatch at the performer's first movement of the two-arm curl and bench press. The timer stops the watch when the performer returns the weight after the last complete or partial repetition of the Indirect 1 RM Test. The timer records the time to the closest whole second. The performer should execute the repetitions at a comfortable pace because the purpose of the power measurement is not to rank and compare the quality of the performer's mean power. If the latter were the goal, the performer would need to execute the maximal repetitions as fast as possible. I am not aware of any norms for such a test. The primary purpose of the mean power "test" is to become familiar with the concept of power and its calculation.[17] Power is calculated according to Equations 1.6a–1.6e (e.g., $P = w/t$) in Chapter 1. The conversions for the various force, work, and power units may need to be reviewed in Table 2.2 of Chapter 2.

Summary of Procedural Steps for Indirect 1 RM and Mean Power

1. The performer lifts the weight as prescribed for the movement and as many times as possible at a comfortable pace, but without a rest interval. The technician starts the stopwatch at the performer's first movement and stops it after the last attempt of a repetition. The technician records the time to the closest second onto Form 4.2.
2. The technician counts and records the number of repetitions maximal (# RM), including the fraction of a possible partial repetition on the last attempt.
3. The technician provides a retrial, after a 5 min to 10 min recovery period, if the performer exceeds or would appear to exceed 20 # RM.
4. The technician calculates and records (Form 4.2) ^+w, w, and $\bar{P}$.
5. The technician (in this case, termed "statistician") compiles the scores and statistics and records onto Forms 4.3 and 4.4.

Calculations

Calculating Indirect 1 RM Based on Linear Relationship
The equation for calculating 1 RM based on the linear rela-tionship between % 1 RM and # RM was presented earlier in Equation 4.1. Table 4.3 substitutes for Equation 4.1 when the number of repetitions maximal (# RM) is 10 or less. For ex-ample, if a performer lifted 40 kg (88 lb) 10 times (10 # RM) then the 1 RM is located by reading down the 10 # RM col-umn to the 40.0 kg number, then reading across this row to the 1 RM column's 50 kg (110 lb).

Calculating Work from Indirect 1 RM Test   Equation 4.2 is used to calculate the **positive work** from the mass lifted (force, F), the displacement of a single **concentric** action (d for one rep$^+$), and the number of maximal repe-titions (# RM). The latter will, presumably, consist of more than one repetition and will include a somewhat subjective estimate of the fractional displacement of the final incomplete attempted repetition. For example, if the performer properly executed nine complete repetitions, but attempted a 10th lift that only went half the proper distance, then record this as 9.5 # RM.

$$^+w = F \times (d \text{ for 1 rep}^+ \times \# RM) \qquad \text{Eq. 4.2}$$

Thus, if a person displaced a load (F) of 50 kg (110 lb) no more than six times (6 # RM), by 0.5 m each lift, then the positive work is calculated as follows:

Table 4.3 **Prediction of One Repetition Maximal (1 RM) from the Number of Repetitions Maximal (# RM)**

	Number of Repetitions Maximal (# RM)									
1 RM	**2 # RM**	**3 # RM**	**4 # RM**	**5 # RM**	**6 # RM**	**7 # RM**	**8 # RM**	**9 # RM**	**10 # RM**
				% 1 RM (kg)						
100 %	98 %	95 %	93 %	90 %	88 %	86 %	84 %	82 %	80 %
lb kg									
25 11.4	11.1	10.8	10.5	10.2	10.0	9.8	9.5	9.3	9.1
30 13.6	13.3	13.0	12.6	12.3	12.0	11.7	11.5	11.2	10.9
35 15.9	15.5	15.1	14.7	14.3	14.0	13.7	13.4	13.0	12.7
40 18.2	17.7	17.3	16.8	16.4	16.0	15.6	15.3	14.9	14.5
45 20.5	19.9	19.4	18.9	18.4	18.0	17.6	17.2	16.8	16.4
50 22.7	22.2	21.6	21.0	20.5	20.0	19.5	19.1	18.6	18.2
55 25.0	24.4	23.8	23.1	22.5	22.0	21.5	21.0	20.5	20.0
60 27.3	26.6	25.9	25.2	24.5	24.0	23.5	22.9	22.4	21.8
65 29.5	28.8	28.1	27.3	26.6	26.0	25.4	24.8	24.2	23.6
70 31.8	31.0	30.2	29.4	28.6	28.0	27.4	26.7	26.1	25.5
75 34.1	33.2	32.4	31.5	30.7	30.0	29.3	28.6	28.0	27.3
80 36.4	35.5	34.5	33.6	32.7	32.0	31.3	30.5	29.8	29.1
85 38.6	37.7	36.7	35.7	34.8	34.0	33.2	32.5	31.7	30.9
90 40.9	39.9	38.9	37.8	36.8	36.0	35.2	34.4	33.5	32.7
95 43.2	42.1	41.0	39.9	38.9	38.0	37.1	36.3	35.4	34.5
100 45.5	44.3	43.2	42.0	40.9	40.0	39.1	38.2	37.3	36.4
105 47.7	46.5	45.3	44.1	43.0	42.0	41.0	40.1	39.1	38.2
110 50.0	48.8	47.5	46.3	45.0	44.0	43.0	42.0	41.0	40.0
115 52.3	51.0	49.7	48.4	47.0	46.0	45.0	43.9	42.9	41.8
120 54.5	53.2	51.8	50.5	49.1	48.0	46.9	45.8	44.7	43.6
125 56.8	55.4	54.0	52.6	51.1	50.0	48.9	47.7	46.6	45.5
130 59.1	57.6	56.1	54.7	53.2	52.0	50.8	49.6	48.5	47.3
135 61.4	59.8	58.3	56.8	55.2	54.0	52.8	51.5	50.3	49.1
140 63.6	62.0	60.5	58.9	57.3	56.0	54.7	53.5	52.2	50.9
145 65.9	64.3	62.6	61.0	59.3	58.0	56.7	55.4	54.0	52.7
150 68.2	66.5	64.8	63.1	61.4	60.0	58.6	57.3	55.9	54.5

$$^+w = 50 \text{ kg} \times (0.5 \text{ m} \times 6 \text{ \# RM})$$

$$= 50 \text{ kg} \times 3 \text{ m}$$

$$= 150 \text{ kg·m}$$

Because force and work are expressed scientifically as newtons (N) and newton meters (N·m) or joules (J), respectively, the conversion of kilograms and kilogram meters (Table 2.2 in Chapter 2) is made as follows:

$$F \text{ (in N)} = 50 \text{ kg} \times 10 = 500 \text{ N}$$

$$^+w \text{ (in N·m or J)} = 150 \text{ kg·m} \times 10 = 1500 \text{ N·m;}$$

$$\text{or } 500 \text{ N} \times 3 \text{ m} = 1500 \text{ N·m}$$

$$= 1500 \text{ J (1.5 kJ)}$$

where:

$$1 \text{ kg} \approx 10 \text{ N (exact } 9.8066)$$

$$1 \text{ N·m} = 1 \text{ J}$$

Positive work, however, accounts only for the concentric muscle action lifting the weight vertically against gravity. To measure the total work of these dynamic exercises, the eccentric muscle action, or **negative work,** must be considered. Although the estimate of negative work is quite variable, it might be assumed to be approximately one-third of positive work for the purposes of appreciating the concept of total work. Thus, using the hypothetical example of 1500 J for positive work, the calculation of **total work** is made by using Equation 1.3b from Chapter 3 ($w = 1.33 \times {}^+w$):

$$w = 1.33 \times 1500 \text{ J} = 2000 \text{ J (2 kJ)}$$

Calculating Mean Power from the Indirect 1 RM Test

If the performer accomplishes 200 kg·m (2000 N·m; 2000 J) of total work in 15 s (or 0.25 min), then **mean power** can be calculated as in any of the four examples listed here in units of (1) kilogram meters per second (#1; kg·m·s^{-1}), (2) kilogram meters per minute (#2; kg·m·min^{-1}), (3) newton meters per second (#3; N·m·s^{-1}), or (4) newton meters per minute (#4; N·m·min^{-1}). Decimal minutes are calculated in #2 and #4 by dividing the number of seconds by 60 (e.g., 15 ÷ 60 = 0.25).

e.g., #1 P (kg·m·s^{-1}) = 200 kg·m ÷ 15 s = 13.3
e.g., #2 P (kg·m·min^{-1}) = 200 kg·m ÷ 0.25 min = 800
e.g., #3 P (N·m·s^{-1}; W) = 2000 N·m ÷ 15 s = 133
e.g., #4 P (N·m·min^{-1}) = 2000 N·m ÷ 0.25 = 8000

Because power is most appropriately expressed scientifically as watts (W), the approximate conversions of kilogram meters per second or minute, and of newton meters per second or minute, are made as follows:

#1 P (W) = 13.3 kg·m·s^{-1} ÷ 0.1 = 133 W
#2 P (W) = 800 kg·m·min^{-1} ÷ 6 = 133 W
#3 P (W) = 133 N·m·s^{-1} ÷ 1 = 133 W
#4 P (W) = 8000 N·m·min^{-1} ÷ 60 = 133 W

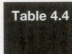

Table 4.4	Optimal Upper Body Free-Weight Strength in Men and Women Based upon the Loads Percentage of Body Weight	
	Two-Arm Curl	**Bench Press**
Men	50%	100%
Women	35%	70%

Source: Percentages derived from Wilmore J. H., & Costill, D. L. (1988). *Training for sport and activity* (p. 377). Dubuque, IA: Wm C. Brown.

where:

$$1 \text{ W} \approx 0.1 \text{ kg·m·s}^{-1}$$

$$1 \text{ W} \approx 6 \text{ kg·m·min}^{-1}$$

$$1 \text{ W} = 1 \text{ N·m·s}^{-1}$$

$$1 \text{ W} = 60 \text{ N·m·min}^{-1}$$

These work and power calculations may appear complicated at first, but they can be simplified quite easily by labeling the lifted weight in newtons (simply adding a zero to the end of the kilogram value). This converts kilograms to approximate newtons; thus, the work units N·m and J (remember, 1 N·m = 1 J) are easily derived. Power units (N·m·s^{-1} or W), can then be easily calculated from Example #3 by dividing the number of seconds (e.g., 15) into the N·m (e.g., 2000). In this example, the watt and N·m·s^{-1} value is 133 W or N·m·s^{-1} (1 W = 1 N·m·s^{-1}). In Example #4, 8000 N·m·min^{-1} is converted to watts by using the conversion: 1 W = 60 N·m·min^{-1}.

Results and Discussion

Strength categories are often selected on the basis of absolute 1 RM and relative 1 RM values. Indeed, a person with a very high absolute 1 RM is strong, but a person of lower body weight and lower 1 RM may also be relatively strong when the 1 RM is related to body weight (mass). Guidelines for the interpretation of strength scores (1 RM) based upon the load's percent of body weight for men and women are found in Table 4.4.[38] These percentages are not based on the necessary data to derive criterion reference standards; nevertheless, they are intended to indicate optimal values. These guidelines suggest that women should achieve a percentage that is 70 % of the men's percentage for the two-arm curl and bench press. For example, if a 60 kg woman's 1 RM for the bench press is 42 kg (≈ 92 lb), then she has met a suggested criterion by benching 70 % of her body weight.

Norms for bench-press strength in adult men and women in three age categories (< 30 y; 30 y–50 y; > 50 y) are presented in Table 4.5.

Persons who know their bench press 1 RM on a **variable resistance machine,** such as the Universal, could

Table 4.5 Percentiles for Free-Weight 1 RM Bench Press Strength (lb and kg) in Adult Men and Women Under 30 y, Between 30 y and 50 y, and over 50 y of Age

%ile	< 30 Men lb	< 30 Men ≈ kg	< 30 Women lb	< 30 Women ≈ kg	30–50 Men lb	30–50 Men ≈ kg	30–50 Women lb	30–50 Women ≈ kg	> 50 Men lb	> 50 Men ≈ kg	> 50 Women lb	> 50 Women ≈ kg
95	203	92	105	48	183	83	95	43	161	73	84	38
90	191	87	100	45	172	78	91	41	151	69	81	37
80	175	80	95	43	158	72	86	39	139	63	76	35
70	164	75	91	41	148	67	83	38	130	59	73	33
60	155	70	88	40	139	63	80	36	122	55	71	32
50	146	66	85	39	131	60	77	35	115	52	68	31
40	137	62	82	37	123	56	74	34	108	49	66	30
30	128	58	79	36	114	52	71	32	100	45	63	29
20	117	53	75	34	104	47	68	31	91	41	60	27
10	101	46	70	32	90	41	63	29	79	36	55	25
5	89	40	65	30	79	36	59	27	69	31	52	24
Mean	146	66	85	39	131	60	77	35	115	52	68	31
SD	35	16	12	5	32	15	11	5	28	13	10	5

Source: R. V. Hockey, *Physical Fitness: The Pathway to Healthful Living,* 1989. Copyright C. W. Mosby Year Book, Inc., St. Louis, MO 63146.
Note: The kilogram values may be converted to newton values by simply attaching a zero at the end of each kilogram value.

compare their scores with those from a large sample of men and women tested at the Cooper Clinic.[19] The women, average age of 39.5 y ($SD = 9.6$), could bench press about 33 kg ($SD = 7.7$), and the men, average age of 41.6 y ($SD = 9.2$) could bench press about 73 kg ($SD = 17.4$). The women's 1 RM represented about 55 % of their body weight, whereas the men's represented about 87 % of their body weight.

Free-weight strength relative to body weight (S:Wt) is the same as the percentage written as a decimal number. For example, if a 25-year-old man, weighing 100 kg (220 lb), benches 120 kg (264 lb), then the strength (S):weight (Wt) ratio is calculated according to Equation 4.3:

$$S:Wt = 1 \ RM / Wt \qquad \text{Eq. 4.3}$$

$$= 120 \ kg \ / \ 100 \ kg = 1.20$$

$$1.20 = 120 \ \% \ Wt$$

Comparative scores for ratios between the two-arm curl 1 RM and body weight have been derived from data on 250 college-age men and women.[11] Table 4.6 categorizes the data into strength categories.

Norms for the power measurement as described here are not available. The mean power values reflect the relationship between force (e.g., load) and speed. The highest loads do not produce the greatest mean power or do the highest speeds. Thus, moderate forces combined with moderate speeds produce optimal mean power.

Prior to the 1980s, strength was not emphasized as a fitness component for middle-aged and older adults. However, due to its effect on retaining muscle mass and preserving bone density, it has attained a greater importance for persons of all ages.[2,4]

Table 4.6 1 RM Two-Arm Curl Strength to Body Weight Ratios (lb:lb; or kg:kg) for College-Age Men and Women

Category	Men	Women
High	0.70	0.50
	0.65	0.45
Above average	0.60	0.42
	0.55	0.38
Average	0.50	0.35
	0.45	0.32
	0.40	0.28
Below average	0.35	0.25
	0.30	0.21
	0.25	0.18

Source: Data from Heywood, V. H. (1991). *Advanced fitness assessment and exercise prescription.* Champaign, IL: Human Kinetics.

References

1. American Academy of Pediatrics. (1983). Weight training and weight lifting: Information for the pediatrician. *The Physician and Sportsmedicine, 11*(3): 157–161.

2. American College of Sports Medicine (ACSM). (2000). *ACSM's guidelines for exercise testing and prescription.* Philadelphia: Lippincott Williams & Wilkins.

3. Berger, R. A., & Smith, K. J. (1991). Effects of the tonic neck reflex in the bench press. *Journal of Applied Sport Science Research, 5,* 188–191.

4. Block, J. E., Smith, R., Friedlander, G., & Genant, H. K. (1989). Preventing osteoporosis with exercise: A review with emphasis on methodology. *Medical Hypotheses, 30*(1): 9–19.

5. Braith, R. W., Graves, J. E., Leggett, S. H., & Pollock, M. L. (1993). Effect of training on the relationship between maximal and submaximal strength. *Medicine and Science in Sports and Exercise, 25*(1), 132–138.

6. Chapman, P. P., Whitehead, J. R., & Brinkhert, R. H. (1996). Prediction of 1-RM bench press from the 225 lbs reps-to-fatigue test in college football players. *Medicine and Science in Sports and Exercise, 28*, Abstract #393, S66.

7. Claiborne, J. M., & Donolli, J. D. (1993). Number of repetitions at selected percentages of one repetition maximum in untrained college women. *Research Quarterly for Exercise and Sports, 64*(Suppl): (Abstract).

8. Clarke, D. H. (1975). *Exercise physiology.* Englewood Cliffs, NJ: Prentice-Hall.

9. Corbin, C. B., & Lindsey, R. (1996). *Physical fitness concepts.* Dubuque, IA: Brown & Benchmark.

10. Cronin, J. B., McNair, P. J., & Marshall, R. N. (2000). The role of maximal strength and load on initial power production. *Medicine and Science in Sports & Exercise, 32*, 1763–1769.

11. Heywood, V. H. (1991). *Advanced fitness assessment and exercise prescription.* Champaign, IL: Human Kinetics.

12. Hislop, H. J., & Perrine, J. J. (1967). The isokinetic concept of exercise. *Physical Therapy, 47*, 144–117.

13. Hockey, R. V. (1989). *Physical fitness: The pathway to healthful living.* St. Louis: Times Mirror/Mosby.

14. Hoeger, W. K., Barette, S. L., Hale, D. F., & Hopkins, D. R. (1987). Relationship between repetitions and selected percentage of one repetition maximum. *Journal of Applied Sports Science Research, 1*, 11–13.

15. Invergo, J. J., Ball, T. E., & Looney, M. (1991). Relationship of push-ups and absolute muscular endurance to bench press strength. *Journal of Applied Sport Science Research, 5*, 121–125.

16. Johnson, P. B., Updyke, W. F., Schaefer, M., & Stollberg, D. C. (1975). *Sport, exercise, and you.* San Francisco: Holt, Rinehart and Winston.

17. Knuttgen, H. G. (1995). Force, work, and power in athletic training. *Sports Science Exchange, 8*(4), 1–5.

18. Knuttgen, H. G., & Kraemer, W. J. (1987). Terminology and measurement in exercise performance. *Journal of Applied Sport Science Research, 1*, 54–68.

19. Kohl, H. W., Gordon, N. F., Scott, C. B., Vaandrager, H., & Blair, S. N. (1992). Musculoskeletal strength and serum lipid levels in men and women. *Medicine and Science in Sports and Exercise, 24*, 1080–1087.

20. Kraemer, R. R., Kilgore, J. L., Kraemer, G. R., & Castracane, V. D. (1992). Growth hormone, IGF-1, and testosterone responses to resistive exercise. *Medicine and Science in Sports and Exercise, 24*, 1346–1352.

21. Kramer, W. J., & Fry, A. C. (1995). Strength testing: Development and evaluation of methodology. In P. J. Maud & C. Foster (Eds.), *Physiological assessment of human fitness* (pp. 115–138). Champaign, IL: Human Kinetics.

22. Kuramoto, A. K., & Payne, V. G. (1995). Predicting muscular strength in women: A preliminary study. *Research Quarterly for Exercise and Sport, 66*, 168–172.

23. Landers, J. (1985). Maximum based on repetitions. *National Strength and Conditioning Association Journal, 6*, 60–61.

24. Liemohn, W. S., et al. (1998). Unresolved controversies in back management. *Journal of Orthopaedic and Sports Physical Therapy, 9*, 239–244.

25. Mayhew, J. L., Ball, T. E., Arnold, M. D., & Bowen, J. C. (1992). Relative muscular endurance performance as a predictor of bench press strength in college men and women. *Journal of Applied Sport Science Research, 6*, 200–206.

26. McArdle, W. D., Katch, F. I., & Katch, V. L. (1996). *Exercise physiology: Energy, nutrition, and human performance.* Baltimore: Williams & Wilkins.

27. McCarthy, J. J. (1991). *Effects of a wrestling periodization strength program on muscular strength, absolute endurance, and relative endurance.* Master's thesis, California State University, Fullerton.

28. McComas, A. J. (1994). Human neuromuscular adaptations that accompany changes in activity. *Medicine and Science in Sports and Exercise, 26*, 1498–1509.

29. Murray, J. A., & Karpovich, P. V. (1956). *Weight training in athletics.* Englewood Cliffs, NJ: Prentice-Hall.

30. National Strength and Conditioning Association. (1985). Position paper on prepubescent strength training. *NSCA Journal, 7*(4), 27–31.

31. *Penn State Sports Medicine Newsletter.* (1992). The RM prescription. *1*(2), 7.

32. Pollock, M. L., Graves, J. E., Leggett, S. H., Braith, R. W., & Hagberg, J. M. (1991). Injuries and adherence to aerobic and strength training exercise programs for the elderly. *Medicine and Science in Sports and Exercise, 23*, 1194–1200.

33. Rikli, R. E., Jones, C. J., Beam, W. C., Duncan, S. J., & Lamar, B. (1996). Testing versus training effects on 1 RM strength assessment in older adults. *Medicine and Science in Sports and Exercise, 28*(5, Suppl.), Abstract #909, S153.

34. Rutherford, W. J., & Corbin, C. B. (1994). Validation of criterion-referenced standards for tests of arm and shoulder girdle strength and endurance. *Research Quarterly for Exercise and Sport, 65*, 110–119.

35. Sale, D. G. (1991). Testing strength and power. In J. D. MacDougal, H. A. Wenger, & H. J. Green (Eds.), *Physiological testing of the high-performance athlete* (pp. 21–106). Champaign, IL: Human Kinetics.

Form 4.3

Group Form for MEN'S Free-Weight Strength (kg), Total Work (w; kJ), and Mean Power (P; W) for Arm Curl (AC) and Bench Press (BP)

Initials or ID #	Direct 1 RM (kg)		Indirect 1 RM (kg)		S:Wt Ratio		w*	Mean P*
	2-AC	BP	2-AC	BP	2-AC	BP	(kJ)	W
1.								
2.								
3.								
4.								
5.								
6.								
7.								
8.								
9.								
10.								
11.								
12.								
13.								
14.								
15.								
16.								
17.								
18.								
M								

*Total work (w) and mean power are calculated from the indirect 1 RM test.

Form 4.4

Group Form for WOMEN'S Free-Weight Strength (kg), Total Work (w; kJ), and Mean Power (P; W) for Arm Curl (AC) and Bench Press (BP)

Initials or ID #	Direct 1 RM (kg)		Indirect 1 RM (kg)		S:Wt Ratio		w*	Mean P*
	2-AC	BP	2-AC	BP	2-AC	BP	(kJ)	W
1.								
2.								
3.								
4.								
5.								
6.								
7.								
8.								
9.								
10.								
11.								
12.								
13.								
14.								
15.								
16.								
17.								
18.								
M								

*Total work (w) and mean power are calculated from the indirect 1 RM test.

The importance of handgrip strength is not just to have an impressive handshake. Good handgrip strength may prevent people from dropping various objects, such as jars, bottles, and cans, in addition to allowing them to open the lid of a jar. Especially for older persons, good handgrip strength may prevent a fall down stairs or in bathtubs by enabling them to grasp a rail; it may also permit them to squeeze the gas pump at the service station. Grip strength also has been used in the occupational setting as a pre-employment device, as a periodic monitoring device, and as a return-to-work rehabilitation device.[18] In summary, handgrip strength is important for successful performance in activities of daily living and occupational activities.

The monitoring of handgrip strength is meaningful in the diagnosis and prognosis of neck and, of course, hand injuries. Thus, the measurement of handgrip strength has implications for people's safety, convenience, and neuromuscular assessment.

Rationale

The rationale for the measurement of strength may be categorized into three areas—anatomical, physiological, and biochemical. All of these are interrelated.

Anatomical Rationale

Grip strength is related ($r = .60$) to muscle mass.[22] Handgrip strength is mainly a function of the muscles in the forearm, in addition to those in the hand. Eight muscles serve as the prime movers and stabilizers for handgrip strength; 11 other muscles within the hand itself assist in the contraction.[6]

Physiological Rationale

Strength is located at the very beginning of the fitness continuum that was described and illustrated in Chapter 1 (Figures 1.1 and 1.2). Some performers can reach their peak force of a static handgrip test of strength in 0.3 s,[5,32] whereas others may take 2.7 s.[3] Similar times to peak force occur in larger muscle groups, such as elbow flexors.[32] Men reach peak force faster than women,[5] possibly because women's more elastic connective tissues require more time to reach the end-point of stretch. Some people may be able to hold the peak force for only 1 s,[21] whereas others might hold it for a few seconds[32] (Figure 5.1).

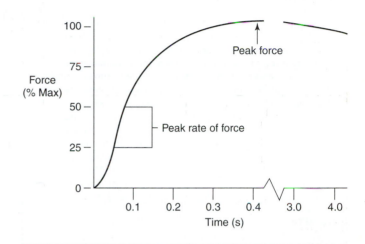

Figure 5.1 A typical force-time curve during a maximal static muscle action of a handgrip strength measurement. The peak force occurs at 100 % max force. The peak rate of force occurs during the steepest portion of the curve.

Biochemical Rationale

Based upon this rapid onset and decay of peak force, it should be obvious that the energy pathway predominantly involved in maximal muscle actions (strength) is the phosphagen system. Thus, the primary biochemical reaction for strength, or any muscle action, is

$$\text{Adenosine triphospate (ATP)} \xrightarrow{\text{ATPase}} \text{ADP} + \text{P} + \text{Energy}$$

Because the need for large amounts of ATP is so urgent, the ATP and its quick rejuvenator, creatine phosphate (CP), must be immediately available for the interacting muscle filaments—actin and myosin. However, the stores of ATP and PC are very limited. Because they cannot be resupplied adequately by the slower glycolytic and oxidative systems, the actin and myosin filaments cannot interact in order to continue contracting forcefully. Consequently, a rapid decay occurs in the peak force despite the physical and mental efforts to sustain it.

Method

The method of field/lab testing of strength is quite simple. The procedures of handgrip dynamometry can be learned quickly by watching a brief demonstration and then practicing

BOX 5.1 Accuracy of Handgrip Strength Testing

Muscular strength is highly affected by the central nervous system. Thus, emotional or mental factors play an important role in strength testing.

If the motivation of the performer is consistent, strength variability should be minimized.

Reliability

One group of investigators reported no significant differences in reliability (Intraclass Correlation Coefficients; ICC) between (1) the maximal force of one trial, (2) the mean maximal force of two trials, (3) the mean maximal force of three trials, and the highest maximal force of three trials.[18] However, another group reported the highest reliability when the mean of three maximal trials was used.[28] Individual daily variations in strength range from 2 % to 12 % in women and 5 % to 9 % in men.[40] Reliability coefficients for strength testing are usually .90 or higher. The grip-handle setting at position #1 of the Jamar dynamometer is significantly less reliable than the other four handle positions.[28] The objectivity, or inter-rater reliability, is very high when two technicians follow standard procedures (r = .97).

Validity

For the average person, handgrip strength correlates moderately (r = .69) with the total strength of 22 other muscles of the body.[10] Static tests of strength are more valid for static muscle actions than they are for dynamic actions.

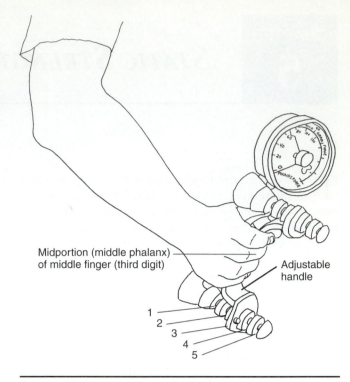

Midportion (middle phalanx) of middle finger (third digit)

Adjustable handle

1
2
3
4
5

Figure 5.2 The proper positioning of the upper arm, forearm, and hand during handgrip strength testing. Numbered slots indicate five different grip size positions of the Jamar™ dynamometer.

for a few minutes. Box 5.1 summarizes the accuracy of handgrip strength testing.

Equipment for Handgrip Strength Testing

In clinical settings, physicians and therapists often evaluate strength by using a manual testing method by which they subjectively determine the resistance they feel when the patient exerts against them. Also, they have used hand-held dynamometers, which they place against the limb of the patient's muscle group, and, again, the test requires both patient and examiner to resist each other.[41]

The word *dynamometer* (dī-na-móm-e-ter) comes from the Greek word meaning *power measure*. Because time is not measured in the strength tests described here, the more apt description of the handgrip dynamometer would be as a force-measuring device, rather than as a power-measuring one. Dynamometers were used as early as 1798.[34]

A common laboratory dynamometer, the Jamar™, uses a sealed hydraulic system to activate its force indicator during static muscle action. For example, the movement of the grip for the Jamar instrument (Fig. 5.2) cannot be perceived; however, grip handles on spring dynamometers, such as the Stoelting™/Smedley™ (Stoelting Co. Wood Dale, IL), the Lafayette™, (Lafayette Instruments, Lafayette, IN), may move more than 1.5 cm during a maximal handgrip contraction.[20]

Strength is usually measured in units of force or torque. The force units for static dynamometry should be expressed, preferably, in newtons (N). Although kilograms (kg) and pounds (lb) are commonly printed on the dials of most handgrip dynamometers, the scientific community encourages the use of newtons.[23] Most handgrip dynamometers provide scales that read up to 200 to 220 lb, or 90 to 100 kg. Most grip dynamometers have dual pointers, one pointer holding the maximal reading until it is reset and the other pointer returning to the zero position. Some have a single floating pointer that holds its position until reset.

Procedures for Handgrip Dynamometry

The procedures for handgrip strength testing are summarized as follows:

1. The performer should be in the standing position (Figure 5.3).
2. The performer's head should be in the midposition (facing straight ahead).
3. The grip size should be adjusted so that the middle finger's (third digit's) midportion (second phalanx) is approximately at a right angle.
   a. Grip adjustments of 1.3 cm (0.5 in) on the Jamar dynamometer (see Box 5.2 for calibration procedure) are made by slipping off the moveable handle and repositioning it into the five manufactured slots:

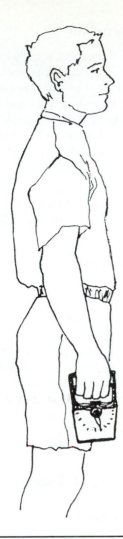

Figure 5.3 The performer squeezes the spring dynamometer maximally from a standing position and facing directly forward with the upper arm hanging straight down and the forearm at any position between 90° angle and 180° angle (straight down).

#1 = the slot at the innermost position for the smallest grip size (see Figure 5.2).

#5 = the slot at the outside position for the largest grip size.[a]

  b. Grip adjustments up to 4 cm for some dynamometers (e.g., Lafayette and Smedley) are made by lifting the hinge, if present, on the side of the fixed outer handle of the dynamometer and then twirling the inner stirrup to the desired setting.

4. The technician should record the grip setting (1 to 5 for Jamar; 10 mm to 40 mm on inner scale for Smedley) on Form 5.1. The same setting should be used for further tests on the same person.

[a]Jamar position #2 spans ≈ 4.4 cm (≈ 1.75 in.).[12]

5. The performer's forearm may be placed at any angle between 90° and 180° (right angle to straight) of the upper arm; the upper arm hangs in a vertical position.
6. The performer's wrist and forearm should be at the midprone position.
7. The performer should exert maximally and quickly after hearing the technician's following instructions:[28]
  a. "Are you ready?"
  b. "Squeeze as hard as you can." As the performer begins:
  c. "Harder! . . . Harder! . . . Relax."
8. The performer should make two[13,30,36] or three[37] trials alternately with each hand, with at least 30 s[26] or up to 1 min[36] between trials for the same hand.
9. The technician should record the force in kg, then convert the circled best score to approximate newtons simply by multiplying the kg value by 10 (9.8066 exact).
10. The technician resets the dynamometer's pointer to zero after each trial.

Comments on the Procedures

The standing position produces higher grip strengths than the sitting position.[1] The midposition of the head is recommended in order to avoid the bias of the tonic neck reflex.[4,17] Although this natural reflex may be diminished in adults, it causes the flexors of the opposite side (contralateral) of the body to be the most strong when the head is turned laterally away from the forearm being tested.[15,16] One group of investigators reported no difference in maximal forces of the dominant hand at 90° elbow flexion or full extension.[9] But other investigators found higher grip strengths with the elbow at full extension.[25,38]

    Grip sizes do not make much difference except in performers with large hands who are tested at small grip settings, or persons with small hands who are tested at large settings.[29] However, when testing many persons without ever adjusting the grip-handle size, it appears that Jamar position #2[12] or #3[19] provides the highest force.

The midpronated arm position was used by investigators whose norms are presented in Tables 5.1–5.3 of this chapter. However, norms are available elsewhere for grip testing in the palm-up position while the forearm rests on a table.[2]

Although performers should make powerful exertions at the start of each trial, they should be careful to avoid jerking the dynamometer. No movement from the initial body position can take place during the trial, nor can the hand touch any other part of the body.

Consistent verbal instruction prior to and during the maximal effort enhances the reliability of the measures.[28] The performer should not gradually approach maximal; in fact, it is counterproductive to take more than five seconds to reach maximal contraction, especially in older persons.[24]

Based on the rapid recovery rate of the phosphagens,[14] 30 s to 1 min should be sufficient as a rest interval between trials for the same hand, especially if each contraction is less than 5 s.

The chosen score has varied among investigators.[2,18,27,30,36,37] Most investigators have used the best of two[13,30,36] or three[37] untimed trials, or the average of the last 2 s of two 3-s trials.[2] I use the best of two trials to compare with the norms of Tables 5.1, and 5.2. Usually (60 % to 66 % of the trials), the first trial of a three-trial protocol will be the highest.[11,33]

Results and Discussion

The norms for grip strength are usually categorized according to age because grip strength is just as strongly correlated with age ($r = -.64$) as with muscle mass.[22] The decline in men's grip strength after the forties follows a curvilinear regression[8] (Eq. 5.1). Women's predictions may be approximated by taking 50 % of the men's values. Based on one pair of researchers' pilot studies, the handgrip test may be contraindicated (not recommended) for persons with arthritic hands.[35]

$$\text{Grip Sum (kg)} = 90.6 + (0.84 \times \text{Age}) \qquad \text{Eq. 5.1}$$
$$- (0.014 \times \text{Age}^2)$$

where:

Grip Sum is the sum of the best right and left grip forces.

Grip strength continues to decrease curvilinearly in men and in women over 60 y of age.[8]

The norms in Tables 5.1 to 5.3 are derived from grip forces measured by spring-type dynamometers. Two of the tables are based on the 1970s epidemiological study of over 6000 persons in Tecumseh, Michigan.[30] The Canadian norms presented in Table 5.2 are based on data from the 1981 Canada Fitness Survey,[13] and show higher values than the Michigan norms.

Table 5.1 **Percentiles (%ile) for Sum (R + L) of Grip Strength (kg) in Men and Women, Ages 18 y to 59 y[a]**

	18	19	20–24	25–29	30–34	35–39	40–44	45–49	50–59
%ile	Men's Grip Strength (kg)								
90	111	110	122	123	124	121	121	110	110
80	106	113	115	115	115	115	115	108	102
70	101	109	110	110	110	109	108	104	96
60	98	104	105	107	106	106	103	99	93
50	96	101	102	103	102	102	100	95	89
40	93	98	99	100	98	98	97	91	85
30	90	94	94	95	95	93	93	82	81
20	86	90	89	90	90	88	87	81	75
10	81	84	80	81	82	79	81	75	66
M	97.1	102.0	102.9	103.6	103.4	101.9	101.4	95.6	89.4
SD	15.5	13.7	16.8	15.6	16.8	17.3	16.1	16.1	16.1

	18	19	20–24	25–29	30–34	35–39	40–44	45–49	50–59
%ile	Women's Grip Strength (kg)								
90	59	63	61	67	65	66	64	64	57
80	55	59	57	62	60	59	58	57	52
70	52	54	53	57	57	55	54	53	48
60	49	50	50	53	53	53	51	52	45
50	46	48	48	49	49	51	49	49	43
40	43	46	45	48	47	49	47	47	40
30	39	42	42	46	44	46	43	44	38
20	36	39	38	43	41	43	40	40	34
10	31	36	34	37	36	36	36	34	30
M	47.1	49.9	48.7	52.2	51.5	51.9	50.0	50.0	44.0
SD	9.7	10.3	9.8	10.7	11.4	11.6	11.1	10.7	9.8

From H. J. Montoye and D. E. Lamphiear, "Grip and arm strength in males and females age 10 to 69," *Research Quarterly,* 48(1), Table 3, p. 113, 1977. Copyright © American Alliance for Health, Physical Education, Recreation and Dance, 1900 Association Dr., Reston, VA 22091.
Note: [a]Spring dynamometer (Stoelting™) and best of two trials.

| Table 5.2 | Percentiles for the Sum of Right and Left Grip Strengths (kg) in Canadian Men (M) and Women (W), Ages 20 y to 69 y[a] | | | | | | | | | |

	20–29		30–39		40–49		50–59		60–69	
	M	W	M	W	M	W	M	W	M	W
%ile										
95	136	78	135	80	128	80	119	72	111	67
90	127	74	127	76	123	76	114	69	106	62
85	124	71	123	73	119	73	110	65	102	60
80	120	70	120	71	117	71	108	63	99	58
75	118	68	117	69	115	69	105	62	96	56
70	115	67	115	68	112	67	103	60	94	55
65	113	65	113	66	110	65	102	59	93	54
60	111	64	111	65	108	64	100	58	91	53
55	109	63	109	63	106	62	99	57	89	52
50	107	62	107	62	104	61	97	56	88	52
45	106	61	105	61	102	59	96	55	86	51
40	104	59	104	60	100	58	94	54	84	50
35	102	58	101	59	98	57	92	53	82	49
30	100	56	99	58	96	56	90	53	81	49
25	97	55	97	56	94	55	87	51	79	48
20	95	53	94	55	91	53	85	50	76	47
15	91	52	91	53	89	51	83	48	73	45
10	87	50	87	51	84	49	80	46	69	43
5	81	47	81	48	76	46	74	42	62	39

Source: Data from Fitness and Amateur Sport, Canada. (1987). *Canadian standarized test of fitness: Operations manual.* (3rd ed.). Ottawa, Ontario, Canada: Fitness and Amateur Sports Directorate.
Note: [a]Best of two trials per hand using spring dynamometer.

| Table 5.3 | Norms for the Ratio of the Sum of Right and Left Grip Strengths to Body Mass (kg·kg^{-1} wt) in Men and Women, Ages 18 y to 59 y[a] | | | | | | | |

	18	19	20–24	25–29	30–34	35–39	40–49	50–59
%ile	Men's Ratios (kg·kg^{-1} body wt)							
90	1.62	1.75	1.73	1.72	1.64	1.62	1.54	1.39
80	1.50	1.54	1.59	1.54	1.52	1.51	1.41	1.30
70	1.47	1.44	1.53	1.47	1.45	1.42	1.34	1.22
60	1.44	1.36	1.45	1.40	1.39	1.35	1.28	1.19
50	1.37	1.33	1.39	1.35	1.33	1.28	1.24	1.14
40	1.33	1.29	1.32	1.28	1.29	1.23	1.19	1.10
30	1.31	1.24	1.26	1.20	1.24	1.17	1.14	1.03
20	1.22	1.17	1.18	1.12	1.18	1.11	1.07	0.98
10	1.16	1.12	1.08	1.01	1.10	1.02	0.99	0.89
M	1.37	1.37	1.39	1.34	1.35	1.30	1.25	1.14

	18	19	20–24	25–29	30–34	35–39	40–49	50–59
%ile	Women's Ratios (kg·kg^{-1} body wt)							
90	1.02	1.10	1.04	1.12	1.05	1.07	1.02	0.90
80	0.95	1.04	0.97	1.02	1.00	1.00	0.93	0.83
70	0.90	0.94	0.91	0.97	0.94	0.93	0.87	0.78
60	0.82	0.85	0.86	0.91	0.89	0.87	0.81	0.71
50	0.78	0.80	0.81	0.86	0.83	0.84	0.77	0.68
40	0.72	0.77	0.77	0.82	0.78	0.80	0.73	0.63
30	0.69	0.74	0.72	0.75	0.72	0.75	0.69	0.69
20	0.65	0.69	0.68	0.68	0.68	0.69	0.68	0.52
10	0.58	0.64	0.61	0.61	0.60	0.60	0.54	0.48
M	0.79	0.85	0.82	0.86	0.83	0.84	0.78	0.68

From H. J. Montoye and D. E. Lamphiear, "Grip and arm strength in males and females age 10 to 69," *Research Quarterly, 48*(1), Table 6, p. 116, 1977. Copyright © American Alliance for Health, Physical Education, Recreation and Dance, 1900 Association Dr., Reston, VA 22091.
Note: [a]Spring dynamometer (Stoelting™) and best of two trials.

For men ages 60–69, 70–79, and 80–89, the mean sums are 88 kg, 75 kg, and 66 kg, respectively.[22] Table 5.3 provides the strength/body weight ratios, whereby the sum of the right and left grip strength scores is divided by the person's body mass (BM) (kg ÷ kg BM). This ratio (relative strength) becomes important when evaluating a person's ability to lift his/her own body weight or to assume and support certain body positions such as hanging from a chin-up bar, or grasping a rail.

The ratio of dominant hand to nondominant hand (D:N) varies slightly with age.[39] Thus, monitoring periodically this ratio may prove helpful in injury or pathological conditions. Mysteriously, right-handers are stronger in their right hand grip (8 % greater force),[7] but professed left-handers show little difference between their left and right handgrip strength.[7,27,31] Perhaps the similarity in right and left handgrip strength in left-handers is because they have more opportunity to use their right hand in mostly a "right-handed world" where tools and appliances are designed for right-handers.[7]

Some conclusions that may be made from these and other norms are as follows: (1) Boys and girls have similar grip strengths until puberty; (2) men's grip sums are between 1.75 and 2.0 times greater than women's for the ages represented in these norms; (3) grip strength increases rapidly with age for males between the onset of puberty and the twenties; (4) grip strength declines slowly with age between the thirties to the fifties but decreases faster after the fifties for both sexes; (5) grip strength decreases curvilinearly in older adults; and (6) it appears that the sum of the right and left grip strengths is about 1.3 times higher than the body mass for the men and about 80 % of the body mass for the women in most of the age groups presented in Table 5.3.[30]

References

1. Balogun, J. A., Akomolafe, C. T., & Amusa, L. O. (1991). Grip strength: Effects of testing posture and elbow position. *Archives of Physical Medicine and Rehabilitation, 72*, 280–283.
2. Baumgartner, T. A., & Jackson, A. S. (1987). *Measurement for evaluation in physical education and exercise science.* Dubuque, IA: Wm. C. Brown.
3. Bemben, M. G., Clasey, J. L., & Massey, B. H. (1990). The effect of the rate of muscle contraction on the force-time curve parameters of male and female subjects. *Research Quarterly for Exercise and Sport, 61*(1), 96–99.
4. Berntson, G. G., & Torello, M. W. (1977). Expression of Magnus tonic neck reflexes in distal muscles of prehension in normal adults. *Physiology and Behavior, 19*, 585–587.
5. Borsa, P. A., & Sauers, E. L. (2000). The importance of gender on myokinetic deficits before and after microinjury. *Medicine and Science in Sports and Exercise, 32*, 891–896.
6. Buck, J. A., Amundsen, L. R., & Nielsen, D. H. (1980). Systolic blood pressure responses during isometric contractions of large and small muscle groups. *Medicine and Science in Sports and Exercise, 12*(3), 145–147.
7. Crosby, C. A., Wehbe, M. A., & Mawr, B. (1994). Hand strength: Normative values. *Journal of Hand Surgery, 19*, 665–670.
8. Desrosiers, J., Bravo, G., Hebert, R., & Dutil, E. (1995). Normative data for grip strength of elderly men and women. *American Journal of Occupational Therapy, 49*, 637–644.
9. Desrosiers, J., Bravo, G., Hebert, R., & Mercier, L. (1995). Impact of elbow position on grip strength of elderly men. *Journal of Hand Therapy, 8*, 27–30.
10. de Vries, H. A. (1980). *Physiology of exercise in physical education and athletics.* Dubuque, IA: Wm. C. Brown.
11. Fess, E. E. (1982). The effects of Jamar dynamometer handle position and test protocol on hand strength. *Journal of Hand Surgery, 1*, 308.
12. Firrell, J. C., & Crain, G. M. (1996). Which setting of the dynamometer provides maximal grip strength? *Journal of Hand Surgery, 21*, 397–401.
13. Fitness and Amateur Sport, Canada. (1987). *Canadian standardized test of fitness: Operations manual* (3rd ed.). Ottawa, Ontario, Canada: Fitness and Amateur Sports Directorate.
14. Foss, M. L., & Keteyian, S. J. (1998). *Fox's physiological basis for exercise and sport.* Boston: McGraw-Hill.
15. George, C. O. (1970). Effects of the asymmetrical tonic neck posture upon grip strength of normal children. *Research Quarterly, 41*, 361–364.
16. George, C. O. (1972). Facilitative and inhibitory effects of the tonic neck reflex upon grip strength of right- and left-handed children. *Research Quarterly, 43*, 157–166.
17. Gesell, A., & Ames, L. B. (1947). The development of handedness. *Journal of Genetic Psychology, 70*, 155–175.
18. Hamilton, A., Balnave, R., & Adams, R. (1994). Grip strength testing reliability. *Journal of Hand Therapy, 7*, 163–170.
19. Harkonen, R., Piirtomaa, M., & Alaranta, H. (1993). Grip strength and hand position of the dynamometer in 204 Finnish adults. *Journal of Hand Surgery, 18*, 129–132.
20. Heyward, V., McKeown, B., & Geeseman, R. (1975). Comparison of the Stoelting handgrip dynamometer and linear voltage differential transformer for measuring maximal grip strength. *Research Quarterly, 46*(2), 262–266.
21. Hislop, H. J. (1963). Quantitative changes in human muscular strength during isometric exercise. *Journal of the American Physical Therapy Association, 43*, 21–38.

22. Kallman, D. A., Plato, C. C., & Tobin, J. D. (1990). The role of muscle loss in the age-related decline of grip strength: Cross-sectional and longitudinal perspectives. *Journal of Gerontology: Medical Sciences, 45,* M82–88.

23. Knuttgen, H. G. (1986). Quantifying exercise performances with SI units. *The Physician and Sportsmedicine, 14*(12), 157–161.

24. Kroll, W., Clarkson, P. M., & Melchionda, A. M. (1981). Age, isometric strength, rate of tension development and fiber type composition. *Medicine and Science in Sports and Exercise, 13,* Abstract, 87.

25. Kuzala, E. A., & Vargo, M. C. (1992). The relationship between elbow position and grip strength. *American Journal of Occupational Therapy, 46,* 509–512.

26. Lind, A. R., & McNicol, G. W. (1967). Circulatory response to sustained handgrip contractions performed during other exercise, both rhythmic and static. *The American Journal of Cardiology, 38,* 46–51.

27. Mathiowetz, V., Kashman, N., Volland, G., Weber, K., Dowe, M., & Rogers, S. (1985). Grip and pinch strength: Normative data for adults. *Archives of Physical Medicine and Rehabilitation, 66,* 69–72.

28. Mathiowetz, V., Weber, K., Volland, G., & Kashman, N. (1984). Reliability and validity of hand strength evaluation. *Journal of Hand Surgery, 9A,* 222–226.

29. Montoye, H. J., & Faulkner, J. A. (1975). Determination of the optimum setting of an adjustable grip dynamometer. *The Research Quarterly, 35,* 30–36.

30. Montoye, H. J., & Lamphiear, D. E. (1977). Grip and arm strength in males and females, age 10 to 69. *Research Quarterly, 48,* 109–120.

31. Montpetit, R. R., Montoye, H. J., & Laeding, L. (1967). Grip strength of school children, Saginaw, Michigan: 1899 and 1964. *Research Quarterly, 38,* 231–240.

32. Morris, A. F., Clarke, D. H., & Dainis, A. (1983). Time to maximal voluntary isometric contraction (MVC) for five different muscle groups in college adults. *Research Quarterly for Exercise and Sport, 54,* 163–168.

33. Patterson, R. P., & Baxter, T. (1988). A multiple muscle strength testing protocol. *Archives of Physical Medicine and Rehabilitation, 69,* 366–368.

34. Regnier, C. (1798). Description and use of the dynamometer, or instrument for ascertaining the relative strength of men and animals. *Philosophical magazine, 1*(1), 399–404.

35. Rikli, R. E., & Jones, C. J. (1999). Development and validation of a functional fitness test for community-residing older adults. *Journal of Aging Physical Activity, 7,* 129–161.

36. Sale, D. G. (1991). Testing strength and power. In J. D. MacDougal, H. A. Wenger, & H. J. Green (Eds.), *Physiological testing of the high-performance athlete* (pp. 21–106). Champaign, IL: Human Kinetics.

37. Stoelting, C. H. (1970). *Smedley instruction manual.* Chicago: Author.

38. Su, C. Y., Lin, J. H., Chien, T. H., Chen, K. F., & Sung, Y. T. (1994). Grip strength in different positions of elbow and shoulder. *Archives of Physical Medicine and Rehabilitation, 75,* 812–815.

39. Thorngren, K. G., & Werner, C. O. (1979). Normal grip strength. *Acta Orthopaedic Scandinavica, 50,* 255–259.

40. Wakim, K. G., Gersten, J. W., Elkins, E. C., & Martin, G. M. (1950). Objective recording of muscle strength. *Archives of Physical Medicine, 31,* 90–100.

41. Wikholm, J. B., & Bohannon, R. W. (1991). Handheld dynamometer measurements: Tester strength makes a difference. *The Journal of Orthopaedic and Sports Physical Therapy, 13,* 191–193.

Form 5.1

Individual Data for Handgrip Strength

Basic Data

Name [   ] Date [   ] Time [   ] a.m. [   ] p.m. [   ] Age [   ] y
    (last)   (first)   (mo/ d / y)

Gender (M or W) [   ] Ht [   ] cm Wt [   ] kg Dominant Hand (check): Right (R) [   ] Left (L) [   ]

Meteorological Data

Tech. Initials [   ] T [   ] °C (closest 0.1 °C) RH % [   ] P_B [   ] mm Hg × 1.333 = [   ] hPa

Instrument

Force (kg) (circle best trial of first two trials of each hand; underline the best of three trials)

	Trial #1	Trial #2	Trial #3
	R L	R L	R L

[Hydraulic (e.g., Jamar)]

Grip Setting Position/#1, #2, #3, #4, #5 (circle):

	R L	R L	R L

[Spring (e.g., Lafayette)] (mm setting on handle): [   ] mm

	R L	R L	R L

[Other type _____]

Best of Two Trials	Right Hand		Left Hand		Sum of R and L			Table %ile 5.1	5.2
Hydraulic	[ ]	+	[ ]	=	[ ]	kg; × 10 = [ ] N		[ ]	[ ]
Spring	[ ]	+	[ ]	=	[ ]	kg; × 10 = [ ] N		[ ]	[ ]
Other	[ ]	+	[ ]	=	[ ]	kg; × 10 = [ ] N		[ ]	[ ]

Ratio of Best Grip Sum to Body Mass (kg·kg^{-1} wt):

Grip Sum [   ] kg ÷ [   ] kg wt = [   ] ratio [   ] %ile (Table 5.3)

Eq. 5.1 (Men): Age-Predicted Grip Sum (kg) = 90.6 + (0.84 × [   ] y) − (0.014 × [   ] y^2)

$$= 90.6 + [\quad] - (0.014 \times [\quad])$$

$$= 90.6 + [\quad] - [\quad]$$

$$= [\quad] \text{ kg} = [\quad] \text{ N}$$

Ratio of Dominant Hand to Nondominant Hand (D:N):

D [   ] kg ÷ N [   ] kg = [   ]

Form 5.2

Group Data for Handgrip Strength

Handgrip Strength[a]

MEN Initials (or ID #)	R kg	L kg	Sum kg	Sum:BM ratio	WOMEN Initials (or ID #)	R kg	L kg	Sum kg	Sum:BM ratio
1.					1.				
2.					2.				
3.					3.				
4.					4.				
5.					5.				
6.					6.				
7.					7.				
8.					8.				
9.					9.				
10.					10.				
11.					11.				
12.					12.				
13.					13.				
14.					14.				
15.					15.				
16.					16.				
17.					17.				
18.					18.				
19.					19.				
20.					20.				
21.					21.				
22.					22.				
Mean					*Mean*				

[a]Best of three trials.

ISOKINETIC STRENGTH

The laboratory test selected for the measurement of leg strength requires the performance of an isokinetic movement on a specially designed machine. The isokinetic measurement of leg strength is classified as a laboratory test because the apparatus does not lend itself to simultaneous testing of individuals; nor is it inexpensive, portable, and simple. Despite the high cost of the isokinetic instrument, the description has been included in this manual because of the prevalence of such machines in many athletic training facilities on college campuses and in sophisticated fitness and rehabilitation clinics. As with many laboratory ergometers and dynamometers, isokinetic machines serve both as fitness testing devices and fitness training devices.

Leg strength diminishes faster than upper body strength as one ages past young adulthood.[29] Thus, leg strength training and periodic monitoring are important for middle-age and older persons if they intend to keep functioning optimally in activities of daily living.

In addition to determining the state of training of the legs, testing the legs may provide insight into the risk of injuring them. Muscle strength asymmetry (difference in strength between right and left legs) may be a predisposing factor in muscle strains,[55] especially in the weaker leg.[22] This asymmetrical leg strength may also lead to knee injuries.[7] Some investigators report that strains are more likely if a **bilateral (contralateral) imbalance** exists. Their criterion for bilateral imbalance is a nondominant-to-dominant ratio of 0.95, 0.90, or less.[33,60] Thus, according to some persons, the nondominant leg should be at least 90 % or 95 % as forceful as the dominant leg. The 90 % (or 0.90 ratio) strength-balance criterion is also recommended as a guide for lower limb stress fracture.[29] This contrasts with the "70 % criterion" reported by a pair of investigators.[26] Adding to the controversy, another group reported no difference in knee injury rate when the ratios of the left leg (assumed nondominant) to right leg (assumed dominant) were less than 0.90.[72]

Similarly, an **ipsilateral imbalance** between the strength of the antagonist (hamstrings) and agonist (quadriceps) of the same leg could lead to a higher risk of leg injury.[36,56] The rationale supporting the lessened risk of injury to the knee's anterior cruciate ligament (ACL) is based on the co-contraction of the less forceful hamstring and the more forceful quadriceps during forceful leg extensions. Stronger co-contraction of the hamstrings reduces the anteriorly directed shear of the tibia relative to the femur due to the high quadriceps force. This, in turn, reduces the strain

(pull) on the ACL.[1,14,67] As with bilateral imbalance, controversy exists over the criteria for the hamstring (H) force to quadriceps force (Q) ratio or percentage and the criteria's validity as an injury predictor.[1] Criteria ratios for H:Q range from 0.50 (50 %)[43] to 0.75 (75 %).[23,42] The wide range is attributed not only to differences of opinion but to the isokinetic velocities of the test, whereby the slower velocities elicit lower ratios than the higher velocities. Not all investigators report a relationship between imbalanced strength and injury susceptibility.[4,28] Confirmation of optimal H:Q ratios still awaits evidence from controlled studies of injury incidence in persons having undergone isokinetic balance testing before their injury.[39]

Rationale for Isokinetic Testing

The rationale for isokinetic testing of leg strength may be categorized into mechanical and anatomical rationales.

Mechanical Rationale for Isokinetic Testing

In 1967, researchers first introduced isokinetics as a type of dynamic muscle action at a constant velocity; thus, no momentum was gained or lost throughout a truly isokinetic movement.[73] Once the performer reaches the set velocity, an increase in force by the performer causes the isokinetic device to counteract this force with an accommodating increase in resistance. Conversely, a decrease in the application of force results in a corresponding decrease in the resistance.[53] Thus, the movement does not change velocity significantly. The testing apparatus controls the angular velocity of the exercise, thus allowing the musculature to elicit maximal tension for each angle within the movement range. Isokinetic movements are rare in most daily, recreational and sports activities.[39] One of those varities occurs when the arms pull through the water in swimming.

The laboratory measurement of isokinetic strength provides torque measurements throughout the active range of motion during this maximal effort. The unit of measure for isokinetic strength is a torque value, commonly referred to as foot-pounds or newton meters (N·m) (see Chapter 1). **Torque** indicates the force rotating about an axis—that is, the turning or twisting force,[31] such as the force produced by a wrench when tightening the nut on a bolt. Because isokinetic devices have lever arms connected to strain gauges, torque is produced and recorded from the

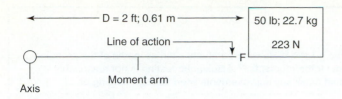

Figure 6.1 Torque production (136 N·m) as a function of the external force (F; 223 N) applied at the end-length of the moment arm (D; 0.61 m).

angular motion. *Peak torque* is the term that indicates muscular strength. Torque (τ), or moment, as presented in Equation 6.1, is the product of force (F) and the perpendicular length (distance; D) of the lever arm.[19]

$$\tau \text{ (ft·lb or N·m)} = F \text{ (lb or N)} \times D^{lever} \text{ (ft or m)} \quad \text{Eq. 6.1}$$

The distance of the lever arm is measured from the center of rotation to the point where the external force is applied (the line of action). This distance is often referred to as the **moment arm.** For example, if a force of 50 lb (22.7 kg or 223 N based on 1 kg = 9.80665; ≈ 9.8 or 10 N) is applied at the end of a moment arm measuring 2 ft (0.61 m) in length (Figure 6.1), then the torque is calculated as

$$\tau \text{ (ft·lb)} = 50 \text{ lb} \times 2 \text{ ft} = 100 \text{ ft·lb}$$

$$\tau \text{ (N·m)} = 223 \text{ N} \times 0.61 \text{ m} = 136 \text{ N·m}$$

The U.S. system's product (ft·lb) could have been converted to the metric unit (N·m) by using the conversion factor (Eq. 6.2):

$$1 \text{ ft·lb} = 1.3560 \text{ N·m} \quad \text{Eq. 6.2}$$

Thus: $1.3560 \times 100 \text{ ft·lb} = 135.6 \text{ N·m}$ (or 136 N·m to the closest whole N·m).[a]

Anatomical Rationale of Isokinetic Leg Flexion and Extension

Although isokinetic dynamometers are capable of measuring the torque of various muscle groups, only those muscles that flex and extend the lower leg are discussed here. Knee extension is represented by the strength of the quadriceps muscle group, which is made up of four muscles—the rectus femoris and the three vasti muscles—vastus medialis, lateralis, and intermedius. The rectus femoris crosses both the knee joint and hip joint, whereas the vasti muscles only cross the knee joint. The vasti contribute much more force (≈ 85 %) than the rectus femoris in a maximal leg extension.[51] Knee flexion is represented by the strength of the hamstring muscle group, which consists of three muscles—the biceps femoris, the semitendinosus, and the semimembranosus.

---

[a]Conversions: 1 ft = 0.3048 m ≈ 0.3 m; 1 lb = 0.454 kg ≈ 4.54 N.

The seated knee extension and knee flexion during isokinetic leg strength testing is an open kinetic chain exercise (OKCE) utilizing single muscle groups, respectively. Also, OKCE are less functional than closed kinetic chain exercise (CKCE).[16,47] CKCE are multi-joint exercises that are more functional because they are similar to running, jumping, squatting, and lunging. An example of OKCE is a leg press on a machine that causes your feet to move forward, but a CKCE leg press would cause your feet to remain stationary while your body moved away from your feet (in other words, the seat went backwards).

Fiber type plays an important role in determining the peak torque and duration of isokinetic contractions. For example, persons with higher percentages of fast-twitch fibers produce more torque ($r = .69$) at moderate ($180°·s^{-1}$) speeds, but have greater fatigability ($r = .86$), than persons with lower percentages.

Method

The methods of testing isokinetic leg strength are much more elaborate than those for testing handgrip strength. Compared with handgrip dynamometers, the equipment for isokinetic testing is very expensive and complex. But no expensive machine can make up for any loss of accuracy by inappropriate procedures of the examiner (see Box 6.1).

Equipment

Various instruments test concentric isokinetic leg strength such as Ariel™, Biodex™, Hydra-Fitness™, LIDO™, Kin-Com™, Merac™, and Cybex II™ (Figure 6.2). Also, they all test static strength, but the Kin-Com™ and Biodex™ machines can test eccentric strength.

Popular isokinetic velocities are $30°·s^{-1}$, $60°·s^{-1}$, $180°·s^{-1}$, and $300°·s^{-1}$; these are often referred to as slow, medium, and fast speeds, respectively. However, the fast velocity may be construed as slow compared with the velocities required in many sports' movements, such as sprinting, throwing, striking, kicking, and jumping. Some models (e.g., Cybex II⁺) provide increments of $15°·s^{-1}$ from $0°·s^{-1}$ to $300°·s^{-1}$ and may be controlled with an electronic remote device. When the velocity is set to $0°·s^{-1}$, static strength is measured. Researchers often express angular velocity as radians per second ($rad·s^{-1}$) by dividing degrees per second by 57.3 (Eq. 6.3).[24,27]

$$rad·s^{-1} = °·s^{-1} \div 57.3 \quad \text{Eq. 6.3}$$

where:

$rad·s^{-1}$ = radial velocity

$rad = 57.3°$

$1° = 0.01745$ radian

radian = the plane angle between two radii of a circle that cut off on the circumference an arc equal in length to the radius.

The conversion of $°·s^{-1}$ to $rad·s^{-1}$ is much simpler than it appears. For example, the calculation for finding the $rad·s^{-1}$ for a velocity of $300°·s^{-1}$ is

$$300°·s^{-1} = 300 \div 57.3$$

$$= 5.24 \text{ rad·s}^{-1}$$

To convert $rad·s^{-1}$ to degrees per second, simply do the reverse by multiplying the $rad·s^{-1}$ by 57.3.

A radian is defined as an angle at the center of a circle described by an arc equal to the length of the radius of the circle.[30] It is important to understand radians, so that readers can interpret the unit used by some researchers and to use the unit for calculating work from the angular movement of isokinetic actions. However, the measurement of isokinetic work is not discussed further in this manual.

Procedures

The procedures for testing the isokinetic strength of the legs include a description of the preparations in addition to the actual testing of the performer. They also include proper reading of the instrument and the graphic recording of torque. Most of the procedures relate to the Cybex II$^+$

(Cybex Medical, Henley International, Sugarland, TX), but are often applicable to the Kin-Com (Chattecx, Chattanooga, TN), and Biodex (Biodex Medical, Shirley, NY). Some differences are noted with respect to the number of trials, rest interval, and activation force. As with most laboratory procedures, adequate preparations include those concerned with the equipment and the performer. See Box 6.2 for calibration procedures.

Instrument Preparations

1. Procedures for periodic calibration are located in the calibration box (6.2) or in the manufacturer's instruction manual.
2. The recording apparatus should be readied for testing by setting the Damp to the No. 2 position; this smooths the printed curve that is generated by the performer's forces.
3. The technician selects an appropriate torque scale on the recorder based upon the estimated output of the performer.

Estimated Force	ft·lb (N·m)
• Low	30 ($\approx$ 41)
• Typical woman	90 (122)
• Typical man	180 (244)
• High	360 (488)

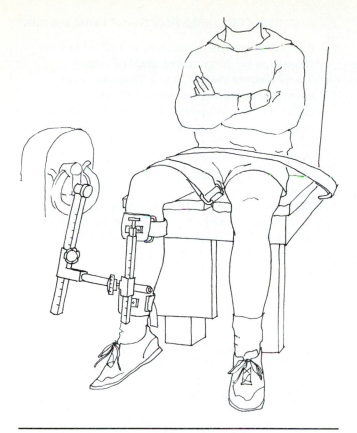

Figure 6.2 The position for isokinetic testing of leg strength with the Cybex II places the performer's hip angle (trunk to upper leg) and knee angle at approximately 90°.

BOX 6.2	Calibration of Isokinetic Machine

The manufacturers' manuals that accompany isokinetic instruments provide detailed calibration procedures. The instrument's torque values, both statically and dynamically, can be checked by attaching known weights to the dynamometer's lever arm at a known distance.[45,48,61] The accuracy of the velocity settings on the Cybex™ can be checked by counting the number of complete turns of the input shaft in one minute.[45,48] Ideally, to correct for the effect of gravity on the Cybex II, the performer should place the tested leg in an extended position and then relax the leg while it passively (no contraction) flexes. The technician will later add this value (N·m) to the extension score and subtract it from the flexion score.[18]

The Kin-Com machine may be set to a certain preload or activation force (e.g., 20–100 N), which means that this preset force must be applied by the performer before the lever arm will move.[38,46]

4. The technician sets the Input Direction to CW (clockwise) for left limb or CCW (counterclockwise) for right limb.

5. The position scale should be placed at the 150° mark, representing the approximate range of motion for testing of knee extension/flexion.

Performer Preparations

1. The performer sits in an upright position with the hips flexed at an angle of 90° (see Figure 6.2). The Kin-Com angle is 80°.
2. The technician uses pelvic and thigh straps to stabilize the hips and thighs, respectively. If available, chest straps are used also.
3. The technician identifies the axis of rotation of the knee joint and visually aligns the input shaft of the dynamometer with this axis of rotation at the lateral epicondyle.
4. The technician adjusts the length of the lever arm so that the inferior rim of the tibia (shin) pad contacts the tibia just above the malleoli of the ankle; the technician secures the shin/ankle strap. It may be advisable to standardize the length of the lever arm at a fixed length to avoid possible alteration of torque output.[68]
5. The performer flexes the knee at a minimum of 90° or as limited by the chair.
6. The performer folds arms across the chest and maintains this position throughout the warm-up and the test.[62,69]
7. The technician explains and demonstrates the leg movements for the strength test. Aside from assuring that the performer understands that maximal efforts are made, no further encouragement during the test is advised so that uniformity in tester-performer interaction is maintained.[52]
8. The performer warms up by making 5 to 10 submaximal repetitions (about 50 % MVC), both during flexion and extension at each speed setting ($30°·s^{-1}$, $60°·s^{-1}$, $180°·s^{-1}$, and $300°·s^{-1}$).
9. The performer then rests for 2 min to 5 min before the initial test, while the technician sets the velocity to $60°·s^{-1}$ and sets the paper recording speed to 5 mm·s^{-1} or 25 mm·s^{-1}.

The Test

1. With the recorder on, the performer makes three (or five)[69] continuous maximal repetitions at $30°·s^{-1}$ [26] or $60°·s^{-1}$.[4,13,36,37,69]
2. After a 30 s[50] to 60 s[65] rest, the performer makes three (or five)[69] maximal repetitions at $180°·s^{-1}$. Instead of consecutive contractions without a pause, technicians may allow rest intervals of 1 min to 3 min for one to five noncontinuous slow velocity ($<180°·s^{-1}$) actions, or 20 s to 30 s between three trials at higher velocities.[68] However, use consistent procedures if comparing performers or repeating tests on a single performer. Performers on the Kin-Com machine may use four alternating test contractions—two concentric and two eccentric—with a 5 s rest between muscle actions.[38]

3. Again after a 30 s to 60 s rest, the performer makes three maximal repetitions at 300°·s⁻¹.

4. The highest torque of each group of three trials is recorded on Form 6.1. See the examples in Figures 6.3 and 6.4.

5. The technician rearranges the apparatus for testing the other leg, and repeats the steps. The dominant leg may be considered as the preferred kicking leg,[80] or simply as the stronger leg.

6. The performer should statically stretch the quadriceps and hamstrings after the testing session.

7. The technician calculates the relative torque ($N \cdot m \cdot kg^{-1}$), and the ratios for ipsilateral (H:Q) and bilateral (L:R; or nondominant:dominant) strength.

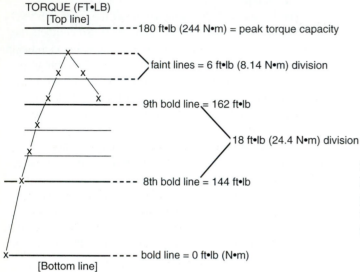

Figure 6.3 Schematic representation of the horizontal lines on the graph paper of an isokinetic recorder (e.g., Cybex II) with a drawn peak torque (x) value of 174 ft·lb (236 N·m).

For estimation of **fast-twitch fiber type of vastus lateralis:**

8. The technician sets the machine to 180°·s⁻¹ and the recorder to the slower paper speed of 5 mm/s.

9. The performer makes 50 to 55 maximal knee extension repetitions; the rest interval between each repetition is about 0.7 s,[75] or about the time required for the submaximal flexion movement (total time ≈ 1 min).

10. The technician counts each repetition and then averages the peak torque for the first to third and 48th to 50th repetitions.

11. The technician obtains the percent fast-twitch (FT %) fibers from Equation 6.4[75] by finding the decline (% ↓) in average peak torque (P-τ) values of the first to third repetitions and 48th to 50th repetitions of maximal knee extensions at 180°·s⁻¹.

$$FT\ \% = (\%\ \tau \downarrow - 5.2) \div 0.90 \qquad \text{Eq. 6.4}$$

where:

$$\%\ \tau \downarrow = \left[\frac{(P\text{-}\tau\ \text{at}\ 1-3) - (P\text{-}\tau\ \text{at}\ 48-50)}{P\text{-}\tau\ \text{at}\ 1-3} \right] \times 100$$

For example, if a person's average peak torques for the first three repetitions and the 48th to 50th repetitions are 200 N·m and 110 N·m, respectively, then the fast-twitch fiber percentage is calculated by first deriving the percentage of torque decrease (% τ ↓) during the trials and then inserting the percentage into Equation 6.4.

$$\%\ \tau \downarrow = [(200\ N \cdot m - 110\ N \cdot m) \div (200\ N \cdot m)] \times 100$$

$$= (90\ N \cdot m \div 200\ N \cdot m) \times 100$$

$$= 0.45 \times 100$$

$$= 45\ \%$$

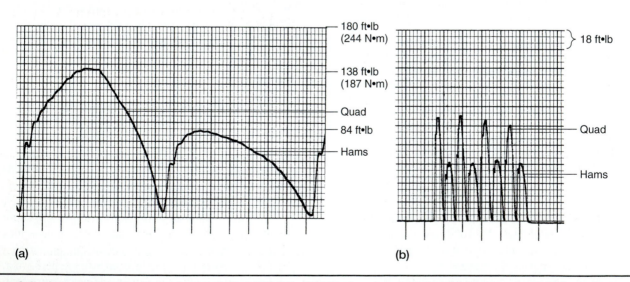

(a) (b)

Figure 6.4 An actual isokinetic tracing scaled at 180 ft·lb (244 N·m) and recorded at (a) 25 mm·s⁻¹, and (b) another person at 5 mm·s⁻¹. Peak torque in (a) for the quadriceps is 138 ft·lb or 187 N·m, and for the hamstrings is 84 ft·lb or 114 N·m. In (b), peak torque for the quadriceps is 96 ft·lb.

Thus,

$$FT \% = (45 \% - 5.2) \div 0.90$$
$$= 39.8 \div 0.90$$
$$= 44.2 \% \text{ (or 44 \% to nearest whole \%)}$$

12. For estimation of **slow-twitch fiber type (% ST),** use Equation 6.5:

$$\% \; ST = 100 - FT \% \qquad \text{Eq. 6.5}$$
$$= 100 - 44.2$$
$$= 55.8 \% \text{ (or 56 \% to the nearest whole \%)}$$

Comments on Isokinetic Procedures

The most common procedures for measuring isokinetic leg strength is at a seated position (80° to 100° angle at hip) and over a range of motion starting at between 100° to 90° knee flexion angle and ending at 0° to 10° knee angle. The performer must maintain the original seated posture throughout all repetitions.

Static strength is measured by performing one repetition at $0°\cdot s^{-1}$ and then resting for about 30 s. The sequence of the testing for leg extension and flexion at different speeds is usually from slowest to fastest (e.g., $30°\cdot s^{-1}$, $60°\cdot s^{-1}$, $180°\cdot s^{-1}$, $240°\cdot s^{-1}$, and $300°\cdot s^{-1}$). Athletes involved in power sports could be tested at the higher speeds. If a detailed analysis of the relationship between torque and angle is desired, then the tracing is usually recorded at a speed of $25 \; mm\cdot s^{-1}$; however, for routine testing the recording speed is usually $5 \; mm\cdot s^{-1}$. The dual tracings provide a recorded replay of the movement, one tracing showing the torque values and another showing the position (angle in degrees) of the lower leg. It is not within the scope of this manual to analyze the strength at the various positions; thus, the angle recording is deleted here.

The recording paper for the torque tracing is divided from top to bottom into 30 divisions with a bold line at every third line and two fainter lines between the bold lines. If the 180 ft·lb (244 N·m) torque scale is selected (Figure 6.3), then the top line represents 180 ft·lb (244 N·m); when 180 is divided by the 30 divisions then each intervening horizontal line is equivalent to 6 ft·lb (8.14 N·m), and the interval between each of the 10 bold lines equivalent to 18 ft·lb (24.4 N·m). In Figure 6.3, the highest "x" on the graph paper represents the peak torque of a hypothetical performer. The peak torque is read as 174 ft·lb (about 236 N·m) because the highest "x" is at the next-to-highest line. Because each line is worth 6 ft·lb and the top line is equivalent to 180 ft·lb, it is apparent that the next-to-highest line represents 174 ft·lb. Figure 6.4 is an actual tracing of the quadriceps during extension (higher curve) and hamstrings during flexion (lower curve).

Results and Discussion

Differences in performers' strengths are affected by such factors as musculotendon architecture, musculoskeletal geometry, muscle fiber types, and voluntary neuromuscular excitation.[64] One of the strongest angles for the measurement of *static* leg extension (quadriceps) is 50°[55] (0° = full extension), whereas the strongest angle for static knee flexion (hamstrings) is 30°.[78] The greatest torque for *dynamic isokinetic* actions is generated at speeds of $30°\cdot s^{-1}$ for both knee extension and flexion. By its very nature, torque is indirectly related to the speed of the movement; that is, the slower the movement, the greater the torque. The hamstring/quadriceps (H/Q), or flexion/extension (Fl/Ex) ratios are lowest at the highest torques, and the highest torques are at the lowest velocities.[56,70,80] The H/Q ratio gets bigger as the velocity increases because the decrease in hamstring torque is less than the decrease in quadriceps torque.

Absolute and Relative Isokinetic Strength

Prior to 1983, no acceptable norms existed for isokinetic testing.[13] However, in 1991 investigators reported the Cybex II™ isokinetic strengths of the knee flexors and extensors on 200 healthy men and women between the ages of 45 y and 78 y.[20] Then in 2000 other investigators reported the Kin-Com™ isokinetic torques of 62 men and women 73 y mean age.[26] The torques in the Kin-Com group were much lower than those of the 65 y to 78 y Cybex group possibly because the Kin-Com group had performers older than 78 y of age (Table 6.1). Table 6.2 provides standard scores (despite only 30 men and 30 women) and torque values for knee extension at $30°\cdot s^{-1}$.[26] Surprisingly, the "50" standard scores are lower in the young adults than the mean scores of the middle-aged adults in Table 6.1.

Comparative torque values at $180°\cdot s^{-1}$ are presented in absolute (N·m) and relative (N·m·kg^{-1} body wt) terms in

| Table 6.1 | Strength of the Knee Extensors and Flexors at an Isokinetic Speed of 60°·s⁻¹ in Middle-Aged Adults |

Age (y)	Extension		Flexion	
	Men			
	(N·m)	(SD)	(N·m)	(SD)
45–54[a]	180	35	100	21
55–64[a]	163	30	94	20
65–78[a]	144	30	78	19
72±9[b]	90	38	56	21
	Women			
	(N·m)	(SD)	(N·m)	(SD)
45–54[a]	108	22	58	14
55–64[a]	98	20	52	10
65–78[a]	89	15	49	10
74±7[b]	56	22	40	15

[a]Adapted from Frontera, W. R., Hughes, V. A., Lutz, K. J., & Evans, W. J. (1991). A cross-sectional study of muscle strength and mass in 45- to 78-yr-old men and women. *Journal of Applied Physiology, 71,* 644–650. [b]From Salem, G. J., Wang, M.-Y., Young, J. T., Marion, M., & Greendale, G. A. (2000). Knee strength and lower- and higher-intensity functional performance in older adults. *Medicine and Science in Sports and Exercise, 32,* 1679–1684.

Table 6.3. The women collegiate athletes' absolute strength was about 60 % as strong as the men's, whereas their relative strength was 80 % of the men's. The ratios for relative strength in flexion ranged from a low of 1.07 in nonathletic women[79] to a high of 1.66 in college football players.[36] The ratios for relative strength in extension ranged from a low of 1.36 in nonathletic women[79] to a high of 2.7 in sprinters and jumpers.[76]

The strength of athletes playing different sports or positions is expected to differ due to the specificity of training. This was demonstrated in differentiating between power performers and endurance performers in elite adolescent female track/field athletes.[37] Also, college football players had greater relative leg extension strength (2.13 $N \cdot m \cdot kg^{-1}$) than sedentary persons (1.9), orienteers (1.7), and racewalkers (2.0).[76] However, the footballers had smaller ratios than elite alpine skiers (2.2),[32] sprinters/jumpers (2.7), and downhill skiers (2.3).[76] The college footballers also were stronger in both absolute and relative terms than high school football players.[21] In both football studies, the linemen were stronger than the backs.

Table 6.2 | **Maximal Torque ($N \cdot m$) at $30° \cdot s^{-1}$ Knee Extension (Quadriceps) in Young Adults**

Standard Score	Men (n = 30)		Women (n = 30)	
	Dominant	Nondominant	Dominant	Nondominant
100	256	239	162	146
90	237	219	152	136
80	219	198	141	125
70	200	178	131	114
60	181	158	120	103
50	162	138	110	92
40	144	117	100	82
30	125	97	89	71
20	106	77	79	60
10	88	56	69	49
0	69	36	58	39

Adapted from Goslin, B. R., & Charteris, J. (1979). Isokinetic dynamometry: Normative data for clinical use in lower extremity (knee) cases. *Scandinavian Journal of Rehabilitation Medicine, 11,* 105–109.

Table 6.3 | **Comparative Isokinetic Values for Knee Extension (Ex;Q) and Flexion (Flex;H) at $180° \cdot s^{-1}$**

Reference/Group	Torque				Ratio		
	$N \cdot m$		$N \cdot m \cdot kg^{-1}$		H/Q	L/R	ND/D[a]
	Flex	Ex	Flex	Ex			
A. Reference #[5]							
Athletic college men			1.36	1.95	0.70		
Athletic college women			1.11	1.58	0.70		
B. Reference #[21]							
High school footballers	105	133	1.42	1.80	0.79		
C. Reference #[32]							
Elite alpine skiers				2.2			
D. Reference #[37]							
Elite adolescent female							
Track/field athletes	80	107	1.29	1.79	0.80		
E. Reference #[36]							
College footballers	157	200	1.66	2.13	0.78	0.97(Q)	
F. Reference #[76]							
Sedentary subjects				1.9			
Orienteers				1.7			
Racewalkers				2.0			
Downhill skiers				2.3			
Sprinters/jumpers				2.7			
G. Reference #[79]							
Nonathletic men	104	133	1.34	1.71	0.78	0.98(Q)	0.97(H)
Nonathletic women	62	61	1.07	1.36	0.79	0.99(Q)	0.99(H)

Adapted from reference numbers 5, 21, 32, 36, 37, 76, and 79.
Note: [a]ND/D = nondominant: dominant ratio; Q = quadriceps; H = hamstrings.

Bilateral (Contralateral) Leg Strength

The strongest leg defined the dominant leg for the data in Table 6.2. The nondominant legs of the young adults were 87 % N·m max of the dominant legs (extension). The investigators suggested a pathological imbalance criterion of one to two standard deviations below the mean, which would be between 57 % and 72 % of the dominant leg's mean maximal torque.[26] These investigators suggested a criterion percentage of 60 % (0.60 ND:D) and others[79] reported 80 % but suggested 95 % before being released from treatment. The 0.60 criterion is based on a velocity of $30°·s^{-1}$, and the 0.95 criterion is based on higher velocities. Each football players' left and right (L/R) legs differed in strength by an average of 3 %, well within either the 5 % or 10 % criterion of acceptability.[33,60] However some authorities advise athletes to seek a zero percent difference between their right and left leg strength.[35]

Ipsilateral (Reciprocal) Leg Strength

The ipsilateral (hams vs. quads; H/Q) ratios of the university football players were 0.77 and 0.89 at $180°·s^{-1}$ and $300°·s^{-1}$, respectively.[36] These values are similar to those reported for collegiate distance runners[56] and high school football players[21] but higher than the 0.64 ratio of male ballet dancers.

The H/Q ratios above were derived from *concentric* isokinetic muscle action. It may be that an H/Q ratio based on isokinetic *eccentric* strength of the hamstrings and concentric strength of the quadriceps is a more valid ratio for estimating muscular stability of the knee joint.[1] However, isokinetic machines, with an eccentric mode (e.g., KinCom, Biodex) would be needed.

Fiber Type

Table 6.4 summarizes various studies[9,12,25,44,76] on fiber type distribution in men and women who are sedentary or participants in various sports. The large variations in percentages within each group testify to the influence of other factors besides fiber type in predicting success for each sport. The prediction of fiber type is enhanced by adding other influencing factors, such as fat-free thigh mass, to the equation.[71]

The fiber type test serves also as a fatigue index for muscular endurance (power endurance and mixed endurance). Some fatigue indexes use the number of repetitions until peak torque is 50 % of the initial peak torque[10,49] or the percentage derived from the last-third of work divided by the first-third of work derived from a Biodex isokinetic machine.[8]

Table 6.4 Fiber Type Distribution in Sedentary and Athletic Men and Women

Men		Women	
Activity	**%Fast Twitch**	**Activity**	**%Fast Twitch**
Sedentary	52	Sedentary	50
Marathoners	19	800 m runners	39
Distance runners	30	X-country skiers	40
X-country skiers	36	Shot-putters	50
Race walkers	40	Cyclists	50
Cyclists	40	Long/high jumpers	52
800 m runners	51	Sprinters	73
Downhill skiers	51	Weightlifters	53
Shot-putters	62	Sprinters/jumpers	63

Source: Based on data from reference numbers 9, 12, 25, 44, and 76.

References

1. Aagaard, P., Simonsen, E. B., Beyer, N., Larsson, B., Magnusson, P., & Kjaer, M. (1997). Isokinetic muscle strength and capacity for muscular knee joint stabilization in elite sailors. *International Journal of Sports Medicine, 18,* 521–525.

2. Abernethy, P. J., & Jurimae, J. (1996). Cross-sectional and longitudinal uses of isoinertial, isometric, and isokinetic dynamometry. *Medicine and Science in Sports and Exercise, 28,* 1180–1187.

3. Abler, P., Foster, C., Thompson, N. N., Crowe, M., Alt, K., Brophy, A., & Palin, W. D. (1986). Determinants of anaerobic muscular performance. *Medicine and Science in Sports and Exercise, 18,* (supplement), Abstract #3, S1.

4. Beam, W. C. (1982). *The influence of body composition, aerobic capacity and muscular strength on the incidence of injury in athletics.* Unpublished doctoral diss., Ohio State University, Columbus.

5. Beam, W. C., Bartels, R. L., Ward, R. W., Clark, N., & Zuelzer, W. A. (1985). Multiple comparisons of isokinetic leg strength in male and female collegiate athletic teams. *Medicine and Science in Sports and Exercise, 17*(2), Abstract #20, 269.

6. Bemben, M. G., Grump, K. J., & Massey, B. H. (1988). Assessment of technical accuracy of the Cybex II isokinetic dynamometer and analog recording system. *Journal of Orthopaedic and Sports Physical Therapy, 19,* 12–17.

7. Bender, J. A. (1964). Factors affecting the occurrence of knee injuries. *Journal of Association of Physical and Mental Rehabilitation, 18,* 130–134.

8. Biodex Medical, Inc. (1994). *Biodex system 2 isokinetic dynamometer applications/operations manual.* Shirley, NY: Author.

9. Burke, E., Cerny, F., Costill, D., & Fink, W. (1977). Characteristics of skeletal muscle in competitive cyclists. *Medicine and Science in Sports and Exercise, 9,* 109–112.

10. Chmelar, R. D., Shultz, B. B., Ruhling, R. O., Fitt, S. S., & Johnson, M. B. (1988). Isokinetic characteristics of the knee in female, professional and university, ballet and modern dancers. *Journal of Orthopaedic and Sports Physical Therapy, 9,* 410–418.

11. Clarkson, P. M., Johnson, J., Dextradeur, D., Leszcyznski, W., Wai, J., & Melchionda, A. (1982). The relationships among isokinetic endurance, initial strength level, and fiber type. *Research Quarterly, 53,* 15–19.

12. Costill, D., Fink, W., & Pollock, M. (1976). Muscle fiber composition and enzyme activities of elite distance runners. *Medicine and Science in Sports and Exercise, 8,* 96–100.

13. Cybex. 1983. *Isolated joint testing and exercise.* Ronkonona, NY: Author.

14. Dragonich, L. F., & Vahey, J. W. (1990). An in vitro study of anterior cruciate ligament strain induced by quadriceps and hamstring forces. *Journal of Orthopedic Research, 8,* 57–63.

15. Elliott, J. (1978). Assessing muscle strength isokinetically. *Journal of the American Medical Association, 240,* 2408–2410.

16. Escamilla, R. F., Fleisig, G. S., Zheng, N., Barrentine, S. W., Wilk, K. E., & Andrews, J. R. (1998). Biomechanics of the knee during closed kinetic chain and open kinetic chain exercises. *Medicine and Science in Sports and Exercise, 30,* 556–569.

17. Farrell, M., & Richards, J. G. (1986). Analysis of the reliability and validity of the kinetic communicator exercise device. *Medicine and Science in Sports and Exercise, 18,* 44–49.

18. Ford, W. J., Bailey, S. D., Babich, K., & Worrell, T. W. (1994). Effect of hip position on gravity effect torque. *Medicine and Science in Sports and Exercise, 26,* 230–234.

19. Fox, E. L. (1984). *Sports physiology.* Philadelphia: W. B. Saunders.

20. Frontera, W. R., Hughes, V. A., Lutz, K. J., & Evans, W. J. (1991). A cross-sectional study of muscle strength and mass in 45- to 78-yr-old men and women. *Journal of Applied Physiology, 71,* 644–650.

21. Gilliam, T. B., Sady, S. P., Freedson, P. S., & Villanacci, J. (1979). Isokinetic torque levels for high school football players. *Journal of Sports Medicine, 60,* 110–114.

22. Gleim, G. W., Nicholas, J. W., & Webb, J. N. (1978). Isokinetic evaluation following leg injuries. *The Physician and Sportsmedicine, 6*(8), 74–82.

23. Glick, J. M. (1980). Muscle strains: Prevention and treatment. *The Physician and Sportsmedicine, 8*(11), 74–82.

24. Golden, C. L., & Dudley, G. A. (1992). Strength after bouts of eccentric or concentric actions. *Medicine and Science in Sports and Exercise, 24,* 926–933.

25. Gollnick, P. D., Armstrong, R. B., Saubert, C. W., et al. (1972). Enzyme activity and fiber composition in skeletal muscle of untrained and trained men. *Journal of Applied Physiology, 33,* 312.

26. Goslin, B. R., & Charteris, J. (1979). Isokinetic dynamometry: Normative data for clinical use in lower extremity (knee) cases. *Scandinavian Journal of Rehabilitation Medicine, 11,* 105–109.

27. Grabiner, M. D., & Hawthorne, D. L. (1990). Conditions of isokinetic knee flexion that enhance isokinetic knee extension. *Medicine and Science in Sports and Exercise, 2,* 235–240.

28. Grace, T. G., Sweetser, E. R., Nelson, M. A., et al. (1984). Isokinetic imbalance and knee-joint injuries. *Journal of Bone and Joint Surgery, 66-A,* 734–740.

29. Grimby, G., & Saltin, B. (1983). The ageing muscle. *Clinical Physiology, 3,* 209–218.

30. Hamill, J., & Knutzen, K. M. (1995). *Biomechanical basis of human movement.* Baltimore: Williams & Wilkins.

31. Hay, J. G. (1978). *The biomechanics of sports technique.* Englewood Cliffs, NJ: Prentice-Hall.

32. Haymes, E. M., & Dickinson, A. L. (1980). Characteristics of elite male and female skiracers. *Medicine and Science in Sports and Exercise, 12,* 153–158.

33. Hinson, M. M. (1977). *Kinesiology.* Dubuque, IA: Wm. C. Brown.

34. Hislop, H. J., & Perrine, J. J. (1967). The isokinetic concept of exercise. *Physical Therapy, 47,* 114–117.

35. Hough, D. O., & Ray, R. (1994). Stress fractures. *Sports Science Exchange, 7*(1), Gatorade Sports Science Institute.

36. Housh, T. J., Johnson, G. O., Marty, L., Eischen, G., Eischen, C., & Housh, D. J. (1988). Isokinetic leg flexion and extension strength of university football players. *Journal of Orthopaedic and Sports Physical Therapy, 9,* 365–369.

37. Housh, T. J., Thorland, W. G., Tharp, G. D., Johnson, G. O., & Cisar, C. J. (1984). Isokinetic leg flexion and extension strength of elite adolescent female track and field athletes. *Research Quarterly for Exercise and Sport, 55,* 347–350.

38. Jensen, R. C., Warren, B., Laursen, C., & Morrissey, M. C. (1991). Static pre-load effect on knee extensor isokinetic concentric and eccentric performance. *Medicine and Science in Sports and Exercise, 23,* 10–14.

39. Kannus, P. (1994). Isokinetic evaluation of muscular performance: Implications for muscle testing and rehabilitation. *International Journal of Sports Medicine, 15* (Suppl 1), S11–S18.

40. Klein, K. K. (1974). Muscular strength and the knee. *The Physician and Sportsmedicine, 2*(12), 29–31.

41. Knapik, J. J., Bauman, C., Jones, B. H., & Vaughan, L. (1989). Preseason screening of female collegiate athletes: Strength measures associated with athletic injuries. *Medicine and Science in Sports and Exercise, 21*(Suppl. 2), Abstract #388, 565.

42. Knapik, J. J., Wright, J. E., Mawdsley, R. H., & Braun, J. M. (1983). Isokinetic, isometric and isotonic strength relationships. *Archives of Physical Medicine and Rehabilitation, 64,* 77–80.

43. Knight, L. K., & Cage, J. B. (1980). Strength imbalance and injury. *The Physician and Sportsmedicine, 8*(3), 140.

44. Komi, P. V., & Karlsson, J. (1977). Physical performance, skeletal muscle enzyme activities, and fiber types in monozygous and dizygous twins of both sexes. *Acta Physiologica Scandinavica, 105,* Suppl. 462.

45. Koutedakis, Y., Frischknecht, R., Vrbova, G., Sharp, N. C. C., & Budgett, R. (1995). Maximal voluntary quadricep strength patterns in Olympic overtrained athletes. *Medicine and Science in Sports and Exercise, 27,* 566–572.

46. Kramer, J. F., Vaz, M. D., & Hakansson, D. (1991). Effect of activation force on knee extensor torques. *Medicine and Science in Sports and Exercise, 23,* 231–237.

47. Lansky, R. C. (1999). Open- versus closed-kinetic chain exercise: Point/counterpoint. *Strength and Conditioning Journal, 21,* 39.

48. Lesmes, G. R., Costill, D. L., Coyle, E. F., & Fink, W. J. (1978). Muscle strength and power changes during maximal isokinetic training. *Medicine and Science in Sports, 10,* 266–269.

49. Lumex Inc. (1975). *Cybex II testing protocol.* Bay Shore, NY: Cybex Division of Lumex, Inc.

50. Marcinik, E. J., Potts, J., Schlabach, G., Will, S., Dawson, P., & Hurley, B. F. (1991). Effects of strength training on lactate threshold and endurance performance. *Medicine and Science in Sports and Exercise, 23,* 739–743.

51. McNair, P. J., Marshall, R. N., & Matheson, J. A. (1991). Quadriceps strength deficit associated with rectus femoris rupture: A case report. *Clinical Biomechanics, 6,* 190–192.

52. Messier, S. P., Edwards, D. G., Martin, D. F., Lowery, R. B., Canon, D. W., James, M. K., Curl, W. W., Read, H. M., & Hunter, D. M. (1995). Etiology of iliotibial band syndrome in distance runners. *Medicine and Science in Sports and Exercise, 27,* 951–960.

53. Moffroid, M., Whipple, R., Hofkosh, J., Lowman, E., & Thistle, H. (1969). A study of isokinetic exercise. *Physical Therapy, 49,* 735–746.

54. Molczyk, L., Thigpen, L. K., Eickhoff, J., Goldgar, D., & Gallagher, J. C. (1991). Reliability of testing the knee extensors and flexors in healthy adult women using a Cybex II isokinetic dynamometer. *Journal of Orthopaedic and Sports Physical Therapy, 14,* 37–41.

55. Morris, A. F. (1974). Myotatic reflex on bilateral reciprocal leg strength. *American Corrective Therapy Journal, 28*(1) 24–29.

56. Morris, A. F., Lussier, L., Bell, G., & Dooley, J. (1983). Hamstring/quadriceps strength ratios in collegiate middle-distance and distance runners. *The Physician and Sportsmedicine, 11*(10), 71, 72, 75–77.

57. Mostardi, R. A., Porterfield, J. A., Greenberg, B., Goldberg, D., & Lea, M. (1983). Musculoskeletal and cardiopulmonary characteristics of the professional ballet dancer. *The Physician and Sportsmedicine, 11,* 53–61.

58. Murray, D. A., & Harrison, E. (1986). Constant velocity dynamometer: An appraisal using mechanical loading. *Medicine and Science in Sports and Exercise, 18,* 612–624.

59. Murray, M. P., Gardner, G. M., Mollinger, L. A., & Sepic, S. B. (1980). Strength of isometric and isokinetic contractions: Knee muscles of men aged 20 to 86. *Physical Therapy, 60,* 412–419.

60. Nicholas, J. A., Strizak, A. M., & Veras, G. (1976). A study of thigh muscle weakness in different pathological states of the lower extremity. *The American Journal of Sports Medicine, 4,* 241–248.

61. Patterson, L. A., & Spivey, W. E. (1992). Validity and reliability of the LIDO active isokinetic system. *Journal of Orthopaedic and Sports Physical Therapy, 15,* 32–36.

62. Pavol, M. J., & Grabiner, M. D. (2000). Knee strength variability between individuals across ranges of motion and hip angles. *Medicine and Science in Sports and Exercise, 32,* 985–992.

63. Perrin, D. H. (1986). Reliability of isokinetic measures. *Athletic Training, 21,* 319–321.

64. Perrin, D. H. (1993). *Isokinetic exercise and assessment.* Champaign, IL: Human Kinetics.

65. Petersen, S. R., Bagnall, K. M., Wenger, H. A., Reid, D. C., Castor, W. R., & Quinney, H. A. (1989). The influence of velocity-specific resistance training on the in vivo torque-velocity relationship and the cross-sectional area of quadriceps femoris. *The Journal of Orthopaedic and Sports Physical Therapy, 10,* 456–462.

66. Pincivero, D. M., Lephart, S. M., & Karunakara, R. A. (1997). Reliability and precision of isokinetic strength and muscular endurance for the quadriceps and hamstrings. *International Journal of Sports Medicine, 18,* 113–117.

67. Renström, P., Arms, S. W., Stanwyck, T. S., Johnson, R. J., & Pope, M. H. (1986). Strain within the anterior cruciate ligament during hamstring and quadriceps activity. *American Journal of Sports Medicine, 14,* 83–87.

68. Sale, D. G. (1991). Testing strength and power. In J. D. MacDougal, H. A. Wenger, & H. J. Green (Eds.), *Physiological testing of the high-performance athlete* (pp. 21–106). Champaign, IL: Human Kinetics.

69. Salem, G. J., Wang, M.-Y., Young, J. T., Marion, M., & Greendale, G. A. (2000). Knee strength and lower- and higher-intensity functional performance in older adults. *Medicine and Science in Sports and Exercise, 32,* 1679–1684.

70. Stafford, M. G., & Grana, W. A. (1984). Hamstring/quadriceps ratios in college football players. A high velocity relationship. *American Journal of Sports Medicine, 12,* 290–311.

71. Suter, E., Herzog, W., Sokolosky, J., Wiley, J. P., Macintosh, B. R. (1993). Muscle fiber type distribution as estimated by Cybex testing and by muscle biopsy. *Medicine and Science in Sports and Exercise, 25,* 363–370.

72. Sweetser, E. R., Grace, T. G., Nelson, M. A., Ydens, L. R., & Skipper, B. J. (1983). Pre-season isokinetic muscle testing in high school athletes and relationship to knee injuries. *Medicine and Science in Sports and Exercise, 15,* Abstract, 154.

73. Thistle, H. G., Hislop, H. J., Moffroid, M. T., & Lowman, E. (1967). Isokinetic contration: A new concept of resistive exercise. *Archives of Physical Medicine and Rehabilitation, 48,* 279–282.

74. Thorstensson, A. (1976). Muscle strength, fibre type and enzyme activities in man. *Acta Physiologica Scandinavica, 98*(Suppl. 443), 1–45.

75. Thorstensson, A., & Karlsson, J. (1976). Fatigability and fiber composition of human skeletal muscle. *Acta Physiologica Scandinavica, 98,* 318–322.

76. Thorstensson, A., Larsson, L., Tesch, P., & Karlsson, J. (1977). Muscle strength and fiber composition in athletes and sedentary men. *Medicine and Science in Sports and Exercise, 9,* 26–30.

77. Tornvall, G. (1963). Assessment of physical capabilities. *Acta Physiologica Scandinavica, 53* (Suppl. 210), 1–102.

78. Williams, M., & Stutzman, L. (1959). Strength variation through the range of motion. *The Journal of Orthopaedic and Sports Physical Therapy, 10,* 456–462.

79. Wyatt, M. P., & Edwards, A. M. (1981). Comparison of quadriceps and hamstring torque values during isokinetic exercise. *Journal of Orthopaedic and Sports Physical Therapy, 3,* 48–56.

Form 6.1

Individual Data for Isokinetic Leg Strength

Name [　　　　　　　　] Date [　　　　] Time [　] a.m. [　] p.m. [　]

Age [　] y Gender (M or W) [　] Ht [　　] cm Wt [　　] kg Technician Initials [　]

Air Temperature [　] °C Barometric Pressure [　] mm Hg Relative Humidity [　] %

Dominant Leg (check): Right (R) [　] Left (L) [　] (Dominant = preferred kicking leg) Calibration date [　　　]

Isokinetic velocity: ($°·s^{-1}$)   30 or 60 (circle one)   180   300

Peak Torque:	N·m		N·m·kg^{-1}		N·m		N·m·kg^{-1}		N·m		N·m·kg^{-1}	
(circle dominant)	L	R	L	R	L	R	L	R	L	R	L	R
Knee Flexion (H)												

	L	R	L	R	L	R	L	R	L	R	L	R
Knee Extension (Q)												

Ratios: 30 or 60 (circle)   180   300

Ipsilateral (Dominant) (Flex:Ex; H/Q) [　] [　] [　]

Ipsilateral (Nondominant) [　] [　] [　]

Bilateral (L:R; H) [　] [　] [　]

(L:R; Q) [　] [　] [　]

(N:D; H) [　] [　] [　]

(N:D; Q) [　] [　] [　]

Fiber Type: <u>Repetition</u>   <u>Average</u>

Peak Torque
(N·m)   1st [____]   2nd [____]   3rd [____]   [____]

Peak Torque 48th [____]   49th [____]   50th [____]   [____]
(N·m)

% Decline = $\left[\dfrac{\text{_____ N·m Ave. of 1 to 3} - \text{_____ N·m Ave. 48 to 50}}{\text{_____ N·m Ave. of 1 to 3}}\right] \times 100$

         = _____ % Decline

(% τ ↓ _____ − 5.2) ÷ 0.90 = _____ %; % ST = 100 − % FT _____ = _____ %

Form 6.2

Group Data for Isokinetic Leg Strength

Isokinetic Speed ($^\circ\cdot s^{-1}$)

MEN Initials (or ID #)	30 or 60 (circle one)				180				300			
	N·m	N·m/kg	H/Q	L/R	N·m	N·m/kg	H/Q	L/R	N·m	N·m/kg	H/Q	L/R
1.												
2.												
3.												
4.												
5.												
6.												
7.												
8.												
9.												
10.												
11.												
Mean												

WOMEN Initials (or ID #)	N·m	N·m/kg	H/Q	L/R	N·m	N·m/kg	H/Q	L/R	N·m	N·m/kg	H/Q	L/R
1.												
2.												
3.												
4.												
5.												
6.												
7.												
8.												
9.												
10.												
11.												
Mean												

ANAEROBIC EXERCISE

The emphasis in Part III is on anaerobic exercise and the tests measuring anaerobic fitness. Traditionally, we have equated anaerobic exercise with muscular endurance. However, I suggested in Chapter 1 that the endurance of the muscles certainly contributes to aerobic activity. Nevertheless, in keeping with tradition, I am placing two of my chosen categories of fitness within the muscular endurance framework—power endurance (15 s to 60 s) and mixed endurance (60 s to 120 s). Quantitatively, one might simply define anaerobic exercise as that which derives more than 50 % of its adenosine triphosphate (ATP) from anaerobic metabolism. Using 50 % as an operational criterion, Chapter 7 shows that strength, power, and power endurance receive more than 50 % of their ATP from anaerobic metabolism. However, it also reveals that all-out exercise within the time zone of the mixed endurance component of fitness receives equally significant ATP contributions from both the anaerobic pathway and the aerobic pathway.

For decades now, researchers have been investigating the percentage contributions of the anaerobic and aerobic pathways to adenosine triphosphate production during various exercise intensities and durations. The anaerobic contribution has been estimated from methods using oxygen deficit, muscle biopsy, and recently radioactive isotope of phosphorus combined with magnetic resonance spectroscopy. Investigators using the muscle biopsy method extract muscle samples with a needle from performers before and after exercise. Then they analyze the samples for their concentrations of such metabolites as lactate, ATP, and creatine phosphate (CrP; CP; PC). One reviewer cautions that the "metabolic response of the biopsied muscle may not be representative of all [muscles involved in the cycle] exercise."[1, a] But he also reports that the oxygen deficit method of determining the anaerobic contribution during whole body exercise may be an underestimation. Thus, the anaerobic contribution may be underestimated in former investigations using the oxygen deficit method. My model (Figure 7.1) is a compromised view of the relative contributions of anaerobic and aerobic pathways to ATP production, whereby it mixes the older oxygen deficit results with the relatively newer biopsy results. For example, in the biopsy studies the glycolytic pathway's ATP contribution is more than the model in Figure 7.1 reveals. The reviewer[1] reported the results of three investigations in which biopsied quadriceps femoris muscle was used to estimate the phosphagenic and glycolytic contributions to the total anaerobic ATP production. During maximal cycling of 6 s, the phosphagenic and glycolytic pathways contributed about equally to the total anaerobic production of ATP.[2,3] For the 30 s cycling bout, the glycolytic pathway contributed more than the phosphagenic pathway.[2,5]

The point of these examples is that we still are not certain what anaerobic pathway dominates in performers of a variety of anaerobic tests. We do know that the dominant pathway depends upon (1) the resistance applied (e.g., power on the cycle ergometer or speed and slope of the treadmill); (2) the duration of the test (e.g., 10 s vs. 30 s vs. 60 s vs. 120 s); and (3) the pacing strategy[20] (e.g., all-out start vs. evenly paced to the finish).

---

[a]All numbered references are found in the References of Chapter 7.

"HORIZONTAL POWER"—SPRINTING

Contrary to aerobic exercise, anaerobic tasks do not rely predominantly upon the transport and extraction of oxygen by the cardiovascular and respiratory systems. Anaerobic fitness and its corresponding anaerobic activities are primarily dependent upon the energy sources already existing within the muscle fibers. Although a popular term for anaerobic fitness is *muscle endurance,* its use is discouraged because muscle endurance may be applied justifiably to the aerobic fitness component.

Although the choice of the dominant pathway depends upon the resistance, duration, and pace,[20] anaerobic fitness may be categorized into three components: (a) power, (b) power-endurance, and (c) mixed endurance. These are based upon the time limits for maximal performance and the predominant energy source(s) for each (see the anaerobic fitness continuum in Figure 7.1).

Power fitness refers to exercise performed at a maximal pace from about 5 s to about 15 s. Power fitness is a dominant fitness component of the principal activities displayed in such popular sports as football, baseball, basketball, and soccer. Performers of such tasks often attempt to accelerate toward 100 % of maximal velocity. Primarily, power is biochemically dependent upon two factors: (1) the muscles' storage capacity (mol) of adenosine triphosphate (ATP) and creatine phosphate (CP) and (2) the muscles' rate (mol·min^{-1}) of resynthesizing and splitting ATP and CP.[4,7,18] The most rapid resynthesis of ATP occurs by energy released from the desynthesis of CP. Secondarily, power fitness is partially dependent upon glycogen energy sources from the glycolytic system.

Power-endurance is a term used to indicate the ability to achieve and sustain maximal efforts that are less intense but slightly longer than those within the power category; however, power-endurance activities are slower (if running) than the power running activities. Thus, maximal efforts ranging from a minimum of 15 to 30 s to a maximum of about 60 s[7,23] are power-endurance activities that rely predominantly upon the anaerobic pathway.[30,31,32,33] For example, some persons running at optimal paces for distances between 200 and 300 m would likely finish between 30 and 60 s, respectively. Biochemically, these power-endurance activities are primarily dependent upon the anaerobic glycolytic system, and, secondarily, upon the anaerobic phosphagenic and aerobic oxidative systems. The power-endurance category includes a 15 s to 30 s division in which the oxidative pathway plays a minor role, and a 30 s to 60 s division when the oxidative pathway plays a moderate role (Figure 7.1).

Mixed-endurances fitness indicates a person's performance for optimally paced activities that can be sustained longer than power-endurance activities. Thus, maximal efforts ranging from a minimum of about 60 s to a maximum of about 2 min are categorized as mixed-endurance fitness on the fitness continuum. "Mixed" fitness is dependent rather equally upon the anaerobic glycolytic pathway and the aerobic pathway for ATP production—with those

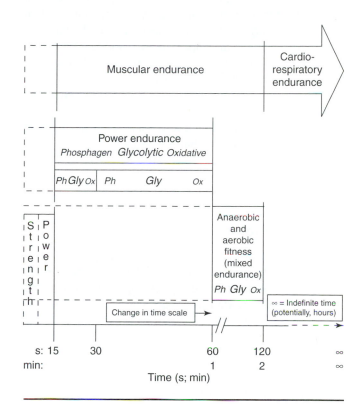

Figure 7.1. This illustration of the fitness continuum emphasizes the power, power-endurance, and mixed endurance components of fitness. Note that the components of power-endurance and mixed endurance are within the fitness component that is traditionally referred to as muscular endurance. As presented in Chapter 1—"Terminology"—the size of the lettering for the bioenergetic pathways—phosphagenic, glycolytic, and oxidative—represents the size of each one's contribution to the production of adenosine triphosphate during all-out effort during the designated time periods.

events closest to 60 s favoring the glycolytic pathway and those closest to 2 min favoring the aerobic pathway.

One of the physiological objectives of anaerobic tests is to hint at the levels of anaerobic substrates, such as ATP and PC, available for successful high-intensity performance. Although noninvasive muscle biopsy measures of substrate concentrations are now possible through nuclear magnetic resonance (NMR) spectroscopy,[8] NMR is much more expensive than other anaerobic field, field/lab, or laboratory tests, such as the Sprint Tests, Wingate Cycle Test, Anaerobic Step Tests, and Anaerobic Treadmill Tests.

Some of the numerous popular anaerobic field tests are (a) sprints or runs of less than 800 m; (b) shuttle runs; (c) standing long jump; (d) sit-ups; and (e) upper body tests, such as pull-ups, pushups, and dips. Ideally, I would have liked to use metric distances, such as 40 m, 50 m, and 60 m, instead of the American equivalents in yards. However, the only comparative scores found were the world records for the 50 m and 60 m sprints and three research reports of either 40 m or 60 m times.[11,22,35] The 40 yd, 50 yd, and 60 yd sprints are popular tests among U.S. college recruiters and professional scouts, who often administer them in order to evaluate or screen baseball and football players. The 60 yd sprint is used by baseball scouts because it is the approximate distance a base runner covers when trying to score from second base on a batter's single. The 40 yd sprint is used by football coaches because it represents the typical punt-coverage distance. Because these two sports are so "American," it is unlikely that in the near future these American units of 40 yd and 60 yd will be changed to their respective metric units rounded off to 37 m and 55 m. We need more metric norms than the mere five published reports presented here in American unit of yards.

Anatomical Rationale

Two investigators suggested that faster sprinters have greater forward propulsion because they have more forceful and powerful hamstrings.[26] Along with the forceful action of the hip extensors and knee flexors during the ground phase, the ankle plantar flexors contribute also to sprint performance.[26] These investigators believe that the principle role of the arms is for balance, not cadence.

Biomechanical Rationale

Technically speaking, anaerobic power is not measured in these sprints. This is because of the lack of a true vertical distance component; only the horizontal distance[a] is known, but it cannot be used to calculate work (or power) as defined by a physicist (w = F × D). However, an esti-

mate of relative "horizontal power"[b] may be made by multiplying the sprint velocity (v) by the body weight (F) of the performer (Eq. 7.1).

$$\text{"Horizontal P"} = \text{"F"} \times \bar{v} \qquad \text{Eq. 7.1}$$

where:

P = power in $kg \cdot m \cdot s^{-1}$ or $N \cdot m \cdot s^{-1}$ (1yd = 0.914 m)

"F" = body weight in kg or N (1 kg ≈ 2.2 lb ≈ 9.8 N)

$\bar{v}$ = average velocity (speed) = D ÷ t = D / t = $m \cdot s^{-1}$

Tests for running speed are not exact estimates of anaerobic power because speed and power are not identical. The contribution of mass (weight) to power may be visualized by comparing the effect of dropping a ping-pong ball versus a golf ball onto a pane of glass. Obviously, the golf ball will have a more powerful effect.

Also, the contribution of velocity may be visualized by comparing the power of two thrown baseballs—one going 50 mph and the other going 100 mph; although they both have the same mass, the faster one is more powerful. The concept of horizontal power is applicable to the collisions often encountered between competitors in such sports as football and ice hockey.

Sprint speed is not only dependent upon muscle power but also upon the elastic component (stiffness) of these muscles. Muscle power is important during the acceleration phase of the sprint and for maintaining maximal velocity, but high leg stiffness enhances rebound and also contributes to maximal velocity.[10,11,34]

Physiological Rationale

The duration of these sprints ranges from a minimum of about 4.3 s in the 40 yd sprint for a world-class runner to about 11 s in the 60 yd sprint for a slow college student. Thus, they are considered anaerobic power tests because they are performed usually in less than 15 s.

Biochemically, the tests are highly dependent upon the capacity and rate of splitting the phosphagens—adenosine triphosphate and creatine phosphate. One group of investigators reported the remaining percentage of creatine phosphate after 40 m and 60 m sprints as 37 % and 38 %, respectively of the pre-sprint concentrations.[22] A submaximal force, but high velocity, activity such as sprinting is probably more dependent upon the *rate* of myosin-actin interactions than upon the *number* of myosin-actin interactions.[19]

Types IIa and IIb muscle fibers predominate in anaerobic activities. Although they fatigue much sooner than the aerobic Type I fibers, they generate the rapid forces that are necessary for anaerobic power activities.

---

[a]Distance and displacement are equal when assuming the runners go in a straight line from start to finish.

[b]Quotation marks emphasize the nontechnical term.

Method

All three of the sprint tests may be administered simultaneously (see Figure 7.2). The facility can be any level terrain—marked-off football field, track, baseball diamond, gymnasium—that has an accurately measured sprint distance. For example, if you are using a baseball diamond, simply add 10, 20, and 30 yd to the distance between the bases in order to create 40, 50, and 60 yd, respectively. There should be a minimum of 25 yd beyond the 60 yd marker in order to provide the sprinter with ample space to slow down; this is called the **coasting, or deceleration, zone.** Box 7.1 discusses the accuracy of sprint tests.

Administrative Procedures

The procedures for administering the sprint tests should include time for prior exercise and cooldown to prevent injuries and muscle soreness. The performers need to know the proper starting technique, while the technicians should become familiar with the timing of the event.

Prior Exercise (PE)

Prior exercise is recommended before all anaerobic tests because they are more apt to cause injury than aerobic tasks. I prefer the term *prior exercise* over the term *warm-up* because of the technical distinction between warm-up and loosening up. When people loosen up, usually by stretching, there is little, if any, change in body temperature; thus, the term *warm-up* is misleading. Table 7.1 provides a prescription (Rx) for prior exercise. The American College of Sports Medicine (ACSM) does not recommend "fast, jerky movements."[2] However, I take the unpopular stance that gradual, progressive, ballistic movements during prior exercise will better prepare the sprinter and better protect the sprinter from injury than static stretching alone.

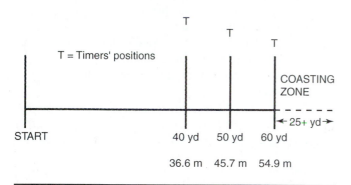

Figure 7.2 The sprint "layout" for measuring the times for the 40 yd (36.6 m), 50 yd (45.7 m), and 60 yd (54.9 m) sprints. 1 yd = 0.914 m; 1 m = 1.0936 yd

Table 7.1	Prior Exercise Prescription (PE-Rx) for the Sprint Tests	
Time (min)	**Activity**	
0:00–3:00	Warm-up—low intensity (1st phase)	
	(1) jogging in place; (2) slow, relaxed jog	
3:00–5:00	Loosen up (stretching)	
	Static stretch: hip-groin area, "gastrocs," "quads," and "hams"	
	Ballistic stretch: same muscle groups as above	
5:00–10:00	Warm-up—moderate intensity (2nd phase)	
	(1) Short hops/jumps; (2) 10 yd, 40 yd, 50 yd runs of moderate speed	
10:00–12:00	Recovery interval between PE-Rx and first trial of sprint test	
	(1) Walking or walking in place; (2) loosening up (ballistic and static)	

BOX 7.1 **Accuracy of Sprint Tests**

Validity

A high correlation (r = .86) was reported between the 40 m (≈ 44 yd) sprint and the 10 m (≈ 11 yd) sprint.[35] The validity of sprint tests is supported by moderate correlations reported between 40 yd[13,29,39] sprint times and other leg-power tests, such as the Vertical Jump (r = −.625, −.50, −.48) and the vertical velocity component of the Margaria Stair-Run Test (r = .711, .88). Moderate to high relationships (r = −.53 to −.91) occur between the 40 m (43.8 yd) sprint and peak anaerobic power of the Wingate Anaerobic Cycle Test (WAnT).[5,13,39] Investigators reported moderate correlations between 50 yd (45.7 m) dash and WAnT power for 5 s (r = −.53) and WAnT capacity for 30 s (r = −.53). The correlations increased to −.69 for both power and capacity when the WAnT scores were divided by body mass in 10-year- to 15-year-old male performers.[39] In nonathletic children, the originators of the Wingate Anaerobic Cycle Test reported correlations of −.84 and −.70 between 50 yd sprint and 5 s anaerobic power and 30 s anaerobic capacity, respectively.[5] It is clear that sprints are more highly correlated with the 5 s Wingate anaerobic power score than with its 30 s anaerobic capacity score. As with many performance tests (e.g., sprint tests) that purport to measure physiological performance, such as phosphagenic ability, the performer's coordination for such activity is a contributing factor.

Reliability

It is possible to test running speed by administering sprints even shorter than 40 yd. However, greater reliability is likely in sprints longer than 20 yd.[6] The reliability of the 40 yd sprint is reported to be as high as .970.[14] Timing errors may range up to 2 % when using a stopwatch.[14, 15]

Sprinter's Starting Technique

In order to reduce the effect of skill or past experience, participants should not use the specialized sprint-start technique of a track athlete. However, the starting position should assume a low center of gravity and a forward lean. Ideally, the performer should have shoes that will not slip upon starting. Starting blocks of any sort, such as using holes in the ground or by bracing against another person's feet, are not prescribed.

Timing of the Sprint

The three timers should use a stopwatch capable of measuring in tenths of a second. If strap-stopwatches are used, the strap should be securely wrapped around the technician's wrist or hung around the neck. After becoming familiar with the stopwatches, the timers should position themselves at the 40 yd, 50 yd, and 60 yd markers to allow an optimal view of the runner when starting and when breaking the plane of the finish line (see Figure 7.2). The timers should acknowledge a "Ready" signal of the runner. As soon as the runner makes the first movement to sprint, all timers start their watches. Thus, a "GO" signal is *not* given because the reaction time of the runner is not a consideration in this power test. As soon as the runner's trunk breaks the plane of the respective finish lines, technicians stop their watches. They record the times to the closest tenth of a second on Form 7.1. The mean time of the two or three trials is used as the sprinter's time for group statistical purposes.[14,28]

Number of Trials

Unless the performer has not been sprint-training, no more than three trials should be performed in one day. Three trials are recommended only if the difference in times between the first two trials is greater than 0.20 s. Regardless of the nonsprint-trained performer's feelings about the muscles or motivational status, strict adherence to the three-trial rule should prevail. Otherwise, delayed onset muscle soreness (DOMS) is likely. To avoid DOMS or injury and to allow restoration of the phosphagens, there should be a rest period between trials of at least 1 min to 2 min if only sprinting 40 m,[3] and 3 min to 8 min if performing 60 m sprints. Two reviewers[40] described a biphasic restoration of creatine phosphate with a fast half-time of $\approx$ 22 s and a slow half-time of $\approx$ 3 min.[21] Using a single muscle fiber, a pair of investigators reported full restoration after 5 min of rest.[38] Active recovery, such as fast walking or slow jogging, is superior to passive recovery, such as sitting or standing, during the relief interval for a supramaximal anaerobic activity, such as sprinting.[36]

Cooldown

Unaccustomed anaerobic activity is conducive to delayed onset muscle soreness, whereby DOMS occurs as early as 6 h, but usually 8 h to 24 h post-exercise.[37] In addition to adhering to the prior exercise prescription and the three-trial maximum, the following two recommendations are made in order to eliminate or minimize stiffness:

1. Immediately following the sprint trials, the sprinter should repeat the first 5 min (warm up and loosen up) of the prior exercise regimen.
2. The sprinter should repeat the static stretching exercises periodically throughout the next three days.[12]

Summary of Procedural Steps for Sprints

1. Sprint participants perform a prior exercise routine similar to the one in Table 7.1.
2. The three timers stand at locations suitable for viewing the single sprinters' start and finish (review Figure 7.2). Thus, one timer is at the 40 yd mark, another at the 50 yd mark and another at the 60 yd mark.
3. The sprinter assumes the starting position by lowering the center of gravity and leaning slightly forward.
4. The sprinter and three timers acknowledge their readiness by (1) the sprinter's yelling, "Ready," and (2) the timers' yelling, "Ready," in return.
5. The timers start their watches at the first starting movement of the sprinter.
6. The sprinter runs as fast as possible through the 40 yd, 50 yd, or 60 yd finish lines, depending upon the yardage comparisons desired by the sprinter or investigators.
7. The timers stop their watches when the sprinter breaks the plane of the respective finish lines; they record the time to the closest tenth of a second onto the Trial 1 box of the individual data form (Form 7.1).
8. The sprinter repeats the trial after a recovery period consisting of a low-intensity activity, such as walking (40 m sprint only = 1 min to 2 min recovery; 50 m = 2 min to 5 min recovery; 60 m = 3 min to 8 min recovery).
9. The sprinter performs a third trial if the difference between the first two trials is greater than 0.2 s.
10. The sprinter performs a proper cooldown by repeating a regimen similar to the first 5 min of the prior exercise prescription (Table 7.1) and by statically stretching the legs periodically during the next three days.

Calculation of Horizontal Power

By using Equation 7.1, "horizontal power" may be calculated from velocity and body mass as follows:

1. Convert the American distances of the sprints into their respective meter units by dividing the yards by 1.0936, or simply by consulting Figure 7.2 or Form 7.1.
2. Calculate the average velocity ($\bar{v}$) by dividing the time (s) into the metric distance ($\bar{v} = m \div s$).
3. Multiply the kilogram body mass by 9.8 to obtain newtons.
4. Multiply newtons (N) by velocity to obtain "horizontal power" expressed as $N \cdot m \cdot s^{-1}$.

Results and Discussion

In general, the norms for the 40 yd and 60 yd sprint tests are ill-defined for the average person. The 50 yd norms are applicable to high school boys and girls (Table 7.2).[1] The average times in the 50 yd sprint for college-aged men and women, including reaction time, have been reported as 6.8 s and 8.2 s, respectively.[24]

The 40 yd sprint times averaged 5.35 s ($SD = 0.30$)[13] and 5.46 s[14] in college football players. Additionally, various criteria have been used often by scouts or coaches of football and baseball organizations that might be helpful in interpreting sprint times. Testimonies of running speed have been presented in such popular media as newspapers, magazines, TV, and radio (examples included in Table 7.3). Cautious interpretation of sprint times for specific sports or positions is warranted, considering the fact that, although football players are often timed in the 40 yd sprint, linemen rarely run 40 yd on any given play. Despite this reservation, however, it appears that the correlation between 5 yd or 15 yd times and 40 yd times is very high.[14]

One pair of investigators reported that their 16-year-old male handball players reached 63 % maximal velocity in 1.6 s and 100 % v_{max} at 5.0 s when running a 40 m sprint[11] (Figure 7.3).

The low creatine phosphate stores remaining after 5 s of sprinting may be responsible for the inability of sprinters to increase maximal velocity after that time.[22] Sprint-training can make any runner faster. Investigators appear to agree that sprint-training does not convert Type I fibers into Type IIb fibers, although it may convert some Type IIa fibers into Type IIb fibers.[9]

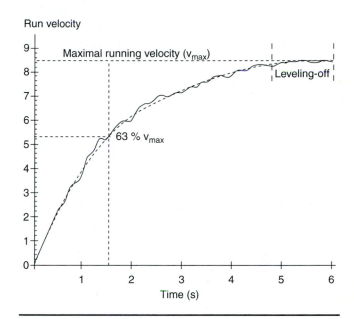

Figure 7.3 This radar-monitored velocity-time curve shows the curvilinear ascent to maximal running velocity (v_{max}) at 8.5 m·s⁻¹ (m/s). As an example, the run velocity at 1.6 s after the start was 5.3 m·s⁻¹, which corresponded to 63 % v_{max}. (Adapted from Chelly, S. M., & Denis, C. (2001). Leg power and hopping stiffness: Relationship with sprint running performance. *Medicine and Science in Sports and Exercise, 33,* 326–333. Reproduced with permission from Lippincott Williams & Wilkins, Hagerstown, MD.)

Table 7.2 AAHPERD Norms for High School Boys and Girls in the 50 yd Sprint

		50 yd Time (s)	
Category	Percentile	Boys	Girls
	95	5.9	6.8
Excellent		6.1	7.0
	75	6.3	7.4
Good		6.4	7.4
Average	50	6.6	7.9
Fair		7.0	8.3
	25	7.0	8.4
Low		7.5	8.9
	5	7.9	9.5

Source: American Alliance for Health, Physical Education, Recreation and Dance. (1976). *AAHPERD youth fitness test manual.* Washington, DC: AAHPERD Publications.

Table 7.3 Comparative Times (s) for the 40 yd, 50 yd, and 60 yd Sprints

40 yd	Time	50 yd	Time	60 yd	Time
Football[a]		Track		Baseball	
College players	5.35[13]	Men's WR[b]	5.15	Top criteria:	
Fast running back[17]	5.44[14]	Women's WR	5.74	High school	7.2
Anaerobic college men athletes	5.87[35]			College	7.0
Fast NFL lineman	4.56	50 m (55 yd)		Professional	6.8 or 6.9
		Men's WR	5.55		
Fast high schoolers		Women's WR	6.06	Track (men's WR in	6.39 (outdoor)
Guards	4.75	College men[24]	6.8	60 m or 65.6 yd)	6.45 (indoor)
Tackles	4.9	College women[24]	8.2		
Pro flanker time[16]	4.4–4.6			Fastest in NFL	6.18
Female college athletes[28]	5.96			55 m (60 yd)	
Gladiator criterion[c]	≤4.8			Men's WR	5.99

Note: [a]NFL scouts sometimes allow "rolling" starts. [b]WR = former world record. [c]Former TV show with battling contestants.

Optional Student Activities

By adding timers at the 10 yd, 20 yd, and 30 yd markers, the velocities for each 10 yd increment can be calculated, then compared. Another option is to add three more timers stationed at metric distances of 40 m, 50 m, and 60 m. Form 7.1 will accommodate such data.

References

1. AAHPERD. (1976). *AAHPERD youth fitness test manual.* Washington, DC: AAHPERD Publications.

2. American College of Sports Medicine. (2000). *ACSM's guidelines for exercise testing and prescription.* Philadelphia: Lippincott Williams & Wilkins.

3. Balsom, P. D., Seger, J. Y., Sjodin, B., & Ekblom, B. (1992). Maximal-intensity intermittent exercise: Effect of recovery duration. *International Journal of Sports Medicine, 13,* 528–533.

4. Bangsbo, J. (1998). Quantification of anaerobic energy production during intense exercise. *Medicine and Science in Sports and Exercise, 30,* 47–52.

5. Bar-Or, O., & Inbar, O. (1978). Relationships among anaerobic capacity, sprint and middle distance running of school children. In R. Shephard & H. Lavalle (Eds.), *Physical fitness assessment* (pp. 142–147). Springfield, IL: Charles C Thomas.

6. Baumgartner, T. A., & Jackson, A. S. (1987). *Measurement for evaluation in physical education and exercise science.* Dubuque, IA: Wm. C. Brown.

7. Boobis, L. H., Williams, C., & Wootton, S. A. (1982). Human muscle metabolism during brief maximal exercise. *Journal of Physiology, 338,* 21–22 P.

8. Brooks, G. A., Fahey, T. D., & White, T. P. (1996). *Exercise physiology: Human bioenergetics and its applications.* Mountain View, CA: Mayfield.

9. Cahill, B. R., Misner, J. E., & Boileau, R. A. (1997). The clinical importance of the anaerobic energy system and its assessment in human performance. *The American Journal of Sports Medicine, 25,* 863–872.

10. Cavagna, G. A., Komarek, L., & Mazzoleni, S. (1971). The mechanics of sprint running. *Journal of Physiology (London), 217,* 709–721.

11. Chelly, S. M., & Denis, C. (2001). Leg power and hopping stiffness: Relationship with sprint running performance. *Medicine & Science in Sports & Exercise, 33,* 326–333.

12. Chen, T. C., & Hsieh, S. S. (1996). The effects of stretching and cryotherapy on delayed onset muscle soreness. *Medicine and Science in Sports and Exercise, 28* (Suppl., 5), Abstract #1077, p. S181.

13. Costill, D. L., Miller, S. J., Myers, W. C., Kehoe, F. M., & Hoffman, W. M. (1968). Relationship among selected tests of explosive leg strength and power. *The Research Quarterly, 39*(3), 785–787.

14. Crews, T. R., & Meadors, W. J. (1978). Analysis of reaction time, speed, and body composition of college football players. *Journal of Sports Medicine and Physical Fitness, 18,* 169–174.

15. deVries, H. A., & Housh, T. J. (1994). *Physiology of exercise for physical education, athletics, and exercise science.* Dubuque, IA: Brown & Benchmark.

16. Dintiman, G. B. (1984). *How to run faster.* Champaign, IL: Leisure Press.

17. Fox, E. L., & Mathews, D. K. (1974). *Interval training: Conditioning for sports and general fitness.* Philadelphia: W. B. Saunders.

18. Gaitanos, G. C., Williams, C., Boobis, L. H., & Brooks, S. (1993). Human muscle metabolism during intermittent maximal exercise. *Journal of Applied Physiology, 75,* 712–719.

19. Green, H. J. (1991). What do tests measure? In J. D. MacDougall, H. A. Wenger, & H. J. Green (Eds.), *Physiological testing of the high performance athlete* (pp. 7–19). Champaign, IL: Human Kinetics.

20. Green, S. (1995). Measurement of anaerobic work capacities in humans. *Sports Medicine, 19,* 32–42.

21. Harris, R. C., Edwards, R. H. T., Hultman, E., Nordesjö, L.-O., & Sahlin, K. (1976). The time course of phosphocreatine resynthesis during recovery of the quadriceps muscle in man. *European Journal of Physiology, 367,* 137–142.

22. Hirvonen, J. S., Rehunen S., Rusko, H., & Härkönen, M. (1987). Breakdown of high-energy phosphate compounds and lactate accumulation during short supramaximal exercise. *European Journal of Applied Physiology, 56,* 253–259.

23. Jacobs, I., Bar-Or, O., Karlsson, J., Dotan, R., Tesch, P., Kaiser, P., & Inbar, O. (1982). Changes in muscle metabolites in females with 30-s exhaustive exercise. *Medicine and Science in Sports and Exercise, 14,* 457–460.

24. Johnson, P. B., Updyke, W. F., Schaefer, M., & Stolberg, D. C. (1975). *Sport, exercise, and you.* New York: Holt, Rinehart and Winston.

25. Kaczkowski, W., Montgomery, D. L., Taylor, A. W., & Klissourous, V. (1982). The relationship between muscle fiber composition and maximal anaerobic power and capacity. *Journal of Sports Medicine and Physical Fitness, 22,* 407–413.

26. Mann, R., & Sprague, P. (1980). A kinetic analysis of the ground leg during sprint running. *Research Quarterly for Exercise and Sport, 51,* 334–348.

27. Mann, R. V. (1981). A kinetic analysis of sprinting. *Medicine and Science in Sports and Exercise, 13,* 325–328.

28. Mayhew, J. L., Bemben, M. G., Rohrs, D. M., & Bemben, D. A. (1994). Specificity among anaerobic power tests in college female athletes. *Journal of Strength and Conditioning Research, 8,* 43–47.

ties of the contractile machinery; and (5) longer time available for force development. The reviewers[5] own findings favor the fifth rationale because the CMJ produces more work during the initial shortening distance.

One must not dismiss the contribution of the arms during a vertical jump. Vertical jumps are enhanced when thrusting the arms upward.[6,7,51] One group of researchers[49] reported that junior elite figure skaters with greater isokinetic strength ($300°·s^{-1}$) of the shoulder adductors were able to jump higher. They speculated that higher jumps would provide the stronger skaters with more time to perform a double axel (two twirls or spins in air). Stronger shoulder *adductors* would permit a tighter spin because weaker muscles would not restrict the high centrifugal forces (91 kg or 200 lb to 136 kg or 300 lb) that cause arms to pull away from the body, which then slows the spin.

Method

The methods of conducting the vertical jump test consider (a) equipment, (b) procedures, (c) prior exercise, (d) body positions and measurements, and (e) calculations. See Box 8.1 for a discussion on the accuracy of vertical jumps.

Equipment

An accurate platform scale may be used to measure the body masses (weights) of the jumpers in their "jumping" clothes and shoes. An anthropometer (stadiometer) may be used to measure stature, which is needed for predicting two subdivisions of power—peak and average. However, adding the jump height, measured at finger tip, to the individual's reaching height (standing) will produce the distance from the floor to the peak jumping point; this would be significant, for example, for basketball and volleyball players. A calculator with square-root capability is convenient for making the power calculations.

The vertical jump test may be conducted with or without special electronic equipment. If the nonelectronic method is used, then a flat measuring scale about 1 ft wide and 3 ft to 4 ft long, with horizontal lines at 1 in. intervals, can be attached to a wall or post (e.g., a basketball backboard). It is possible to use a simple yard/meter stick as the measuring scale, but this is not preferred due to a greater likelihood of making visual errors when observing the jump mark. If the flat scale is used, the gymnast's chalk, chalk dust, or water (not saliva) on the jumper's fingers may be used to mark the peak jump of the performer.

The flat scale is not necessary if using a commercial jump scale (e.g., Vertec™; Sports Imports, Columbus, OH; Figure 8.1). This non-electronic standing scale resembles a volleyball standard and has red, white, and blue markers (vanes) spaced 0.5 in. apart; the red markers are spaced every 6.0 in., the blue ones every 1.0 in., and the white ones every 0.5 in. except where there is a red or a blue one. The sweep of the jumper's hand causes the several vanes to

swivel near the peak height of the jump. Thus, the highest vane that is moved represents the height of the jump.

Electronic scales calculate vertical jump distance from various methods. Some make the calculation from the time spent in the air (Verti-Leaper™; Country Technology, Gays Mills, WI), some use sonar echo (Vertisonic™, Lafayette Instruments, Lafayette, IN) and some use the take-off force (Quattro Jump™, Kistler Corp., Amherst, NY).

Procedures for Vertical Jump

The emphasis in this manual is upon nonelectronic methods for measuring vertical jump. Regardless of the technical

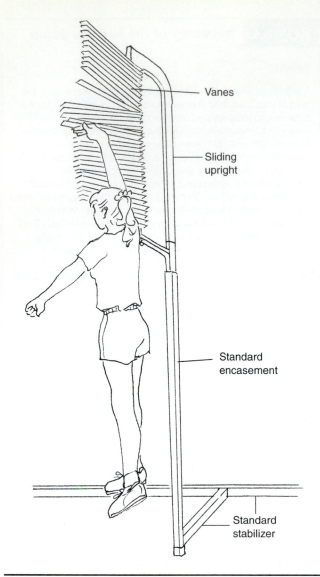

Figure 8.1 An example of a commercial jump test instrument (Vertec®) showing the jumper descending after displacing the swatted vanes.

Labels in figure: Vanes; Sliding upright; Standard encasement; Standard stabilizer

Body Positions and Measurements

The jump distance is calculated from the two vertical measurements for the vertical jump test—the standing reach and the jump reach. These may be made in inches (in.) or centimeters (cm) to the closest 0.5 in. or 1 cm.[30]

Standing Reach

The standing reach (Figure 8.2a) is measured as the jumper stands with the feet together and the dominant arm near (≈ 4 in.) the wall or standard of the commercial apparatus (Vertec™). The jumper then reaches as high as possible with the dominant arm so that the palm of the hand is against the measurement scale[32] or the wall. The highest point of the reach (usually tip of the middle finger) is observed and then recorded onto Form 8.1. If using the Vertec, adjust the standard so that the tip of the tallest finger during the reach is at the bottom surface of the lowest vane on the Vertec. If the jumper is not likely to jump more than 24 in. (61 cm), then the Vertec standard can be adjusted so that the lowest vane is at the jumper's standing reach height. In this case, the standing height can be considered the zero point and can be recorded as such on Form 8.1. The Vertec sliding upright may remain in place but with the lower vanes pivoted out of the way before making the jump. If the jumper is likely to jump more than 24 in., then the sliding upright must be raised accordingly after the standing-reach zero. The inch scale on the upright will be added to the inches indicated by the highest dislocated vane.

Jumping Reach

After the standing reach is measured, the jumper moves the feet to a jumping position. The feet cannot change from this position prior to jumping, nor are any preparatory movements permitted other than one quick dip (countermovement) of the knees and one swing of the arms.

The performer makes the jump while touching or swatting the measurement scale or vanes at the peak of the jump (Figure 8.2b). The chalk or water mark on the wall scale is observed by a technician, who stands on a higher platform (e.g., a chair or a table) near eye level to the jump mark.

Three jump trials are usually given and the best trial used for group statistics. If using the Vertec, then all the vanes below the highest vane displaced can be pivoted out of the way for the subsequent trials. If a jumper continues to improve on the third trial, then subsequent trials can be given. However, comparisons are less valid because the norms were developed from only three trials. Due to the rapid recovery of the relatively small volume of phosphagens used for performing one vertical jump, the several seconds taken to observe and record the height of the jump are adequate for recovery between trials.

sophistication, a prior exercise routine is recommended. The procedures should also include standardized body positions before and during the jump.

Prior Exercise

Prior exercise need not be quite so extensive as that typically recommended for sprint running. However, a "warm-up" appears to enhance jumping performance.[18] About 5 min to 10 min of loosening up and warming up, with the latter including a few vertical jumps at one-half to three-quarter effort, should be sufficient. The loosening up exercises should include shoulder stretches because the arm reach requires a full range of motion.

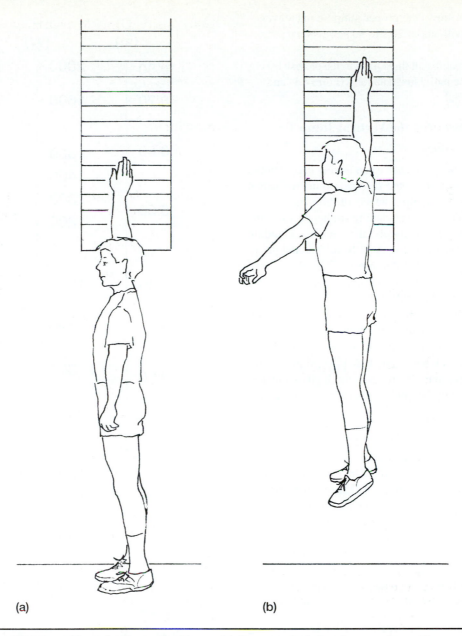

(a)   (b)

Figure 8.2 The significant positions for the vertical jump: (a) the recorded standing-reach position and (b) the recorded jump position.

Summary of Procedural Steps for Vertical Jumps

1. The performer executes a 5 min to 10 min prior exercise regimen.
2. The technician explains and demonstrates the proper position for the standing reach:
   a. Stand with feet together and dominant side near the wall or apparatus.
   b. Reach as high as possible with the dominant arm but keep feet flat on the floor.
   c. Place the palm of the hand against the flat measurement scale on the wall or place the tip of the highest finger against the bottom of the Vertec vane nearest to the finger tip.

3. The performer follows the proper body positioning and the technician records the reach height onto Form 8.1.
4. The technician explains and demonstrates the vertical jump and reach.
   a. Move the feet to a comfortable jumping take-off position; the feet cannot move from this original position.
   b. Make one countermovement (dip) of the legs and hips plus one swing of the arms immediately prior to the push-off phase of the jump.
   c. While in the air, reach as high as possible and swat the wall's scale or the vanes of the commercial apparatus.
   d. Land with knees bent in order to enhance the absorption of forces.

5. The performer follows the proper jumping maneuver for three trials with about 20 s to 30 s of recovery between trials.
6. The technician records all three trials to the closest 1.0 cm or 0.5 in. onto the individual data form (Form 8.1) and circles the best trial.

Calculation of Power for the Vertical Jump Test

Jump Distance (Difference)

The first step in calculating power when having used devices such as the wall scale and Vertec is to determine the actual distance of the jump. The jump distance, or difference (D), is calculated by subtracting the standing reach height from the jumping reach height. For example, if a person's standing reach touches the measurement scale at 10 in., and the jumping height is 32 in., then the difference is 22 in. When converted to centimeters by dividing by 0.3937, or multiplying by 2.54, the metric jump height becomes 56 cm to the closest whole centimeter, or 0.56 m. If using the commercial apparatus, technicians should calculate the number of inches (to closest 0.5 in.) to the highest vane that was moved. If the Vertec sliding upright's lowest vane was adjusted to zero for anticipated jumps less than 24 in., then the highest touched vane represents the jump height. In this case, no subtraction is necessary.

Mean Power

Mean power, not instantaneous (peak) power, can be estimated by knowing the work accomplished over a measured time period. The anaerobic power of this test may be derived without any calculations by using the modified Lewis nomogram (Figure 8.3). Equation 8.2 calculates the same power (P) value as the nomogram by considering the duration of the ascending phase of the flight, not the total thrust (push-off) duration. In actuality, the flight time is not measured but is derived from a constant based upon the rate of falling bodies.

$$P\ (\text{kgm·s}^{-1}) = 2.21 \times BM \times \sqrt{VJ\ D} \qquad \text{Eq. 8.2}$$

where:

$\quad$ 2.21 = a constant; $\sqrt{4.9}$

$\quad$ BM = body mass (kg) in jump clothes

$\quad$ VJ D = difference (distance) between standing reach (m) and vertical jump (VJ) height (m)

For example, if the difference in reach height and jump height was 20 in. (51 cm or 0.51 m) in a person with a body mass of 67 kg, then the following calculation would provide the anaerobic power in kilogram meters per second (kg·m·s⁻¹):

$$P\ (\text{kg·m·s}^{-1}) = 2.21 \times 67\,\text{kg} \times \sqrt{0.51\,\text{m}}$$
$$= 148 \times 0.714$$
$$= 106$$

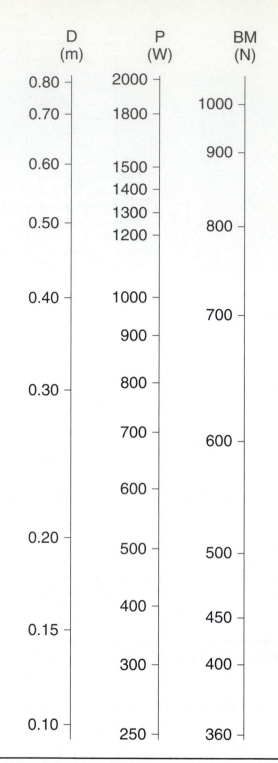

Figure 8.3 The Lewis nomogram for approximating the power (P; W) from the jump height difference (D; m) and body mass (BM; N). Adapted from Mathews, D. K., & Fox, E. L. (1976). *The physiological basis of physical education and athletics.* Philadelphia: W. B. Saunders.

Because the International System of measuring units requires power units to be expressed in newton meters per second (N·m·s⁻¹) or watts (W), the rounded-conversions[b] become

$$10 \times 106 \text{ kg·m·s}^{-1} = 1060 \text{ N·m·s}^{-1} \text{ and } 1060 \text{ W}$$

The term *absolute power* is appropriate when the power unit is expressed only as watts (W). The term *relative power* (*relative P*) is appropriate when absolute watts is divided by body mass (W·kg⁻¹), as in Equation 8.3. The positive relationship is linear ($r = .99$) between peak power output expressed as watts per kilogram body mass and the vertical distance of the center of gravity during the jump from a force platform.[16] The following calculation produces the relative power for the person with a body mass of 67 kg and an absolute power of 1060 W, as in our prior example:

$$\text{Relative P (W·kg}^{-1}) = W \div kg \text{ BM} \qquad \text{Eq. 8.3}$$

where:

W = absolute power in watts

BM = body mass

Example:

Relative P = 1060 W ÷ 67 kg

= 15.8 W·kg⁻¹

Nomogram Mean Power

An approximate estimate of anaerobic power may be made from the modified Lewis nomogram in Figure 8.3.[40] This is done by placing a straightedge on the jump-distance (D) line (the difference between the reach height and the jump height in meters) and then pivoting the straightedge to the body mass (BM; N). Where the straightedge crosses the power line is the anaerobic power (N·m·s⁻¹ or W). This is an approximate estimate because of "eye-ball" error.

Time-in-Air Calculation of Jump Distance

If using a timing device to measure the jumper's time in air, then Equations 8.4 and 8.5 derive the height of the jump.[7] The first step is to calculate the vertical velocity (V_v) of the center of gravity (g); the second step is to calculate the height (h) of the rise in center of gravity.

$$V_v \text{ (m·s}^{-1}) = 0.5 \times t_{air} \times g \qquad \text{Eq. 8.4}$$

where:

g = acceleration of gravity (9.81 m·s⁻¹) Eq. 8.5

The sensing-mat timer of some devices (e.g., Verti-Leaper™) automatically converts the time in the air to the jump height.

[b]The other multiplication factors to convert kg·m·s⁻¹ to N·m·s⁻¹—the approximate 9.8 or the exact 9.80665—can replace the approximate conversion 10.

Results and Discussion

Two different aspects of power during the vertical jump can be predicted for college men and women athletes by using Equations 8.6 and 8.7,[34] which were derived from an electronic force platform. One aspect—peak power (P_{pk})—reflects the highest power output during a single moment of the push-off phase of the jump. The other aspect—average power (P_{ave})—represents the average power output over the entire duration of the push-off phase.

$$P_{pk} \text{ (W)} = [78.5 \times VJ \text{ (cm)}] + [60.6 \times BM \text{ (kg)}]$$
$$- [15.3 \times ht \text{ (cm)}] - 1308 \qquad \text{Eq. 8.6}$$

$$P_{ave} \text{ (W)} = [41.4 \times VJ \text{ (cm)}] + [31.2 \times BM \text{ (kg)}]$$
$$- [13.9 \times ht \text{ (cm)}] + 431 \qquad \text{Eq. 8.7}$$

where:

VJ = vertical jump; jump-reach minus standing-reach

BM = body mass (wt)

ht = height; body stature

The peak power will be almost double that of the average power. The average power from the force platform equation (Eq. 8.6) is almost twice the power derived from the Lewis nomogram. Vertical jump tests are often administered to track and field athletes and to basketball and volleyball players. Some of the high scores reported in the popular media (TV, radio, newspapers, and magazines) were not produced under the same procedures as the vertical jump described in this manual. For example, some measures were made while the jumper took two or more preparatory steps. In various scientific studies, some low vertical jump scores are the result of using a *more* restrictive method than the one presented here. For example, the jumper's reaching arm may have been restricted to remain in the elevated position during the preparatory and jump phases[23] or countermovements were disallowed.[25] Countermovements and arm swings combine to improve vertical jumps by more than 10 %,[6,7] possibly due to the contributions of the stored elastic energy of the tendon-muscle complex and the neural facilitation of the stretch reflex, but more likely from the longer time available for force development, thus more work initially.[5] If timed optimally, the forward and upward thrusting of the arms enhances the momentum and, hence, the height of the jump.[51]

Some of the scores that have been accumulated under a variety of methods are presented in Table 8.1. It is not unusual for a heavier performer to have greater absolute power than a lighter jumper even when the latter jumps higher. For example, the highest power value in our laboratory was 2060 W by a heavier person who jumped 85 cm, but the power of a lighter person was only 1760 W despite jumping 99 cm. Thus, a heavier person generates more power if jumping a given height. However, the lighter person's relative power is higher.

Table 8.1 Jump-Reach Height and Power on Various Vertical Jump Tests

Method of Testing	Jump Height		Power	
	in.	cm	W	W·kg⁻¹
Unknown				
Michael Jordan[33]	41	104		
UCLA 1963–64 basketball team[54]	27–36	69–91		
Facing Wall, 2-Arm Reach				
Average college male	20	51		
Average college female[35]	13	33		
Method Described in This Text				
Highest P in CSUF laboratory	33.5	85	2060	20.3
Highest jump height at CSUF	39	99	1760	21.5
College football players[13]	20.9	53		
50th %ile 17-year-old boys[4]	19.5	50		
50th %ile 17-year-old girls[4]	13.0	33		
50th %ile 17- to 18-year-old boys[1]	20	51		
50th %ile 17- to 18-year-old girls[2]	13	33		
50th %ile 18- to 34-year-old men[32]	16	41		
50th %ile 18- to 34-year-old women[32]	8	20		
Average male college students[13,22]	21.3; 21.6	54		
50th %ile male college students[47]	16	41		
Active men college students[42]		53	1240	
Active women college students[42]		36	792	
Female college athletes[43]	15.7	40	877	13.8
50th %ile women college students[47]	8	20		
Average woman kinesiology major (CSUF)			750	
Average man kinesiology major (CSUF)			1340	
U.S. rugby team forwards[41]			1570	
CSUF baseball team	26	66	1500	18.1
Italian men's volleyball team (static)[8]		44[a]	1240	
Soldiers of India (38 y to 43 y)[39]	12.5			

[a]Lower jump height due to hands-on-hips jump position.

Table 8.2 Vertical Jump-Reach Scores of College Men and Women

	Jump-Reach Height Difference					
	Men			Women		
Percentile	in.	cm	m	in.	cm	m
90	25	64	0.64	14	36.0	0.360
80	24	61	0.61	13	33.0	0.330
70	23	58	0.58	12	30.0	0.300
60	19	48	0.48	10	25.0	0.250
50	16	41	0.41	8	20.0	0.200
40	13	33	0.33	6	15.0	0.150
30	9	23	0.23	4	10.0	0.100
20	8	20	0.20	2	5.0	0.050
10	2	5	0.05	1	2.5	0.025

Modified from H. J. Montoye, *Living Fit*, page 53. Copyright © 1988 Benjamin/Cummings Publishing, Menlo Park, CA.

Table 8.3 Vertical Jump-Reach Height[a] in Finnish Men and Women (*n* = 670)

	Men			Women		
Age (y)	cm	SD	in.	cm	SD	in.
25	32.5	5.0	12.8	20.9	3.9	8.2
35	28.4	5.2	11.2	18.6	3.6	7.3
45	25.1	4.9	9.9	15.7	3.5	6.2
55	21.1	4.4	8.3	12.5	2.4	4.9

Note: [a]Similar jump technique as in *Exercise Physiology Laboratory Manual*, but calculated from flight time of center of gravity as described in reference #7. Adapted from Table 2 on p. 891 of Kujala et al. (1994). Physical activity, VO₂ max, and jumping height in an urban population. *Medicine and Science in Sports and Exercise, 26,* 889–895. © ACSM, 1994, Indianapolis, IN.

References

1. AAHPER. (1966). *Skills test manual: Basketball for boys.* Washington, DC: Author.

2. AAHPER. (1966). *Skills test manual: Basketball for girls.* Washington, DC: Author.

3. Bannister, E. W., & Mekjavic, I. B. (1987). *Experiments in human performance.* Philadelphia: W. B. Saunders.

4. Baumgartner, T. A., & Jackson, A. S. (1987). *Measurement for evaluation in physical education and exercise science.* Dubuque, IA: Wm. C. Brown.

The norms in Tables 8.2[47] and 8.3[37] are based upon larger samples but do not include power values. The values in Table 8.3 clearly show an age-related decline in jumping ability. For men and women, vertical jumps decrease about 4 cm and 3 cm, respectively, for every 10 y after the age of 25.[7,37]

The P_{pk} and P_{ave} for college athletes were 5782 W and 3037 W, respectively, for men, and 2385 W and 1828 W, respectively, for women.[34]

5. Bobbert, M. F., Gerritsen, K. G. M., Litjens, M. C., & Van Soest, A. J. (1996). Why is countermovement jump height greater than squat jump height? *Medicine and Science in Sports and Exercise, 28,* 1402–1412.

6. Bosco, C., & Komi, P. V. (1979). Mechanical characteristics and fiber composition of human leg extensor muscles. *European Journal of Applied Physiology, 41,* 275–284.

7. Bosco, C., & Komi, P. V. (1980). Influence of aging on the mechanical behavior of leg extensor muscles. *European Journal of Applied Physiology, 45,* 209–219.

8. Bosco, C., Mognoni, P., & Luhtanen, P. (1983). Relationship between isokinetic performance and ballistic movement. *European Journal of Applied Physiology, 51,* 357–364.

9. Bosworth, J. M. (1964). *The effect of isometric training and rebound tumbling on performance in the vertical jump.* Master's thesis, Springfield College, MA.

10. Bowers, P., Coleman, A., & Oshiro, T. (1993). Measuring anaerobic power of aged men and women. *Sports Medicine, Training, and Rehabilitation, 4,* 304 (Abstract).

11. Clarke, H. H. (1957). Relationships of strength and anthropometric measures to physical performances involving the trunk and leg. *Research Quarterly, 28,* 223.

12. Clutch, D., Wilton, M., McGown, C., & Bryce, G. R. (1983). The effect of depth jumps and weight training on leg strength and vertical jump. *Research Quarterly for Exercise and Sport, 54,* 5–10.

13. Considine, W. J., & Sullivan, W. J. (1973). Relationship of selected tests of leg strength and leg power on college men. *Research Quarterly, 44,* 404–416.

14. Costill, D. L., Miller, S. J., Myers, W. C., Kehoe, F. M., & Hoffman, W. M. (1968). Relationship among selected tests of explosive leg strength and power. *Research Quarterly, 39,* 785.

15. Cureton, T. K. (1941). Fitness of feet and legs. *Research Quarterly, 12,* 368.

16. Davies, C. T. M., & Young, K. (1984). Effects of external loading on short term power output in children and young male adults. *European Journal of Applied Physiology, 52,* 351–354.

17. de Vries, H. A. (1971). *Laboratory experiments in physiology of exercise.* Dubuque, IA: Wm. C. Brown.

18. de Vries, H. A., & Housh, T. J. (1994). *Physiology of exercise for physical education, athletics, and exercise science.* Dubuque, IA: Brown & Benchmark.

19. Garhammer, J. (1993). A review of power output studies of Olympic and powerlifting: Methodology, performance prediction, and evaluation tests. *Journal of Strength and Conditioning Research, 7,* 76–89.

20. Garhammer, J., & Gregor, R. (1992). Propulsion forces as a function of intensity for weightlifting and vertical jumping. *Journal of Applied Sport Science Research, 6,* 129–134.

21. Genuario, S. E., & Dolgener, F. A. (1980). The relationship of isokinetic torque at two speeds to the vertical jump. *Research Quarterly for Exercise and Sport, 51,* 593–598.

22. Glencross, D. J. (1966). The nature of the vertical jump test and the standing broad jump. *Research Quarterly, 37,* 353–359.

23. Gray, R. K., Start, K. B., & Glencross, D. J. (1962). A test of leg power. *Research Quarterly, 33,* 44.

24. Hakkinen, K. (1991). Force production characteristics of leg extensor, trunk flexor and extensor muscles in male and female basketball players. *Journal of Sports Medicine and Physical Fitness, 31,* 325–331.

25. Harman, E. A., Rosenstein, M. T., Frykman, P. N., & Rosenstein, R. M. (1990). The effects of arms and countermovement on vertical jumping. *Medicine and Science in Sports and Exercise, 22,* 825–833.

26. Harman, E. A., Rosenstein, M. T., Frykman, P. N., Rosenstein, R. M., & Kraemer, W. J. (1989). Evaluation of the Lewis power output test. *Medicine and Science in Sports and Exercise, 21* (Suppl.), Abstract #305, S51.

27. Harman, E., Rosenstein, M., Frykman, P., Rosenstein, R., & Kraemer, W. (1991). Estimation of human power output from vertical jump. *Journal of Applied Sport Science Research, 3,* 116–120.

28. Harman, E. A., & Sharp, M. A. (1989). Prediction of power output during vertical jumps using body mass and flight time. *Medicine and Science in Sports and Exercise, 21* (Suppl. 2), Abstract #306, S51.

29. Hay, J. G., & Reid, J. G. (1982). *The anatomical and mechanical bases of human motion.* Englewood Cliffs, NJ: Prentice-Hall.

30. Henry, F. M. (1959). Influence of measurement error and intra-individual variation on the reliability of muscle strength and vertical jump tests. *Research Quarterly, 30,* 155.

31. Hortobagyi, T., Houmard, J. A., Stevenson, J. R., Fraser, D. D., Johns, R. A., & Israel, R. G. (1993). The effects of detraining on power athletes. *Medicine and Science in Sports and Exercise, 25,* 929–935.

32. Johnson, B. L., & Nelson, J. K. (1974). *Practical measurements for evaluation in physical education.* Minneapolis: Burgess.

33. Johnson, C. (1966, March). Bodies of evidence. *Outside,* pp. 58–63.

34. Johnson, D. L., & Bahamonde, R. (1996). Power output estimate in university athletes. *Journal of Strength and Conditioning Research, 10,* 161–166.

35. Johnson, P. B., Updyke, W. F., Schaefer, M., & Stolberg, D. C. (1975). *Sport, exercise, and you.* New York: Holt, Rinehart & Winston.

36. Kraemer, W. J., & Newton, R. U. (1994). Training for improved vertical jump. *Sports Science Exchange, 7*(6), 1–5.

37. Kujala, U. M., Viljanen, T., Taimela, S., & Viitasalo, J. T. (1994). Physical activity, $\dot{V}O_2$ max, and jumping height in an urban population. *Medicine and Science in Sports and Exercise, 26,* 889–895.

38. Latchaw, M. (1954). Measuring selected motor skills in fourth, fifth, and sixth grades. *Research Quarterly, 25,* 439.

39. Malhotra, M. S., Ramaswamy, S. S., Dua, G. L., & Sengupta, J. (1966). Physical work capacity as influenced by age. *Ergonomics, 9,* 305–316.

40. Mathews, D. K., & Fox, E. L. (1976). *The physiological basis of physical education and athletics.* Philadelphia: W. B. Saunders.

41. Maud, P. J., & Shultz, B. B. (1984). The U.S. National Rugby Team: A physiological and anthropometric assessment. *The Physician and Sportsmedicine, 12* (9), 86–94, 99.

42. Maud, P. J., & Shultz, B. B. (1986). Gender comparisons in anaerobic power and anaerobic capacity tests. *British Journal of Sports Medicine, 20,* 51–54.

43. Mayhew, J. L., Bemben, M. G., Rohrs, D. M., & Bemben, D. A. (1994). Specificity among anaerobic power tests in college female athletes. *Journal of Strength and Conditioning Research, 8,* 43–47.

44. McArdle, W. D., Katch, F. I., & Katch, V. L. (1996). *Exercise physiology: Energy, nutrition, and human performance.* Baltimore: Williams & Wilkins.

45. Mero, A., & Komi, P. V. (1986). Force-, EMG-, and elasticity-velocity relationships at submaximal, maximal and supramaximal running speeds in sprinters. *European Journal of Applied Physiology, 55,* 553–561.

46. Misner, J. E., Boileau, S. A., Plowman, S. A., Elmore, B. G., Gates, M. A., Gilbert, J. A., & Horswill, C. (1988). Leg power of female firefighter applicants. *Journal of Occupational Medicine, 30,* 433–437.

47. Montoye, H. J., Christian, J. L., Nagle, F. J., & Levin, S. M. (1988). *Living fit.* Menlo Park, CA: Benjamin/Cummings.

48. O'Shea, P. (1999). Toward an understanding of power.

49. Podolsky, A., Kaufman, K. R., Cahalan, T. D., Aleshinsky, S. Y., & Chao, E. Y. (1990). The relationship of strength and jump height in figure skaters. *American Journal of Sports Medicine, 18,* 400–405.

50. Sargent, D. A. (1921). The physical test of a man. *American Physical Education Review, 26,* 188.

51. Semenick, D. M., & Adams, K. O. (1987). The vertical jump: A kinesiological analysis with recommendations for strength and conditioning programming. *National Strength and Conditioning Association Journal, 8,* 9–13.

52. Tharp, G. D., Newhouse, R. K., Uffleman, L., Thorland, W. G., & Johnson, G. O. (1985). Comparison of sprint and run times with performance on the Wingate anaerobic test. *Research Quarterly for Exercise and Sport, 56,* 73–76.

53. Viitasalo, J. T. (1988). Evaluation of explosive strength for young and adult athletes. *Research Quarterly, 59,* 9–13.

54. Wooden, J. (1972). *They call me coach.* Waco, TX: Word Books.

Form 8.1

Individual Data for the Vertical Jump Test

Name [＿＿＿＿＿＿＿＿＿＿＿] Date [＿＿＿＿] Time [＿＿] a.m. [＿] p.m. [＿]

Age [＿] y   Gender (M or W) [＿]   Ht [＿＿] cm   Wt [＿＿] kg

Wt (body mass plus jump clothes) [＿＿] kg   [＿＿] N (acts as a Force unit)   Tech. Initials [＿]

Meteorological Data

T [＿] °C (closest 0.1 °C)   RH % [＿] P_B [＿] mm Hg × 1.333 = [＿] hPa (mbar)

Jump Data

Reach Position[a] [＿＿＿＿] in. (to closest 0.5 in.); ÷ 0.3937 = [＿＿＿＿] (closest cm)

Jump Height
(Circle best trial)   Trial #1 [＿] in. [＿] cm   Trial #2 [＿] in. [＿] cm   Trial #3 [＿] in. [＿] cm

Jump Ht Minus Reach Ht (VJ D) [＿＿＿] in. [＿＿] cm [＿＿] m

Power = 2.21 × [＿] kg × $\sqrt{\text{VJ D}}$ ＿＿＿ m (From Eq. 8.2: P (kg·m·s^{-1})=2.21 × BM × $\sqrt{\text{VJ D}}$)

= [＿＿] × [＿＿] m = [＿＿] kg·m·s^{-1}; × 10^b = [＿＿] N·m·s^{-1}; W

P_{pk} (W) = 78.5 × VJ D [＿] cm + 60.6 × BM [＿] kg – 15.3 × ht [＿] cm – 1308 (From Eq. 8.6)

P_{ave} (W) = 41.4 × VJ D [＿] cm + 31.2 × BM [＿] kg – 13.9 × ht [＿] cm + 431 (From Eq. 8.7)

[a]The height of the reach position does not need to be measured if it is simply used as a zero reference point.
[b]The conversion factors 9.8 or 9.80665 can be substituted for 10.

Form 8.2

Group Data for Vertical Jump

MEN Initials	Jump Ht (D) (m)	Absolute P (W)	Relative P (W·kg⁻¹)	WOMEN Initials	Jump Ht (D) (m)	Absolute P (W)	Relative P (W·kg⁻¹)
1.				1.			
2.				2.			
3.				3.			
4.				4.			
5.				5.			
6.				6.			
7.				7.			
8.				8.			
9.				9.			
10.				10.			
11.				11.			
12.				12.			
13.				13.			
14.				14.			
15.				15.			
16.				16.			
17.				17.			
18.				18.			
19.				19.			
20.				20.			
M				*M*			
Minimum				*Minimum*			
Maximum				*Maximum*			

CHAPTER 9

ANAEROBIC CYCLING

The most popular anaerobic cycling test is the Wingate Anaerobic Test (WAnT), named after a university in Israel. The original test[18] was designed for adolescents but became popular for adults in the late 1970s.[5] It fulfilled the need for a precisely measured anaerobic power test. It may be used to test either arm or leg power but is most commonly used to test the legs.

This anaerobic test can determine the performer's **peak anaerobic power, average (mean) anaerobic power, total work,** and **fatigue index.** *Peak power* is based on the highest power level averaged usually over a 5 s period during the test, whereas *mean power* refers to the average power during the entire 30 s of the test. The total work represents the product of the cycle distance and the force or resistance during the 30 s test. The fatigue index measures the rate of power decrease from the point of peak anaerobic power to the finish of the test.

Physiological Rationale for the Wingate Test

Despite the anaerobic nature of the WAnT, the cardiovascular and respiratory systems are challenged during this supramaximal test. Peak heart rates for persons in their early twenties range from 170 b/min in nonelite athletic men and women[67] to 181 b/min in U.S. elite cyclists.[40] Peak ventilations may average 110 L/min.[13]

The Wingate Anaerobic Test is truly a supramaximal test when maximal oxygen consumption serves as the maximal reference point, because the WAnT usually requires a power level that, in turn, would require two to four times the participant's maximal oxygen consumption.[7] Thus, the physiological basis of the Wingate Test is best understood by focusing mainly on the contributions of the anaerobic pathway to the major components of the Wingate Test. One reviewer of anaerobic tests concluded that 30 s is an optimal duration for an all-out test of anaerobic work or mean anaerobic power.[27] The first several seconds of the WAnT represents anaerobic power, thus is logically placed in the anaerobic power category of the fitness continuum described in Chapter 1. The total work during the 30 s WAnT reflects the mean anaerobic power and is categorized as power endurance in the fitness continuum. Hence, the performers of the WAnT test may receive from 60 %[50] or 66 %[13] up to 85 %[23] of their ATP from the powerful phosphagenic component and the

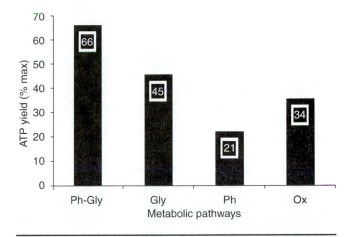

Figure 9.1 The percentage of total ATP contributed by the anaerobic pathway (66 % max ATP) is nearly twice the percentage contributed by the aerobic pathway (34 % max ATP) when performing a 30 s sprint on a cycle ergometer based on muscle biopsies of the vastus lateralis muscle. Figure adapted from data of Bogdanis, G. C., Nevili, M. E., Boobis, L. H., & Lakomy, H. K. A. (1996). Contribution of phosphocreatine and aerobic metabolism to energy supply during repeated sprint exercise. *Journal of Applied Physiology, 80,* 876–884.[13]

enduring glycolytic component of the anaerobic pathway (see Figure 9.1).

Peak Anaerobic Power (Pk-AnP)

The peak anaerobic power reflects the participant's ability to use the phosphagenic system at a rapid rate because peak AnP is usually determined within the first 2 s,[27] 5 s,[30, 59, 64] 8 s[36] or 10 s[64] of the Wingate test.[a] One group of investigators determined the ATP contribution of the phosphagenic pathway during the first 10 s of all-out cycling in 24-year-old men recreational athletes by sampling biopsied muscle.[13] Discounting the ATP stores, they reported that the phosphagenic pathway contributed 43 % of the *anaerobic* energy supply. Contrary to earlier reports,[43,44] even in the first 10 s, the glycolytic pathway makes a significant contribution based on lactate values after 10 s that may be four times the resting value.[35]

---

[a]Differences in time to peak power are attributed to the pedal revolutions at the rolling start and the chosen time interval, such as each second or every 5 s.

Mean Anaerobic Power (M-AnP) and Total Work

Mean anaerobic power (M-AnP) often has been referred to its equivalent as anaerobic capacity,[27] but the promoter of the test, Dr. Bar-Or,[7] and I prefer the term mean anaerobic power when watts is the unit of measure. M-AnP mainly reflects the ability to transform energy from the anaerobic glycolytic pathway. Whereas the phosphagenic pathway is the main contributor of ATP to pk-AnP, the glycolytic pathway contributes most to a performer's mean anaerobic power and total work in the 30 s test. Based on vastus lateralis biopsies of recreational athletes who cycled all-out for 30 s, the phosphagenic pathway contributed 32 % of the total *anaerobic* ATP production and 21 % of the total *anaerobic plus aerobic* production[13] (Figure 9.1). The latter percentage agrees with earlier reports of 23 % on aerobically trained men.[59] Despite contributing as much as 45 %,[13] or 49 %[59] of all the ATP, and, therefore, being the main contributor during the Wingate Test, the glycolytic capacity is not fully utilized due to the short (30 s) duration of the test.[33] Thus, some investigators suggest that the term *anaerobic capacity* may be misleading,[34] despite the report[6] of its correlation with maximal oxygen debt. The 30 s duration of the Wingate test is certainly shorter than the 40 s[43] or 2 min[49] that may be required to exhaust the anaerobic capacity or maximize the lactate production volume. However, it is possible that the maximal *rate,* not total amount, of lactate production, which indicates anaerobic power[48] or power-endurance, may occur sometime during the Wingate test. The anaerobic glycolytic production of ATP is evidenced by the moderate-to-high blood lactate values (ranging from 6 to 15 times the resting value) measured in Wingate-test performers by various investigators.[34,53,56,61,62,65]

The phosphagenic contribution to the entire 30 s of the test was substantiated by investigators[34] who found that female participants reduced their phosphagen levels to 70 % of their original adenosine triphosphate values and 40 % of their original creatine phosphate values after performing the Wingate Test. Recreational men athletes reduced their creatine phosphate stores to 17 % of pre-exercise levels.[13]

Although the aerobic source of energy accounts for a lesser amount than the combined anaerobic sources, it also contributes from 9 % to 19 %,[30,37] or 28 %,[30,59] or as high as 34 %[13] or 40 %,[49] depending upon assumptions regarding efficiency, oxygen consumption time delay, and oxygen stores.[30]

It is appropriate to affix a higher role during the WAnT by Type II (fast-twitch) fibers than to Type I (slow-twitch) fibers because of the significant correlation between type II fibers and mean anaerobic power.[22] Therefore, because the Wingate Test is a maximal-effort exercise bout for 30 s, it relies principally upon the two anaerobic pathways and secondarily upon the oxidative (aerobic) metabolic pathway to produce ATP.[32,59] Figure 9.1 illustrated the primary role of the anaerobic pathway during the WAnT.

Method

The methodology for the Wingate Test includes a brief description of the equipment, such as ergometer, counter, and timer; it also includes a description of the test procedures and calculations. For a discussion on the accuracy of the Wingate Test, see Box 9.1.

Equipment

Ergometer

Although isokinetic ergometers have been used,[42] mechanically braked cycle ergometers, such as Monark™ and Fleisch™, usually are used to perform the WAnT. These ergometers utilize a constant force concept, meaning that the resistance does not change during the course of the test. Thus, the speed of pedaling determines the power in the mechanically braked ergometers, whereas the force produced on the pedals by the performer determines the power on the isokinetic ergometers.[8] Constant power ergometers do not facilitate Wingate testing because the power on these cycles does not change throughout the course of the test. Probably the best type of mechanically braked ergometer is one in which the force (kg; N) can be applied immediately and accurately. Some ergometers (e.g., Monark #814E, 824E, and 834E) have a peg or basket-type device (0.5 kg or 1 kg) onto which the desired weights can be dropped (Figure 9.2), thus eliminating the oscillation that occurs in the swinging force-pendulum of some ergometers (see Figure 14.1 in Chapter 14). Some Monark™ cycles have a knob, which the technician turns to the proper force setting, and others can be controlled electronically (e.g., 839E).

The popularity of the WAnT has inspired various corporations (e.g., International Tapetronics, Sports Medicine Industries, Medical Graphics) to either modify or computerize ergometers (e.g., CardiO$_2$™; WATCycle™) so that their software facilitates the procedures and calculations required of the test. Some of these systems have inexpensive software, but complete packages of ergometer, computer, and software can be expensive. If a laboratory is fortunate enough to have such systems, then a separate revolutions counter and a timer are not needed. Sophisticated automation allows electromagnets to feed pedal counts into the port of a microcomputer that can calculate online all of the test indices.

Revolutions Counter

Ideally, the cycle ergometer should have a device that automatically counts the pedal revolutions. An inexpensive mechanical counter works by extending a lever out to the circuitous path of the pedal, whereby it is "tripped" with each pedal revolution. Also, more sophisticated electronic and magnetic counters can be assembled on the ergometer rather inexpensively. If the cycle ergometer does not have an automatic counter, then a technician must count and record the revolutions.

The accuracy of all exercise physiology tests is mainly dependent upon their validity, variability, and reliability.

Validity

There is no "gold standard" anaerobic performance test by which to compare the scores of the Wingate Test. It might be argued that for the Wingate Test to have physiological validity, the performers with the highest lactate values after the Wingate Test would be expected to have the highest glycolytic or anaerobic capacities. In a validation study,[62] only a moderate relationship (r = .55 and .60) was reported between mean anaerobic power (W and W·kg⁻¹) and blood lactates; the relationship between mean anaerobic power and maximal oxygen debt was slightly lower. These researchers concluded that the test's validity was tenuous. Another research group, using the accumulated oxygen deficit as a measure of anaerobic energy release, agrees that the WAnT "may not be a proper anaerobic capacity test" because it does not exhaust the anaerobic capacity.[50] However, because of the contributions of the phosphagenic and oxidative systems, the Wingate's validity should not be dependent upon its ability to incur maximal lactates or on its ability to exhaust anaerobic energy sources. For example, investigators supported the test's physiological validity by finding a significant relationship between both the peak anaerobic power (Pk-AnP for 5 s) and the total work versus the fast-twitch fiber area and percentage.[35]

Its performance validity was supported by the high relationship between Pk-AnP and the time for the 50 m run (r = −.91),[35] and the vertical jump.[44] Low to moderate correlations have been reported between mean AnP and 50 m time (r = −.79)[52] and 300 m cycling time (r = −.75).[56] Low and moderate correlations also were reported between total work and the 300 m run (r = −.64; −.83).[11,56] Lean body mass and peak isokinetic torque are positively related to anaerobic mean power.[1] Further evidence of the test's validity is provided by the higher power outputs found in more elite cyclists than less elite cyclists.[63] It seems logical that the WAnT would relate more closely to anaerobic cycling events than to anaerobic running events.[24] However, the WAnT improves the predictability of run performance when power is divided by body mass (W·kg⁻¹).[64]

Finally, a brief comment on the mechanical validity of the WAnT is in order, but the details are beyond the scope of this laboratory manual. In the mid 1980s, it became apparent that corrections for acceleration and deceleration of the flywheel were necessary to produce valid power outputs.[17] The power outputs derived from WAnT on a mechanically braked (friction) cycle ergometer (e.g., Monark™ 324E), which provided much of the published data, included only the braking resistance (force) and flywheel velocity. Power outputs on such cycle ergometers are much lower than the corrected power outputs for peak power and slightly lower for mean power.[57] Fortunately, electrically braked ergometers reduce the inertial effects. Additionally, computer software makes corrections more practical. For more information, the reader is referred to detailed descriptions of the corrections.[16,57]

Reliability

It appears that the day-to-day variability of anaerobic power tests is similar to aerobic tests—that is, about 5 % to 6 %.[15,66] The variability of the Wingate Test is partly attributed to its reliability. Reliability coefficients (test-retest comparisons) for maximal anaerobic power/capacity are very high, usually ranging from a low of .89 in elderly pulmonary patients[10] to as high as .95 to .98.[5,9,23,32,35] The retesting reliability of the fatigue index can range from such low values near .43 to moderate values near .73.[66] The intraclass correlation coefficient (ICC) for repeat WAnT within one week of each other was r = .98 for mean anaerobic power.[67]

Timing Apparatus

At least three types of timers can be used to administer the Wingate Test: a laboratory set-timer, a stopwatch, or the timer attached to the ergometer. Any of these can monitor the 5 s time intervals and the total 30 s duration of the test.

The laboratory set-clock can be used to measure either elapsed time (i.e., continuous running time) or time remaining by setting it to buzz at the end of the test. Laboratory set-timers (e.g., Figure 9.3) are preferable to wall clocks for monitoring either the time remaining or the elapsed time for any interval from 1 s to 60 min. The minute hand (hooked-end) of the set-timer and its seconds hand make one counterclockwise revolution in 60 min and 60 s, respectively.

Elapsed time is the typical perception of time in an event. Thus, at the start and end of the WAnT, the timer displays 0 s and 30 s, respectively. Both hands of the elapsed timer are read on the inner circle of small numerals.

The set-timer is set for elapsed time by moving both hands in a clockwise direction until they both rest on the small inside 0 and the large 55.

Wall or built-in ergometer clocks may be used as elapsed timers. Also, the stopwatch mode on a wristwatch is an acceptable timer for the WAnT. Most laboratory facilities have wall clocks with seconds hands; however, these are recommended only if set-clocks are not available. Some ergometers have clocks built into the dashboard chassis. If stopwatches are used, technicians should secure them with a neck or wrist strap, and treat them as an expensive camera.

Remaining time simply means that the timer displays 30 s at the start of the WAnT and 0 s at the finish. The set-timer is set for remaining time by manually moving the minute hand in a clockwise direction to the outer-zero mark and the seconds hand to the outer-number 30; then the switch or knob is set to the buzzer label so that the sound occurs at the finish.

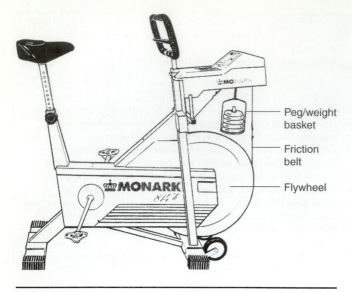

Figure 9.2 This older model of a weight ergometer clearly shows the peg/weight basket that holds the small weights producing the force or resistance on the friction belt surrounding the flywheel. Courtesy of Monark AB, Sweden.

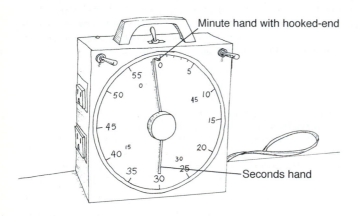

Figure 9.3 Laboratory set-clock (e.g., Gralab Universal Timer®).

Weight Scale

Use an accurate platform beam scale or electronic digital scale to weigh the performer. Although body mass was not considered in the original Wingate Test, it is now often used as the divisor to calculate the relative (e.g., $W \cdot kg^{-1}$) anaerobic power indices.[29]

Test Procedures

Teamwork among technicians is essential for the accurate administration of the WAnT; thus, the test procedures should be rehearsed prior to the actual test. Some of the factors to consider in the test procedures are (a) preparation, (b) Wingate Test protocol, and (c) the roles of timer, force-setter, revolutions counter, and recorder.

Preparation

Basic data, such as the performer's body mass, should be measured as described in Chapter 3. The performer's nude weight, weight in scanty attire, or weight derived by subtracting the weight of the attire, should be recorded onto Form 9.1, along with the other basic data variables.

Meteorological data should be recorded on Form 9.1 even though environmental temperature, relative humidity, and the hydration of the performer do not affect the WAnT results.[20,33] High altitude, and its associated low barometric pressure, may be slightly influential, as hypoxia was shown to affect marginally peak anaerobic power.[38]

Calibration of the mechanically braked cycle ergometer is presented in Box 14.2 of Chapter 14.

Force (F) Setting. The body mass (BM) is not only necessary to derive the relative power and work scores but to prescribe the force (kg; N) setting on the arm or the cycle ergometer. The force selection varies with such factors as the general anaerobic fitness of the performer, gender, age, and the type of ergometer.[8,26] Obtaining the optimal force for each person would require testing that person several times. Thus, for practical reasons, equations are presented that may approximate the optimal force setting for a person. The first equation (Eq. 9.1) converts body mass in kilograms to newtons (N).

$$BM\ (N) \approx 10 \times kg \qquad \text{Eq. 9.1a}$$

$$\approx 9.8 \times kg \qquad \text{Eq. 9.1b}$$

$$= 9.80665 \times kg \qquad \text{Eq. 9.1c}$$

For leg ergometry by active adult women and men on a Monark™ cycle, Equations 9.2 and 9.3 are recommended.[7,14,21,66] For anaerobically fit males and females, Equation 9.4 is recommended, whereby the force setting may range from 9.0 %[60] or 9.4 %[55] or 9.5 %[63] to 10 %[60] of body mass. For sedentary persons, or children and older adults, the traditional equations can be used for leg (Eq. 9.5) and arm[b] (Eq. 9.6) ergometry, respectively.[5,23,36,51]

Active Adult Women:

$$\text{Leg Force (N)} = BM\ (N) \times 0.086 \qquad \text{Eq. 9.2}$$

Active Adult Men:

$$\text{Leg Force (N)} = BM\ (N) \times 0.090 \qquad \text{Eq. 9.3}$$

Anaerobically Fit Persons (Athletes):

$$\text{Leg Force (N)} = BM\ (N) \times 0.090 \text{ to } 0.10 \qquad \text{Eq. 9.4}$$

Children, Older Adults, and Sedentary Persons:

$$\text{Leg Force (N)} = BM\ (N) \times 0.075 \qquad \text{Eq. 9.5}$$

$$\text{Arm Force (N)} = BM\ (N) \times 0.05 \qquad \text{Eq. 9.6}$$

---

[b]Monark *arm* ergometers have wheel perimeters of 1 m; the wheel covers a distance of 2.5 m per pedal revolution.

For example, if the body mass of a sedentary person is 67.7 kg ≈ (677 N), then the load (F) setting for leg ergometry is calculated as

$$\text{Leg F (N)} = 677 \text{ N} \times 0.075 = 50.7 = 51 \text{ N (or 5.1 kg)}^c$$

Whereas the leg-force setting in children, older adults, and sedentary persons (Eq. 9.5) represents about 7.5 % of kilogram body mass (0.75 % N), the force setting in Equation 9.2 represents 9.0 % to 10 % kilogram body mass. Force settings between 8.5 % and 9.5 % of kilogram body mass are likely to elicit greater anaerobic indices for young men[12,55] and female softball players.[60] However, it appears that resistance settings greater than 10 % of body mass do not enhance Wingate scores.[19] Although nothing short of having to perform two trials at different force settings to rectify it, the force necessary to yield optimal peak power in the WAnT is greater than the force necessary to yield optimal mean power.[21,55]

Seat height affects the efficiency, thus the power output of the WAnT. After the performer's force setting is recorded onto Form 9.1, the technician should adjust the seat height so that the performer's knee is slightly bent when the ball of the foot is on the pedal (see Chapter 14 for details). Most cycle ergometers have seat posts labeled with heights, which then can be recorded onto the individual data collection form (Form 9.1).

Wingate Test Protocol

The Wingate protocol (Table 9.1) has five distinct time periods: (1) prior exercise, (2) recovery interval, (3) acceleration period, (4) Wingate Test,[6,8] and (5) cooldown period.

As with the other anaerobic tests, **prior exercise** is recommended for both safety (e.g., muscle injury and ischemic heart prevention)[3,4] and performance reasons.[47] The warm-up includes 5 min of low to moderate intensity pedaling at about 50 rpm to 60 rpm, interspersed by four or five all-out sprints of 4 s to 6 s duration; the sprints should progressively increase in resistance (force) so that by the fourth or fifth sprint the prescribed resistance for the Wingate Test is reached.[8,31]

The **recovery interval** between the end of the prior exercise and the beginning of the Wingate Test should not be less than 2 min after the prior exercise or more than 5 min after the warm-up portion of the prior exercise. The 2 min minimum provides adequate recovery time from any possible fatigue that the performer may have incurred during the warm-up. The 5 min maximum recovery still retains muscle temperature and blood flow to a significant extent. The activity during the recovery interval may consist of simply resting while seated on the bike or pedaling at a minimal resistance (e.g., 1 kg or ≈ 10 N at 10 rpm and 20 rpm; about 10 W to 20 W).

The **acceleration period** consists of two brief phases beginning immediately after the recovery interval. In the first phase, the performer pedals at about 20 rpm to 50 rpm for about 5 s to 10 s at a resistance that is about one-third of that prescribed from one of the chosen equations. In the second phase, the performer increases the rpm to a near-maximal rate while the technician loads the prescribed force (F) setting immediately, if using a basket-loaded ergometer, or within 2 s to 5 s if using a pendulum-loaded ergometer. The total acceleration period, therefore, may last for as little as 7 s or as long as 15 s.

The actual **Wingate Test duration** of all-out cycling is 30 s. It begins at the end of the acceleration period and divides the 30 s into six continuous time intervals of 5 s each. The performer continuously tries to obtain the highest number of revolutions during each 5 s interval. For example, the performer does not pace the effort so that the last 5 s contains as many revolutions as the previous 5 s intervals. Thus, the test can be described as a rush to the peak power and a fading to the lowest power.

The **cooldown** period lasts for 2 min to 3 min[8] and consists of pedaling at a low to moderate power level on the cycle ergometer immediately after the Wingate Test. Thus, the force setting can be set between 5 N and 20 N, and the revolutions at 50 rpm to produce between 25 W and 100 W. If for some reason a repeat test on the same person and on the same day is necessary, then about 10 min of recovery is recommended.[2,28]

The Roles of Timer, Force-Setter, Revolutions-Counter, and Recorder

One technician is needed to serve as the timer for the Wingate protocol time periods, especially the 5 s intervals and the duration of the test. At least three other technicians and the performer must pay close attention to the timer technician in order to perform their roles effectively. These other technicians may be called the force-setter, the revolutions-counter, and the recorder.

Timer   After coordinating the Wingate protocol periods for prior exercise, recovery interval, and the acceleration period, the timer officially begins the test itself as soon as the force-setter finishes setting the prescribed resistance. The timer yells, "Start!" or "Go!" when the prescribed load is set. The timer begins the clock, and the performer begins pedaling as fast as possible for a 30 s period while remaining seated on the ergometer during this time. The timer shouts the time every 5 s. At the end of 30 s the timer yells, "End!" or "Stop!" or the buzzer of the laboratory set-timer signals the end of the test.

Force Setter   The force-setter maintains the prescribed setting on the ergometer. At the end of 30 s, the force-setter lowers the force setting to a cooldown recovery setting (usually between 10 N and 20 N; 1 kg to 2 kg) while the performer continues pedaling comfortably at about 50 rpm for 2 min to 3 min.

---

cThe weights for loading weight ergometers (pegged-basket type) usually are labeled in kilograms. It may be helpful to paint the newton value on these.

Counter   The counter shouts the number of pedal revolutions for the respective 5 s intervals by observing the number of times the left or right pedal makes a complete rotation from the original pedal position at the "GO" signal. The counter gives the whole, not fractional, number of revolutions for each 5 s interval. For example, when the timer yells "five seconds," if the pedal is at half of a complete rotation after having made 10 complete revolutions, the counter tells the recorder, "Ten," not "Ten and a half." The counter then counts the completion of that half-rotation as a whole revolution for the next 5 s interval. Usually, the count starts over at "one," but sometimes the number can be continued, for example, as "eleven" for the next interval.

Recorder   The recorder records each 5 s value onto Form 9.1, then circles the highest revolutions and sums the revolutions.

It should be evident why computers can enhance the accuracy of the WAnT by precisely recording the exact pedal position at the exact time. If an inexpensive automatic counter is attached to the ergometer, then the counter technician can simply record the observed number at the Start or Go command of the timer and the subsequent numbers at 5 s intervals.

Summary of Preparation and Procedural Steps

Preparation

1. Body mass is measured and recorded as described in Chapter 3.
2. The force (resistance) is prescribed using the appropriate equation (Eqs. 9.2 to 9.6).
3. The ergometer seat is adjusted so that the performer has a slight bend at the knee.
4. The technician tells the performer that the test requires an all-out effort but lasts for only 30 s.
5. The Wingate protocol for (1) prior exercise, (2) recovery interval, and (3) acceleration period follows fairly close to Table 9.1.

Procedures

1. The force-setter dictates the start of the WAnT by applying the prescribed force.
2. The timer shouts, "GO!" or "Start!"; the performer pedals at an all-out rate.
3. The revolutions-counter mentally notes the position of the performer's pedal at the timer's "GO" signal and starts counting pedal revolutions.
4. The timer shouts the elapsed time every five seconds: "5," "10," "15," etc.
5. The counter tells the recorder how many revolutions occurred during each 5 s interval during the 30 s test; the recorder records these values onto Form 9.1.
6. The force-setter ensures that the prescribed force is sustained throughout the test.
7. Recorder and force-setter motivate the performer throughout the test.
8. At the 30th second, the force-setter lowers the resistance to about 10 N to 20 N (1 kg to 2 kg) as the performer pedals at about 50 rpm for 2 min to 3 min.
9. Calculations are made to derive the peak anaerobic power, total work, mean anaerobic power, and fatigue index.

Calculations

Although data collection and calculations can be performed by a computer interfaced with the appropriate hardware and software,[52] the calculations described here are performed without such means. Calculations are made to derive such indices of the WAnT as (1) peak anaerobic power (pk-AnP) expressed in watts (W) and relative watts (W·kg^{-1}); (2) total work (w) expressed in joules (J) or kilo-joules (kJ) and relative joules (J·kg^{-1}); (3) mean anaerobic power (M-AnP) expressed the same as pk-AnP; and (4) fatigue index (FI) expressed as a percentage (%) of pk-AnP.

Peak Anaerobic Power (Pk-AnP)

Peak anaerobic power should be expressed in the scientifically accepted unit of watts. To facilitate this, it is probably best to use the newton (N) unit as the expression for force (F), the newton meter (N·m) or joule (J) as the expression for work (w), and the newton meter per minute or per second (N·m·min^{-1}; N·m·s^{-1}) because of the ease in converting them to the watts power unit. Although automated systems can derive the peak power for a specific second, the hand-calculated method derives the average peak power for a 5 s interval (N·m–5 s). Thus, Equation 9.7 is used, based on power as the rate of work ($P = w \cdot t^{-1}$). The work component is represented by the first part of the equation whereby the force (F) setting (N) is multiplied by the distance traveled in 5 s. Distance is the product of the highest number of revolutions (rev$_{max}$) among the 5 s intervals (usually the first or second 5 s interval) and six—the rounded-off distance in meters that the Monark cycle's

Table 9.1   Wingate Test Protocol

Period	Time Length	Activity
Prior exercise	5 min	Cycle at low to moderate intensity; intersperse with four or five sprints of 4 s to 6 s at prescribed force (F).
Recovery interval	2 min to 5 min	Rest or cycle slowly against minimal F.
Acceleration period	7 s to 15 s	1st phase: Cycle for 5 s to 10 s at one-third prescribed F at 20 rpm to 50 rpm.
		2nd phase: Cycle 2 s to 5 s against F; approaching prescribed F at near-maximal rpm.
Wingate Test	30 s	Cycle at highest rpm possible against prescribed F.
Cooldown period	2 min to 3 min	Cycle at low to moderate aerobic power level (e.g., 25 W to 100 W).

wheel[d] travels for each pedal revolution (rev). The product of these two products is then divided by the time component, 5 s.

$$\text{Power} \quad = \quad \text{work} \div \text{time}$$

$$\text{Force} \times \text{Distance}$$

$$\text{Pk-AnP (N·m·s}^{-1}; \text{W}) = [\text{N} \times (\text{rev}_{max} \times 6)] \div 5 \quad \text{Eq. 9.7}$$

For example, if a person's highest 5 s interval was 12 revolutions at a force setting of 45 N on a Monark cycle ergometer in which the wheel's perimeter travels 6 m per pedal revolution, then a Pk-AnP of 648 W would be calculated from Equation 9.7 as follows:

$$\text{Pk-AnP (N·m·s}^{-1}; \text{W}) = [45 \text{ N} \times (12 \text{ rev}_{max} \times 6 \text{ m})] \div 5$$

$$= (45 \text{ N} \times 72 \text{ m}) \div 5$$

$$= 3240 \text{ N·m} \div 5$$

$$= 648$$

Relative Peak Anaerobic Power (rel-pk-AnP)

Because relative anaerobic power is often more important than absolute power,[29] Wingate scores that are expressed in watts are often divided by body mass (Eqs. 9.8 and 9.10). Thus, the score to indicate relative (rel) pk-AnP is expressed in units of W·kg^{-1}.

$$\text{rel-pk-AnP (W·kg}^{-1}) = \text{W} \div \text{kg} \quad \text{Eq. 9.8}$$

If the person in our previous example weighed 60 kg, then rel-pk-AnP is calculated simply by dividing the respective watts by the 60 kg body mass. Thus, the rel-pk-AnP of 10.8 W·kg^{-1} is found by dividing 648 W by 60 kg.

Total Work (w)

Total work is based upon the total number of revolutions at the end of the 30 s. If an automated counter is reset to zero at the start of the test, then the counter's display at the end of 30 s is the total number of revolutions. But if the counter is not reset to zero, then the number on the counter at the start of the test must be subtracted from the final 30 s total. If the revolutions are counted by a technician's observation, then the total number of revolutions is the sum of the six 5 s revolutions. Equation 9.9 uses the same principle as the work portion of Equation 9.7, except that the number of revolutions in 30 s replaces the number in 5 s.

$$\text{w (N·m; J)} = \text{N} \times (\text{rev in 30 s} \times 6 \text{ m}) \quad \text{Eq. 9.9}$$

Using the same person as an example, if a total of 52 revolutions in 30 s were made, then total work would be calculated from Equation 9.9 as follows:

$$\text{w (N·m; J)} = 45 \text{ N} \times 52 \text{ rev in 30 s} \times 6 \text{ m}$$

$$= 14\,040 \text{ N·m} = 14\,040 \text{ J} = 14.04 \text{ kJ}$$

$$= 14.0 \text{ to closest tenth kilojoule}$$

Relative Total Work (rel-w)

Relative total work (J·kg^{-1}) can be normalized for weight by dividing the total work by body mass (BM) as dictated by Equation 9.10.

$$\text{rel-w} = \text{w (J)} \div \text{BM (kg)} \quad \text{Eq. 9.10}$$

For example, that same 60 kg person accomplishing 14 040 J in 30 s would have a relative total work of 234 J·kg^{-1} based on the following calculation:

$$\text{rel-w} = 14\,040 \text{ J} \div 60 \text{ kg}$$

$$= 234 \text{ (J·kg}^{-1})$$

Mean Anaerobic Power (M-AnP)

The average anaerobic power (W) during the test is calculated from Equation 9.11 simply by dividing the total work (J) by 30 s.

$$\text{M-AnP (W; J·s}^{-1}) = \text{total w (J)} \div 30 \text{ s} \quad \text{Eq. 9.11}$$

For example, the person accomplishing 14 040 J in 30 s would have a M-AnP of 468 W based on the following calculation:

$$\text{M-AnP (W; J·s}^{-1}) = 14\,040 \text{ J} \div 30 \text{ s}$$

$$= 468 \text{ J·s}^{-1} = 468 \text{ W}$$

Relative Mean Anaerobic Power (rel-M-AnP)

The relative mean anaerobic power (W·kg^{-1}) is calculated by dividing the M-AnP (W) by the body mass (kg) as in Equation 9.12.

$$\text{rel-M-AnP (W·kg}^{-1}) = \text{M-AnP (W)} \div \text{BM (kg)} \quad \text{Eq. 9.12}$$

For example, the 60-kg person with an M-AnP of 468 W would have a rel-M-AnP of 7.8 W·kg^{-1} based on the following calculation:

$$\text{rel-M-AnP (W·kg}^{-1}) = 468 \text{ W} \div 60 \text{ kg}$$

$$= 7.8 \text{ W·kg}^{-1}$$

Fatigue Index (FI)

The fatigue index indicates the decrease in power from the pk-AnP to the lowest AnP. The higher the person's percentage value, the greater is the decrease. The power output may decline due to fatigue by 40 %[30] or more from the first 5 s to the last 5 s. Equation 9.13 shows that FI (%) is calculated by dividing the difference between the pk-AnP (W) and the lowest AnP (W) by the pk-AnP and then multiplying by 100 to get a percentage. Usually the lowest AnP is calculated from the last 5 s because it has the lowest number of revolutions.

$$\text{FI (\%)} = [(\text{pk-AnP} - \text{lowest AnP}) \quad \text{Eq. 9.13}$$
$$\div \text{pk - AnP}] \times 100$$

---

[d]The precise circumference of the Monark cycle's flywheel is 1.62 m. The flywheel makes 3.7 circuits for each pedal revolution, producing a distance of 6 m per pedal revolution.

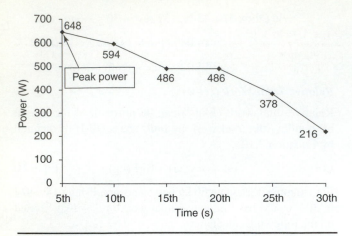

Figure 9.4 The plot of power vs. time produces a graphic negative curvilinear relationship. In the example, which is taken from the text, the cyclist pedaled against a force of 45 N for 12 pedal revolutions in the first five seconds (12 rev/5 s), producing the highest power (648 W) during the 30 s Wingate Test. During the subsequent five-second periods, the performer's pedal revolutions decreased to 11, 9, 9, 7, and 4 rev/5 s, respectively.

For example, if the pk-AnP is 648 W and the lowest AnP is 300 W, then the FI % is 54 % based on the following calculation:

$$FI\ (\%) = [(648\ W - 300\ W) \div 648] \times 100$$

$$= (348\ W \div 648\ W) \times 100$$

$$= 54\ \%$$

Hence, this person's power declined by 54 % from the pk-AnP early in the test to the lowest AnP at or near the end of the test.

Summary of Calculations

Although these calculations and indices can be quite intimidating at first, they can serve as another way to become familiar with a few physical principles and the common terms and expressions used by exercise physiologists. It can be helpful to visualize a person's WAnT performance by plotting the power values (vertical axis) for the six 5 s time intervals (horizontal axis) using the graph on Form 9.2 (see Figure 9.4).

Results and Discussion

High scores on the WAnT are meant to indicate high anaerobic fitness. Some of those anaerobic factors reportedly[66] associated with higher scores are (1) greater capacity to produce lactic acid; (2) greater stores of the phosphagens; (3) greater buffering capacity; and (4) a combination of greater motivation and greater tolerance to discomfort. As mentioned in the introduction to this test, however, aerobic metabolism, thus aerobic fitness, plays a small but significant part in this all-out exercise bout that lasts for 30 s.

Although it would be impossible for persons to maintain their peak or mean Wingate anaerobic power for an entire minute, these anaerobic indices make for an interesting comparison with minute-based power levels that are frequently prescribed for aerobic cycle ergometry. For example, 200 W might be considered a heavy aerobic intensity for typical males, whereas the mean anaerobic powers may range from 450 W[31] to 563 W[46] on the WAnT.

The scores presented in Table 9.2 are for comparative purposes. They should not be used to classify people because they are not based upon large representative samples or equal force settings. Also, some studies may have used toe stirrups, which may increase peak and mean anaerobic power by 5 % to 12 %.[39] When comparing genders, there are large differences between average men and women when peak and mean anaerobic power are expressed in absolute terms, but these differences are reduced when expressed in relative terms of body mass or fat-free mass.[45] Scores for male children and adolescents are available,[31] as are those for the men's U.S. Olympic volleyball team.[62] The Olympians were tested with the force setting at 10 %, instead of the original 7.5 %, of the body mass. The Olympians averaged 46.5 pedal revolutions in the 30 s period. By varying the force setting for the female softball players, higher peak powers were elicited for the higher settings (9 % and 10 % of body mass) than for the lower ones (7 % and 8 %).[60] Some values in the table are based upon a force setting of 9.5 % body mass.[30] The percentiles listed in Tables 9.3, 9.4, and 9.5 are based on men and women between the ages of 18 y and 28 y at a force setting of 7.5 % BM. The average men's and women's peak anaerobic powers are about 700 W and 454 W, respectively; their relative peak anaerobic powers are about 9.2 W·kg^{-1} and 7.6 W·kg^{-1}, respectively. The mean anaerobic powers are about 563 W and 381 W, respectively; their relative mean anaerobic powers are about 7.3 W·kg^{-1} and 6.3 W·kg^{-1}, respectively.

Anaerobic power and work values in a wide age range of adults are scarce in the literature. However, the values from one group of investigators[42] may be helpful despite their use of an isokinetic cycle ergometer, which makes comparisons with the traditional mechanically braked ergometer's scores less valid. Their participants, aged 15 y to 71 y, pedaled with maximal effort for 30 s at a constant 60 rpm. The torque exerted on the pedals, which allowed the calculation of peak power, mean power, and total work, showed a 6 % decrease in these indices for each age decade, but not for the fatigue index. (The participants' peak and mean powers were also related to lean thigh volume.) As with the norms in Tables 9.3 and 9.4 the values in this wider age group demonstrated that the women's anaerobic indices were about two-thirds of the men's values (see Figure 9.5).

A question sometimes asked by students is "Would I accumulate more work if I paced myself throughout the 30 s instead of going all-out at the start?" Two researchers answered this question by concluding there is no significant difference (all-out = 772 W vs. paced = 787 W) between the two approaches.[41]

Table 9.2 Comparative Scores for the Wingate Anaerobic Cycle Test

Group	F-Set	Pk-AnP	Rel-Pk-AnP	Total w	M-AnP	Rel-M-AnP
Males	(%wt)	(W)	(W·kg⁻¹)	(kJ)	(W)	(W·kg⁻¹)
Normals						
18 y–24.9 y[31]	7.5	540	8.2	13.5	450	7.0
25 y–34 y[31]	7.5	700	9.2	16.2	540	7.2
35 y–44 y[31]	7.5	660	8.6		500	6.6
18 y–28 y[46]	7.5	700	9.2		563	7.3
Nonathletic[25]		650		15.6	465	
Athletes[36]	7.5		11.8			
U.S. Olympic kilo cyclists[25]		1075		27.5	917	
U.S.C.F. Cyclists[63]						
Category I and II	10.0	1125	14.7	27.1	903	11.8
Category II–IV	9.5	963	13.3	23.5	783	10.8
Ice Hockey[39]	7.5			15.6		
Volleyball Olympians[62]	10.0			23.9	797	9.1
Sprinters[58]	9.0		14.2	23.9		
Nondesignated[30]	9.5	1064		25		
Females						
Average[46] 18 y to 28 y	7.5	454	7.6		381	6.3
Nonathletes[14] Mix F		576	9.8	12.3	411	6.9
PE Majors[33]	≈ 7.7	561	9.0		453	7.2
Softball Players[60]	7.0		9.1			
	8.0		9.6			
	9.0		10.8			
	10.0		11.1			

Table 9.3 Percentile (%ile) Norms for Pk-AnP (W) and Rel-Pk-AnP (W·kg⁻¹) for the Wingate Test in Physically Active Men ($n = 62$) and Women ($n = 68$), Ages 18 y to 28 y

%ile Rank	Pk-Anaerobic Power (W)		Relative-Pk-AnP (W·kg⁻¹)	
	Men (W)	Women (W)	Men (W·kg⁻¹)	Women (W·kg⁻¹)
95	867	602	11.1	9.3
90	822	560	10.9	9.0
85	807	530	10.6	8.9
80	777	527	10.4	8.8
75	768	518	10.4	8.6
70	757	505	10.2	8.5
65	744	493	10.0	8.3
60	721	480	9.8	8.1
55	706	464	9.5	7.8
50	689	449	9.2	7.6
45	678	447	9.0	7.2
40	671	432	8.9	7.0
35	662	418	8.6	7.0
30	656	399	8.5	6.9
25	646	396	8.3	6.8
20	618	376	8.2	6.6
15	594	362	7.4	6.4
10	570	353	7.1	6.0
5	530	329	6.6	5.7
M	699.5	454.5	9.18	7.61
SD	94.7	81.3	1.43	1.24
Minimum	500	239	5.3	4.6
Maximum	927	623	11.9	10.64

From P. J. Maud and B. B. Shultz, Norms for the Wingate Anaerobic Test with comparison to another similar test. *Research Quarterly for Exercise and Sport, 60*(2), p. 147, 1989. Copyright © 1989 AAHPERD, 1900 Association Dr., Reston, VA 22091.[46]

%ile Rank	M-Anaerobic Power (W)		Relative-M-AnP (W·kg⁻¹)	
	Men (W)	Women (W)	Men (W·kg⁻¹)	Women (W·kg⁻¹)
95	677	483	8.63	7.5
90	662	470	8.24	7.3
85	631	437	8.09	7.1
80	618	419	8.01	7.0
75	604	414	7.96	6.9
70	600	410	7.91	6.8
65	592	402	7.70	6.7
60	577	391	7.59	6.6
55	575	386	7.46	6.5
50	565	381	7.44	6.4
45	553	377	7.26	6.2
40	548	367	7.14	6.15
35	535	361	7.08	6.13
30	530	353	7.00	6.0
25	521	347	6.79	5.9
20	496	337	6.59	5.7
15	485	320	6.39	5.6
10	471	306	5.98	5.3
5	453	287	5.56	5.1
M	562.7	381	7.28	6.35
SD	66.5	56.4	0.88	0.73
Minimum	441	235	4.6	4.5
Maximum	711	529	9.1	8.1

From P. J. Maud and B. B. Shultz, Norms for the Wingate Anaerobic Test with comparison to another similar test. *Research Quarterly for Exercise and Sport, 60*(2), p. 146, 1989. Copyright © 1989 AAHPERD, 1900 Association Dr., Reston, VA 22091.[46]

%ile	Fatigue Index (%)	
	Men (%)	Women (%)
95	55	48
90	52	47
85	47	44
80	46.7	43.6
75	45	42
70	43	40
65	42	39
60	40	38
55	39	38
50	38	35
45	37	34
40	35	33.7
35	34	31
30	31	29
25	30	28
20	29.5	26
15	27	25
10	23	25
5	21	20
M	37.7	35.0
SD	9.9	8.3
Minimum	15	18
Maximum	58	49

From P. J. Maud and B. B. Shultz, Norms for the Wingate Anaerobic Test with comparison to another similar test. *Research Quarterly for Exercise and Sport, 60*(2), p. 148, 1989. Copyright © 1989 AAHPERD, 1900 Association Dr., Reston, VA 22091.[46]

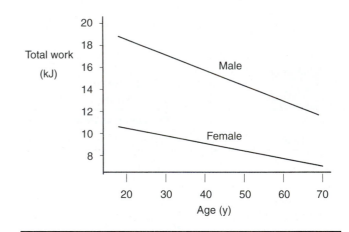

Figure 9.5 The relationship between age and total work (kJ) in males and females 15 y to 70 y of age on an isokinetic cycle ergometer. Modified from Makrides, L., Heigenhauser, G. J. F., McCartney, N., & Jones, N. L. (1985). Maximal short term exercise capacity in healthy subjects aged 15–70 years. *Clinical Science, 69,* 200.

References

1. Abler, P., Foster, C., Thompson, N. N., Crowe, M., Alt, K., Brophy, A., & Palin, W. D. (1986). Determinants of anaerobic muscular performance. *Medicine and Science in Sports and Exercise, 18,* Abstract #3, S1.

2. Ainsworth, B. E., Serfass, R. C., & Leon, A. S. (1993). Effects of recovery duration and blood lactate level on power output during cycling. *Canadian Journal of Applied Physiology, 18,* 19–30.

3. Barnard, R. J. (1975). Warm-up is important for the heart. *Sports Medicine Bulletin, 10*(1), 6.

4. Barnard, R. J., Gardner, G. W., Diaco, N. V., MacAlpin, R. N., & Kattus, A. A. (1973). Cardiovascular responses to sudden strenuous exercise—Heart rate, blood pressure, and ECG. *Journal of Applied Physiology, 34,* 833–837.

5. Bar-Or, O. (1978). A new anaerobic capacity test: Characteristics applications. Proceedings of the 21st World Congress in Sports Medicine at Brasilia.

6. Bar-Or, O. (1981). Le test anaerobie de Wingate. *Symbiosis, 13,* 157–172.

7. Bar-Or, O. (1987). The Wingate Anaerobic Test: An update on methodology, reliability, and validity. *Sports Medicine, 4,* 381–394.

8. Bar-Or, O. (1994). *Testing of anaerobic performance by the Wingate Anaerobic Test.* Bloomington, IL: ERS Tech, Inc.

9. Bar-Or, O., Berman, L., & Salsberg, A. (1992). An abbreviated Wingate. Anaerobic Test for women and men of advanced age. *Medicine and Science in Sports and Exercise, 24,* Abstract, S22.

10. Bar-Or, O., Dotan, R., & Inbar, O. (1977). A 30-second all-out ergometric test: Its reliability and validity for anaerobic capacity. *Israel Journal of Medical Science, 13,* Abstract, 326.

11. Bar-Or, O., & Inbar, O. (1978). Relationships among anaerobic capacity, sprint and middle distance running of school children. In R. J. Shephard & H. Lavallee (Eds.), *Physical fitness assessment—Principles, practice and application,* (pp. 142–147). Springfield, IL: Charles C Thomas.

12. Beld, K., Skinner, J. S., & Tran, Z. V. (1989). Load optimization for peak and mean power output on the Wingate Anaerobic Test. *Medicine and Science in Sports and Exercise, 21* (Suppl., 2), Abstract #164, S28.

13. Bogdanis, G. C., Nevill, M. E., Boobis, L. H., & Lakomy, H. K. A. (1996). Contribution of phosphocreatine and aerobic metabolism to energy supply during repeated sprint exercise. *Journal of Applied Physiology, 80,* 876–884.

14. Bradley, A. L., & Ball, T. E. (1992). The Wingate Test: Effect of load on the power outputs of female athletes and nonathletes. *Journal of Applied Sport Science Research, 6,* 193–199.

15. Coggan, A. R., & Costill, D. L. (1983). Day-to-day variability of three bicycle ergometer tests of anaerobic power. *Medicine and Science in Sports and Exercise, 15,* Abstract #1, 141.

16. Coleman, S. G. S., & Hale, T. (1998). The effect of different calculation methods of flywheel parameters on the Wingate Anaerobic Test. *Canadian Journal of Applied Physiology, 23,* 409–417.

17. Coleman, S. G. S., Hale, T., & Hamley, E. J. (1986). Correct power output in the Wingate Anaerobic Test. In *Kinanthropometry III* (pp. 308–309). London: E. & F. N. Spon.

18. Cumming, G. (1972). Correlation of athletic performance and aerobic power in 12 to 17-year old children with bone age, calf muscle, total body potassium, heart volume and two indices of anaerobic power. *Proceedings of the Fourth International Symposium on Pediatric Work Physiology,* pp. 109–134.

19. Davy, K., Pizza, F., Guastella, P., McGuire, J., & Wygand, J. (1989). Optimal loading of Wingate power testing in conditioned athletes. *Medicine and Science in Sports and Exercise, 21* (Suppl., 2), Abstract #160, S27.

20. Dotan, R., & Bar-Or, O. (1980). Climatic heat stress and performance in the Wingate Anaerobic Test. *European Journal of Applied Physiology, 44,* 237–243.

21. Dotan, R., & Bar-Or, O. (1983). Load optimization for the Wingate Anaerobic Test. *European Journal of Applied Physiology, 51,* 409–417.

22. Esbjornsson, M., Sylven, C., Holm, I., & Jansson, E. (1993). Fast twitch fibers may predict anaerobic performance in both females and males. *International Journal of Sports Medicine, 14,* 257–263.

23. Evans, J. A., & Quinney, H. A. (1981). Determination of resistance settings for anaerobic power testing. *Canadian Journal of Applied Sport Science, 6,* 53–56.

24. Falk, B., Weinstein, Y., Dotan, R., Abramson, D. R., Mann-Segal, D., & Haffman, A. (1996). A treadmill test for sprint running. *Scandinavian Journal of Medicine and Science in Sports, 6,* 259–264.

25. Foss, M. L., & Keteyian, S. J. (1998). *Fox's physiological basis for exercise and sport.* Boston: WCB McGraw-Hill.

26. Gledhill, N., & Jamnik, R. (1995). Determining power outputs for cycle ergometers with different sized flywheels. *Medicine and Science in Sports and Exercise, 27,* 134–135.

27. Green, S. (1995). Measurement of anaerobic work capacities in humans. *Sports Medicine 19,* 32–42.

28. Hebestreit, H., Mimura, K., & Bar-Or, O. (1993). Recovery of anaerobic muscle power following 30 s supramaximal exercise: Comparison between boys and men. *Journal of Applied Physiology, 74,* 2875–2880.

29. Henrich, T. W., Hasson, S. M., Gadberry, W. G., Fang, F., & Barnes, W. S. (1986). The relationship between absolute and relative leg power. *Medicine and Science in Sports and Exercise, 18* (2), Abstract, S6–7.

30. Hill, D. W., & Smith, J. C. (1992). Calculation of aerobic contribution during high intensity exercise. *Research Quarterly for Exercise and Sport, 63,* 85–88.

31. Inbar, O., & Bar-Or, O. (1986). Anaerobic characteristics in male children and adolescents. *Medicine and Science in Sports and Exercise, 18,* 264–269.

32. Inbar, O., Dotan, R., & Bar-Or, O. (1976). Aerobic and anaerobic component of a thirty-second supramaximal cycling test. *Medicine and Science in Sports, 8,* 51.

33. Jacobs, I. (1980). The effects of thermal dehydration on performance of the Wingate Anaerobic Test. *International Journal of Sports Medicine, 1,* 21–24.

34. Jacobs, I., Bar-Or, O., Karlsson, J., Dotan, R., Tesch, P., Kaiser, P., & Inbar, O. (1982). Changes in muscle metabolites in females with 30-s exhaustive exercise. *Medicine and Science in Sports and Exercise,14*(6), 457–460.

35. Jacobs, I., Tesch, P. A., Bar-Or, O., Karlsson, J., & Dotan, R. (1983). Lactate in human skeletal muscle after 10 and 30 s of supramaximal exercise. *Journal of Applied Physiology: Respiratory, Environmental, Exercise Physiology, 55,* 365–367.

36. Kaczkowski, W., Montgomery, D. L., Taylor, A. W., & Klissourous, V. (1982). The relationship between muscle fiber composition and maximal anaerobic power and capacity. *Journal of Sports Medicine and Physical Fitness, 22,* 407–413.

37. Kavanagh, M. F., & Jacobs, I. (1988). Breath-by-breath oxygen consumption during performance of the Wingate Test. *Canadian Journal of Sport Sciences, 13,* 91–93.

38. Kavanagh, M. F., Jacobs, I., Pope, J., Symons, D., & Hermiston, A. (1986). The effects of hypoxia on performance of the Wingate Anaerobic Power Test (WAnT). *Canadian Journal of Applied Sport Sciences, 11,* Abstract 22P.

39. LaVoie, N. F., Dallaire, J., Brayne, S., & Barrett, D. (1984). Anaerobic testing using the Wingate and Evans-Quinney protocols with and without toe stirrups. *Canadian Journal of Applied Sport Sciences, 9,* 1–5.

40. Lemmer, J. T., Fleck, S. J., Wallach, J. M., Fox, S., Burke, E. R., Kearny, J. T., & Storms, W. W. (1995). The effects of albuterol on power output in nonasthmatic athletes. *International Journal of Sports Medicine, 16,* 243–249.

41. MacIntosh, B. R., & MacEachern, P. (1997). Paced effort and all-out 30-second power tests. *International Journal of Sports Medicine, 18,* 594–599.

42. Makrides, L., Heigenhauser, G. J. F., McCartney, N., & Jones, N. L. (1985). Maximal short term exercise capacity in healthy subjects aged 15–70 years. *Clinical Science, 69,* 197–205.

43. Margaria, R., Cerretelli, P., & Mangili, F. (1964). Balance and kinetics of anaerobic energy release during strenuous exercise in man. *Journal of Applied Physiology, 19,* 623–628.

44. Margaria, R., Oliva, D., DiPrampero, P. E., & Cerretelli, P. (1969). Energy utilization in intermittent exercise of supramaximal intensity. *Journal of Applied Physiology, 26,* 752–756.

45. Maud, P. J., & Shultz, B. B. (1986). Gender comparisons in anaerobic power and capacity tests. *British Journal of Sports Medicine, 20,* 51–54.

46. Maud, P. J., & Shultz, B. B. (1989). Norms for the Wingate Anaerobic Test with comparison to another similar test. *Research Quarterly for Exercise and Sport, 60*(2), 144–151.

47. McKenna, M. J., Green, R. A., Shaw, P. F., & Meyer, A. D. (1987). Tests of anaerobic power and capacity. *Australian Journal of Science and Medicine in Sport, 19,* 13–17.

48. Medbo, J. I., & Burgers, S. (1990). Effect of training on the anaerobic capacity. *Medicine and Science in Sports and Exercise, 22,* 501–507.

49. Medbo, J. I., Mohn, A. C., Tabata, I., Bahr, R., Vaage, O., & Sejersted, O. M. (1989). Anaerobic capacity determined by maximal accumulated O_2 deficit. *Journal of Applied Physiology, 64,* 50–60.

50. Medbo, J. I., & Tabata, I. (1993). Anaerobic energy release in working muscle during 30 s to 3 min of exhaustive bicycling. *Journal of Applied Physiology, 75,* 1654–1660.

51. Montgomery, D. L. (1982). The effect of added weight on ice hockey performance. *The Physician and Sportsmedicine, 10,* 91–95, 99.

52. Nicklin, R. C., O'Bryant, H. S., Zehnbauer, T. M., & Collins, M. A. (1990). A computerized method for assessing anaerobic power and work capacity using maximal cycle ergometry. *Journal of Applied Sports Science Research, 4,* 135–140.

53. Pate, R. R., Goodyear, L., Dover, V., Dorociak, J., & McDaniel, J. (1983). Maximal oxygen deficit: A test of anaerobic capacity. *Medicine and Science in Sports and Exercise, 15*(2), Abstract, 121–122.

54. Patton, J. F., & Duggan, A. (1987). An evaluation of tests of anaerobic power. *Aviation Space, and Environmental Medicine, 58,* 237–242.

55. Patton, J. F., Murphy, M. M., & Frederick, F. A. (1985). Maximal power outputs during the Wingate Anaerobic Test. *International Journal of Sports Medicine, 6,* 82–85.

56. Perez, H. R., Wygand, J. W., Kowalski, A., Smith, T. K., & Otto, R. M. (1986). A comparison of the Wingate Power Test to bicycle time trial performance. *Medicine and Science in Sports and Exercise, 18* (Suppl., 2), Abstract #1, S1.

57. Reiser, R. F., Broker, J. P., & Peterson, M. L. (2000). Inertial effects on mechanically braked Wingate power calculations. *Medicine and Science in Sports and Exercise, 32,* 1660–1664.

58. Scott, C. B., Roby, F. B., Lohman, T. G., & Bunt, J. C. (1991). The maximally accumulated oxygen deficit as an indicator of anaerobic capacity. *Medicine and Science in Sports and Exercise, 23,* 618–624.

59. Serresse, O., Lortie, G., Bouchard, C., & Boulay, M. R. (1988). Estimation of the contribution of the various energy systems during maximal work of short duration. *International Journal of Sports Medicine, 9,* 456–460.

60. Shaw, K., Davy, K., Coleman, C., & Kamimukai, C. (1988). Optimal resistance loading of the Wingate Power Test in female softball players. *Medicine and Science in Sports and Exercise, 20* (Suppl., 2), Abstract #105, S18.

61. Song, T. K., Serresse, O., Ama, P., Theriault, G., Boulay, M. R., & Bouchard, C. (1988). Effects of three anaerobic tests on venous blood values. *Medicine and Science in Sports and Exercise, 20* (Suppl., 2), Abstract #229, S39.

62. Tamayo, M., Sucec, A., Phillips, W., Buono, M., Laubach, L., & Frey, M. (1984). The Wingate anaerobic power test, peak blood lactate, and maximal oxygen debt in elite volleyball players: A validation study. *Medicine and Science in Sports and Exercise, 16*(2), Abstract #10, 126.

63. Tanaka, H., Bassett, D. R., Swensen, T. C., & Sampredo, R. M. (1993). Aerobic and anaerobic power characteristics of competitive cyclists in the United States Cycling Federation. *International Journal of Sports Medicine, 14,* 334–338.

64. Tharp, G. D., Newhouse, R. K., Uffelman, L., Thorland, W. G., & Johnson, G. O. (1985). Comparison of sprint and run times with performance on the Wingate Anaerobic Test. *Research Quarterly for Exercise and Sport, 56,* 75–76.

65. Thompson, N. N., Foster, C., Crowe, M., Rogowski, B., & Kaplan, K. (1986). Serial responses of anaerobic muscular performance in competitive athletes. *Medicine and Science in Sports and Exercise, 18* (Suppl.), Abstract, S1.

66. Vandewalle, H., Peres, G., & Monod, H. (1987). Standard anaerobic exercise tests. *Sports Medicine, 4,* 268–289.

67. Weinstein, Y., Bediz, C., Dotan, R., & Falk, B. (1998). Reliability of peak-lactate, heart rate, and plasma volume following the Wingate Test. *Medicine and Science in Sports and Exercise, 30,* 1456–1460.

Form 9.1

Individual Data for Wingate Cycle Test

Name ⬚ Date ⬚ Time ⬚ a.m. ⬚ p.m. ⬚

Age ⬚ y Gender (M or W) ⬚ Ht ⬚ cm Wt ⬚ kg

Meteorological Data

T ⬚ °C (closest 0.1 °C)   RH % ⬚ P_B ⬚ mm Hg × 1.333 = ⬚ hPa (mbar)

Toe Clips: Yes ⬚ No ⬚ seat ht. ⬚ Technician's Initials: ⬚ Force Setter ⬚ Timer ⬚ Counter ⬚

BM (N): Select from Eqs. 9.1a, 9.1b, 9.1c (circle selection)

Eq. 9.1a: BM (N) ≈ 10 × kg; 10 × ⬚ kg ≈ ⬚ N

Eq. 9.1b: BM (N) ≈ 9.8 × kg; 9.8 × ⬚ kg ≈ ⬚ N

Eq. 9.1c: BM (N) = 9.80665 × kg; 9.80665 × kg = ⬚ N

Force (F) Setting: Select from Eqs. 9.2, 9.3, 9.4, 9.5, 9.6 (circle selection)

Eq. 9.2 (Women): F (N) = BM (N) × 0.086 = ⬚ N

Eq. 9.3 (Men): F (N) = BM (N) × 0.090 = ⬚ N

Eq. 9.4 (Anaerobic Athletes): F (N) = BM (N) × 0.090 to 0.10 = ⬚

Eq. 9.5: Leg F (N) = BM (N) × 0.075 = ⬚ N Children, Older Adults, Sedentary.

Eq. 9.6: Arm F (N) = BM (N) × 0.05 = ⬚ N Also used for leg-injured persons.

Time Interval (5 s)	0–5	5–10	10–15	15–20	20–25	25–30	Total
Pedal Revolutions (rev$_{max}$; circle highest)							

Pk-AnP (N·m·s⁻¹; W)

Eq. 9.7: Pk-AnP $(N \cdot m \cdot s^{-1}; W)$ = F-setting (N) × $\dfrac{(rev_{max} \times 6 \text{ m}^a)}{5 \text{ s}}$

=

Relative-pk-AnP (W·kg⁻¹)

Eq. 9.8: rel-pk-AnP $(W \cdot kg^{-1})$ = W ÷ kg BM =

Total Work (w):

Eq. 9.9: w $(N \cdot m; J)$ = N × rev in 30 s × 6 m; kJ = J ÷ 1000 = ☐ kJ (to closest tenth)

=

Relative Total Work (rel-w):

Eq. 9.10: rel-w $(J \cdot kg^{-1})$ = w (J) ÷ BM (kg); kJ·kg⁻¹ = ☐

Mean Anaerobic Power (M-AnP):

Eq. 9.11: M-AnP $(W; J \cdot s^{-1})$ = w (J) ÷ 30 s =

Relative Mean Anaerobic Power (rel-M-AnP):

Eq. 9.12: rel-M-AnP $(W \cdot kg^{-1})$ = M-AnP (W) ÷ BM (kg) =

Fatigue Index (FI):

Eq. 9.13: FI (%) = $\dfrac{(\text{pk-AnP–lowest AnP})}{\text{pk-AnP}} \times 100$

(see pk–AnP at top of this form) lowest AnP (W) = $\dfrac{\text{F-setting (N)} \times rev_{lowest} \times 6 \text{ m}}{5 \text{ s}}$

=

FI (%) =

ᵃ Use 2.5 m if the ergometer is a Monark arm ergometer.

Form 9.2

Graphic Relationship Between an Individual's Power Output and Time during Wingate Test

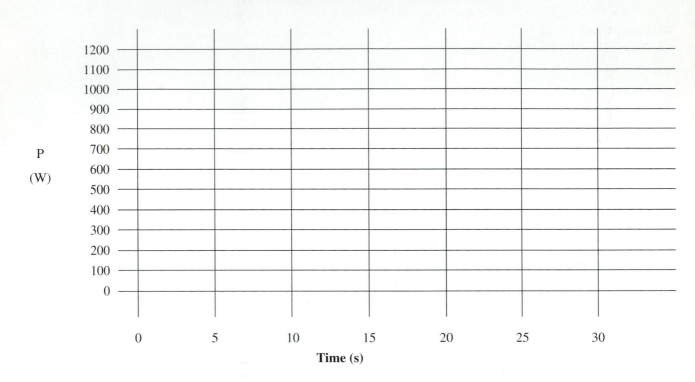

AnP for 0 s to 5th s $= \dfrac{\text{F-setting (N)} \times \text{rev} \times 6\text{m}}{5\text{ s}} =$

AnP for 5th s to 10th s =

AnP for 10th s to 15th s =

AnP for 15th s to 20th s =

AnP for 20th s to 25th s =

AnP for 25th s to 30th s =

Form 9.3

Group Data for Wingate Cycle Test

Initials	Pk-AnP	Rel-Pk-AnP	Total w	M-AnP	Rel-M-AnP	FI
Men	W	W·kg⁻¹	kJ	W	W·kg⁻¹	%
1.						
2.						
3.						
4.						
5.						
6.						
7.						
8.						
9.						
10.						
11.						
M						
Women	W	W·kg⁻¹	kJ	W	W·kg⁻¹	%
1.						
2.						
3.						
4.						
5.						
6.						
7.						
8.						
9.						
10.						
11.						
M						

The anaerobic field/lab step test may be categorized as a power endurance test because the test duration is 60 s at maximal effort. Power endurance activities were defined in Chapter 1 as all-out events lasting from a minimum of 15 s to a maximum of 60 s. The performance of the anaerobic step test is primarily dependent upon the glycolytic pathway (lactate system) of metabolism, but also receives ATP contributions from the phosphagenic system and the oxidative system. Åstrand and Rodahl suggested that maximal efforts involving large muscle groups of one-minute duration require metabolic contributions of about 30 % to 35 % aerobic and 65 % to 70 % anaerobic.[1] They also stated that the highest lactate values occur "in well-trained athletes at the end of competitive events of 1–2 minutes duration." Blood lactates in elite athletes engaging in all-out efforts of power endurance activities have been reported as high as 17 times (16.7 mmol·L^{-1}) the resting values.[4] Thus, the anaerobic step test is expected to elicit moderately high lactate values because of its duration of 1 min.

However, because only one leg is used predominantly during the Anaerobic Step Test, the lactate values are less than maximal. Thus, despite presumably high lactate levels in the local muscle mass of the dominant leg, the lactate levels are diluted in the general circulation because of the smaller muscle mass compared with two-legged exercise. Indeed, the post-anaerobic step test values of finger-pricked blood lactate were about six times greater (~6 mmol·L^{-1}) than resting values (~1 mmol·L^{-1}).[9]

Method

The Method section in the description of most exercise physiology tests includes descriptions of equipment, preparations, procedures, and calculations. The accuracy of the Anaerobic Step Test is described in Box 10.1.

Equipment

The equipment for the Anaerobic Step Test is inexpensive. It requires only a bench (step), a watch with a seconds indicator, a calculator, and an accurate body weighing scale. The step or bench is lower than the 18 in. (45.7 cm) used by the investigators in the original study[3] who adopted the same height as used for the Skubic and Hodgkins[7] aerobic step test. The height of 40 cm (15.75 in.) is the same as that used by males who perform the Forestry Aerobic Step Test.[6]

BOX 10.1 Accuracy

Validity

The number of steps performed by ninth-grade girls in the earlier version of the Anaerobic Step Test was highly correlated ($r = -.824$) with the time for the 600 yd run.[3] In the earlier test, however, they were allowed to change support legs during the test; this would lead, presumably, to higher anaerobic scores. Anaerobic Step Test power (W) for NCAA basketball players increased during their preseason training.[10] This shows that the Anaerobic Step Test is sensitive to the effects of heavy anaerobic training. There appears to be a strong relationship ($r = .87$) between the anaerobic power of the anaerobic step test and lean body mass; there is a moderate relationship ($r = .61$) between the anaerobic step test score and dominant-leg strength.[5] A report from a master's project indicated no relationship between the time in the 400 m run and mean anaerobic power ($r = -.08$), but a significant relationship ($r = -.79$) with the number of steps in 1 min.

Reliability

The test-retest reliability of the Anaerobic Step Test is high ($r > .90$) based upon two tests, each administered no more than one week apart to 30 university students.[9] However, significantly higher scores on the second trials indicate a likely learning effect.

A watch with a seconds indicator (digital or sweep) can be used for timing the test. Laboratory set-clocks are excellent for this test because a buzzer may be sounded at the end of the test. A basic pocket calculator is convenient for making all of the calculations for the Anaerobic Step Test. An accurate platform scale should be used to weigh the performer in stepping attire.

Preparation

In preparation for the Anaerobic Step Test, the stepper should follow the basic plan of the prior exercise regimen. The prior exercise also familiarizes the stepper with the proper stepping technique. The performer should avoid becoming fatigued at any time during the prior exercise.

• 0:00–2:00 min   Walk-in-place at a moderate rate; lift thighs to 90°.

- 2:00–3:00 min   Loosen up (stretch): (1) groin; (2) quadriceps; (3) calf.
- 3:00–5:00 min   Step up and down on a step, stool, or bench using both legs in a traditional four-count cadence at a moderate pace (15 to 20 steps per minute).
- 5:00–7:00 min   Relief interval: Mild walking in place and/or loosening up.

Procedures

The Anaerobic Step Test is a modification of three other step tests—the Forestry[6] and Skubic and Hodgkins[7] *aerobic* step tests and an earlier *anaerobic* step test.[3] There are four major differences between the anaerobic step test and the aerobic step tests—one concerned with the position of the stepper, another concerned with cadence, another concerned with the primary leg, and, finally, another concerned with calculation of power or capacity. Also, the newer anaerobic step test provides more information than the original 18-in. anaerobic step test, because body mass is used to calculate anaerobic power.

Stepping Technique

The stepping technique is different from any of the common aerobic stepping techniques. The technique for the Anaerobic Step Test places a greater emphasis on one leg than the other. The initial position of the stepper is standing alongside the bench, not in front of it. The preferred (dominant leg) rests on the top of the step (bench) in preparation for the start of the test (Figure 10.1a). The other leg, called the free leg, need not touch the bench when the test leg lifts the body (Figure 10.1b).

During the test, each concentric muscle action of the top leg raises the body to the top of the step. The free leg dangles in a straight position during the ascent, and its heel reaches the height of the bench. The foot of the free leg can push off when it contacts the floor. The foot on the step remains there for the duration of the test. The legs and the back must be straightened with each step. In fact, the back should start in a straight position and remain so throughout the test. The arms may be used for balance but cannot be pumped vigorously during the test. Ideally, the arms should be abducted to a penguinlike position at about 30° to 45° from the sides (Figure 10.1b).

The cadence for the test is at a one-two count; "one" is up and "two" is down. This is different from the typical four-count cadence of aerobic step tests. An additional difference is that the performer goes as fast as possible at a pace designed to give a maximum number of steps during the one-minute time period. Thus, the stepper should barely be able to perform another step at the end of one minute.

Measurements

Measurements are made on only three items: (a) the body mass of the performer, (b) the performer's number of steps, and (c) the duration of the test.

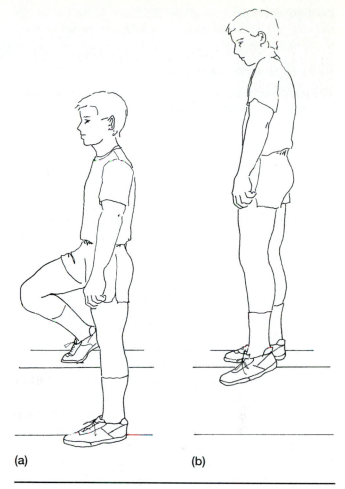

(a)   (b)

Figure 10.1   The positions for the Anaerobic Step Test: (a) the starting position with the body alongside the bench; (b) the "up" position.

Body Mass (BM)   The performer should be weighed to the closest tenth of a kilogram in the same clothes and shoes that are worn for the step test. The total mass is important because the kilograms will be converted to newtons for the calculations of anaerobic power.

Number of Steps   A step is counted for each time the stepper's support leg is straightened and then returned to the starting position. Steps are not counted if the support leg does not straighten or if the back is bent. Technicians count aloud in order to give immediate feedback to the participant. The counting should be as follows: "up-1, up-2, up-3, up-4, up-5," etc. Thus, a full step is considered to be a return to the starting position (down) after the ascent. The technician records the number of steps fully completed in 60 s onto Form 10.1.

Duration   The duration of the test is the same for everyone—1 min. The time begins with the first upward movement of the stepper. The technician should call out the time every 15 s or allow the timer to be visible for the stepper. The laboratory set-clock can be set to buzz at the end of the test.

Recovery from the Anaerobic Step Test

The performer's support leg is likely to be very weak at the end of this test, perhaps, causing a few "buckled" walking steps. The quadriceps of the test leg and the calf of the free leg are the most likely muscle groups to become sore within about 12 h. In order to prevent or minimize delayed onset muscle soreness (DOMS), static stretching exercises should be repeated periodically after the test throughout the day. Based on the enhanced subsequent performance of 60 s events and lactate removal, active recovery, such as walking, mild jogging, or walking in place, is recommended immediately after the test.[11]

Summary of the Procedures

1. Weigh the performer in stepping attire.
2. Convert the body mass to newtons ($\approx N = 10 \times kg$ or $9.8 \times kg$) and record onto Form 10.1.
3. The performer stands alongside the bench with the foot of the dominant leg on the bench.
4. The time begins when the performer starts.
5. The technician counts aloud the number of correct steps.
6. The technician reminds the performer to keep the back straight and the arms in a penguinlike position.
7. The technician states the time every 15 s.
8. At the end of 1 min, the last repetition of a complete step is recorded.
9. The technicians encourage the performer to actively recover immediately and to stretch the leg muscles periodically throughout the day.

Calculations

The norms in Table 10.1 are based on the performers' pacing themselves during the entire 60 s of the test, in contrast to an immediate all-out effort, such as in the Wingate Test. Thus, peak anaerobic power is not measured, only mean/anaerobic power. Also, the work term *anaerobic capacity* may represent total work in 1 min.

By using Equation 10.1, mean anaerobic power (M-AnP) is calculated from the work accomplished in 1 min. The first part of Equation 10.1 represents a person's total work in 1 min. The second part ($\div t$) represents M-AnP, hence the unit of measure watts (W). Eccentric exercise (negative work) is accounted for by the 1.33 factor of bench stepping (see Chapter 2). There is no need to calculate the backward and forward component of work because there is little, if any, such motion in this step test. There is a slight lateral movement in most performers.

$$\text{M-Anp (W)} = (^+w \times 1.33) \div t \qquad \text{Eq. 10.1}$$

Table 10.1 Norms for Anaerobic Step Test in Active Men ($n = 130$) and Women ($n = 70$) Between 18 y and 30 y of Age

Percentile	Men's Power (W)	Women's Power (W)
99	730	490
95	608	407
90	584	391
85	554	370
80	536	358
75	520	348
70	507	339
65	495	331
60	483	322
55	472	315
50	460	307
45	448	299
40	438	292
35	425	283
30	413	275
25	400	266
20	384	258
15	366	244
10	336	223
5	312	207

Source: Petersen, M. (1989). AnP Norms and the relationship between anaerobic power versus leg strength and lean body mass. Master's thesis, California State University, Fullerton, p. 22.

where:

$$^+w = \text{positive work (Force} \times \text{Distance) in 1 min}$$
$$\text{force} = \text{body mass in N}$$
$$\text{distance} = \text{height of step (0.40 m)} \times \text{steps in 1 min}$$
$$1.33 = \text{factor to convert } ^+w \text{ to total work (N·m; J)}$$
$$t = 60 \text{ s}$$

For example, if a 68 kg (680 N) person stepped 50 times in 60 s, then the following calculation would produce the mean anaerobic power:

$$\text{M-AnP (W; N·m·s}^{-1}) = (680 \text{ N} \times 0.40 \text{ m} \times 50 \times 1.33) \div 60 \text{ s}$$
$$= 18\,088 \text{ N·m} \div 60 \text{ s}$$
$$= 301 \text{ N·m·s}^{-1} \text{ or W}$$

Results and Discussion

The mean anaerobic powers of self-selected adults between the ages of 18 y and 30 y ($M = 23$ y) attending a fitness center were 460 W for men and 307 W for women.[5] (See Table 10.1.) In a master's project, a student reported a significant difference between mean anaerobic power of the dominant leg (405 W) versus non-dominant leg (385 W) of high school athletes.

Table 10.2 provides comparative scores from various groups, such as high school athletes, NCAA basketball play-

here. However, roads at 20 % slope or grade are rarely found; for example, interstate highway regulators discourage the construction of roads with more than a 6 % slope. Good treadmills are very expensive, especially research-precision ones. Treadmills with front and side handrails are required for the An-TM tests. A novel treadmill (Gymrol™, France), combined with software, is capable of directly measuring peak and mean anaerobic power.[5] It utilizes a pivoting bar that measures vertical displacement of the runner's center of gravity and a strain gauge to measure horizontal force.

Timer

A seconds-watch, not necessarily one that is capable of measuring tenths of a second, is needed to measure the duration of the performance to the closest second.

Treadmill Protocol

The protocol for the treadmill tests should include a prior exercise and familiarization period, along with a cooldown period (Table 11.1). The prior exercise should consist of a warm-up and loosening-up regimen that mimics the movements of running and stretches the running muscles, respectively. The warm-up should not cause fatigue; some investigators[4,8] did not allow a warm-up for the treadmill runners in their research studies.

The An-TM tests are constant load tests because each one's speed and slope never change throughout the run. The Fast (F) Test should be performed first if two tests are given within one hour. This is because recovery from this shorter test is quicker than the others. However, it is probably wiser to do the tests on separate days so that the Slow Test can be administered first. This gives the performers and technicians some input into the runner's capabilities for the more intimidating Fast Test. For example, if runners in the longer test cannot continue longer than 30 s, they may not be able to run without the use of the handrails at the least, and only a few seconds at the most, on the faster treadmill test. For these latter performers, the speed of the Fast Test might be reduced from 8 mph (12.9 km/h) to the moderate test's 7 mph (11.3 km/h). One or two trials may be run for each performer, depending upon the fatigue of the performer and the administrative considerations of the lab director.

The cooldown period should be done off the treadmill and begin with fast walking and gradually slower walking for a combined time of about 3 min to 5 min.

Procedures

As with all test procedures, technicians must be concerned with the safety and psychological well-being of the participants prior to and during the treadmill test. As with all tests, basic data and meteorological data should be recorded. The key measurement for these tests is the total time that the performer can continue running at the given speed and slope.

Safety

These treadmill tests can induce more psychological distress than any other tests described in this manual. A fast-moving treadmill belt can be intimidating, even to experienced

---

Table 11.1   Protocols for the Slow (S), Moderate (M), and Fast (F) Anaerobic Treadmill Tests (An-TM)

Period	Time (min)	Activity
Prior exercise and familiarization	0:00–10:00	(1) Jog in place; (2) slow jogging; (3) short bouts on level TM: (a) one walk bout at 2 mph (3.2 km/h) and another bout at 4 mph (6.4 km/h) for 10s each; enter and exit the treadmill for each bout; (b) one jogging bout at 6 mph (9.7 km/h) and another bout at 8 mph (12.9 km/h) for 10 s each; enter and exit the treadmill for each bout; (4) short bouts on sloped treadmill: (a) one walk bout at 2 mph (3.2 km/h) at 5 % slope and a walk/jog bout at 4 mph (6.4 km/h) at 10 % slope for 10 s each; enter and exit the treadmill for each bout; (b) one jog/run at 6 mph (9.7 km/h) and at 15 % slope and a run bout at 8 mph (12.9 km/h) at 20 % slope for 5 s each; enter and exit the treadmill for each bout.
Relief interval	10:00–11:00	Slow walking or walking in place

Treadmill Test	Time (min)	Slope (%)	Speed
Slow		20	6 mph (9.6 km·h⁻¹; 160 m·min⁻¹; 2.67 m·s⁻¹; 10 min per mile pace)
Moderate		20	7 mph (11.3 km·h⁻¹; 188 m·min⁻¹; 3.13 m·s⁻¹; 8.6 min per mile pace)
Fast		20	8 mph (12.9 km·h⁻¹; 215 m·min⁻¹; 3.58 m·s⁻¹; 7.5 min per mile pace)
CoolDown	3:00–5:00		Gradually slower jogging and walking; stretching

treadmill users. Thus, the technician's sensitivity to the performers' fears should include a sincere effort to familiarize them with the safe and proper technique of using the handrails to get on and off the fast-moving treadmill belt. Participants should be given time to practice this procedure. The key to the runners' mental security is their contact with the handrails. If a person is too fearful to let go of the handrail, then the test should be modified to a speed that the performer selects. The technician in control of the treadmill should be prepared to stop the treadmill as soon as the runner touches the handrails in preparation of exiting, while a spotter at the rear end of the treadmill should be prepared to support the runner if necessary. A hip-belt harness attached from the runner to the treadmill rails or the ceiling is ideal for maximizing safety and promoting uninhibited efforts.

Measurements

Except for the basic and meteorological data, there is only one measurement—the time (to the closest second) spent at the prescribed speed and slope of the treadmill. The timer starts the clock as soon as the performer, while running, releases the handrails. The timer stops the watch when the runner takes hold of the handrails in preparation for exiting from the treadmill belt. If two trials are given, the better time is used for statistical purposes. In summary, the checklist of procedures is as follows:

1. Record the performer's weight in running attire onto Form 11.1.
2. The runner follows an appropriate prior exercise and familiarization regimen similar to the one presented in Table 11.1.
3. A technician (*protocoller*) places the treadmill at the prescribed speed for the selected test (slow = 6 mph or 2.67 m·s⁻¹; moderate = 7 mph or 3.13 m·s⁻¹; fast = 8 mph or 3.58 m·s⁻¹) and slope (20 %).
4. With hands on the rails, the performer either straddles the treadmill's belt or stands with both feet on one side of the treadmill belt.
5. With hands still holding onto the rails, the performer steps onto the moving treadmill belt.
6. A technician (timer) starts the watch as soon as the runner's hands release the handrail.
7. The timer stops the seconds-watch as soon as the runner touches the handrails.
8. Also at this time, the protocoller stops the treadmill.
9. The time is recorded to the closest second on Form 11.1.
10. The performer cools down (see Table 11.1).

Calculations

The field of exercise physiology qualifies as a science because it quantifies exercise. The calculation of anaerobic work may be made from the time spent on the treadmill, the slope and speed of the treadmill, and the mass of the attired runner. The percent grade or slope is defined as the pro-

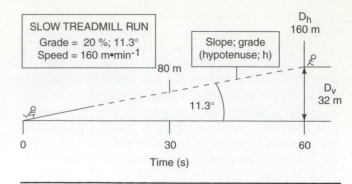

Figure 11.1 If a runner continues to run at a grade of 20 % and a speed of 160 m·min⁻¹ until exhaustion at the 60th s, the projected vertical distance (D_v) of the runner is 20 % of the covered distance of the treadmill belt/runner (hypotenuse; D_h = 160 m). Thus, the runner in this case would be projected vertically to a height of 32 m. If the runner stopped in 30 s, then the hypotenuse distance would be 80 m and the vertical distance would be 20 % of 80 m, which is equal to 16 m.

jected distance of the vertical rise (D_v) per 100 units of the belt's travel. Running up a 20 % slope simply means that, for every 100 m traveled by the treadmill's belt, hence runner, there will be a vertical rise of 20 m (see Figure 11.1). Sometimes the slope is expressed in degrees, but the value is not the same as the percent value. The degree number is always less than the percent number.

Equation 11.1 for calculating the work on a treadmill is similar to the work equation in Chapter 1, except that the vertical distance factor has been emphasized by the subscript *v*:

$$w = F \times D_v \qquad \text{Eq. 11.1}$$

where:

w = work in N·m or J

F = force (mass of attired performer) in N

where:

1 kg ≈ 10 N

≈ 9.8 N

= 9.80665 N

D_v = projected vertical distance in m

The projected vertical distance (D_v) of the runner is found trigonometrically by dividing the % slope by 100 and then multiplying by the hypotenuse distance (D_h), as in Equation 11.2[a] (see Figure 11.1).

---

[a]Trigonometry is the mathematical study of triangles. A right triangle is formed when the runner's projected vertical distance (side "a" of the triangle) is connected to the top of the hypotenuse (slope; side "c") and the horizontal baseline (side "b"). The angle (theta) formed by the slope (grade) determines the percent slope. The percent slope equals the sine (sin) of angle theta multiplied by 100. The sine equals the ratio of side "a" (projected vertical distance) to side "c" (hypotenuse); thus sine theta = D_v/D_h.

$$D_v = (\% \text{ slope} / 100) \times D_h \qquad \text{Eq. 11.2}$$

The hypotenuse distance is found by multiplying the speed by the total time, as in Equation 11.3.

$$D_h = \text{mph or km·h}^{-1} \text{ or m·min}^{-1} \qquad \text{Eq. 11.3}$$
$$\text{or m·s}^{-1} \times t \text{ (h; min; s, respectively)}$$

where t = time in decimal hours or minutes or whole seconds.

For anaerobic treadmill tests, it is simpler to convert mph to m·min^{-1} or m·s^{-1} by using the conversion factors:

$$1 \text{ mph} \approx 27 \text{ m·min}^{-1} \approx 0.45 \text{ m·s}^{-1}$$

$$1 \text{ mph} = 26.8 \text{ m·min}^{-1} = 0.447 \text{ m·s}^{-1}$$

The calculation of anaerobic work (An-w) for a 68-kg person running at a 20 % grade and 8 mph (12.9 km·h^{-1} or 216 m·min^{-1} or 3.6 m·s^{-1}) for 60 s (1.0 min) is made as follows when using approximate conversions:

$$\text{An-w} = F \times D_v = F \times \text{decimal slope} \times D_h$$

$$= 680 \text{ N} \times (0.20 \times 216 \text{ m·min}^{-1}) \times 1.0 \text{ min}$$

$$\text{or } 680 \text{ N} \times (0.20 \times 3.6 \text{ m·s}^{-1}) \times 60 \text{ s}$$

$$= 680 \text{ N} \times 43.2 \text{ m·min}^{-1} \times 1.0 \text{ min}$$

$$\text{or } 680 \text{ N} \times 0.72 \text{ m·s}^{-1} \times 60 \text{ s}$$

$$= 29\ 376 \text{ N·m or J; or } 29.4 \text{ kJ}^{b}$$

Results and Discussion

Norms, especially expressed in total work units, are needed for these treadmill tests. Table 11.2 presents unpublished percentiles from a master's project (2000) for time and anaerobic work in men ages 18 y to 24 y who performed the Fast An-TM Test. The men averaged 34 s ($n = 105$) for the 8 mph (12.9 km·h^{-1}) test and accomplished an average work total of 18.6 kJ ($n = 71$). Those presented in Table 11.3 are not *true* norms due to the small samples from the typical population and the lack of true work units. Thus, they are presented for comparative, not classification, purposes. Men appear to endure about two times longer than women on the Slow Anaerobic Test and about three times longer than women on the Fast Anaerobic Treadmill Test.

Running performance for such competitive distances as the 200 m, 300 m, and 400 m are predominantly anaerobic events. A pair of investigators used the accumulated oxygen deficit (AOD) to estimate the energy contribution by the aerobic pathway for treadmill simulated 200 m, 400 m, and 800 m run events in highly trained runners.[18] AOD is calculated by subtracting the accumulated oxygen consumption from the accumulated oxygen demand for the duration of each run. For the 200 m run, the aerobic

---

[b]If using the exact conversions for N and m·min^{-1} or m·s^{-1}, then the total work is 28 677 J or 28.7 kJ.

| Table 11.2 | Percentiles for Time ($n = 105$) and Anaerobic Work ($n = 71$) for Men, Ages 18 y to 24 y, Performing the Fast An-TM Test |

Percentile	Time (s)	Anaerobic Work (kJ)	Fitness Category
95	54	28.2	High
90	50	25.3	
85	46	23.8	
80	42	22.4	
75	41	21.5	Above average
70	39	21.1	
65	37	20.4	
60	36	19.8	
55	35	19.4	Average
50	33	18.6	
45	32	17.7	
40	30	17.3	
35	29	16.4	Below average
30	28	15.6	
25	27	15.2	
20	23	15.0	
15	21	12.6	Low
10	19	10.9	
5	18	10.2	
Mean	33.6	18.64	
SD	11.3	5.73	

Source: Calmelot, R. (2000). Unpublished master's project at California State University, Fullerton.

| Table 11.3 | Comparative Scores for the Anaerobic Treadmill Tests |

Reference	Group	Time(s)
	Slow Test (6 mph; 9.6 km·h^{-1})	
($n = 46$)[a]	Men PE majors	78.4 ($R = 49–167$)
($n = 34$)[a]	Women PE majors	36.8 ($R = 20–58$)
#11	Dinghy sailors	65; $SD = 16$
	Fast Test (8 mph; 12.9 km·h^{-1})	
($n = 38$)[a]	Men PE majors	33 ($R = 18–66$)
($n = 14$)[a]	Women PE majors	14[b] ($R = 8–22$)
($n = 105$)	College men[c]	33.6; $SD = 11.3$ $R = 6–62$
#1 ($n = 10$)	National alpine skiers	77
($n = 22$)	Less elite club skiers	56
#4 ($n = 8$)	Normal males	
	Pretraining:	52; $SD = 13$
	Posttraining:	64
#8 ($n = 11$)	College ice hockey forwards	54; $SD = 15$
#6 ($n = 16$)	Elite jr. ice hockey	
	Preseason	64
	Postseason	75
#10 ($n = 6$)	Elite 800 m runners	114
#13 ($n = 6$)	Elite athletes	82; $SD = 20$
#14	Olympic soccer players	92; $SD = 10$ ($R = 68–102$)
	Moderate Test (7 mph; 11.3 km·h^{-1})	
($n = 15$)[a]	Women kines. majors	20.4
#15 (7 mph)	Female basketball players	39; $SEM = 2.2$

Note: [a]Unpublished data. [b]Some women were not included because of zero seconds. [c]Unpublished master's project (2000). R = range

pathway contributed 29 % of the energy; hence, the anaerobic pathway contributed 71 %. The aerobic contribution for the 400 m run was 43 %—hence, 57 % by the anaerobic pathway. For the 800 m run, the aerobic pathway contributed 84 % of the energy; hence, the anaerobic pathway contributed only 16 % of the total energy. The treadmill tests described in this chapter often produce run times that presumably would require anaerobic contributions falling between the percentages of 16 % and 71 % reported for the 800 m and 200 m runs, respectively. The lower percentage (16 %), which was equivalent to a time of 113 s by the elite runners, was quite lower than the 40 % contribution determined by another group of investigators.[17] One reviewer mentioned a maximum duration of 60 s as a criterion to qualify as a valid anaerobic test.[7] He suggested that times beyond 60 s would likely exceed 50 % energy contribution by the aerobic pathway. Thus, it appears that, if runners exceed 60 s on any of the An-TM tests, then the speed and/or the slope should be increased in order to get a true anaerobic fitness evaluation of power endurance. However, times between 60 s and 120 s should be a valid indicator of mixed endurance, which I define as all-out activities lasting between 60 s and 120 s.

References

1. Bouchard, C., Taylor, A. W., Simoneau, J. A., & Dulac, S. (1991). Testing anaerobic power and capacity. In J. D. MacDougall, H. A. Wenger, & H. J. Green (Eds.), *Physiological testing of the high performance athlete.* Champaign, IL: Human Kinetics.

2. Brown, S. L., & Wilkinson, J. G. (1983). Characteristics of national, divisional, and club male Alpine ski racers. *Medicine and Science in Sports and Exercise, 15,* 491–495.

3. Costill, D. L., Barnett, A., Sharp, R., Fink, W. J., & Katz, A. (1983). Leg muscle pH following sprint running. *Medicine and Science in Sports and Exercise, 15,* 325–329.

4. Cunningham, D. A., & Faulkner, J. A. (1969). The effect of training on aerobic and anaerobic metabolism during a short exhaustive run. *Medicine and Science in Sports and Exercise, 1,* 65–69.

5. Falk, B., Weinstein, Y., Dotan, R., Abramson, D. A., Mann-Segal, D., & Hoffman, J. R. A treadmill test of sprint running. *Scandinavian Journal of Medicine and Science in Sports, 6,* 259–264.

6. Green, H. J., & Houston, M. E. (1975). Effect of a season of ice hockey on energy capacities and associated functions. *Medicine and Science in Sports and Exercise, 7,* 299–303.

7. Green, S. (1995). Measurement of anaerobic work capacities in humans. *Sports Medicine, 19,* 32–42.

8. Houston, M. E., & Green, H. J. (1976). Physiological and anthropometric characteristics of elite Canadian ice hockey players. *Journal of Sportsmedicine and Physical Fitness, 16,* 123–128.

9. Mackova, E. V., Melichna, J., Vondra, K., Jurimae, T., Tomas, P., & Novak, J. (1985). The relationship between anaerobic performance and muscle metabolic capacity and fibre distribution. *European Journal of Applied Physiology, 54,* 413–415.

10. McKenzie, D. C., Parkhouse, W. S., & Hearst, W. D. (1982). Anaerobic performance characteristics of elite Canadian 800 meter runners. *Canadian Journal of Applied Sports Science, 7,* 158–160.

11. Niinimaa, V., Wright, G., Shephard, R. J., & Clarke, J. (1977). Characteristics of the successful dinghy sailor. *Journal of Sportsmedicine and Physical Fitness, 17,* 83–96.

12. Paavolainen, L. M., Nummela, A. T., & Rusko, H. K. (1999). Neuromuscular characteristics and muscle power as determinants of 5-km running performance. *Medicine and Science in Sports and Exercise, 31,* 124–130.

13. Parkhouse, W. S., & McKenzie, D. C. (1983). Anaerobic capacity assessment of elite athletes. *Medicine and Science in Sports and Exercise, 15,* Abstract, 142.

14. Rhodes, E. C., Mosber, R. E., McKenzie, D. C., Franks, J. M., Potts, J. E., & Wenger, H. A. (1986). Physiological profiles of the Canadian Olympic Soccer Team. *Canadian Journal of Applied Sport Sciences, 11,* 31–36.

15. Rlezebos, M. L., Paterson, D. H., Hall, C. R., & Yuhasz, S. (1983). Relationship of selected variables to performance in women's basketball. *Canadian Journal of Applied Sports Sciences, 8,* 34–40.

16. Rusko, H., Nummela, A., & Mero, A. (1993). A new method for the evaluation of anaerobic running power in athletes. *European Journal of Applied Physiology, 66,* 97–101.

17. Scott, C. B., Roby, F. B., Lohman, T. G., & Bunt, J. C. (1991). The maximally accumulated oxygen deficit as an indicator of anaerobic capacity. *Medicine and Science in Sports and Exercise, 23,* 618–624.

18. Spencer, M. R., & Gastin, P. B. (2001). Energy system contribution during 200- to 1500-m running in highly trained athletes. *Medicine and Science in Sports and Exercise, 33,* 157–162.

19. Thomson, J. M., & Garvie, K. J. (1981). A laboratory method for determination of anaerobic energy expenditure during sprinting. *Canadian Journal of Applied Sport Science, 6,* 21–26.

Form 11.1

Individual Data for Treadmill Anaerobic Tests

Name [ ] Date [ ] Time [ ] A.M. [ ] P.M. [ ]

Age [ ] y   Gender (M or W) [ ]   Ht [ ] cm   Wt [ ] kg   [ ] N   Tech. Initials [ ]

Meteorological Data

T [ ] °C (closest 0.1 °C)   RH % [ ] P_B [ ] mm Hg × 1.333 = [ ] hPa

Slow-Test Time
(6 mph; 9.6 km·h⁻¹)

Trial 1 [ ] s (closest s)

Trial 2 [ ] s (Optional)

Moderate-Test Time
(7 mph; 11.3 km·h⁻¹)

[ ] s

[ ] s (Optional)

Fast-Test Time
(8 mph; 12.9 km·h⁻¹)

[ ] s

[ ] s (Optional)

Slow-Test Work (N·m; J): w = F × D$_v$ (Eq 11.1)

D_h = 2.67 m·s⁻¹ × [ ] s = [ ] m (Eq. 11.3)[a]

D_v = 0.2 × [ ] m = [ ] m D_v = 20 % slope/100 × D_h (Eq. 11.2)

w = F [ ] N × D$_v$ [ ] m = [ ] N·m; J ÷ 1000 = [ ] kJ (closest tenth)

Moderate-Test Work (N·m; J): w = F × D$_v$ (Eq 11.1)

D_h = 3.13 m·s⁻¹ × [ ] s = [ ] m (Eq. 11.3)[a]

D_v = 0.2 × [ ] m = [ ] m D_v = 20 % slope/100 × D_h (Eq. 11.2)

w = F [ ] N × D$_v$ [ ] m = [ ] N·m; J ÷ 1000 = [ ] kJ (closest tenth)

Fast-Test Work (N·m; J): w = F × D$_v$ (Eq 11.1)

D_h = 3.58 m·s⁻¹ × [ ] s = [ ] m (Eq. 11.3)[a]

D_v = 0.2 × [ ] m = [ ] m D_v = 20 % slope/100 × D_h (Eq. 11.2)

w = F [ ] N × D$_v$ [ ] m = [ ] N·m; J ÷ 1000 = [ ] kJ (closest tenth)

[a] Speed values are based on exact conversion.

Form 11.2

Group Data for Anaerobic TM Tests

MEN Initials	Slow Test (6 mph)	Moderate Test (7 mph; 11.3 km·h⁻¹)	Fast Test (8 mph)	WOMEN Initials	Slow Test (6 mph)	Moderate Test (7 mph; 11.3 km·h⁻¹)	Fast Test (8 mph)
1.				1.			
2.				2.			
3.				3.			
4.				4.			
5.				5.			
6.				6.			
7.				7.			
8.				8.			
9.				9.			
10.				10.			
11.				11.			
12.				12.			
13.				13.			
14.				14.			
15.				15.			
16.				16.			
17.				17.			
18.				18.			
19.				19.			
20.				20.			
M				M			
R				R			

The men's and women's TIME (s) headers span the Slow Test, Moderate Test, and Fast Test columns respectively.

Aerobic tests measure aerobic power, a term that is often used synonymously with *cardiovascular endurance and cardiorespiratory fitness.* Aerobic power is of primary importance in performing exercise that continues beyond 2 min and contributes substantially to mixed endurance, those continuous activities lasting between 1 min and 2 min. Most aerobic power tests require submaximal bouts of exercise that vary in duration. Some aerobic tests, however, require the participant to progress to maximal or supramaximal intensities—that is, intensities at or above maximal oxygen consumption. For example, some stepping tests conclude in 3 min. Other aerobic tests, such as the Texas Steady-State Run test, may require up to 30 min.[3] Direct measures of maximal oxygen consumption ($\dot{V}O_2$max) usually take from 5 min to 9 min. Surprisingly, valid estimates of aerobic power are available that require no exercise testing at all of low to moderately fit persons. These estimates usually consider such factors as gender, age, percent fat (or body mass index), and a questionnaire that allows a rating for habitual physical activity.[1,5,6]

Questionnaires may also help ensure that exercise testing is safe for the participant. For example, the Physical Activity Readiness Questionnaire (PAR-Q, 1994; see Appendix E) asks seven questions pertaining to

1. The doctor's assessment of the prospective participant's heart condition and any subsequent doctor's limitations of the participant's physical activity
2. Chest pain at exercise
3. Chest pain during the previous month without exercising
4. Loss of balance due to dizziness or loss of consciousness
5. Bone or joint problems
6. Current use of prescription drugs
7. Participant's opinion of any possible problems associated with exercise.[8]

The importance of aerobic fitness is accentuated by the reported association of low cardiovascular (aerobic) endurance fitness and increased coronary heart disease risk factors.[4,7] This association is especially disheartening in light of reports that most Americans (> 60 %) do not exercise regularly.[2] The existing norms for the run/walk tests allow us to classify the aerobic fitness level of persons and to enhance the individuality of a possible exercise prescription.

References

1. Ainsworth, B. E., Richardson, M. T., Jacobs, D. R., & Leon, A. S. (1992). Prediction of cardiorespiratory fitness using physical activity questionnaire data. *Medicine, Exercise, Nutrition Health, 1,* 75–82.
2. American College of Sports Medicine. (2000). *ACSM's guidelines for exercise testing and prescription.* Philadelphia: Lippincott Williams & Wilkins.
3. Baumgartner, T. A., & Jackson, A. S. (1991). *Measurement for evaluation in physical education and exercise science.* Dubuque, IA: Wm C. Brown.
4. Blair, S. N., & Morrow, M. S. (1997). Surgeon general's report on physical fitness: The inside story. *ACSM's Health & Fitness Journal, 1*(1), 14–18.
5. Heil, D. P., Freedson, P. S., Ahlquist, L. E., Price, J., & Rippe, J. M. (1995). Nonexercise regression models to estimate peak oxygen consumption. *Medicine and Science in Sports and Exercise, 27,* 599–606.
6. Jackson, A. S., Blair, S. N., Mahar, M. T., Wier, L. T., Ross, R. M., & Stuteville, J. E. (1990). Prediction of functional aerobic capacity without exercise testing. *Medicine and Science in Sports and Exercise, 22,* 863–870.

7. Pate, R. R., Pratt, M., Blair, S. N., Haskell, W. L., Macera, C. A., Bouchard, C., Buchner, D., Ettinger, W., Heath, G. W., King, A. C., et al. (1995). Physical activity and public health: A recommendation from the Centers for Disease Control and Prevention and the American College of Sports Medicine. *JAMA: The Journal of the American Medical Association, 273,* 402–407.

8. Thomas, S., Reading, J., & Shephard, R. J. (1992). Revision of the Physical Activity Readiness Questionnaire (PAR-Q). *Canadian Journal of Sport Science, 17,* 338–345.

AEROBIC RUNNING AND WALKING

Chapter 12 discusses three popular field tests—the 1.5 Mile/12 Minute Test, the AAHPERD Run Test, and the Rockport Walk Test. These are good examples of field tests due to the use of minimal equipment, their application to large groups, and their ease of administration. Aerobic run/walk tests are the most common field tests of cardiorespiratory fitness.[26] Despite their value in measuring functional fitness, these field tests are not usually considered replacement tests for the direct measurement of oxygen consumption in research studies. A portion of this chapter includes a discussion of some physiological measures, such as heart rate and breathing frequency, that can be estimated or measured while performing the aerobic run tests.

Dr. Kenneth Cooper developed the 12 Minute Test from Balke's[10] original 15 Minute Run Test. Cooper's test includes the 12 min and 1.5 mi versions. The 1.5 Mile/12 Minute Test is routinely used by such organizations as the U.S. Navy, U.S. Air Force, and the American Alliance for Health, Physical Education, Recreation and Dance (AAHPERD).

The AAHPERD Run Test includes both versions of Cooper's Test, in addition to the 1.0 Mile and 9 Minute Run Tests[2] (Table 12.1). The short versions of the AAHPERD Run Tests are recommended for children between the ages of 5 y and 12 y, whereas adolescents 13 y to 17 y and college students have the option of performing any of the four versions of the AAHPERD Aerobic Run Test.

Tests that prescribe walking may be most prudent for middle-age and older adults because walking is a moderate exercise that is less stressful to the joints. The Ameri-can College of Sports Medicine does not feel a need to recommend a medical examination for apparently healthy older adults prior to performing tests of moderate exercise.[5] The Rockport 1.0 Mile Walk Test predicts aerobic fitness for ages ranging from 30 y to 69 y.[45] This test incorporates the time to finish the walk, exercise heart rate, body mass, age, and gender into an equation to predict aerobic fitness. Although not discussed here, the George-Fisher Jogging Test utilizes the same factors as the Rockport Test but applies them more specifically to physically fit college-age persons.[34,35,36]

Purpose of the Aerobic Run/Walk Tests

The purpose of Aerobic Run Tests as performed in *Exercise Physiology Laboratory Manual* is slightly different from what Dr. Cooper originally intended for the general public. He sought to enhance the exercise habits of the population.

Our laboratory objectives also include Cooper's objective but add objectives related to the physiological effects of running and walking, as well as those related to the administrative aspects of the tests.

Physiological Rationale for the Aerobic Run/Walk Tests

Oxidative metabolism predominates for events that last for about two or more minutes. A pair of investigators estimated that highly trained runners performing the 1500 m ($\approx$ 100 m short of one mile) in 3 min 55 s received 84 % of their energy from the aerobic pathway.[61] Thus, the aerobic pathway would dominate in the times required for the one mile and 1.5 mile tests. Oxygen is transported first by the respiratory (pulmonary) system to the cardiovascular system, and then from there to the contracting muscles. The muscles consume the oxygen in order to provide sufficient amounts of adenosine triphosphate (ATP) for the myosin filaments to pull the actin filaments; the pulling within the muscles causes muscle action. Without a sufficient amount of oxygen, there is not enough ATP produced to sustain muscular action beyond a couple minutes. Thus, other factors being equal, the runner who can supply the highest rate of oxygen to the muscles will be able to perform aerobic exercise at a faster speed. The highest possible rate of oxygen consumption is called the maximal oxygen consumption ($\dot{V}O_2max$).

Table 12.1	Suitability of Different Versions of Aerobic Run/Walk Tests
Age (y) and Fitness Status	**Aerobic Run/Walk Test**
All ages if apparently healthy and habitual exerciser	1.5 Mile Run for time or 12 min Run for distance (Cooper's test)
All ages if apparently healthy (no medical exam required)	Rockport Walk Test (1.0 mi)
College age or 13 y to 17 y	1.5 Mile/12 Min or 1.0 Mile/9 Min Run (AAHPERD test)
	George-Fisher Jogging Test
5 y to 12 y	1.0 Mile Run for time or 9 Min Run for distance (AAHPERD test)

Method

The Method section includes descriptions of the (1) facility, (2) equipment, and (3) procedures and calculations. Comments pertaining to the accuracy of run/walk tests are in Box 12.1.

Facility

The facility requires a level terrain that has accurately measured distances. Most new track facilities are ovals of 400 m, which means that each lap on the metric track is 2.5 yd shorter than the older 440 yd American ovals (Figure 12.2). This means that if performing on a metric track, the runner or walker must go 10 yd (9 m) beyond 4 laps for the 1.0 Mile Test, and 15 yd (14 m) beyond for the 1.5 Mile Test. The two straightaways and the turns of a quarter-mile (440 yd) track are usually 110 yds. Thus, any distance halfway between any one of the four intervals is 55 yd. Also, keep in mind that the 400 m or 440 yd distance for one lap applies only to the inside lane (about 1 ft from the curb). A treadmill is optional when performing the Rockport Walk Test.[51,66]

Equipment

The only piece of equipment that is absolutely necessary to conduct the Aerobic Run/Walk Tests is a watch with a seconds indicator. For greater accuracy in measuring heart rate for the Rockport Test, electronic monitoring using miniature transmitters and receivers (e.g., Polar™) are practical[47] and inexpensive (about $120). These monitors have a transmitting device and chest electrodes built into the chest strap. A receiver, which also serves other functions, digitally displays the updated heart rate every five seconds. The runner or walker wears the strap and the "wristwatch" receiver, or the technician, within five feet of the participant, can hold the receiver ("wristwatch"). Another practical device is the hand-held baton, which can be grasped by a runner crossing the finish line. It provides a digital display of the heart rate within a few seconds (Instapulse™).

    Large groups may be tested easily on these tests. At the "Go!" signal, all participants begin running or walking, and the timer starts the clock. At the end of either the prescribed time or the prescribed distance, the timer yells out the times so that the participants or recorders can write down their times or distances.

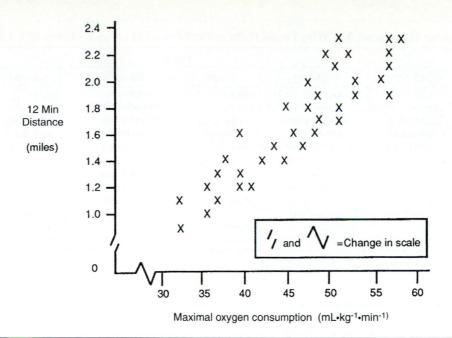

Figure 12.1 The relationship between the distance run in 12 minutes and maximal oxygen consumption is direct (positive; linear).

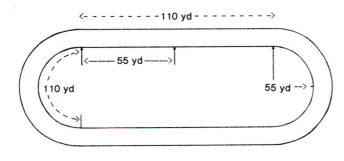

Figure 12.2 Layout of a quarter-mile (440 yd; 402.3 m) track. The straightaways and turns are 110 yd each; thus, the midpoints between these are 55 yd each (1 yd = 0.914 m; 1 m = 1.0936 yd).

Procedures and Calculations for the Aerobic Run/Walk Tests

It is probably prudent to administer the PAR-Q questionnaire (see Appendix E), or other non-exercise predictors of cardiorespiratory endurance, prior to any of the run/walk tests. The questionnaires may disclose persons who deserve cautionary measures or special guidance.[7,64] Also, the data from the questionnaires can be compared to the run/walk results.[1,41,42]

The primary measurement for both the 1.5 Mile Run Test and the 1.0 Mile Run Test is time in minutes and seconds. Based on performance time, each participant's aerobic fitness category, percentile, or maximal oxygen consumption ($\dot{V}O_2$max) may be estimated (Tables 12.2–12.5). The primary measurement for the 9 Min and 12 Min Tests is distance in yards or meters. Runners of the 9 Minute and

Table 12.2	1.5 Mile Times and Fitness Categories for Active College Males and Females 17 y to 35 y of Age	
Fitness Category	**Time (min:s), Ages 17 y to 25 y**	**Time (min:s), Ages 26 y to 35 y**
Superior		
Females	< 10:30	< 11:30
Males	< 8:30	< 9:30
Excellent		
Females	10:30–11:49	11:30–12:49
Males	8:30–9:29	9:30–10:29
Good		
Females	11:50–13:09	12:50–14:09
Males	9:30–10:29	10:30–11:29
Moderate		
Females	13:10–14:29	14:10–15:29
Males	10:30–11:29	11:30–12:29
Fair		
Females	14:30–15:49	15:30–16:49
Males	11:30–12:29	12:30–13:29
Poor		
Females	> 15:49	> 16:49
Males	> 12:29	> 13:29

Source: Draper D. O., & Jones, G. L. (1990). The 1.5 mile run revisited—An update in women's times. *Journal of Physical Education Recreation, & Dance, 61* (9), 78–80. Reston, VA: AAHPERD.

12 Minute Tests may be troubled by estimating the distance of their run. Ideally, the distances should be estimated as closely as possible in order to accommodate the available norms (e.g., at least the nearest 40 m for the 12 Minute Test). The norms in Table 12.4 and Table 12.6 (12 Min Test), are presented in about 175 yd and 40 m to 60 m increments,

Table 12.3 Aerobic Fitness vs. 1.5 Mile Times (min:s) for Males (M) and Females (F), 13 y to 60+ y of Age

Fitness Level		13–19	20–29	30–39	40–49	50–59	60+
Very poor	M	> 15:30	> 16:00	> 16:30	> 17:30	> 19:00	> 20:00
	F	> 18:30	> 19:00	> 19:30	> 20:00	> 20:30	> 21:00
Poor	M	12:11–15:30	14:01–16:00	14:44–16:30	15:36–17:30	17:01–19:00	19:01–20:00
	F	16:55–18:30	18:31–19:00	19:01–19:30	19:31–20:00	20:01–20:30	20:31–21:00
Fair	M	10:49–12:10	12:01–14:00	12:31–14:45	13:01–15:35	14:31–17:00	16:16–19:00
	F	14:31–16:54	15:55–18:30	16:31–19:00	17:31–19:30	19:01–20:00	19:31–20:30
Good	M	9:41–10:48	10:46–12:00	11:01–12:30	11:31–13:00	12:31–14:30	14:00–16:15
	F	12:30–14:30	13:31–15:54	14:31–16:30	15:56–17:30	16:31–19:00	17:31–19:30
Excellent	M	8:37–9:40	9:45–10:45	10:00–11:00	10:30–11:30	11:00–12:30	11:15–13:59
	F	11:50–12:29	12:30–13:30	13:00–14:30	13:45–15:55	14:30–16:30	16:30–17:30
Superior	M	< 8:37	< 9:45	< 10:00	< 10:30	< 11:00	< 11:15
	F	< 11:50	< 12:30	< 13:00	< 13:45	< 14:30	< 16:30

Source: Adapted from Table 14 with permission from Kusinitz, I., & Fine, M. (1991). *Your guide to getting fit.* Mountain View, CA: Mayfield Publishing.

Table 12.4 AAHPERD Percentile (%ile) Norms for the 1 Mile Run and 9 Min Run

Percentile (%ile)	College Men			College Women		
	1 Mile Run (min:s)	9 Min (yd)	Distance (m)	1 Mile Run (min:s)	9 Min (yd)	Distance (m)
99th	5:06	3035	2775	6:04	2640	2414
75th	6:12	2349	2148	8:15	1870	1710
50th	6:49	2200	2012	9:22	1755	1605
25th	7:32	1945	1779	10:41	1460	1335
5th	9:47	1652	1511	12:43	1101	1007

Reprinted by permission of the American Alliance for Health, Physical Education, Recreation and Dance. (1985). *Norms for college students.* 1900 Association Dr., Reston, VA 22091.

Table 12.5 The Relationship Between 1.5 Mile Time and Maximal Oxygen Consumption ($\dot{V}O_2$max)

1.5 Mile Time (min:s)	$\dot{V}O_2$max (mL·kg^{-1}·min^{-1})	1.5 Mile Time (min:s)	$\dot{V}O_2$max (mL·kg^{-1}·min^{-1})
< 7:31	75	12:31–13:00	39
7:31–8:00	72	13:01–13:30	37
8:01–8:30	67	13:31–14:00	36
8:31–9:00	62	14:01–14:30	34
9:01–9:30	58	14:31–15:00	33
9:31–10:00	55	15:01–15:30	31
10:01–10:30	52	15:31–16:00	30
10:31–11:00	49	16:01–16:30	28
11:01–11:30	46	16:31–17:00	27
11:31–12:00	44	17:01–17:30	26
12:01–12:30	41	17:31–18:00	25

From Wilmore J. H., & Bergfeld, J. A. A comparison of sports: Physiological and medical aspects, Table 24-6, p. 363, 1979, in *Sports Medicine and Physiology,* edited by R. H. Strauss. Copyright © 1979 W. B. Saunders Company, Philadelphia, PA.

respectively.[3] When distances are estimated and rounded off, fitness differences may become obscured.

The estimated maximal oxygen consumption (mL·kg^{-1}·min^{-1}) is needed in order to categorize performers of the 12 min distance run or the Rockport Walk Test. Performers in the 12 min distance run can obtain their $\dot{V}O_2$max values from Table 12.6[68] or the transposition of Cooper's[20,22] original equation (Eq. 12.1).

The Rockport walkers obtain their values from Equation 12.2, which includes the time to complete 1.0 mile and the heart rate. Charts depicting the fitness levels for Rockport Walk performers are available from The Rockport Company™ and other sources.[40]

The 1.0 Mile or 1.5 Mile Run Test

1. Participants run on a level terrain for the prescribed distance of one mile (1609 m; 1.6 km) or 1.5 mi[a] (2414 m; 2.4 km).

---

[a]The National Institute of Standards and Technology use the abbreviation mi to indicate miles when accompanied by a number.[63]

Table 12.6 — The Relationship between Maximal Oxygen Consumption and 12 Min Distance

Distance (miles)	1/4 Mile Laps	Distance m	$\dot{V}O_2$max mL·kg^{-1}·min^{-1}	Distance (miles)	1/4 Mile Laps	Distance m	$\dot{V}O_2$max mL·kg^{-1}·min^{-1}
<1.0	<4	<1609	25.0	1.500	6	2414	42.6
1.000	4	1609	25.0	1.530	. . .	2462	43.8
1.030	. . .	1658	26.0	1.565	6.25	2519	45.0
1.065	4.25	1714	27.0	1.590	. . .	2559	46.0
1.090	. . .	1754	28.2	1.625	6.5	2615	47.2
1.125	4.5	1811	29.0	1.650	. . .	2655	48.0
1.150	. . .	1851	30.2	1.687	6.75	2715	49.2
1.187	4.75	1910	31.6	1.720	. . .	2768	50.2
1.220	. . .	1963	32.8	1.750	7	2816	51.6
1.250	5	2012	33.8	1.780	. . .	2865	52.6
1.280	. . .	2060	34.8	1.817	7.25	2924	53.8
1.317	5.25	2120	36.2	1.840	. . .	2961	54.8
1.340	. . .	2157	37.0	1.875	7.5	3018	56.0
1.375	5.5	2213	38.2	1.900	. . .	3058	57.0
1.400	. . .	2253	39.2	1.937	7.75	3117	58.2
1.437	5.75	2313	40.4	1.970	. . .	3170	59.2
1.470	. . .	2366	41.6	2.000	8	3219	60.2

Adapted from Wilmore, J. H. & Costill, D. L. *Training for sport and activity*, 3d ed. Copyright ©1988 Wm. C. Brown Communications, Inc., Dubuque, Iowa. All Rights Reserved. Reprinted by permission.

2. The timers record the participants' times to the closest second onto Form 12.1. As a recommended optional measure, the timers record the heart rate for 15 s immediately after the participants cross the finish line.
3. The fitness level based upon the 1.5 mi run time is determined by consulting Table 12.2 for collegians and Table 12.3 for the general population. Table 12.4 is consulted for collegians running 1.0 mi.
4. For the 1.5 Mile Test, the $\dot{V}O_2$max is estimated by consulting Table 12.5 or using Equation 12.1.[18]

$$\dot{V}O_2\text{max (mL·kg}^{-1}\text{·min}^{-1}) = (483 \div t) + 3.5 \qquad \text{Eq. 12.1}$$

where:

t = time to the closest 0.1 min; e.g., 30/60 = 0.5 min

3.5 = resting metabolism in mL·kg^{-1}·min^{-1}; one MET

Sample Calculation: If a performer runs 1.5 miles in 13:30, then the calculation proceeds as follows:

$$\dot{V}O_2\text{max (mL·kg}^{-1}\text{·min}^{-1}) = (483 \div 13.5) + 3.5$$
$$= 35.8 + 3.5 = 39.3$$

The 9 Min or 12 Min Run Tests

1. Participants run for 9 min or 12 min.
2. Runners and their assistants estimate the distance to the nearest 40 m or less.[b] As a recommended optional measure, record heart rate for 15 s immediately after the participant finishes the 9 min run or 12 min run.
3. The fitness percentiles of collegians for the 9 Min Test are determined by consulting Table 12.4.
4. The fitness level for the 12 Min Test requires first an estimation of $\dot{V}O_2$max by consulting Table 12.6 or by using Equation 12.2 (men and women).

[b] 1 m = 3.281 ft = 1.0936 yd; 1 km = 0.62137 mi; 1 mi = 1609.35 m.

5. $\dot{V}O_2$max is calculated by inserting the distance (mi) into Equation 12.2a or by inserting kilometers into Eq. 12.2b.

$$\dot{V}O_2\text{max (mL·kg}^{-1}\text{·min}^{-1}) \qquad \text{Eq. 12.2a}$$
$$= (D \text{ in miles} - 0.3138) \div 0.0278$$

$$= (D \text{ in km} - 0.505) \div 0.0447 \qquad \text{Eq. 12.2b}$$

For example, if the distance in 12 min is 1.25 mi (2.011 km), then the maximal oxygen consumption can be calculated as follows:

$$\dot{V}O_2\text{max (mL·kg}^{-1}\text{·min}^{-1}) = (1.25 - 0.3138) \div 0.0278$$
$$= 0.936 \div 0.0278$$
$$= 33.7 \text{ mL·kg}^{-1}\text{·min}^{-1}$$

6. Record the fitness category onto Form 12.1 by referring to Table 12.7 (men) and Table 12.8 (women).[58]

The Rockport Walk Test

1. Technicians weigh the participants in their running attire.
2. Participants walk as fast as possible for one mile on any level terrain.
3. Heart rates (HR) are taken by technicians or the participants by pulse palpation or electronic monitoring for 10 s or 15 s immediately upon crossing the 1 mi mark or during the last quarter mile.[7]
4. Technicians multiply the last minute of the number of beats in 10 s by six, or the 15 s value by four, and record the product onto Form 12.1.
5. Timers record the participants' times to the closest second and later convert them to the nearest hundredth minute onto Form 12.1. For example, if the participant finishes in 13:30, then the recorded time is converted to the nearest hundredth minute by dividing the seconds—30—by 60 s. Thus, the time is 13.50 min.

6. Calculate $\dot{V}O_2$max $(mL \cdot kg^{-1} \cdot min^{-1})$ according to Equation 12.3a[45] for the general population and according to Eq. 12.3b[30,34] for collegians:

$$\dot{V}O_2\text{max } (mL \cdot kg^{-1} \cdot min^{-1}) = 132.85 \qquad \text{Eq. 12.3a}$$
$$- (0.0769 \times \text{lb BM or } 0.1692 \times \text{kg BM})$$
$$- (0.3877 \times \text{age}) + (6.315 \times \text{gender})$$
$$- (3.2649 \times t \text{ in 100th of min})$$
$$- (0.1565 \times \text{HR in b} \cdot min^{-1})$$

$$\dot{V}O_2\text{max } (mL \cdot kg^{-1} \cdot min^{-1}) \qquad \text{Eq. 12.3b}$$
$$= 88.768 + 8.892 \text{ (gender)}$$
$$- 0.0957 \text{ BM lb} - 1.4537 \, t$$
$$- 0.1194 \text{ HR}$$

where:

gender = 0 for women, and 1 for men

BM = body mass in walking clothes

Example of calculating $\dot{V}O_2$max $(mL \cdot kg^{-1} \cdot min^{-1})$:

Age = 30 y   BM = 150 lb   time (t) to walk 1 mi = 13.50

Gender = male   HR = 145 b·min^{-1}

$$\dot{V}O_2\text{max } (mL \cdot kg^{-1} \cdot min^{-1}) = 132.85 - (0.0769 \times 150 \text{ lb})$$
$$- (0.3877 \times 30 \text{ y}) + (6.315 \times 1) - (3.2649 \times 13.50)$$
$$- (0.1565 \times 145 \text{ b} \cdot min^{-1})$$
$$= 132.85 - 11.535 - 11.631 + 6.315 - 44.076 - 22.693$$
$$= 49.23$$

7. Charts depicting the fitness levels for Rockport Walk performers are available from The Rockport Company™ and other sources.[40] If these are not easily obtained, fitness levels are presented in Tables 12.7 and 12.8.[58]

Results and Discussion

This section includes comments and tables to help interpret the results of the Aerobic Run/Walk Tests. Thus, norms are included, along with some physiological measures that are

Table 12.7   Aerobic Fitness Categories for Men, 18 y to 75 y of Age

	Fitness Category Maximal Oxygen Consumption (mL·kg⁻¹·min⁻¹)[a]						
Age (y)	Excellent	Very Good	Good	Average	Fair	Poor	Very Poor
18–20	> 63	62–57	56–51	50–46	45–39	38–33	< 33
21–25	> 62	62–56	55–51	50–45	44–38	37–32	< 32
26–30	> 59	59–55	54–48	47–42	41–36	35–30	< 30
31–35	> 56	56–52	51–47	46–40	39–35	34–29	< 29
36–40	> 54	54–49	48–45	44–38	37–33	32–28	< 28
41–45	> 51	51–47	46–42	41–36	35–31	30–26	< 26
46–50	> 49	49–45	44–40	39–35	34–30	29–25	< 25
51–55	> 46	46–42	41–37	36–33	32–28	27–24	< 24
56–60	> 44	44–39	38–35	34–31	30–26	25–22	< 22
61–65	> 41	41–37	36–33	32–29	28–25	24–21	< 21
66–70	> 38	38–35	34–31	30–27	26–24	23–19	< 19
71–75	> 35	35–32	31–28	27–24	23–21	20–17	< 17

Note: Table derived from graphs in Shvartz, E., & Reibold, R. C. (1990). Aerobic fitness norms for males and females aged 6 to 75 years: A review. *Aviation, Space, and Environmental Medicine, 61,* 31–11.
[a]Reading error in transition from graph to table is ±1–2 mL·kg⁻¹·min⁻¹.

Table 12.8   Aerobic Fitness Categories for Women, 18 y to 75 y of Age

	Fitness Category[a] Maximal Oxygen Consumption (mL·kg⁻¹·min⁻¹)[a]						
Age (y)	Excellent	Very Good	Good	Average	Fair	Poor	Very Poor
18–20	> 53	53–48	47–43	42–38	37–33	32–28	< 28
21–25	> 50	50–46	45–42	41–36	35–32	31–27	< 27
26–30	> 48	48–44	43–40	39–35	34–31	30–26	< 26
31–35	> 46	46–42	41–37	36–33	32–29	28–25	< 25
36–40	> 43	43–39	38–35	34–31	30–27	26–23	< 23
41–45	> 40	40–36	35–33	32–29	28–26	25–22	< 22
46–50	> 37	37–35	34–31	30–27	26–24	23–20	< 20
51–55	> 36	36–32	31–28	27–25	26–24	23–20	< 20
56–60	> 33	33–30	29–26	25–23	22–20	19–17	< 17
61–65	> 30	30–27	26–24	23–21	20–18	17–15	< 15
66–70	> 27	27–25	24–22	21–19	18–16	15–14	< 14
71–75	> 25	25–23	22–20	19–17	16–15	14–13	< 13

Table derived from graphs in Shvartz, E., & Reibold, R. C. (1990). Aerobic fitness norms for males and females aged 6 to 75 years: A review. *Aviation, Space, and Environmental Medicine, 61,* 3–11.
Note: [a] Reading error in transition from graph to table is ±1–2 mL·kg⁻¹·min⁻¹.

associated with the test. Data collection forms at the end of the chapter allow us to compile the statistics, which, in turn, allow us to make a concluding statement.

Prior to 1987, little information *directly* related aerobic fitness to health or disease.[26] But now the Surgeon General's Report on Physical Activity and Health reinforces the message that inactivity is a serious health threat.[13,14,54,59] The interpretation of the aerobic fitness norms should consider other contributing factors to aerobic performance besides $\dot{V}O_2max$:[60] (1) differences in body composition, (2) running economy (efficiency), (3) fractional utilization (%) of maximal oxygen consumption—that is, the ability to run or walk continuously at a high percentage of maximal oxygen consumption, and (4) motivation. Also, these run/walk tests measure fitness for distances and times more indicative of *short* aerobic fitness than *long* aerobic fitness. (See Figure 1.3 in Chapter 1.) Thus, a longer test, such as the Texas Steady State Run Test,[11] would be more appropriate for long aerobic fitness (continuous activities ≥ 60 min).

Norms for 1.5 Mile Time

Norms are usually categorized into different levels of fitness ranging from poor (low $\dot{V}O_2max$) to superior (high). The norms in Table 12.2 are based upon over 1500 active college students.[31] Its six fitness categories represent a bell curve with three areas delineated by three standard deviations (*SD*) above and below the mean. Thus, the good, excellent, and superior categories are in the area within 1, 2, and 3 *SD* from the mean, respectively. The investigators[31] present a convincing argument for replacing the former Cooper norms[24,25,46] (e.g., Table 12.3), which have much easier criteria, with the norms in Table 12.2, which reflect a more active population, especially for women.

The traditional norms in Table 12.3 are based upon data collected in the 1970s.[23] The values between *fair* and *good* fitness categories in Table 12.3[46] are considered *average* for men and women from ages 13 y to over 50 y. In order to qualify for the *good* fitness category, men and women between 20 y and 29 y of age must run 1.5 mi in less than 12:01 and 15:55, respectively; this compares to the more stringent "good" category criteria in Table 12.2 of 10:30 and 13:10 that were derived from testing active college men and women 25 y of age.

The derived $\dot{V}O_2max$ values in Tables 12.4 and 12.5 may be used to compare with another set of norms in Tables 12.6 (men) and 12.7 (women). The latter set of norms classifies fitness for a wider age group and a more general population.

Norms for the 12 Minute Distance Test

Fitness categories for men and women ages 18 y to 75 y may be derived by using Table 12.6 or Equations 12.2a or 12.2b in conjunction with Tables 12.7 (men) and 12.8 (women).[58]

Norms for the AAHPERD Health-Related Test

Table 12.4 presents the norms for college men and women performing the AAHPERD 1 Mile Run Test or 9 Minute Run Test.[3] There are no age distinctions because of the similarity of scores for the typical college-age range. The norms are presented as percentiles (%ile) for each gender. Percentile values are simple and practical. For example, if a 21-year-old man ran 1 mi in 6 min 49 s (6:49), he would be at the 50th %ile, meaning that he runs the mile faster than 50 % of all college-aged men from whom these norms were extracted. Some authorities suggest criterion reference (CR) norms (standards) with the *minimal acceptable* percentile as the 25th (men 7:32; women 10:41) and the *minimal goal* percentile as the 50th.[12] Decisively superior scores might be those above the 80th %ile. The AAHPERD 9 Minute Run Test recommends that distances be estimated to the closest 10 yd (11 m) in order to interpret the test to the closest percentile when using their original percentile table[3] but the table is not included here.

Interpretation of Norms

Running 1.5 mi in less than 12 min is consistent with a maximal oxygen consumption above 43 mL·kg⁻¹·min⁻¹ (Table 12.5). As of 1992, the Air Force ROTC standards for the 1.5 Mi Run for men and women between 17 y and 29 y of age were 12:00 and 14:00, respectively. For ROTC personnel over 29 y of age, the standards for men and women were 12:30 and 14:52, respectively. The U.S. Navy requires its recruits to run 1.5 mi in 14 min or less.

Two reviewers[27] stated that Cooper[21] suggested a $\dot{V}O_2max$ of 42 mL·kg⁻¹·min⁻¹ as being consistent with good health and functional capacity for daily living in men, and that only 35 mL·kg⁻¹·min⁻¹ was necessary in women due to their greater essential fat and lower blood hemoglobin concentration. These criteria values were adopted also by FITNESSGRAM of the Institute for Aerobics Research (1987) and represent the means of young adults,[8,70] and are associated with a reduced risk of all-cause mortality.[13] If the 1.5 mi run is performed at a location between 1524 m (5000 ft) and 2439 m (8000 ft), then the times listed in Table 12.3 should be adjusted by an additional 30 s.

The *AAHPERD Physical Best* criterion-referenced standards for the 1 mile run are 50 and 43 mL·kg⁻¹·min⁻¹ for 20-year-old men and women, respectively.[4] Thus, they are 8 mL·kg⁻¹·min⁻¹, or one standard deviation, higher than Cooper's criteria. Cooper's criteria seem applicable to middle-aged persons, whereas the AAHPERD criteria are applicable to young adults.[27]

Summary of the Aerobic Run Tests

Five versions of walk/run tests were presented as aerobic field tests of fitness. The 1.5 Mile Test, 12 Minute Test, 1.0 Mile Run Test, 9 Minute Run Test, and Rockport Walk

Test are all *field tests* because they require accessible facilities, minimal equipment, and simple procedures, and they may be administered to many persons simultaneously. They are aerobic fitness tests because they measure performance in large-muscle, rhythmic, continuous activities. They are physiologically meaningful because they allow the estimation of aerobic power in units of maximal oxygen consumption, an indicator of cardiovascular endurance. Norms are available that allow participants to be categorized according to their fitness level.

Optional Physiological Measures for the Run/Walk Tests

Some physiological variables that lend themselves to simple measurement before, during, and after the run/walk tests are (a) heart rate, (b) respiration, and (c) subjective responses.

Heart Rate

The recording of heart rate can provide insights into such factors as (a) the degree of anxiety preceding the run test (the anticipatory effect), (b) the degree of effort and motivation during the test, and (c) the fitness comparisons among individuals and in the same individual when repeating the test.

In order to measure heart rate accurately, electronic monitoring or the best palpatory site should be selected. Additionally, the timing and counting technique should be mastered.

Palpation

The feeling of a pulse or vibration is called palpation. Pulses are generated by the whiplike action of the aorta artery, whereas the vibration pulse (apical beat) is generated by the left ventricle hitting against the chest wall (precordium) near the fifth rib. The arterial pulses that may be felt most easily are the radial, carotid, and temporal. When palpating the carotid artery in the neck, press lightly to avoid bradycardia (slowing of heart rate) via a sensitive baroreceptor reflex in some persons.[7] The apical beat can be quite prominent in lean persons immediately after exercise. It can be palpated by the entire hand held as in the pledge of allegiance over the left side of the chest.

Counting Technique

Count the number of pulses or beats in 10 s or 15 s by using a stopwatch or digital watch. If a partner is timing, then the voice command should be one-syllable words, such as *Count* and *Stop*. The heart rate in beats per minute (b·min^{-1}) is obtained by multiplying the 10 s count by six or the 15 s count by four. The heart rate that represents the exercise heart rate is taken immediately after exercise. Thus, as soon as the run test is completed, the performer should palpate the pulse or beat within 5 s. To avoid pooling of blood in the lower extremities, the performer should walk slowly or in place while taking the heart rate. The runner or walker should tell the partner the number of beats in 10 s or 15 s so that the partner can record it on Form 12.2. Students are encouraged to practice the palpation and counting of heart rate before collecting the actual walk/run test data.

Heart Rate (HR) Data Prior to the Run/Walk Test (Preexercise)

Form 12.2 can be used to record your **resting heart rate (HR)** under two conditions: (1) in the standing position under relaxed conditions in the laboratory before arrival at the test field (or track) and (2) in the standing position at the starting line immediately prior to the Go! signal for the run test. If a warm-up does not precede the measurement of the latter heart rate, it may be designated as the anticipatory (or excitatory) heart rate.

Exercise Heart Rate

The exercise and recovery heart rates are also recorded onto Form 12.2. The 15 s count is started within 5 s of completing the run/walk test. The number of beats is recorded by the same partner who recorded the time or distance of the run/walk.

The heart rate derived from the 5th to 20th s postexercise pulse count is approximately 90 % of the actual peak exercise rate.[49] Equation 12.4 shows that the 15 s count is first multiplied by 4; then the product is multiplied by 1.10 in order to account for the slight decrease during the 15+ s it took to measure it.

$$\text{Exercise HR (b·min}^{-1}) = (4 \times 15\text{s count}) \times 1.10 \quad \text{Eq. 12.4}$$

For example, if the 15 s count is 40 beats, then multiplying this by 4 gives the product, 160; 160 multiplied by the constant, 1.10, gives the actual exercise heart rate of 176 b·min^{-1}.

Recovery Heart Rate

The heart rates of most run/walk participants at the fifth minute into recovery often drop about 50 beats from their peak exercise heart rates. For example, if a person's heart rate upon crossing the finish line for the 1.5 mile run is 190 b·min^{-1}, then it is likely that the 5 min recovery heart rate will drop to less than 140 b·min^{-1}. A heart rate that drops no more than 12 b·min^{-1} at one minute postexercise has a bad prognosis for coronary heart disease risk.[19]

Heart Rate and Motivation

An approximate indication of motivation during the Aerobic Run Tests may be made by comparing the finish-line heart rate with the known or predicted maximal heart rate of the participant. Those who are closer to their maximal heart rate are considered to have given a greater effort. This should be interpreted cautiously, however, if using *predicted* maximal heart rates because of the 10-beat variation in age-group maximal heart rates.[9]

Maximal heart rate is best determined by monitoring the electrocardiogram at the exhaustive point of a progressive exercise test. The most common estimate of maximal heart rate (HRmax) subtracts age (y) from 220 (Eq. 12.5). Higher maximal heart rates may exist in women; thus, some reviewers recommend subtracting the woman's age from 226.[32]

$$\text{HRmax (b·min}^{-1}) = 220 - \text{age (y)} \qquad \text{Eq. 12.5}$$

Respiration During the Run/Walk Test

Both the cardiovascular and respiratory systems play prominent roles during the performance of aerobic run/walk tests. Previously, the heart rate's role in the cardiovascular system was examined. Now, breathing frequency and breathing depth are examined as respiratory variables during the run/walk tests. Prior to these tests, however, students should practice observing breathing frequency and depth by recording on Form 12.2 the values at rest and while jogging in place for 3 min.

Breathing Frequency (f)

The rate of breathing, of course, increases as the intensity of exercise increases. Breathing frequency can be influenced voluntarily, but this influence during exercise is minimized. The expected breathing frequencies will range from about 25 to 45 breaths per min (br·min⁻¹) for most persons during the run/walk tests. Breaths should be counted for one minute during the fifth or sixth minute in order to assure that steady state has been attained.

Depth of Breathing (Tidal Volume; V_T or TV)

The size of each breath is called the tidal volume. Under laboratory conditions, it is measured in liters (L) or milliliters (mL) by special respiratory instruments. Although subject to considerable error, an approximation of tidal volume can be made by subjectively comparing the tidal volume during the run/walk test with that at rest. Thus, the runner simply judges how much greater the depth of the exercise breath is than the resting breath. The depth of the exercise breath is an estimated multiple of the resting value. In many cases, the multiple will be between three and five.

Subjective Responses to the Run/Walk Tests

Exercise physiology students can apply their newly acquired knowledge by being aware of various physiological symptoms as they perform their daily routines or, as in this case, as they perform the run/walk tests. Thus, it is not always necessary to have instruments by which to measure these symptoms or responses. Subjective responses are those that are estimated by the participant; they may include such factors as thermal, muscular, and psychological responses. Each timer/recorder should remind his or her running partner to express verbally the state of these factors as they occur or at designated times during the run.

Thermal Response—Perspiration

The sweating response is influenced not only by exercise but also by such factors as the environmental temperature, the relative humidity, convection (breezes), clothing, and the state of hydration. Students are encouraged to make a mental note as to the chronology of sweating—that is, the time of onset for sweating and the length of time it continues after exercise. The site of perspiration should be noted also.

Muscle Response

Obviously, the muscles are responsible for the movement of the limbs while performing these tests. Muscles may be perceived to alter their state of smoothness (efficiency) or tightness at various times throughout the test due to such factors as warm-up, fatigue, and psychological factors (perception). It is also possible that uncommon episodes, such as cramps and side stitch, may occur along with the expected muscle fatigue.

Rating of Perceived Exertion (RPE)

The rating of perceived exertion[15,16,17] integrates a variety of strain signals into a general whole sensation. Thus, signals coming from the body as a whole—cardiovascular, respiratory, muscular, and nervous systems—provide the performer with a perception of the intensity of exertion. The original Borg RPE category scale ranges from the lowest degree of exertion, 6, to the highest degree, 20; thus, it is sometimes referred to as the Borg 15-category RPE scale.[17] Borg chose the number 6 to start his linear scale because, when 6 was multiplied by 10, producing 60, it represented a low resting heart rate.[39] Odd numbers are given anchor descriptions, such as *very, very light* for 7 and *very, very hard (heavy)* for 19. For example, 7 describes the exertion while pedalling a cycle ergometer slowly at zero resistance, and 19 describes the most physically exhaustive exercise ever encountered by the performer.[55]

The original RPE scale, based on the linear relationship among RPE, power output, and heart rate,[52] was revised with ratio properties based on the nonlinear (exponential or power function) properties of psychophysical and some physiological variables, such as blood lactate and ventilation.[6] For example, the original Borg RPE scale (6–20) would not indicate that lactate is really increasing about three times more at the top (16–17) of the scale than at the bottom. Thus, Borg's newer scale sets the semantic descriptions (e.g., weak, moderate, and strong) to a positively accelerating function.[52] This newer category-ratio (CR-10) scale may be more suitable for determining subjective symptoms associated with breathing, aches, and pains; it also has a high correlation with lactate.[17,62] Although Borg favored his original, 6–20 scale for simple applied studies, the editors of *ACSM's Guidelines for Exercise Testing and Prescription* (2000) state that the newer 0–10 ratio scale is easier for the performer to understand and, thus, more valid.[7] However, either scale has been recommended for the

Table 12.9 The Rating of Perceived Exertion

The 15-Category Scale (6–20)[a]	The Category Ratio (CR-10) Scale[b]
6	0 Nothing at all
7 Very, very light	0.5 Very, very (extremely) weak; (just noticeable)
8	1 Very weak
9 Very light	2 Weak (light)
10	3 Moderate
11 Light	4 Somewhat strong
12	5 Strong (heavy)
13 Somewhat heavy (hard)	6
14	7 Very strong
15 Heavy (hard)	8
16	9
17 Very heavy (hard)	10 Very, very (extremely) strong (almost maximal)
18	10+ Maximal (strongest ever)
19 Very, very heavy (hard)	
20	

Sources: [a]From Borg, G. A. V. (1970). Perceived exertion as an indicator of somatic stress. *Scandinavian Journal of Rehabilitative Medicine, 2,* Table 1, p. 93. [b]From Borg, G. A. V. Psychophysical bases of perceived exertion in *Medicine and Science in Sports and Exercise, 14*(5), 377–381, Table 2, p. 380. Copyright ©1982 Williams & Wilkins Publishers. Reprinted by permission of Lea & Febiger.
Note: I substituted the word *heavy* for *hard* to provide an English parallel descriptor for the word *light*. The same logic applies to the words *weak* and *strong* for the CR-10 scale.

run/walk tests and can be used to prescribe and monitor exercise training programs.[29,38]

One researcher suggests that heart rates between 110–150 b·min^{-1} would elicit in most people RPE values between 3 ("moderate") and 5 ("strong"; "hard").[51] CR-10 ratings between 4 and 7 correspond to exercise intensities between 50 % and 85 % of maximal oxygen consumption,[11] whereas the original RPE scale's ratings between 11 and 16 represent about 50 % to 75 % of maximal.[5]

All run/walk performers must be oriented in RPE terminology (Table 12.9) in order to use the RPE scale effectively. The performers should read the instructions while in the laboratory prior to testing. Again, someone should read the instructions aloud just prior to the Go! signal for the tests. Specific instructions for the CR-10 scale are in other sources[6,7,11] but are similar to those for the original RPE scale.[50] The instructions are read aloud to the performer as follows:

> You are now going to take part in a work test. We want you to try to estimate how hard you feel the exercise is; that is, we want you to rate the degree of perceived exertion you feel. By perceived exertion we mean the total amount of exertion and physical fatigue, combining all sensations and feelings of physical stress, effort and fatigue. Don't concern yourself with any one factor such as leg pain, shortness of breath, or exercise intensity, but try to concentrate on your total, inner feeling of exertion. Try to estimate as honestly and objectively as possible. Don't underestimate the degree of exertion you feel, but don't overestimate it either. Just try to estimate as accurately as possible p. 401.[50, c]

---

[c]Morgan, W. P. (1981). Psychophysiology of self-awareness during vigorous physical activity. *Research Quarterly for Exercise and Sport, 52,* 385–427.

As an optional RPE method, the category 6–20 scale may be differentiated into three distinctive categories:[48] (1) local, (2) central, and (3) overall. The local category represents the participant's rating of strain in the exercising muscles and joints; the central rating reflects ventilatory strain; and the overall rating integrates local and central factors.

Recording the Data

Individual data forms (12.1 and 12.2) provide spaces for inserting basic data, meteorological data, performance (times and distances) data, and physiological data. Form 12.3 provides columns for inserting the group data of run/walk times, distances, and maximal oxygen consumptions.

References

1. Ainsworth, B. E., Richardson, M. T., Jacobs, D. R., & Leon, A. S. (1992). Prediction of cardiorespiratory fitness using physical activity questionnaire data. *Medicine, Exercise, Nutrition Health, 1,* 75–82.
2. American Alliance for Health, Physical Education, Recreation and Dance. (1980). *Health related physical fitness test manual.* Washington, DC: Author.
3. American Alliance for Health, Physical Education, Recreation and Dance. (1985). *Norms for college students.* Washington, DC: Author.
4. American Alliance for Health, Physical Education, Recreation and Dance. (1988). *Physical best.* Reston, VA: Author.
5. American College of Sports Medicine. (1991). *Guidelines for exercise testing and prescription.* Philadelphia: Lea & Febiger.
6. American College of Sports Medicine. (1995). *ACSM's guidelines for exercise testing and prescription.* Philadelphia: Williams & Wilkins.
7. American College of Sports Medicine. (2000). *ACSM's guidelines for exercise testing and prescription.* Philadelphia: Lippincott Williams & Wilkins.
8. American Heart Association. (1972). *Exercise testing and training of apparently healthy individuals: A handbook for physicians.* New York: Author.
9. Åstrand, P.-O., & Rodahl, K. (1977). *Textbook of work physiology.* New York: McGraw-Hill.
10. Balke, B. (1963). *A simple field test for the assessment of physical fitness.* (CARI Report 63-18). Oklahoma City: Civil Aeromedical Research Institute, Federal Aviation Agency.
11. Baumgartner, T. A., & Jackson, A. S. (1991). *Measurement for evaluation in physical education and exercise science.* Dubuque, IA: Wm. C. Brown.
12. Blair, S. N., Falls, H. B., & Pate, R. R. (1983). A new physical fitness test. *The Physician and Sportsmedicine, 11*(4), 87–91, 94–95.

13. Blair, S. N., Kohl, H. W., Paffenbarger, R. S., Clark, D. H., Cooper, K. H., & Gibbons, L. W. (1989). Physical fitness and all-cause mortality. A prospective study of healthy men and women. *Journal of American Medical Association, 262,* 2395–2401.

14. Blair, S. N., & Morrow, M. S. (1997). Surgeon general's report on physical fitness: The inside story. *ACSM's Health and Fitness Journal, 1*(1), 14–18.

15. Borg, G. A. V. (1962). *Physical performance and perceived exertion.* Lund, Sweden: Gleerup.

16. Borg, G. A. V. (1970). Perceived exertion as an indicator of somatic stress. *Scandinavian Journal of Rehabilitative Medicine, 2,* 92–98.

17. Borg, G. A. V. (1982). Psychophysical bases of perceived exertion. *Medicine and Science in Sports and Exercise, 14,* 377–381.

18. Brooks, G. A., Fahey, T. D., White, T. P., & Baldwin, K. M. (2000). *Exercise physiology: Human bioenergetics and its applications.* Mountain View, CA: Mayfield.

19. Cole, C. R., Blackstone, E. H., Pashkow, F. J., Snader, C. E., & Lauer, M. S. (1999). Heart-rate recovery immediately after exercise as a predictor of mortality. *New England Journal of Medicine, 341,* 1351–1357.

20. Cooper, K. H. (1968). A means of assessing maximal oxygen intake. *Journal of the American Medical Association, 203,* 135–138.

21. Cooper, K. H. (1968). *Aerobics.* New York: M. Evans & Bantam Books.

22. Cooper, K. H. (1968). Testing and developing cardiovascular fitness within the United States Air Force. *Journal of Occupational Medicine, 10,* 636–639.

23. Cooper, K. H. (1970). *The new aerobics.* New York: Bantam Books.

24. Cooper, K. H. (1982). *The aerobics program for total well-being.* New York: M. Evans & Co.

25. Cooper, K. H., Pollock, M. L., Martin, R. P., White, S. R., Linnerud, A. C., & Jackson, A. (1976). Physical fitness levels vs. selected coronary risk factors. *Journal of American Medical Association, 236,* 166–169.

26. Cureton, K. J. (1987). Commentary on children and fitness: A public health perspective. *Research Quarterly for Exercise and Sport, 58,* 315–320.

27. Cureton, K. J., & Warren, G. L. (1990). Criterion-referenced standards for youth health-related fitness tests: A tutorial. *Research Quarterly for Exercise and Sport, 61,* 7–19.

28. deVries, H. A., & Housh, T. J. (1994). *Physiology of exercise.* Dubuque, IA: Brown & Benchmark.

29. Dishman, R. K., Patton, R. W., Smith, J., Weinberg, R., & Jackson, A. (1987). Using perceived exertion to prescribe and monitor exercise training heart rate. *International Journal of Sports Medicine, 8,* 208–213.

30. Dolgener, F. A., Hensley, L. D., Marsh, J. J., & Fjelstul, J. K. (1994). Validation of the Rockport Fitness Walking Test in college males and females. *Research Quarterly for Exercise and Sport, 65,* 152–158.

31. Draper, D. O., & Jones, G. L. (1990). The 1.5 mile run revisited—An update in women's times. *JOPERD, Journal of Physical Education, Recreation, & Dance, 61*(9) 78–80.

32. Edington, D. W., & Cunningham, L. (1975). *Biological awareness.* Englewood Cliffs, NJ: Prentice-Hall.

33. Fenstermaker, K. L., Plowman, S. A., & Looney, M. A. (1992). Validation of the Rockport Fitness Walking Test in females 65 years and older. *Research Quarterly for Exercise and Sport, 63,* 322–327.

34. George, J. D., Fellingham, G. W., & Fisher, A. G. (1998). A modified version of the Rockport Fitness Walking Test for college men and women. *Research Quarterly for Exercise and Sport, 69,* 205–209.

35. George, J. D., Fisher, A. G., & Vehrs, P. R. (1994). *Laboratory experiences in exercise science.* Boston: Jones and Bartlett.

36. George, J. D., Vehrs, P. R., Allsen, P. E., Fellingham, G. W., & Fisher, A. G. (1993). $\dot{V}O_2$max estimation from a submaximal 1-mile track jog for fit college-age individuals. *Medicine and Science in Sports and Exercise, 25,* 401–406.

37. Getchell, L. H., Kirkendall, D., & Robbins, G. (1977). Prediction of maximal oxygen uptake in young adult women joggers. *Research Quarterly, 48,* 61–67.

38. Glass, S. C., Knowlton, R. G., & Becque, M. D. (1992). Accuracy of RPE from graded exercise to establish exercise training intensity. *Medicine and Science in Sports and Exercise, 24,* 1303–1307.

39. Golding, L. A. (2000). From the editor. *ACSM's Health and Fitness Journal, 4*(5), 1.

40. Hastad, D. N., & Lacy, A. C. (1994). *Measurement and evaluation in physical education and exercise science.* Scottsdale, AZ: Gorsuch Scarisbrick.

41. Heil, D. P., Freedson, P. S., Ahlquist, L. E., Price, J., & Rippe, J. M. (1995). Nonexercise regression models to estimate peak oxygen consumption. *Medicine and Science in Sports and Exercise, 27,* 599–606.

42. Jackson, A. S., Blair, S. N., Mahar, M. T., Wier, L. T., Ross, R. M., & Stuteville, J. E. (1990). Prediction of functional aerobic capacity without exercise testing. *Medicine and Science in Sports and Exercise, 22,* 863–870.

43. Jackson, A. S., & Coleman, A. E. (1976). Validation of distance run tests for elementary school children. *Research Quarterly, 47,* 86–94.

44. Kline, G. M., Porcari, J. P., Freedson, P. S., Ward, A., Ross, J., Wilke, S., & Rippe, J. (1987). Does aerobic capacity affect the validity of the one-mile walk $\dot{V}O_2$max prediction? *Medicine and Science in Sports and Exercise, 19,* Abstract #172, S29.

45. Kline, G. M., Porcari, J. P., Hintermeister, R., Freedson, P. S., Ward, A., McCarron, R. F., Ross, J., & Rippe, J. (1987). Estimation of $\dot{V}O_2$max from a one-mile track walk, gender, age, and body weight. *Medicine and Science in Sports and Exercise, 19,* 253–259.

46. Kusinitz, I., & Fine, M. (1991). *Your guide to getting fit.* Mountain View, CA: Mayfield.

47. Leger, L., & Thivierge, M. (1988). Heart rate monitors: Validity, stability, and functionality. *The Physician and Sportsmedicine, 16*(5), 143–151.

48. Maresh, C. M., Deschenes, M. R., Seip, R. L., Armstrong, L. E., Robertson, K. L., & Noble, B. J. (1993). Perceived exertion during hypobaric hypoxia in low- and moderate-altitude natives. *Medicines and Science in Sports and Exercise, 25,* 945–951.

49. McArdle, W. D., Zwiren, L., & Magel, J. R. (1969). Validity of postexercise heart rate as a means of estimating heart rate during work of varying intensities. *Research Quarterly, 40,* 523–529.

50. Morgan, W. P. (1981). Psychophysiology of self-awareness during vigorous physical activity. *Research Quarterly for Exercise and Sport, 52,* 385–427.

51. Nieman, D. C. (1995). *Fitness and sports medicine.* Palo Alto, CA: Bull.

52. Noble, B. J., Borg, G. A. V., Jacobs, I., Ceci, R., & Kaiser, P. (1983). A category-ratio perceived exertion scale: Relationship to blood and muscle lactates and heart rate. *Medicine and Science in Sports and Exercise, 15,* 523–528.

53. O'Hanley, S., Ward, A., Zwiren, L., McCarron, R., Ross, J., & Rippe, J. M. (1987). Validation of a one-mile walk test in 70–79 year olds. *Medicine and Science in Sports and Exercise, 19,* Abstract #167, S28.

54. Pate, R. R., Pratt, M., Blair, S. N., Haskell, W. L., Macera, C. A., Bouchard, C., Buchner, D. Ettinger, W., Heath, G. W., King, A. C., et al. (1995). Physical activity and public health: A recommendation from the Centers for Disease Control and Prevention and the American College of Sports Medicine. *Journal of the American Medical Association, 273,* 402–407.

55. Perkins, K. A., Sexton, J. E., Solberg-Kassel, R. D., & Epsteing, L. H. (1991). Effects of nicotine on perceived exertion during low-intensity activity. *Medicine and Science in Sports and Exercise 23,* 1283–1288.

56. The Rockport Walking Institute. (1986). *Rockport fitness walking test.* Marlboro, MA: The Rockport Company.

57. Safrit, M. J., Hooper, L. M., Ehlert, S. A., Costa, M. G., & Patterson, P. (1988). The validity generalization of distance run tests. *Canadian Journal of Sport Science, 13,* 188–196.

58. Shvartz, E., & Reibold, R. C. (1990). Aerobic fitness norms for males and females aged 6 to 75 years: A review. *Aviation, Space, and Environment Medicine, 61,* 3–11.

59. Simons-Morton, B. G., O'Hara, N. M., Simons-Morton, D. G., & Parcel, G. S. (1987). Children and fitness: A public health perspective. *Research Quarterly for Exercise and Sport, 58,* 295–302.

60. Sparling, P. B., & Cureton, K. J. (1983). Biological determinants of the sex difference in 12-minute run performance. *Medicine and Science in Sports and Exercise, 15,* 218–223.

61. Spencer, M. R., & Gastin, P. B. (2001). Energy system contribution during 200- to 1500-m running in highly trained athletes. *Medicine and Science in Sports and Exercise, 33,* 157–162.

62. Sylven, C., Borg, G., Holmgren, A., & Astrom, H. (1991). Psychophysical power functions of exercise limiting symptoms in coronary heart disease. *Medicine and Science in Sports and Exercise, 23,* 1050–1054.

63. Taylor, B. N. (1995). *Guide for the use of the International System of Units (SI).* United States Department of Commerce. (NIST Special Publication 811, 1995 Edition). Gaithersburg, MD: NIST.

64. Thomas, S., Reading, J., & Shephard, R. J. (1992). Revision of the Physical Activity Readiness Questionnaire (PAR-Q). *Canadian Journal of Sport Science, 17,* 338–345.

65. Warren, B. J., Dotson, R. G., Nieman, D. C., & Butterworth, D. E. (1993). Validation of a 1-mile walk test in elderly women. *Journal of Aging and Physical Activity, 1,* 3–21.

66. Widrick, J., Ward, A., Ebbeling, C., Clemente, E., & Rippe, J. M. (1992). Treadmill validation of an overground walking test to predict peak oxygen consumption. *European Journal of Applied Physiology, 64,* 304–308.

67. Wilmore, J. H., & Bergfeld, J. A. (1979). A comparison of sports: Physiological and medical aspects. In R. H. Strauss (Ed.), *Sports medicine and physiology* (pp. 353–372). Philadelphia: W. B. Saunders.

68. Wilmore, J. H., & Costill, D. L. (1988). *Training for sport and activity.* Dubuque, IA: Wm. C. Brown.

69. Zingraf, S. A., & McClendon, T. (1986). An alternative index for cross-validating regression equations. *Abstract of Research Papers, 1986, AAHPERD Convention, Cincinnati,* p. 28. Reston, VA: American Alliance for Health, Physical Education, Recreation and Dance. (Abstract)

70. Zuti, W. B., & Corbin, B. (1977). Physical fitness norms for college students. *Research Quarterly, 48,* 499–503.

71. Zwiren, L. D., Freedson, P. S., Ward, A., Wilke, S., & Rippe, J. M. (1991). Estimation of $\dot{V}O_2$max: A comparative analysis of five exercise tests. *Research Quarterly for Exercise and Sport, 62,* 73–78.

Example: 70 kg man performing Forestry Step Test

$$\dot{V}O_2 = (0.2 \times 22.5 \,/\, min) + [1.33 \times (1.8 \times 0.40 \\ \times 22.5 \,/\, min)] + 3.5$$

$$= 4.5 + (1.33 \times 0.72 \times 22.5 \,/\, min) + 3.5$$

$$= 4.5 + 21.5 + 3.5$$

$$= 29.5 \text{ mL·kg}^{-1}\text{·min}^a$$

Although the test was originally designed for forestry firefighters, it is applicable for most apparently healthy persons. The moderate exercise intensity required for this test should enable most younger adults and middle-aged adults to complete the prescribed duration of the test (5 min). The intensity is probably high enough to raise the heart rates of fit persons above those rates that might possibly be influenced by emotional factors. However, the test may be too severe for persons of extremely low fitness and for many persons over 60 years of age.

Fitness Classification

The Forestry Step Test classifies the fitness status of its participants and provides an indirect measure of maximal oxygen consumption. As do many aerobic fitness tests, the Forestry Test demonstrates the importance of maximal oxygen consumption in aerobic fitness. By relating this predicted value of maximal oxygen consumption to the requirements of certain occupations, it is possible to predict the job suitability of either the candidate or a present employee.

Because the final score derived from the Forestry Step Test is a maximal oxygen consumption value, the score may be related to norms for maximal oxygen consumption that have been adjusted according to age categories for aerobic fitness. Although there are age and gender modifications for the fitness categories of this test, it is recommended that they be disregarded if the primary purpose of the test is to screen persons for occupational suitability.

In addition to classifying the fitness level, this test may be used to develop a prescription for exercise. Periodic testing of the exercise participant will allow for evaluation of both the prescription and the participant.

Summary of Purposes

The purposes of the Forestry Step Test are related to its importance. The primary purpose is to measure the aerobic (cardiovascular endurance) fitness of persons. Second, the test may be used to screen potential employees for their physical aptitude in an occupation. Third, it may be used to monitor the fitness progress of exercise trainees.

---

[a]1 MET = 3.5 mL·kg^{-1}·min^{-1}; thus, 29.5 mL·kg^{-1}·min^{-1} ÷ 3.5 = 8.4 MET.

Physiological Rationale

All tests in exercise physiology should be based upon a valid physiological rationale. The Forestry Step Test is based upon the direct relationships among oxygen consumption, heart rate, and power. Dr. Sharkey, who developed the present version of the Forestry Step Test, wanted a simple test that would predict the success of wilderness firefighters. He determined that direct field measurements of wilderness firefighting tasks averaged 22.5 mL·kg^{-1}·min^{-1}.[19] Given the intermittent nature of firefighting tasks, Sharkey reasoned that a physically fit individual could sustain work rates not more than 50 % of capacity over an 8-h period. Therefore, he concluded that an aerobic capacity of at least 45 mL·kg^{-1}·min^{-1} would be required for forestry firefighters. This criterion has been adopted by the U.S. Forest Service.[24]

As with oxygen consumption, most of the heart rate range is linearly and positively related to exercise power. This also means that steady-state heart rate and oxygen consumption are directly related. Heart rates are not measured *during* the Forestry Test but at *recovery* from the stepping exercise. Therefore, it is important that the recovery heart rate be relatively indicative of the exercise heart rate. There appears to be ample evidence to support a high relationship between exercise recovery heart rate and the actual exercise heart rate.[14,17,22]

The fitness of a person is related to both maximal oxygen consumption and submaximal exercise heart rate response. Low recovery heart rates reflect a low stress level by the performer, whereas high rates reflect a high stress level. This cardiovascular stress, as reflected by recovery heart rate, indicates the degree of aerobic fitness of the individual. Obviously, low stresses, or low heart rates, at any given exercise power equate with higher predicted maximal oxygen consumption values, which indicate a higher aerobic fitness level.

Method

Some of the factors described for the Forestry Test under the heading *Method* are (a) equipment, (b) preparation, and (c) testing. A discussion of the Forestry Step Test's accuracy is presented in Box 13.1.

Equipment

The recommended pieces of equipment are presented in Table 13.2. The obvious pieces of equipment are the step apparatus and a timing device for measuring the duration of the test and the performer's heart rate. A stadiometer and scale measure the performer's stature and body mass. The portability of the testing apparatus lends to testing under a variety of environmental conditions. Some meteorological instruments may be expensive, such as a single unit that combines automated wet/dry, bulb/globe thermometers with an anemometer for measuring wind speed.

All laboratories should have a good barometer for measuring the barometric pressure. Environmental temperature (T) and relative humidity (RH) are especially important meteorological readings for step tests performed in the field or in facilities without thermostatic control. Both temperature and humidity will influence heart rate when they are outside a certain range. For example, the norms for the Forestry Step Test are based upon environmental temperatures between 20 °C and 26.3 °C (68 °F to 79 °F).[20] Relative humidity may be calculated from an inexpensive sling psychrometer's wet and dry bulb temperatures or may be measured directly with a hygrometer.

The ergometric equipment—the step itself—is simple, inexpensive, and often portable. Step benches may be built to accommodate one or more persons. Sometimes sturdy benches are elevated to the prescribed height by simply inserting appropriately sized blocks under the supports of the bench. Electronically programmed step ergometers are available but are not commonly used to perform standard step tests.[12]

A field/lab test, such as the Forestry Step Test, is converted into a laboratory test by controlling meteorological variables and by enhancing the sophistication of the physiological measurements. For example, greater sophistication occurs when replacing finger palpation of pulse rate with electrocardiograph monitoring of heart rate.

Preparation

Administration of any step test requires appropriate preparations on the part of both the participant (performer) and the technician (tester). The preparation of the participant for this test applies to most field/lab tests.

Performer

1. Refrain from exercise the day of testing.[2]
2. Relax 5 min immediately preceding the test.
3. Loosen up (stretch), but do not warm up, prior to testing.
4. Take no food, stimulants (tobacco, "uppers," coffee, tea, colas, chocolate, etc.), or depressants (alcohol, "downers") 3 h preceding the test.[2] A longer abstinence from drugs may be necessary, depending upon the strength and amount of the particular drug dosage.
5. The performer should not have gone more than 5 h without food.
6. Be euhydrated, meaning normal hydration, which is neither hypohydrated nor hyperhydrated.

BOX 13.1 Accuracy of the Forestry Step Test

Obviously, predictive tests such as the aerobic run tests and the step tests are not as valid as making actual measurements of maximal oxygen consumption. The validity correlations based on the relationship between various step test scores and directly measured $\dot{V}O_2$max are reported to range from .46 to .66.[13] In general, step tests have standard errors of estimate (SEE) ranging from about 12 % to 15 %.[8] This means that the predicted score may overestimate or underestimate the directly measured maximal oxygen consumption in two-thirds of the population by as much as 12 % to 15 %; thus, the error in one-third of the population is even larger. If an error of 12 % is assumed, and an individual's directly measured maximal oxygen consumption is 50 mL·kg^{-1}·min^{-1}, then the estimated values from the step test would likely fall between 44 and 56 "mL's" (calculated as 50 mL $\pm$ [0.12 $\times$ 50]). A significant part of the error in predicting $\dot{V}O_2$max from submaximal step testing is due to the within-subject variation in oxygen demand when tested on different days.[23] This may also contribute to the daily variation of heart rate at submaximal exercise, which is reported to vary by about 5 b·min^{-1}.[14]

Finally, the efficiency of stepping may affect the accuracy of the test. Although the length of the performer's legs (or stature) is sometimes presumed to affect the results of stepping, there has been only weak,[23] or U-shaped,[18] or no relationship.[7] One general guideline is that, if the top of the bench is no higher than the performer's knee, there is no disadvantage in the efficiency of stepping. An additional error may be attributed to habituation, whereby performers improve their stepping efficiency as a result of the first or second test.[21] As with all heart-rate based fitness tests, the differences in maximal heart rates contribute to the standard error of prediction.

Table 13.2 Equipment for Forestry Step Test

Type of Measure	Type of Instrument
Meteorological	
Environmental temperature (°C)	Dry bulb; wet bulb;[a] globe[a]
Relative humidity (RH %)	Hygrometer;[a] sling psychrometer[a]
Barometric pressure (mm Hg)[b]	Mercury barometer;[a] aneroid[a]
Basic Data	
Body mass (kg)	Platform scale
Stature (cm; m)	Anthropometer; stadiometer
Ergometric	
Step ergometer (cm; m)	Bench, stool, box, or bleacher/stadium step **Men:** 40 cm (15.75 in.) **Women:** 33 cm (13 in.)
Timing	
Minutes; seconds (min:s)	Laboratory timer;[a] stopwatch; watch; clock
Metronome	Mechanical or electronic; audio recording of cadence
Heart Rate Monitoring	
Stethoscope[a]	Bell or diaphragm shape
Electrocardiograph[a]	Single-lead only
Wrist/chest monitor[a]	Polar™, etc.

Notes: [a]Optional instruments for more controlled testing. [b]The hectopascal (hPa) is the accepted SI unit of measure for barometric pressure. The hPa is the same pressure as the meteorologists' millibar. However, because most U.S. laboratory barometers have scales only in units of millimeters of mercury (mm Hg)—the same as torr—then it is suggested that hPa units be recorded in parentheses following the mm Hg unit. 1 mm Hg = 1 torr = 1.333 hPa or mbar; 760 mm Hg = 1013 hPa or mbar (sea level).

7. Have no distension of the urinary bladder.[10]
8. Wear lightweight shoes and lightweight/loose clothing (preferably, tennis shoes and shorts). An exception to this might be if the objective is to determine the stress response under occupational or athletic conditions (e.g., firefighters, cross-country skiers, etc.).

Technician

The technician's preparations for many lab/field tests usually consider four major factors: (1) calibration (see Box 13.2), (2) the gathering of basic and meteorological data, (3) the orientation of the participant to the testing procedure, and (4) the selection of the best palpatory sites and verification of the performer's and technician's practice of pulse counts.

Basic and meteorological data are important in interpreting the test. For example, a very small stature or excess body mass of a performer may influence the efficiency of stepping. The body mass of the performer includes the exercise clothes and shoes.[20] Contrary to most normative data, this clothed weight should be used to calculate the relative maximal oxygen consumption ($\dot{V}O_2$max divided by body mass in kilograms).

A meteorological factor might consider if a fan is used during the test. If so, it should be noted on the test form. A good fan might allow an additional 2 °C to the upper limit of temperature for any exercise tests in the laboratory.[3]

Orientation makes the performer aware of the purpose of the test. Second, it provides instructions and information that may satisfy legal or ethical requirements for informed consent. Third, it may enhance the accuracy and validity of the test.

The technician emphasizes the importance of keeping proper cadence and of straightening the back and legs at the top of the step (Figure 13.1). The cadence may be kept with the aid of the metronome, which is set to a 90 b·min^{-1} in order to produce the prescribed step rate (f·min^{-1}) of 22.5·min^{-1} for the Forestry Step Test. The four-count cadence is as follows:

"Up-one": One foot goes to top of step.
"Up-two": The other foot follows to top of step.
"Down-one": One foot descends to floor.
"Down-two": The other foot follows to floor.

The performer's leading foot (first foot on step) may be changed a few times during the test. The technician reminds the performer to sit down on the bench immediately following the test.

Upon being seated, both the performer and technician palpate the performer's pulse at the predesignated sites. Both persons practice heartbeat palpation prior to the test. The pulse may be palpated at various sites. Try all four palpatory sites and rank from best to worst on Form 13.1. The radial pulse is on the thumb side of the wrist; contrary to popular belief, it is acceptable to palpate your *own* pulse with your thumb. It is not acceptable to palpate someone

---

BOX 13.2   Calibration for the Step Test

Calibration of some instruments does not have to be repeated on every test occasion. For example, after the initial verification of the step ergometer's height, it may never need to be measured again. The calibration of the platform weight scale was discussed in Chapter 2. The metronome should be checked for accuracy by counting the number of beats for 1 min at the prescribed test setting. For example, the setting for the Forestry Step Test is 90 b·min^{-1}. Thus, when starting a watch with a seconds hand simultaneously with a beat (sound) on the metronome and then counting the next beat as one, the 90th beat should occur at the end of 1 min.

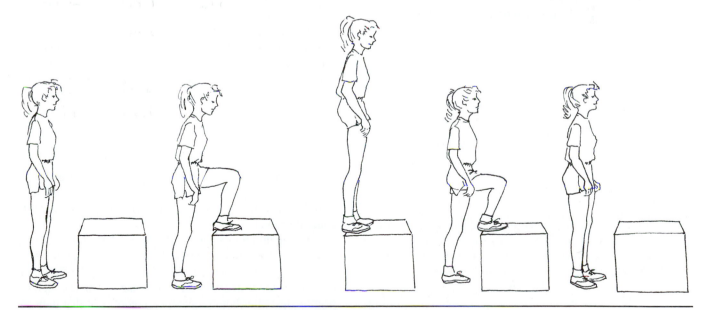

Figure 13.1   The four-count stepping technique for the step-test performer.

else's pulse with your thumb; use the joined index and middle fingers instead.

The carotid pulse may be palpated on either side of the neck. There is some controversy over the bradycardiac (slowing) effect of carotid palpation. However, in a well-controlled study, the investigators reported no significant difference between carotid and radial palpation of heart rate.[17] They cautioned, however, against unnecessary pressure against the carotid artery. The temporal pulse or the apical (chest) beat may also be convenient sites.

The technician's preparatory steps for many field/lab tests are as follows:

1. Calibrate the instruments prior to on-site orientation of the performer (review Box 13.2).
2. Set metronome to proper cadence (90 b·min⁻¹).
3. Record meteorological data:
   a. Environmental temperature (°C)
   b. Relative humidity (% RH)
   c. Barometric pressure (P_B; mm Hg; convert to hPa)
4. State the purpose of the test to the performer, e.g., ". . . to record post-exercise heart rate in order to estimate your aerobic fitness."
5. Question the performer regarding drugs, physical activity, meal time, or any possible medical factors that might contraindicate (argue against) exercise testing at the present time.
6. Record basic data—date, time of day, gender, and age; measure and record stature (cm) and body mass (kg).
7. Explain and briefly demonstrate the test:
   a. Exercise protocol
      1. Exercise mode—step ergometer
      2. Timing—cadence, rate, and duration
      3. Intensity—submaximal (low to moderate)
   b. Technique of exercising—proper stepping
   c. Physiological measures
      1. The variable and method: pulse count by palpation
      2. Timing of variable: onset and duration of pulse count
8. Ask performer if there are any questions.
9. Obtain performer's informed consent (agreement to be tested; see Appendix E).
10. Provide a nonfatiguing practice period for the performer that includes stepping and palpating of pulse.

Testing

The testing procedures for various step tests are similar. The exercise protocol (Table 13.3) for the Forestry Step Test includes such factors as height of step, rate of stepping, duration of stepping, and time period of the pulse count. The procedures for the Forestry Step Test include such factors as paying attention to warning signs, timing and palpating the pulses, and cooling down.

Table 13.3	Protocol for the Forestry Step Test[a]
Step Height	
Men:	40 cm (15.75 in.)
Women:	33 cm (13 in.)
Step Rate	22.5 steps per min; (metronome = 90 b·min⁻¹)
Stepping Duration	5 min
Pulse count time period	15 s (5:15–5:30)

Note: [a]Same protocol as for Åstrand-Ryhming Step Test.[4,16]

Table 13.4	Stop-Test Indicators from Unmonitored Performer during Exercise Testing

Indicator	Performer Characteristics
1. Request[a]	Makes request to end the test
2. Pallor[a]	Skin becomes pale, cyanotic
3. Ataxia[a]	Lacks coordination; e.g., fails to keep proper cadence for *20 consecutive seconds*
4. Confusion[a]	Inability to focus attention; e.g., time disorientation
5. Syncope	Faintness, dizziness, or light-headedness
6. Nausea[a]	Sick to the stomach; vomiting symptoms
7. Dyspnea	Undue shortening of breath
8. Angina	Chest pain
9. Muscular problem	Side stitch, cramp, strain, undue fatigue
10. Facial disorder	Panic look, blank stare, unresponsive

[a] Adapted from The American College of Sports Medicine, *Guidelines for Graded Exercise Testing and Prescription*, p. 72, 1991. Copyright © 1991 Lea & Febiger Publishers, Malvern, PA. Reprinted by permission.[1]

Warning Signs

If the performer cannot complete the test due to fatigue or any stop-test characteristics listed in Table 13.4, then the technician should record the actual total time of the test in addition to the reason for terminating the test (e.g., fatigue, pallor, dyspnea). Stopping an exercise test for *specific* indications, such as a drop in blood pressure, are not applicable for the Forestry Step Test because the performer usually is not monitored for that variable. Therefore, the stop-test signs listed in Table 13.4 are general signs that are likely to indicate a deficiency in an *unmonitored* physiological system.

Timing the Pulse Count

The laboratory clock should continue to run after the 5th min; the time for counting pulses begins at 5:15 and ends at 5:30. The metronome is stopped at the fifth minute, however, because it may be disconcerting while trying to count heartbeats.

The technician's and performer's 15 s pulse counts should not differ by more than two beats. (It is quite likely that only the performer will count the pulse under field conditions.) If the difference is greater than two beats, then repeat the test after both palpators are confident that they are palpating correctly.

It is very important to get accurate pulse counts. They will be used for estimating the individual's maximal oxygen consumption. In general, palpation errors are those of *underestimation* because people are more likely to miss pulses than add extra ones.[11]

Cooldown

To alleviate possible delayed muscle stiffness or dizziness, the performer should walk for about three minutes immediately following the test. After mild walking, the performer should stretch the calves (e.g., wall-lean exercise) and quadriceps on three or four occasions for 3 s to 60 s with 2 min relief intervals. The quadriceps stretch can be performed from the standing position by flexing the lower leg toward the buttocks, then grabbing the flexed leg's ankle with the opposite hand. You may need a wall, chair, or table to hold onto for balance.

Summary of Procedures for the Forestry Step Test

The sequence of procedures may be summarized in 12 steps as follows:

1. Performer stands facing 40 cm (men) or 33 cm (women) step bench.
2. Technician starts metronome, which is set for 90 b·min^{-1}.
3. Technician requests performer to start stepping at any metronome beat.
4. Technician starts timer as soon as performer makes first movement.
5. Technician helps with cadence initially by counting aloud: "up-one, up-two, down-one, down-two."
6. Technician encourages performer to straighten the back and the legs at top of step.
7. Technician encourages completion of the test while keeping aware of stop-test indicators (Table 13.4).
8. Technician stops test and metronome at 5th min.
9. Performer sits down immediately upon completion of test.
10. Technician and performer immediately palpate pulse and count silently for 15 s, starting the count at 5:15 (15 s after the test) and stopping at 5:30.
11. The technician records the 15 s pulse count on Form 13.1.
12. Performer cools down by walking and statically stretching the gastrocnemius and quadriceps for the next 5 min to 8 min.

Derivation of Aerobic Fitness from the Forestry Step Test

The unit of measure derived from the heart rate response from the Forestry Step Test is a maximal oxygen consumption value (milliliters of oxygen per kilogram body weight per minute; mL·kg^{-1}·min^{-1}). Tables 13.5 (men), 13.6 (women), and 13.7 (age adjustment) minimize mathemati-

cal calculations.[20] The body mass and 15 s pulse count are needed to find the *nonadjusted* value of maximal oxygen consumption in the tables for men and women, respectively. Age and the nonadjusted value are needed to find the age-adjusted aerobic fitness for men and women 15 y to 65 y of age.

Body Mass (BM)

The bottom two rows of Tables 13.5 and 13.6 are presented in 10 lb and 4.5 kg increments. The columns above each body mass (BM) represent the predicted maximal oxygen consumption ($\dot{V}O_2$max) for any given row of pulse counts that intersects the BM column. Because the efficiency of stepping (mL·kg^{-1}·min^{-1}) changes very little for any given change in body mass (especially for men), there is no need to interpolate the BM columns for those who lie between the columns. Hence, the $\dot{V}O_2$max changes insignificantly between paired BM columns.

Pulse Count

The far left columns in Tables 13.5 and 13.6 represent the post-step test heartbeats (15 s) from 20 to 45. The value at the intersection of the row for the pulse counts and the column for the body mass is the nonadjusted fitness score ($\dot{V}O_2$max in mL·kg^{-1}·min^{-1}) for the Forestry Step Test. The tables must be used because no regression equation has been derived from the original Sharkey data.

It is not essential to calculate heart rate in order to derive the aerobic fitness score. It should be recognized that the actual exercise heart rate during the last minute of the Forestry Step Test is really higher than that represented by the 15 s pulse count even after the 15 s count is converted to a minute rate. This is because heart rate would continue to decrease from the 15th to 30th s of post-exercise.

As an example of using the nonadjusted fitness tables, suppose the number of pulse counts between the 15th and 30th s following the step test is 30 for a 50.0 kg (110 lb) woman. By reading horizontally along the 30 pulse-count row (or marking lightly with a pencil) to the point where it intersects the 50.0 kg column (may also be marked with a pencil), the value 44 is found. This value represents a maximal oxygen consumption of 44 mL·kg^{-1}·min^{-1}. If a man weighing 68.2 kg (150 lb) has a pulse count response of 30, his nonadjusted maximal oxygen consumption is 49 mL·kg^{-1}·min^{-1}. However, both the woman's and the man's values need to be adjusted for age.

Age-Adjusted Aerobic Fitness

In order to derive a valid aerobic fitness score for persons 30 y of age or more, it is necessary to account for the natural decrease in maximal heart rate due to aging. This decrease was presented in Chapter 12 as follows: maximal HR equals 220 minus age.

Table 13.5 Forestry Nonadjusted Aerobic Fitness ($\dot{V}O_2$max) for Men

Pulse Count (15 s) 5:15–5:30	Maximal Oxygen Consumption (mL·kg^{-1}·min^{-1})												
45	33	33	33	33	33	32	32	32	32	32	32	32	32
44	34	34	34	34	33	33	33	33	33	33	33	33	33
43	35	35	35	34	34	34	34	34	34	34	34	34	34
42	36	35	35	35	35	35	35	35	35	35	35	34	34
41	36	36	36	36	36	36	36	36	36	36	36	35	35
40	37	37	37	37	37	37	37	37	35	35	35	35	35
39	38	38	38	38	38	38	38	38	38	38	38	37	37
38	39	39	39	39	39	39	39	39	39	39	39	38	38
37	41	40	40	40	40	40	40	40	40	40	40	39	39
36	42	42	41	41	41	41	41	41	41	41	41	40	40
35	43	43	42	42	42	42	42	42	42	42	42	42	41
34	44	44	43	43	43	43	43	43	43	43	43	43	43
33	46	45	45	45	45	45	44	44	44	44	44	44	44
32	47	47	46	46	46	46	46	46	46	46	46	46	46
31	48	48	48	47	47	47	47	47	47	47	47	47	47
30	50	49	49	49	48	48	48	48	48	48	48	48	48
29	52	51	51	51	50	50	59	50	50	50	50	50	50
28	53	53	53	53	52	52	52	52	51	51	51	51	51
27	55	55	55	54	54	54	54	54	54	53	53	53	52
26	57	57	56	56	56	56	56	56	56	55	55	54	54
25	59	59	58	58	58	58	58	58	58	56	56	55	55
24	60	60	60	60	60	60	60	59	59	58	58	57	
23	62	62	61	61	61	61	61	60	60	60	59		
22	64	64	63	63	63	63	62	62	61	61			
21	66	66	65	65	65	64	64	64	62				
20	68	68	67	67	67	67	66	66	65				
BM (lb)	120	130	140	150	160	170	180	190	200	210	220	230	240
BM (kg)	54.5	59.1	63.6	68.2	72.7	77.3	81.8	86.4	91	95.4	100	104.5	109

From Sharkey, B. J. *Physiology of Fitness,* Table B.1, p. 258, 1984. Copyright © 1984 Human Kinetics Publishers, Champaign, IL.[20]

Table 13.6 Forestry Nonadjusted Aerobic Fitness Values (mL·kg^{-1}·min^{-1}) for Women

Pulse Count 5:15–5:30	Maximal Oxygen Consumption ($\dot{V}O_2$max)											
45										29	29	29
44								30	30	30	30	30
43							31	31	31	31	31	31
42			32	32	32	32	32	32	32	32	32	32
41			33	33	33	33	33	33	33	33	33	33
40			34	34	34	34	34	34	34	34	34	34
39			35	35	35	35	35	35	35	35	35	35
38			36	36	36	36	36	36	36	36	36	36
37			37	37	37	37	37	37	37	37	37	37
36		37	38	38	38	38	38	38	38	38	38	38
35	38	38	39	39	39	39	39	39	39	39	39	39
34	39	39	40	40	40	40	40	40	40	40	40	40
33	40	40	41	41	41	41	41	41	41	41	41	41
32	41	41	42	42	42	42	42	42	42	42	42	42
31	42	42	43	43	43	43	43	43	43	43	43	43
30	43	43	44	44	44	44	44	44	44	44	44	44
29	44	44	45	45	45	45	45	45	45	45	45	45
28	45	45	46	46	46	47	47	47	47	47	47	
27	46	46	47	48	48	49	49	49	49			
26	47	48	49	50	50	51	51	51				
25	49	50	51	52	52	53	53					
24	51	52	53	54	54	55						
23	53	54	55	56	56	57						
BM (lb)	80	90	100	110	120	130	140	150	160	170	180	190
BM (kg)	36.4	40.9	45.4	50.0	54.5	59.1	63.6	68.2	72.7	77.3	81.8	86.4

From Sharkey, B. J. *Physiology of Fitness,* Table B.2, p. 259, 1984. Copyright © 1984 Human Kinetics Publishers, Champaign, IL.[20]

Table 13.7 Age-Adjusted Fitness Scores for the Forestry Step Test

Age (y)	Nonadjusted Fitness Score																				
	30	31	32	33	34	35	36	37	38	39	40	41	42	43	44	45	46	47	48	49	50
	Age-Adjusted Score (mL·kg^{-1}·min^{-1})																				
15	32	33	34	35	36	37	38	39	40	41	42	43	44	45	46	47	48	49	50	51	53
20	31	32	33	34	35	36	37	38	39	40	41	42	43	44	45	46	47	48	49	50	51
25	30	31	32	33	34	35	36	37	38	39	40	41	42	43	44	45	46	47	48	49	50
30	29	30	31	32	33	34	35	36	37	38	39	40	41	42	43	44	45	46	47	48	49
35	27	28	29	31	32	33	34	35	36	37	38	39	40	41	42	43	44	45	46	47	48
40	26	27	28	30	31	32	33	34	35	36	37	38	39	40	41	42	43	44	45	46	47
45	25	26	27	29	30	31	32	33	34	35	36	37	38	39	40	41	42	43	44	45	46
50	24	25	26	28	29	30	31	32	33	34	35	36	37	38	39	40	41	42	43	44	45
55	23	24	25	27	28	29	30	31	32	33	34	35	36	37	38	39	40	40	41	42	43
60	22	23	24	25	26	27	28	30	31	32	33	34	35	36	37	37	38	39	40	41	42
65	21	22	23	24	25	26	27	28	29	30	31	32	33	34	35	36	37	38	38	39	40

Example: If your age is 40 years and you score 50 on the step test, your age-adjusted score is 47 mL·kg^{-1}min^{-1}.

Age (y)	Nonadjusted Fitness Score																					
	51	52	53	54	55	56	57	58	59	60	61	62	63	64	65	66	67	68	69	70	71	72
	Age-Adjusted Score (mL·kg^{-1}·min^{-1})																					
15	54	55	56	57	58	59	60	61	62	63	64	65	66	67	68	69	70	71	72	74	75	76
20	52	53	54	55	56	57	58	59	60	61	62	63	64	65	66	67	68	69	70	71	72	73
25	51	52	53	54	55	56	57	58	59	60	61	62	63	64	65	66	67	68	69	70	71	72
30	50	51	52	53	54	55	56	57	58	59	60	61	62	63	64	65	66	67	68	69	70	71
35	49	50	51	52	53	54	55	56	57	58	59	60	60	61	62	63	64	65	66	67	68	69
40	48	49	50	51	52	53	54	55	55	56	57	58	59	60	61	62	63	64	65	66	67	68
45	47	48	49	50	51	52	52	53	54	55	56	57	58	59	60	61	62	63	64	65	65	66
50	45	46	47	48	49	50	51	52	53	53	54	55	56	57	58	58	59	61	61	62	63	64
55	44	45	46	46	47	48	49	50	51	52	53	53	54	55	56	57	58	59	59	60	61	62
60	42	43	44	45	46	46	47	48	49	50	51	51	52	53	54	55	56	57	57	58	59	60
65	41	42	42	43	44	45	46	46	47	48	49	50	50	51	52	53	54	54	55	56	57	58

From B. J. Sharkey, *Physiology of Fitness,* Table B.3, 260–1, 1984. Copyright © 1984 Human Kinetics Publishers, Champaign, IL.[20]

For example, if a 20-year-old man and 50-year-old man have the same pulse count after the step test, they do not have equal aerobic fitness levels. Theoretically, the 30 pulse counts (120 b·min^{-1}) for the 20-year-old represent only 120/200th (60 %) of his maximal rate (200 b·min^{-1}), whereas 30 counts represent 120/170th (70 %) of the 50-year-old's maximal rate (170 b·min^{-1}). Thus, the degree of stress for the older person is relatively greater during the step test because he is working closer to his maximal heart rate.

To find the age-adjusted fitness score, the first step is to round off the performer's age to the closest fifth year (y). For example, if the person is 33 y of age, then locate the 35-year row originating at the far left of Table 13.7;[20] if the performer is 32 y of age, then locate the 30 y row. Then read horizontally along the *age* row to where the age intersects with the nonadjusted fitness score. If the nonadjusted $\dot{V}O_2$max is 44 mL·kg^{-1}·min^{-1}, then the age-adjusted $\dot{V}O_2$max is 43 mL·kg^{-1}·min^{-1} for the 32 y old man. This age-adjusted fitness score should be used to categorize the aerobic fitness level found in Table 13.8.[20]

Results and Discussion

The interpretation of the predicted maximal oxygen consumption from the Forestry Step Test is made by consulting the aerobic fitness norms in Table 13.8. The fitness categories distinguish between gender and age groups. For example, the 30-year-old man or woman whose age-adjusted $\dot{V}O_2$max is 43 mL·kg^{-1}·min^{-1}, are categorized as "good" and "very good," respectively. Neither of these scores meets the criterion of 45 mL·kg^{-1}·min^{-1} suggested by Sharkey for wilderness firefighters. However, it requires only 15 mL·kg^{-1}·min^{-1} to perform daily independent-living tasks by older adults.[5]

Table 13.8 Aerobic Fitness Categories in Men (M) and Women (W) for the Forestry Step Test

		Fitness Categories						
		Superior	Excellent	Very Good	Good	Fair	Poor	Very Poor
Age (y)		Maximal Oxygen Consumption (mL·kg⁻¹·min⁻¹)						
15	M	57+	56–52	51–47	46–42	41–37	36–32	< 32
	W	54+	53–49	48–44	43–39	38–34	33–29	< 29
20	M	56+	55–51	50–46	45–41	40–36	35–31	< 31
	W	53+	52–48	47–43	42–38	37–33	32–28	< 28
25	M	55+	54–50	49–45	44–40	39–35	34–30	< 30
	W	52+	51–47	46–42	41–37	36–32	31–27	< 27
30	M	54+	53–49	48–44	43–39	38–34	33–29	< 29
	W	51+	50–46	45–41	40–36	35–31	30–26	< 26
35	M	53+	52–48	47–43	42–38	37–33	32–28	< 28
	W	50+	49–45	44–40	39–35	34–30	29–25	< 25
40	M	52+	51–47	46–42	41–37	36–32	31–27	< 27
	W	49+	48–44	43–39	38–34	33–29	28–24	< 24
45	M	51+	50–46	45–41	40–36	35–31	30–26	< 26
	W	48+	47–43	42–38	37–33	32–28	27–23	< 23
50	M	50+	49–45	44–40	39–35	34–30	29–25	< 25
	W	47+	46–42	41–37	36–32	31–27	26–22	< 22
55	M	49+	48–44	43–39	38–34	33–29	28–24	< 24
	W	46+	45–41	40–36	35–31	30–26	25–21	< 21
60	M	48+	47–43	42–38	37–33	32–28	27–23	< 23
	W	45+	44–40	39–35	34–30	29–25	24–20	< 20
65	M	47+	46–42	41–37	36–32	31–27	26–22	< 22
	W	44+	43–39	38–34	33–29	28–24	23–20	< 20

From Sharkey, B. J. *Physiology of Fitness,* Tables B.4 and B.5, p. 262, 1984. Copyright © 1984 Human Kinetics Publishers, Champaign, IL.[20]

References

1. American College of Sports Medicine. (1991). *Guidelines for graded exercise testing and prescription.* Philadelphia: Lea & Febiger.
2. American College of Sports Medicine. (2000). *ACSM's guidelines for graded exercise testing and prescription.* Philadelphia: Lippincott Williams & Wilkins.
3. Andersen, K. L., Shephard, R. J., Denolin, H., Varnauskas, E., & Masironi, R. (1971). *Fundamentals of exercise testing.* Geneva: World Health Organization.
4. Åstrand, P.-O., & Ryhming, I. (1954). A nomogram for calculation of aerobic capacity (physical fitness) from pulse rate during submaximal work. *Journal of Applied Physiology, 7,* 218–221.
5. Blair, S. N., Brill, P. A., & Kohl, H. W. (1989). Physical activity patterns in older individuals. In W. W. Spirduso & H. M. Eckert (Eds.), *Physical activity and aging* (pp. 120–130). Champaign, IL: Human Kinetics.
6. Brouha, L. (1943). The Step Test: A simple method of measuring physical fitness for muscular work in young men. *Research Quarterly, 14,* 30–35.
7. Cicutti, N., Jette, M., & Sidney, K. (1991). Effect of leg length on bench stepping efficiency in children. *Canadian Journal of Sport Science, 16,* 58–63.
8. deVries, H. A. (1971). *Lab experiments in exercise physiology.* Dubuque, IA: Wm. C. Brown.
9. Fox, E. L., Bowers, R. W., & Foss, M. L. (1993). *The physiological basis for exercise and sport.* Dubuque, IA: Brown & Benchmark.
10. Frohlich, E. D., Grim, C., Labarthe, D. R., Maxwell, M. H., Perloff, D., & Weidman, W. H. (1987). *Recommendations for human blood pressure determination by sphygmomanometers: Report of a special task force appointed by the steering committee, American Heart Association.* Dallas: National Center, American Heart Association.
11. Greer, N. L., & Katch, F. I. (1982). Validity of palpation recovery pulse rate to estimate exercise heart rate following four intensities of bench step exercise. *Research Quarterly for Exercise and Sport, 53,* 340–343.
12. Howley, E. T., Colacino, D. L., & Swensen, T. C. (1992). Factors affecting the oxygen cost of stepping on an electronic stepping ergometer. *Medicine and Science in Sports and Exercise, 24,* 1055–1058.
13. Johnson, J., & Siegel, D. (1981). The use of selected submaximal step tests in predicting change in the maximal oxygen intake of college women. *Journal of Sports Medicine and Physical Fitness, 21,* 259–264.
14. McArdle, W. D., Katch, F. I., & Katch, V. L. (1996). *Exercise physiology: Energy, nutrition, and human performance.* Baltimore: Williams & Wilkins.
15. Nagle, F. J., Balke, B., & Naughton, J. P. (1965). Gradational step tests for assessing work capacity. *Journal of Applied Physiology, 20,* 745–748.

16. Ryhming, I. (1953). A modified Harvard step test for the evaluation of physical fitness. *Arbeitsphysiologie, 15,* 235–250.

17. Sedlock, D. A., Knowlton, R. G., Fitzgerald, P. I., Tahamont, M. V., & Schneider, D. A. (1983). Accuracy of subject-palpated carotid pulse after exercise. *The Physician and Sportsmedicine, 11*(4) 106–108, 113–116.

18. Shahnawaz, H. (1978). Influence of limb length on a stepping exercise. *Journal of Applied Physiology, 44,* 346–349.

19. Sharkey, B. J. (1977). *Fitness and work capacity.* (Report FS-315.) Washington, DC: U.S. Department of Agriculture.

20. Sharkey, B. J. (1984). *Physiology of fitness.* Champaign, IL: Human Kinetics.

21. Shephard, R. J. (1969). Learning, habituation, and training. *Internationale Z. Angew. Physiologi, 28,* 38–48.

22. Shephard, R. J. (1971). Standard test of aerobic power. In R. J. Shephard (Ed.), *Frontiers in fitness* (pp. 133–165). Springfield, IL: Charles C Thomas.

23. Thomas, S. G., Miller, I. M. R., & Cox, M. H. (1993). Sources of variation in oxygen consumption during a stepping task. *Medicine and Science in Sports and Exercise, 25,* 139–144.

24. Washburn, R. A., & Safrit, M. J. (1982). Physical performance tests in job selection—A model for empirical validation. *Research Quarterly for Exercise and Sport, 53*(3), 267–270.

Form 13.1

Individual Data for Forestry Step Test

Name [　　　　　　　　　　　　] Date [　　　　　] Time [　　　] A.M. [　] P.M. [　]

Age [　] y   Gender (M or W) [　]   Ht [　　] cm   Wt (in exercise clothes) [　　] kg [　　] N

Meteorological Data

Tech. Initials [　] T [　] °C (closest 0.1 °C)   RH % [　] P_B [　] mm Hg × 1.333 = [　] hPa (mbar)

Fan: Yes [　]   No [　]

Palpatory Site (Rank from best—1st—to worst—4th):

Radial [　]   Carotid [　]   Temporal [　]   Apical [　]

Test Data

Proper Cadence (check one):   Always [　]   Usually [　]   Seldom [　]

Proper Technique (check one):   Always [　]   Usually [　]   Seldom [　]

Comment, if applicable, on cadence, duration, and technique: _____

15 s Pulse Count (5:15–5:30) [　　]

Aerobic Fitness (mL·kg⁻¹·min⁻¹):   Nonadjusted (Table 13.5; Men) (Table 13.6; Women)   Age Adjusted (Table 13.7)

[　　　　] [　　　　]

Aerobic Fitness Category (Table 13.8; check one):

Superior [　]   Excellent [　]   Very Good [　]   Good [　]

Fair [　]   Poor [　]   Very Poor [　]

Qualification as Wilderness Firefighter (45⁺ mL·kg⁻¹·min⁻¹):   Yes [　]   No [　]

Step $\dot{V}O_2$ (mL·kg⁻¹·min⁻¹) = 29.5 (from Eq. 13.1)

Absolute $\dot{V}O_2$ (L·min⁻¹) = (29.5 × BM [　] kg) ÷ 1000 = [　] L·min⁻¹

Form 13.2

Group Data for Forestry Step Test

M E N

Initials/I.D.	$\dot{V}O_2$max $(mL \cdot kg^{-1} \cdot min^{-1})$
1.	
2.	
3.	
4.	
5.	
6.	
7.	
8.	
9.	
10.	
11.	
12.	
13.	
14.	
15.	
16.	
17.	
18.	
19.	
20.	
21.	
22.	
M	
Minimum	
Maximum	

W O M E N

Initials/I.D.	$\dot{V}O_2$max $(mL \cdot kg^{-1} \cdot min^{-1})$
1.	
2.	
3.	
4.	
5.	
6.	
7.	
8.	
9.	
10.	
11.	
12.	
13.	
14.	
15.	
16.	
17.	
18.	
19.	
20.	
21.	
22.	
M	
Minimum	
Maximum	

AEROBIC CYCLING

The Åstrand Cycle Test is one of the most popular sub-maximal exercise tests in exercise physiology laboratories and fitness clinics. It is a more sophisticated field/lab test than the step test, partially due to its more complicated procedures and its more expensive and less portable ergometer. Group testing is severely restricted due to the need for numerous cycle ergometers. It nearly qualifies as a laboratory test because heart rate can be measured *during* exercise by more sophisticated methods (e.g., ECG and auscultation) than by palpation, such as in most step tests. However, it probably does not qualify as a laboratory test because it is not a direct measure of maximal oxygen consumption.

Purpose of the Åstrand Cycle Test

The purpose of this submaximal exercise test is similar to the run tests and the step tests—that is, to estimate a person's aerobic fitness. Additionally, I have expanded the designers'[3,4,6] original purposes to include educational objectives, such as familiarization with cycle ergometry, achievement of the skill in auscultation of heartbeats, and the understanding of the rationale for the test.

Physiological Rationale

All submaximal cycle ergometer tests are designed to rely predominantly upon the oxidative metabolic pathway (aerobic) to supply the majority of the ATP to the muscles. As is typical of exercise meant to promote aerobic fitness, the muscles used in cycling are relatively large. For example, the extension of the hip and knee joints for the downstroke in cycling is accomplished mainly by the gluteus maximus, rectus femoris, and the vastus lateralis. Knee flexion, on the other hand, is accomplished by the biceps femoris and the gastrocnemius during the upstroke, while hip flexion is accomplished by the rectus femoris during the latter part of the upstroke.[14]

The Åstrand Test *predicts* maximal oxygen consumption ($\dot{V}O_2max$) based upon the steady-state heart rate of a person exercising at a submaximal power level for 6 min. Thus, the rationale is similar to that of step tests in that the test is dependent upon the direct relationships among power level, oxygen consumption, and heart rate. The positive relationship between heart rate and oxygen consumption is most linear between 50 % and 90 % of maximal heart rate.[13] Expressed in terms of the respective units of mea-

sure, the physiological rationale for the Åstrand Test can be stated as the following: A prediction of maximal oxygen consumption ($L \cdot min^{-1}$) based upon the performer's heart-rate response at a given power (W; $N \cdot m \cdot min^{-1}$) or submaximal oxygen consumption. Åstrand and Ryhming observed that the heart rates for men and women at 50 % $\dot{V}O_2max$ were 128 $b \cdot min^{-1}$ and 138 $b \cdot min^{-1}$, respectively. Thus, if a man exercised at a power level that required an oxygen consumption of 2.1 L/min and his heart rate was 128 $b \cdot min^{-1}$ then his predicted $\dot{V}O_2max$ based on the assumed linear relationship would be 4.2 L/min.

Method

As with all field or laboratory tests, the methodology of the Åstrand Cycle Test includes such factors as (a) equipment, (b) technician preparations, (c) test procedures, and (d) calculations of $\dot{V}O_2max$. Many of these methods apply to other cycle ergometer tests that predict aerobic fitness, such as the YMCA Test.[16] The description of the accuracy of the Åstrand Cycle Test is in Box 14.1, and the calibration procedures are in Box 14.2.

Equipment

The equipment for administering the Åstrand Cycle Test varies according to the purposes of the investigator, technician, teacher, or student. For example, no equipment is necessary to palpate the pulse; however, if the goal of students is to develop auscultatory (listening to heart sounds) skills, then stethoscopes will be needed. Additionally, if assured accuracy is required, then an investigator would need an electrocardiogram to measure heart rate. Also, heart-rate telemetry may be used, whereby chest electrodes send electrocardiographic signals to an FM radio transmitter, which relays the heart rate to an external display or receiver "wristwatch."

The equipment needed for the purposes presented in this manual are (a) a cycle ergometer, (b) a seconds stopwatch, (c) laboratory timers, (d) a metronome or tachometer, (e) a stethoscope, and (f) a calculator.

Cycle Ergometer

There are various types of cycle ergometers. Most ergometers may be classified in two ways, either according to their braking method or according to the constancy of the power

BOX 14.1 Accuracy of the Åstrand Cycle Test

Reliability

The test-retest reliability coefficients were acceptable for older men (r = .835)[9] and college women (r = .87)[40] who twice performed the Åstrand Cycle Test. When heart rates are taken daily on a person exercising at the same exercise power level, they vary by about ±5 b·min^{-1}.[26]

Validity

All *predictive* tests should be interpreted with caution, especially if the original data from the test were from a different type of population. For example, both age and fitness are characteristics that may influence the interpretation of a test. With respect to age, low validity coefficients (approximately .60) were reported between the Åstrand Cycle Test and the directly measured maximal oxygen consumption of middle-aged men.[19] With respect to fitness, untrained persons are more likely to be underestimated by the Åstrand Cycle Test, whereas the highly trained are more likely to be overestimated in their maximal oxygen consumptions.[5]

The ability of the Åstrand Test to predict or estimate the actual measured maximal oxygen consumption varies considerably. The standard error of the estimate *(SEE)* has ranged from as low as 6 % to 10 %[38] to as high as 15 % to 20 %.[19,25,27]

One investigator reported a validity coefficient of .74 between the Åstrand predicted values and the directly measured maximal oxygen consumption values.[10] In a review of 13 studies, validity coefficients ranged from as low as .34 to as high as .94, with the average being .64.[19] The rationale of the Åstrand Cycle Test assumes that the heart rate versus oxygen consumption relationship remains linear to maximal levels. This has been contested by some investigators[31,41] and is likely to contribute to the underestimation of $\dot{V}O_2$max in persons of average or low fitness. Although researchers report a linear increase in optimal pedalling rate with increased power output in cycle ergometry,[7] the 50 r·min^{-1} prescribed for the Åstrand Cycle Test was the original rate in the development of the test's predictions and norms.

BOX 14.2 Calibration of the Cycle Ergometer

Mechanically Braked Ergometers

The mechanically braked (friction belt) ergometer (Figure 14.1) can be statically (no pedalling) calibrated based upon the movement of the pendulum to a given reading on the force scale (Figure 14.2) which corresponds to the amount of weight suspended from the friction belt. Fortunately, Monark ergometers rarely need recalibration.

Zero

1. Remove the belt from the spring-belt junction at the front of the ergometer.
2. Adjust the "winged-bolt" screw at the front rim of the Force scale "quadrant" so that the zero point of the scale coincides with the red index mark on the pendulum weight.
3. Tighten the lock nut of the thumb screw.

Range

1. Hang a known weight from the spring or suspension hook where the friction belt attaches.
2. The pendulum weight should move to the corresponding marker on the Force scale (e.g., a 4 kg weight moves the pendulum to the 40 N or 4 kp [kilopond] marker). *Note:* kp is essentially the same as kg.
3. If not in agreement, adjust the weight pin inside the pendulum disk with the lock screw in the center of the backside of the disk.
4. A less sophisticated adjustment can be made by taping over the present numbers on the scale and writing in the correct values.[a]

Electronically Braked Constant-Power Cycle Ergometer

Although these cycle ergometers are calibrated by the manufacturer, they can lose their calibration with constant use. Advertisers of electronic calibrators claim that the typical accuracy of the power setting is 5 % to 20 %. These cycles require either a technician's expertise in interfacing the cycle's electronic output to a volt/watt meter or the purchase of an expensive special calibrating dynamometer (e.g., Quinton, model 805; Vacu·Med). The calibrators can measure the accuracy of powers up to 600 W from 40 rpm to 120 rpm (Vacu·Med®). Some dynamometric calibrators are capable of detecting power variations of about 1 W. Manufacturers may perform the calibration periodically; however, this can be expensive. Rough checks of the accuracy can be made with a conventional torque wrench, following instructions from the manufacturer.

Note: [a]The friction in the transmission (mainly the chain) of the Monark cycle increases the stated power level by 9 %. Most tables relating power to oxygen consumption disregard this frictional contribution to the listed power levels. Thus, the stated and calculated (F × D) power level of 600 kg·m·min^{-1} is really 650 kg·m·min^{-1}; a power of 1200 kg·m·min^{-1} is 1300 kg·m·min^{-1}. Consequently, 1.5 L·min^{-1} of oxygen consumption is actually atained at 109 W and 650 kg·m·min^{-1}, not at 100 W or 600 kg·m·min^{-1}, as listed in the Monark operations manual.[4]

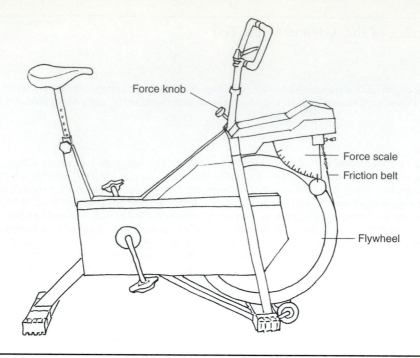

Figure 14.1 A mechanically braked cycle ergometer; the force (load) remains constant at its setting regardless of pedal revolutions.

level. There are usually two types of braking methods—mechanical or electrical; similarly, there are two types of power controls—one that is constant regardless of pedal speed and one that changes power according to pedal speed.

Mechanically braked cycles (e.g., Monark™) in laboratories are usually of a superior quality, compared with most of the mechanically braked ones sold in department stores or used in fitness centers. The resistance to the wheel of a mechanically braked bike is based upon the tightening (friction) of the belt that surrounds the flywheel. The typical force settings range from 5 N (0.5 kg) to a high of 70 N (7.0 kg). The popular Monark™ ergometer has a force scale with gradations marked in kiloponds (kp)[a] and newtons (N). The scale uses approximate conversions from kp (kg) to newtons, where 1 kp is equivalent to 1 kg.

- 1 kp = 1 kg
- 1 kg ≈ 10 N
- 1 kg = 9.80665 N

Mechanically braked ergometers provide a constant force, but a nonconstant power at varying pedal revolutions. Thus, any increase in the rate of pedal revolutions (r·min^{-1}; rpm) causes an increase in work (w) and power (P). This is because any change in pedal revolutions (r) changes the dis-

tance (D) factor of the work and power equations. The Monark™ ergometer's flywheel has a circumference of 1.62 m (often stated in rounded figures as 2 m) and travels 6 m in 3.7 circuits (often stated as 3 circuits) with each pedal revolution.[15] Thus, in mechanically braked ergometers, any change in pedal revolutions per minute (r·min^{-1}; rpm) will alter the work (w) and power (P) as presented in Equation 14.1.

Constant **Force** Ergometer:

$$\text{Change in r·min}^{-1}; \text{rpm} = \text{change in D} \qquad \text{Eq. 14.1}$$
$$= \text{change in w and P}$$

When combining the force (F) component with the distance (D) per minute component, the product becomes a power unit—that is, work rate. Although watts (W) is the preferred expression of the power unit by the International System, kilogram meters per minute (kg·m·min^{-1}; "kgm/min") is often seen in early research publications. Newton meters per minute (N·m·min^{-1}), may be used also but is a more cumbersome abbreviation than the *W* for watts. Thus, the power for any force or distance can be calculated from Equation 14.2.

$$P = F \times D / t \qquad \text{Eq. 14.2}$$

For example, if the force setting is 20 N (or 2 kg) and the distance traveled in 1 min is 300 m, then the power is

$$20 \text{ N} \times 300 \text{ m·min}^{-1} = 6000 \text{ N·m·min}^{-1}$$

or

$$2 \text{ kg} \times 300 \text{ m·min}^{-1} = 600 \text{ kg·m·min}^{-1}$$

---

[a]One kilopond represents the force at normal acceleration of gravity that is dependent upon the global latitude. For example, a person's body mass is greater at the North Pole (90° latitude) than at the Equator (0° latitude) due to the greater pull of gravity at the pole. However, the difference between kilogram and kilopond has little practical significance for exercise laboratories.

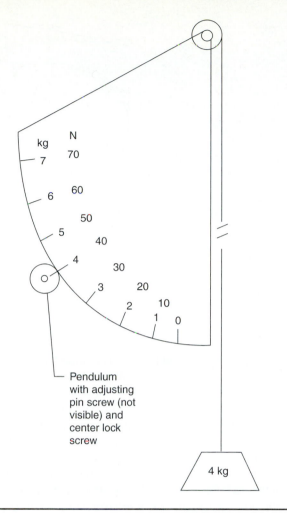

Figure 14.2 The force scale indicates by its pendulum the accuracy of a mass of 4 kg representing a force of 40 N on the friction belt of the mechanically braked cycle ergometer.

Because 1 W is equal to 60 N·m·min⁻¹ and approximately 6 kg·m·min⁻¹, the watt value is 100 W.

- $1 \text{ W} \approx 6 \text{ kg·m·min}^{-1}$
- $1 \text{ W} = 6.118 \text{ kg·m·min}^{-1}$
  $= 1 \text{ N·m·s}^{-1}$
  $= 60 \text{ N·m·min}^{-1}$

Electromagnetically braked cycle ergometers (e.g., Tectrix™, Biodex™, and Sensor Medics™ and some computer-controlled ergometers (Monark 839E™) do not require strict attention to pedal frequency. If the distance (D) changes because the pedal revolutions increase or decrease on a constant-power ergometer, the force (F) factor compensates electronically to maintain a constant power level (Eq. 14.3).

Constant **Power** Ergometer:

$$\text{Change in rpm} = \text{change in D but compensating change in F}$$

$$= \text{no change in work (w)} \quad \text{Eq. 14.3}$$
$$\text{and power (P)}$$

Obviously, these constant power ergometers simplify matters. However, the relationships among force, distance, work, time, and power are more easily conceptualized by students of exercise physiology when using the constant force ergometer. It should be noted for the pure measure of work these calculations do not consider the internal work from the rotation of the lower limbs themselves during cycling.[39]

Timing Mechanisms

Three types of timers can be used to administer the Åstrand Cycle Test. Stopwatches (or wristwatches capable of measuring tenths of a second) are mandatory for measuring heart rate, while either a laboratory set-clock or wall clock is acceptable for elapsed time—that is, the continuous running time.

Metronome or Tachometer

Metronomes are probably more accurate than most cycle tachometers. The purpose of the metronome for the cycle test is the same as that for the step tests—to provide the prescribed cadence for the exerciser.

The Åstrand Test often prescribes a pedal frequency of 50 r·min⁻¹ when using mechanically braked, nonconstant-power ergometers (e.g., Monark™). This 50 r·min⁻¹ is equivalent to a metronome setting of 100 b·min⁻¹ based upon either foot of the cyclist being at the bottom of the stroke at each beat of the metronome. The tachometer on the ergometer should display a speed of 18 km·h⁻¹ (11.2 mph) at a setting of 50 r·min⁻¹.

The Monark ergometer's flywheel has a circumference of 1.62 m and travels 6 m in 3.7 circuits with each pedal revolution. Equation 14.4 states that the cycling distance is a function of pedal rate and flywheel circumference and flywheel circuits per pedal revolution.

$$D \text{ (m·min}^{-1}) = \text{r·min}^{-1} \times \text{wheel} \quad \text{Eq. 14.4}$$
$$\text{circumference (m)} \times \text{flywheel}$$
$$\text{circuits per pedal r}$$

The calculation of total distance (D) for mechanically braked cycles in 1 min for the Åstrand Test uses the simplified Equation 14.5.

$$D \text{ (m·min}^{-1}) = 50 \text{ r·min}^{-1} \times 6 \text{ m} \quad \text{Eq. 14.5}$$
$$= 300 \text{ m·min}^{-1}$$

where:

$$50 \text{ r·min}^{-1} = \text{commonly prescribed pedal rate for}$$
$$\text{Åstrand Test}$$

$$6 \text{ m} = 1.62 \text{ m} \times 3.7 \text{ circuits}$$

Stethoscope

Heart rates can be determined by palpation, stethoscope, heart-rate monitors, or electrocardiograph. Auscultatory (by ear) heart rates are preferred over palpatory ones (by pulse or apical beat) for some tests when performed by experienced technicians.[16] The standard error between auscultation by

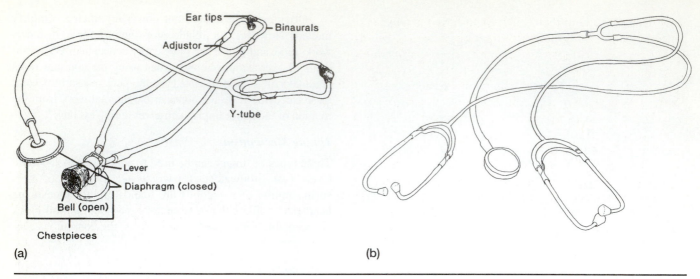

Figure 14.3 (a) Stethoscopes for auscultation of heart rate have two different chestpieces. The chestpiece to the left is the diaphragm type and the one to the right has a lever to direct sound to either a diaphragm or a bell chestpiece. (b) A double-binaural stethoscope.

stethoscope and recording by electrocardiograph for measuring heart rate was less than 2 b·min^{-1} in one unpublished study. The chestpiece of a stethoscope (Figure 14.3a) may be an open (bell-shaped) or closed diaphragm. The flatter and larger closed diaphragm is preferred for auscultating heart rates. Double-binaural stethoscopes can be purchased or improvised that enable two persons to listen simultaneously (Figure 14.3b).

The basic purpose of the stethoscope—to bring the ear of the listener closer to the source of the sound—has not changed since a one-piece hollow tube first was used in 1819.[22] Typical stethoscopes do not amplify sounds, although some battery-powered ones may amplify by 100 times. The length of the tubing makes little, if any, practical difference in the sound intensity unless it exceeds three feet.[29] Heart-rate monitors are accurate as long as electrical interference from other heart-rate monitors or computerized equipment is avoided.[2,20]

Technician Preparations

Adequate preparation for the administration of the Åstrand Cycle Test consists of (1) periodic calibrations of equipment as described in Box 14.2, (2) orientation of the performer (3) recording of basic and meteorological data, (4) development of the technician's auscultatory and timing skills, (5) adjustment of the ergometer's seat height, and (5) prescription of the performer's exercise protocol.

Orientation of the Performer (Participant)

The orientation of the performer by the technician includes such factors as (1) the establishment of the standard and neutral conditions of the performer and environment, respectively, and (2) the explanation of the purpose and basic features of the test.

The performer should be in a condition that is standard for laboratory testing. This means that he or she is relaxed, drug free, euhydrated (normal hydration), appropriately attired and is neither hungry nor full. The facility should be environmentally controlled so that the air temperature (T_a) is not higher than 23 °C (≈ 74 °F).[2] Ideally, some investigators suggest an environmental temperature as low as 17 °C (≈ 62 °F) for the best prediction of maximal oxygen consumption in trained persons.[31] The air's water vapor content should produce less than 60 % relative humidity (RH).[1] Natural barometric pressures above 630 mm Hg (> 840 hPa)—equivalent to altitudes less than 1500 m or 5000 ft—will not affect the results of the exercise test.

The technician's explanations of the performer's exercise task (e.g., intensity of the exercise) and the associated risks should satisfy most of the questions a performer might have regarding the Åstrand Cycle Test. For classroom purposes a verbal assent should be adequate, but for tests administered outside the classroom, a written consent should be obtained (see the Informed Consent information in Appendix E).

Recording of Basic Data and Meteorological Data

Most of the considerations for recording these data were presented in Chapters 2 and 3. Contrary to the Aerobic Step Test procedures in Chapter 13, however, the nude body mass measurement is recommended for the calculations of relative V̇O$_2$max for the Åstrand Cycle Test. Also, it is not unusual for some laboratory personnel to turn on a fan during cycle ergometry. Thus, the use of the fan should be noted on Form 14.1.

Auscultation of Heartbeats

The vibrations of the heart valves and blood are responsible for the heart sounds. Their sounds are of low frequency and low decibel, making them difficult to hear for inexperienced technicians. The two distinct heart sounds heard under resting conditions are often referred to as *lub-dup*. The first sound, *lub*, is a systolic (ventricles contract) sound, and the second sound, *dup*, is the diastolic (ventricles relax) sound. The sound of systole is due primarily to the closing of the atrioventricular valves (mitral and tricuspid) and secondarily to the opening of the semilunar valves (aortic and pulmonic). *Lub* is heard best at the 4th to 5th intercostal space near the midclavicular line.[21,22] The *dup* sound of diastole is due mainly to the closing of the semilunar valves[23] and is heard best at the pulmonic area near the base of the heart, which is externally marked between the 2nd and 3rd intercostal space at a point about 2 cm to 3 cm left of the sternum.[8,21,22] Under exercise conditions, the duration between the *lub* and *dup* is usually too short to distinguish as two separate sounds. Thus, at exercise, each sound is equivalent to one heartbeat.

Stethoscopes have binaurals, which sometimes curve near the ear tips; the direction of the binaurals should point toward the nose because the ear canals point in that direction. By tapping gently on the diaphragm, the listener can assure that the sound is being transmitted adequately. The diaphragm of a stethoscope should not be used over cloth and should be flush with the skin (i.e., no air spaces between it and the skin surface).

In general, the heartbeat is heard best at the apical region just below the pectoralis major muscle and the left nipple. Occasionally, it is more convenient to auscultate heartbeat at its base area just below and to the left of the sternum's manubrium (Figure 14.4).

Technicians should learn to feel comfortable testing members of the opposite sex. For example, the participant should not be asked to hold the diaphragm of the stethoscope in position while the technician listens. The technician should not be shy about placing the diaphragm of the stethoscope against skin at the appropriate site even if that site is near the breasts. Because heart sounds cannot be heard well through breast tissue, there is no need to place the diaphragm on the breasts. Participants should avoid talking while the technician is listening to their heartbeats.

The following procedures for timing the heartbeats and converting the number of beats to heart rate in the Åstrand Cycle Test are different from those commonly prescribed for run tests and step tests.

1. Start the watch on a heartbeat while silently saying "zero."
2. Count 30 heartbeats (30 b).
3. Stop the watch on the 30th beat.
4. Record the time (*t*) to closest 0.1 s for the 30 beats (30 b *t*).
5. Calculate the heart rate (HR) by using Equation 14.6a or 14.6b.

$$\text{HR (b·min}^{-1}) = 60\ s \times (30\ b \div 30\ b\ t) \qquad \text{Eq. 14.6a}$$

$$= 1800 \div 30\ b\ t \qquad \text{Eq. 14.6b}$$

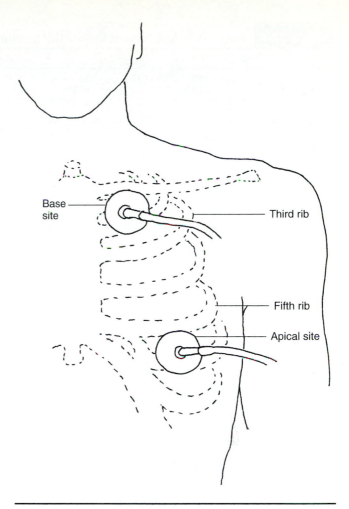

Figure 14.4 Two practical stethoscopic sites are at the base and apical regions of the heart.

Because 30 b and 60 s are constants for one form of the equation (14.6a), the equation may be simplified by using the value 1800 in the second form (Eq. 14.6b). As an example, suppose that the time for 30 b under resting conditions is 26.0 s. The heart rate, then, is 69 b·min^{-1}, found by dividing 1800 by 26.0. A table can be derived from the equations, but often it is faster to perform the calculation on a hand calculator.

This 30 b method of obtaining heart rate is considered more exact than the 15 s method prescribed for some field tests.[4] This is due to the elimination of partial intervals between beats at the start and finish of a timing period. Only whole intervals are in the 30 b method, because the stopwatch is started and stopped on the respective beats, not on a go and stop signal or the movement of a seconds hand or display digit.

By auscultating heart rate while the performer sits at rest on the ergometer prior to the test, the technician may be alerted to any difficulties associated with hearing the heartbeat. Heart rate may also reveal any anxiety in the participant. The resting heart rate, however, is not used to estimate the maximal oxygen consumption, but it can serve as

rpm km·h⁻¹		40 14.4		50 18.0		60 21.6		70 25.2		80 28.8	
Force kg (kp)	N	kg·m·min⁻¹	W	kg·m·min⁻¹	W	Power kg·m·min⁻¹	W	kg·m·min⁻¹	W	kg·m·min⁻¹	W
0.5	5	120	20	150	25	180	30	210	35	240	40
1.0	10	240	40	300	50	360	60	420	70	480	80
1.5	15	360	60	450	75	540	90	630	105	720	120
2.0	20	480	80	600	100	720	120	840	140	960	160
2.5	25	600	100	750	125	900	150	1050	175	1200	200
3.0	30	720	120	900	150	1080	180	1260	210	1440	240
3.5	35	840	140	1050	175	1260	210	1470	245	1680	280
4.0	40	960	160	1200	200	1440	240	1680	280	1920	320
4.5	45	1080	180	1350	225	1620	270	1890	315	2160	360
5.0	50	1200	200	1500	250	1800	300	2100	350	2400	400
5.5	55	1320	220	1650	275	1980	330	2310	385	2640	440
6.0	60	1440	240	1800	300	2160	360	2520	420	2880	480
6.5	65	1560	260	1950	325	2340	390	2730	455	3120	520
7.0	70	1680	280	2100	350	2520	420	2940	490	3360	560

a starting point if graphing the relationship between exercise heart rate and elapsed time.

In cases where auscultation is difficult, it is helpful to get second opinions from more experienced technicians or to use a double-binaural stethoscope or an amplifying stethoscope. Also, heart rate monitors have been perfected to provide accurate and practical measures.[20]

Seat Adjustment

The position of the cycle seat affects the efficiency of the rider.[33] Mechanical efficiency may vary by ± 6 % on the cycle ergometer even when appropriate seat adjustments are made.[5] For example, at a power level of 100 W, two-thirds of the population will consume oxygen at a rate between 1.41 L·min⁻¹ and 1.59 L·min⁻¹ [1.5 ± (6 % × 1.5)]. In order to assure that the efficiency remains within this narrow range, or is optimal for the performer, the seat adjustment should be based upon various accepted criteria.[2,11,28]

With the ball of the cyclist's foot on the pedal, the leg should have a bend of only 5° at the bottom of the stroke[1] (see Figure 14.5a). The leg should be straight if the heel of the foot is on the pedal at the bottom of the stroke (Figure 14.5b). A quick guideline for preventing seat heights from being too high is for the performer to try backpedalling while the technician observes the hips.[b] If the hips rock or if the heels slip off the pedals, then the seat is too high.

Most seat posts have numbers at intervals of about 2 cm to 3 cm. Once the proper seat height has been established, the seat setting should be recorded onto the individual's data collection form (Form 14.2).

Power Prescription for Exercise Protocol

A constant power ergometer simplifies the process of applying the power level and pedal revolutions because the technician does not have to supply a force, per se, or be so attentive to the performer's pedal revolutions. Usually, all the technician does to set the power is press the appropriate button on the ergometer's console. On the other hand, the technician must understand the relationship among force (F), work (w), and power (P) in order to make the proper exercise prescription on mechanically braked cycle ergometers. The force component of work is often displayed on the ergometer as kg, kp, or N. For practical purposes, the kg and kp are identical. The power units are often expressed as kg·m·min⁻¹ ("kgm/min") or watts (W). Table 14.1 shows the relationship between these units when the mechanically braked ergometer's rpm range is from 40 to 80; special attention should be given to the 50 rpm column because it is the originally prescribed rpm for the Åstrand Cycle Test.[6]

The original and most common cycling cadence is 50 rpm. However, any cadence between 50 rpm and 80 rpm appears valid for predicting $\dot{V}O_2$max (peak) in a wide range of performers.[37] Experienced cyclists tend to be more economical at the higher end of this range (e.g., 70 rpm to 80 rpm) at the high power levels.[7,17,36]

An estimation of the appropriate power dosage for the participant can be made by following the guidelines in Table 14.2. It prescribes the power based on (1) age and/or (2) the best guess or estimate ("guesstimate") of the participant's fitness level.

Ideally, for persons under 30 years of age, the power level of the protocol should elicit a heart rate between 150 and 160 beats per minute (b·min⁻¹). This target heart rate may be reduced by about one-half beat per minute for each year over 30 years of age (Eq. 14.7).

---

[b]Avoid backpedalling on Monark™ *basket-loaded* ergometers because the cord tends to slip off the flywheel.

| Table 14.2 | Guidelines for Target Heart Rate (HR) Zones and Initial Power Levels for the Åstrand Cycle Test |

| Age (y) | Target HR (b·min⁻¹) | Power (kg·m·min⁻¹; W) | |
		Average Man	Average Woman
< 30	150–160	900–1050; 150–175	750–900; 125–150
30–39	145–155	750–900; 125–150	600–750; 100–125
40–49	140–150	600–750; 100–125	600; 100
50–59	135–145	600; 100	450–600; 75–100
60–69	130–140	450–600; 75–100	300–450; 50–75
70–79	125–135	300–450; 50–75	300; 50

Note: For the average person, a general guideline is to prescribe 1.65 W (10 kg·m·min⁻¹) for each kilogram body mass. Highly trained persons, especially of high body mass, require higher power levels.

$$\text{Target HR} = 150 - [0.5 \times (\text{Age} - 30)] \qquad \text{Eq.14.7}$$

For example, the target heart rate (within 5 b·min⁻¹) for a 50-year-old person would be calculated as follows:

$$150 - [0.5 \times (50{-}30)] = 140 \text{ b·min}^{-1}$$

Table 14.2 also shows that the prescribed power level for *sedentary* persons may be based upon a general rule of 10 kg·m·min⁻¹ ($\approx$ 1.65 W) per kilogram of body mass. For example, if a sedentary person weighs 75 kg, then the prescribed power level is 750 kg·m·min⁻¹; if expressing it in watts, then 1.65 × 75 is equal to 123.75 W, or approximately 125 W.

Summary of Technician's Preparatory Steps for the Åstrand Cycle Test

1. Calibrate the cycle ergometer and metronome (review Box 14.2). The instructor may have done this already.
2. Orient the performer by
   (a) Stating the purpose of the test to the performer— i.e., ". . . to record heart rate during cycling exercise so that aerobic power ($\dot{V}O_2$max) may be estimated"
   (b) Explaining the protocol of the test (e.g., duration, intensity, mode, and technique)
   (c) Assuring the performer's informed consent (Appendix E) and ascription to all preparatory guidelines as outlined here and in Chapter 13.
3. Measure and record the basic data and the meteorological data (Form 14.1).
4. Practice auscultating the performer's heart rate while he or she is seated comfortably in a chair; record quality and rate onto Form 14.1, thus establishing the diaphragm site of auscultation (review Figure 14.4).
5. Measure heart rate while performer is seated at rest on the cycle ergometer; record onto Form 14.2.
6. Adjust the seat height so that the cyclist's leg is nearly straight with the ball of the foot on the down pedal (review Figure 14.5).
7. Record the seat-post number onto Form 14.2.

8. Establish the cycling cadence (100 b·min⁻¹) or speed (18 km/h) of cycling:
   (1) Show how one foot is at the bottom of the stroke with each metronome beat.
   (2) Show where the tachometer indicates 18 km/h or 50 r·min⁻¹.
9. Establish the power (W; N·m·min⁻¹; kg·m·min⁻¹) level for the exercise protocol. Record power level onto Form 14.2.

Test Procedures

The normal duration of the single-stage Åstrand Cycle Test is six minutes. During this time, the technicians are mainly responsible for auscultating heartbeats, calculating and recording heart rates, adjusting the power level, and observing the performer for any "stop-test" indicators. The procedures during the test are summarized as follows:

1. Start the metronome if using a constant-force ergometer.
2. Ask the performer to begin cycling at the proper cadence, using the metronome or tachometer as an aid.
3. Once the performer has achieved the proper cadence, increase the power level to the prescribed setting (review Table 14.2).
4. Start the timer.
5. Auscultate and time 30 heartbeats starting between 1:30 and 1:45 of the test; repeat this at 1 min intervals through the last minute (sixth) of the test.
6. Record the 30 beat time on the data form; while waiting for the next auscultation period, calculate the heart rate using Equation 14.6b.
7. Readjust the power level after the 3 min heart rate if the heart-rate target zone is unlikely to be achieved. Use Table 14.3 and Eq. 14.7 as guides.
8. After the 6th min, if no power adjustments were made, set the force level to 0.5 kg (5 N) and ask the performer to continue cycling for recovery/cooldown purposes until the heart rate is less than 100 b·min⁻¹.

Power Adjustments during the Test

The power levels of some mechanically braked ergometers cannot be adjusted precisely to the prescribed level unless the performer is cycling. Additionally, the flywheel tension may slip or drift upward occasionally during the test,[32] requiring readjustment and periodic monitoring.

Table 14.3 and Figure 14.6 provide guides for changing the original power level after the third minute of the cycle test if it appears that the target heart rate is unlikely to be obtained. For example, if a 30-year-old's heart rate (HR) is less than 110 b·min⁻¹ at the end of the third minute (2:30–3:00), then the power level should be raised by 50 W or 75 W (300 kg·m·min⁻¹ or 450 kg·m·min⁻¹) to enhance the probability of reaching the target heart-rate zone. On the other hand, if the heart rate at the end of the third minute is

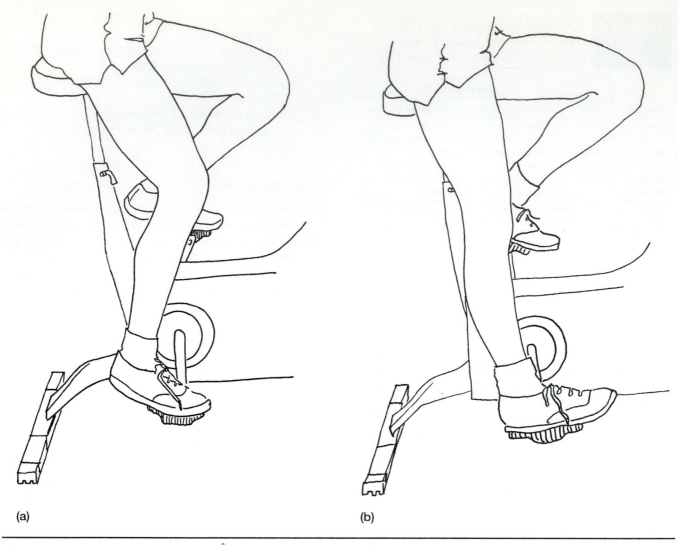

(a)   (b)

Figure 14.5 Adjusting the seat for the Åstrand Cycle Test: (a) slight bend in knee when the ball of the foot is on the pedal at the bottom of the pedal stroke; (b) straight leg when the heel is on the pedal. The cycling movement occurs with the ball of the foot on the pedal.

Table 14.3 **Possible Power Adjustments after 3.5 min of the Åstrand Cycle Test[a]**

kg·m·min⁻¹	W	Heart Rate b·min⁻¹	Force kg	N
A. Raise power level by:				
300–450	50–75	If HR is < 110	1.0–1.5	10–15
150–300	25–50	If HR is 110–129	0.5–1.0	5–10
≤ 150	≤ 25	If HR is 130–139	≤ 0.5	≤ 5
B. Lower power level by:				
150–300	25–50	If HR is 160	0.5–1.0	10
≤ 150	≤ 25	If HR is 150–159	≤ 0.5	≤ 5

Note: [a]Subtract (> 30 y) or add (< 30 y) one-half beat per minute for each year above or below 30 years of age, respectively.

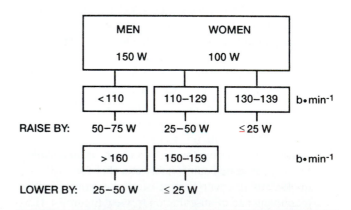

Figure 14.6 Schematic of possible power adjustments after 3 min of the Åstrand Cycle Test. Also adjust for age by subtracting or adding 0.5 b·min⁻¹ for each year above or below 30 y of age, respectively.

160 b·min^{-1} or more, then the power should be decreased by 25 W or 50 W. The ideal goal is for the 30 y old performer to reach a steady state heart rate between 145 b·min^{-1} and 155 b·min^{-1} by the 6th min or soon after. If a change is made immediately after the third minute, a steady state will likely be achieved by the end of the 6 min test. Any change in power level after 3.5 min requires an extension of one minute to the typical 6 min test.

Time Adjustments During the Test

If the difference between the heart rates during minutes 5 and 6 exceeds 10 beats, then the performer should continue to exercise until the difference between the final two heart rates is 10 or less. One group of investigators suggested that, if the difference between the final two heart rates is between 6 and 10 beats, then ignore the earlier minute's rate and use only the final minute's heart rate to make the calculation for predicting maximal oxygen consumption.[12]

Cooldown

It is important that the cyclist be given a low-intensity exercise level after the regular test protocol. This will prevent the pooling of blood in the legs, which could lead to fainting if the performer were to stand still immediately after finishing the test. In general, the recovery exercise can be terminated when the heart rate is 100 b·min^{-1} or less (18.0 s for 30 beats). Muscle soreness is unlikely in performers of this aerobic submaximal test.

Calculation of $\dot{V}O_2$max

The prediction of the maximal oxygen consumption ($\dot{V}O_2$max) can be made by equation, table, or nomogram (not presented here), all of which are based on the heart rate at the steady state of exercise during the Åstrand Test. This is a single stage submaximal test unless the power needs to be changed to reach the target heart-rate zone.

Equation Method of Calculating $\dot{V}O_2$max

Unless, the final two heart rates of the exercise test differ by 6 to 10 beats, they are averaged in order to determine the steady state heart rate in the calculations. The averaged rate is then used with either the Åstrand-Ryhming nomogram[3,4] or derived equations; both are based on the ratio between submaximal oxygen consumption ($\dot{V}O_2$SM) and maximal oxygen consumption. This ratio is expressed in terms of maximal (HRmax) and submaximal (HRsm) heart rates and put in equation form.[34,35] The generalized form of that equation is presented in Equation 14.8. The prediction of maximal oxygen consumption is more accurate if the popular formula for predicting maximal heart rate (220 – age) substitutes[24] for the original HR Range values. Thus, Equations 14.9 and 14.10 are suggested for calculating maximal oxygen consumption for men and women, respectively. Presumably, it would be best to use the individual's known maximal heart rate if such data are available from previous maximal exercise testing.

$$\dot{V}O_2\text{max (L·min}^{-1}) = \dot{V}O_2 \times \frac{\text{HR Range}}{\text{HRsm Range}} \qquad \text{Eq. 14.8}$$

$$\text{Men: } = \dot{V}O_2 \times \frac{(220 - \text{age}) - 61}{\text{HRsm} - 61} \qquad \text{Eq. 14.9}$$

$$\text{Women: } = \dot{V}O_2 \times \frac{(220 - \text{age}) - 72}{\text{HRsm} - 72} \qquad \text{Eq. 14.10}$$

where:

$\dot{V}O_2$ = L of oxygen required for the Åstrand power level (Eq. 14.11, 14.12, or 14.13) used during the Åstrand Test.[c] $\dot{V}O_2$ (L·min^{-1}) =

$$[P \text{ (in N·m·min}^{-1}) \times 0.0002] + 0.3 \qquad \text{Eq. 14.11}$$

$$[P \text{ (in kg·m·min}^{-1}) \times 0.002] + 0.3 \qquad \text{Eq. 14.12}$$

$$[P \text{ (in W)} \times 0.012] + 0.3 \qquad \text{Eq. 14.13}$$

HR Range = HRmax (known value or 220 – age) minus resting HR (men = 61; women = 72)
HRsm = the steady – state heart rate (b·min^{-1}) during the Åstrand Test

Thus, to calculate maximal oxygen consumption, one needs to insert three values into Equation 14.9 or 14.10: (1) age, (2) the submaximal heart rate (HRsm) elicited during the Åstrand Cycle Test, and (3) the submaximal oxygen consumption ($\dot{V}O_2$) value for the power level eliciting the submaximal heart rate.

For example, if a 25-year-old man's heart rate (HRsm) is 155 b·min^{-1} at 150 W (900 kg·m·min^{-1}), then the submaximal and maximal oxygen consumption, respectively, may be calculated as follows:

Submaximal

$$\dot{V}O_2 \text{ (L·min}^{-1}) = (0.002 \times 900 \text{ kg·m·min}^{-1}) + 0.3$$

$$= 2.1 \text{ L·min}^{-1} \text{ (from Eq. 14.12)}$$

$$\text{or} = (0.012 \times 150 \text{ W}) + 0.3$$

$$= 2.1 \text{ L·min}^{-1} \text{ (from Eq. 14.13)}$$

Maximal

$$\dot{V}O_2 \text{ max (L·min}^{-1}) = 2.1 \times \frac{(220 - 25) - 61}{155 - 61}$$

$$= 2.1 \times \frac{134}{94}$$

$$= 2.1 \times 1.43$$

$$= 3.0 \text{ L·min}^{-1} \text{ (from Eq. 14.9)}$$

---

[c]These simplified equations for converting power to oxygen consumption are appropriate for power levels ≤ 900 kg·m·min or ≤ 150 W. For power levels > 150 W to 200 W use $\dot{V}O_2$ (mL·min^{-1}) = 1.8 × P × BM in kg + 7.[2]

Table Method for Predicting V̇O₂max

The same $\dot{V}O_2$max value (3.0 L·min⁻¹) as in the example of the 25-year-old man could have been determined by using Table 14.4 (men). Accordingly, Table 14.5 (women) may be used to predict maximal oxygen consumption (L·min⁻¹) from the steady-state heart rates of women at given power levels (kg·m·min⁻¹; W) of the Åstrand Cycle Test.[4] For example, if a 20-year-old woman has a heart rate of 168 b·min⁻¹ at 125 W (750 kg·m·min⁻¹), then Table 14.5 shows that the maximal oxygen consumption is 2.4 L·min⁻¹.

Age-Adjusted V̇O₂max for Table Method

When the maximal oxygen consumptions of persons over 25 y of age are derived from the tables, but not from Equations 14.9 or 14.10, an adjustment needs to account for the decrease in maximal heart rate with increased age. The maximal oxygen consumptions derived from the tables are based upon a constant maximal heart rate of 195 b·min⁻¹, regardless of age. Because maximal heart rate decreases with age, a proper correction must be used unless the performer is 25 y of age. In the latter case, the correction factor (CF) is 1.0, i.e., no correction at all. The correction factors (HRmax CF) for various ages are listed in Table 14.6.[3] The appropriate correction factor from Table 14.6 is then inserted into Equation 14.14 to calculate the age-adjusted maximal oxygen consumption (Age $\dot{V}O_2$max).

$$\text{Age } \dot{V}O_2\text{max (L·min}^{-1}) \qquad \text{Eq. 14.14}$$
$$= \text{HRmax CF} \times \text{Table } \dot{V}O_2$$

Thus, if a 40-year-old man has a table-derived maximal oxygen consumption value of 3.0 L·min⁻¹, then 3.0 multiplied by the HRmax CF 0.83 provides an adjusted value of 2.49 L·min⁻¹.

Calculations for Body Mass Adjusted V̇O₂max

The equations and the nomogram value may also be adjusted to account for differences in body mass. The nomogram is not presented here but is in various texts of exercise physiology[10,30] and the original source.[4] Maximal oxygen consumption, expressed as liters per minute, is closely related to body size; it is sometimes referred to as the raw or absolute value. However, maximal oxygen consumption is usually expressed relative to body mass when predicting performance in activities that require the performer to lift his or her own body mass. The unit of measure denoting relative oxygen consumption is milliliters per kilogram per minute (mL·kg⁻¹·min⁻¹). To convert the raw score to the relative score, Equation 14.15 is used, whereby the absolute value is multiplied by 1000 (1 L = 1000 mL) and the product is divided by the body mass (kg).

Table 14.4 Prediction of Maximal Oxygen Consumption from Heart Rate (HR) and Cycling Power (Men)

Maximal Oxygen Consumption (L·min⁻¹)						Maximal Oxygen Consumption (L·min⁻¹)				
HR b/min	Power (kg·m·min⁻¹; W)					HR bpm	Power (kg·m·min⁻¹; W)			
	300; 50	600; 100	900; 150	1200; 200	1500; 250		600; 100	900; 150	1200; 200	1500; 250
120	2.2	3.5	4.8			146	2.4	3.3	4.4	5.5
121	2.2	3.4	4.7			147	2.4	3.3	4.4	5.5
122	2.2	3.4	4.6			148	2.4	3.2	4.3	5.4
123	2.1	3.4	4.6			149	2.3	3.2	4.3	5.4
124	2.1	3.3	4.5	6.0		150	2.3	3.2	4.2	5.3
125	2.0	3.2	4.4	5.9		151	2.3	3.1	4.2	5.2
126	2.0	3.2	4.4	5.8		152	2.3	3.1	4.1	5.2
127	2.0	3.1	4.3	5.7		153	2.2	3.0	4.1	5.1
128	2.0	3.1	4.2	5.6		154	2.2	3.0	4.0	5.1
129	1.9	3.0	4.2	5.6		155	2.2	3.0	4.0	5.0
130	1.9	3.0	4.1	5.5		156	2.2	2.9	4.0	5.0
131	1.9	2.9	4.0	5.4		157	2.1	2.9	3.9	4.9
132	1.8	2.9	4.0	5.3		158	2.1	2.9	3.9	4.9
133	1.8	2.8	3.9	5.3		159	2.1	2.8	3.8	4.8
134	1.8	2.8	3.9	5.2		160	2.1	2.8	3.8	4.8
135	1.7	2.8	3.8	5.1		161	2.0	2.8	3.7	4.7
136	1.7	2.7	3.8	5.0		162	2.0	2.8	3.7	4.6
137	1.7	2.7	3.7	5.0		163	2.0	2.8	3.7	4.6
138	1.6	2.7	3.7	4.9		164	2.0	2.7	3.6	4.5
139	1.6	2.6	3.6	4.8		165	2.0	2.7	3.6	4.5
140	1.6	2.6	3.6	4.8	6.0	166	1.9	2.7	3.6	4.4
141		2.6	3.5	4.7	5.9	167	1.9	2.6	3.5	4.4
142		2.5	3.5	4.6	5.8	168	1.9	2.6	3.5	4.3
143		2.5	3.4	4.6	5.7	169	1.9	2.6	3.5	4.3
144		2.5	3.4	4.5	5.7	170	1.8	2.6	3.4	4.3
145		2.4	3.4	4.5	5.6					

Modified from nomogram in I. Åstrand, *Acta Physiologica Scandinavica, 49,* (suppl. 169), 1960, by P.-O. Åstrand in *Work Test with Bicycle Ergometer,* Varberg, Sweden, Monark, 1988.

Table 14.5 Prediction of Maximal Oxygen Consumption from Heart Rate (HR) and Cycling Power (Women)

Maximal Oxygen Consumption (L·min⁻¹)						Maximal Oxygen Consumption (L·min⁻¹)					
HR b/min	Power (kg·m·min⁻¹; W)					HR b/min	Power (kg·m·min⁻¹; W)				
	300; 50	450; 75	600; 100	750; 125	900; 150		300; 50	450; 75	600; 100	750; 125	900; 150
120	2.6	3.4	4.1	4.8		146	1.6	2.2	2.6	3.2	3.7
121	2.5	3.3	4.0	4.8		147	1.6	2.1	2.6	3.1	3.6
122	2.5	3.2	3.9	4.7		148	1.6	2.1	2.6	3.1	3.6
123	2.4	3.1	3.9	4.6		149		2.1	2.6	3.0	3.5
124	2.4	3.1	3.8	4.5		150		2.0	2.5	3.0	3.5
125	2.3	3.0	3.7	4.4		151		2.0	2.5	3.0	3.4
126	2.3	3.0	3.7	4.4		152		2.0	2.5	2.9	3.4
127	2.2	2.9	3.5	4.2		153		2.0	2.4	2.9	3.3
128	2.2	2.8	3.5	4.2		154		2.0	2.4	2.8	3.3
129	2.2	2.8	3.4	4.1		155		1.9	2.4	2.8	3.2
130	2.1	2.7	3.4	4.0	4.7	156		1.9	2.3	2.8	3.2
131	2.1	2.7	3.4	4.0	4.6	157		1.9	2.3	2.7	3.2
132	2.0	2.7	3.3	4.0	4.5	158		1.8	2.3	2.7	3.1
133	2.0	2.6	3.2	3.8	4.4	159		1.8	2.2	2.7	3.1
134	2.0	2.6	3.2	3.8	4.4	160		1.8	2.2	2.6	3.0
135	2.0	2.6	3.1	3.7	4.3	161		1.8	2.2	2.6	3.0
136	1.9	2.5	3.1	3.6	4.2	162		1.8	2.2	2.6	3.0
137	1.9	2.5	3.0	3.6	4.2	163		1.7	2.2	2.6	2.9
138	1.8	2.4	3.0	3.5	4.1	164		1.7	2.1	2.5	2.9
139	1.8	2.4	2.9	3.5	4.0	165		1.7	2.1	2.5	2.9
140	1.8	2.4	2.8	3.4	4.0	166		1.7	2.1	2.5	2.8
141	1.8	2.3	2.8	3.4	3.9	167		1.6	2.1	2.4	2.8
142	1.7	2.3	2.8	3.3	3.9	168		1.6	2.0	2.4	2.8
143	1.7	2.2	2.7	3.3	3.8	169		1.6	2.0	2.4	2.8
144	1.7	2.2	2.7	3.2	3.8	170		1.6	2.0	2.4	2.7
145	1.6	2.2	2.7	3.2	3.7						

Modified from nomogram in I. Åstrand, *Acta Physiologica Scandinavica, 49,* (suppl. 169), 1960, by P.-O. Åstrand in *Work Test with Bicycle Ergometer,* Varberg, Sweden, Monark, 1988.

Table 14.6 Age Correction Factors (CF) for Age-Adjusted Maximal Oxygen Consumption

Age	CF	Age	CF	Age	CF	Age	CF	Age	CF
15	1.10	25	1.00	35	0.87	45	0.78	55	0.71
16	1.10	26	0.99	36	0.86	46	0.77	56	0.70
17	1.09	27	0.98	37	0.85	47	0.77	57	0.70
18	1.07	28	0.96	38	0.85	48	0.76	58	0.69
19	1.06	29	0.95	39	0.84	49	0.76	59	0.69
20	**1.05**	30	**0.93**	40	**0.83**	50	0.75	60	**0.68**
21	1.04	31	0.92	41	0.82	51	0.74	61	0.67
22	1.03	32	0.91	42	0.81	52	0.73	62	0.67
23	1.02	33	0.90	43	0.80	53	0.73	63	0.66
24	1.01	34	0.88	44	0.79	54	0.72	64	0.66

Table adapted from Åstrand, I. (1960). Aerobic work capacity in men and women with special reference to age. *Acta Physiologica Scandinavica, 49* (Suppl. 169), 45–60.
Note: Correction factors between boldface values were derived by interpolation by the present author. Mnemonic: age 65 y = CF 0.65.

Relative $\dot{V}O_2$ max   Eq. 14.15

$$(mL \cdot kg^{-1} \cdot min^{-1}) = \frac{\dot{V}O_2 max\ (L \cdot min^{-1}) \times 1000}{BM\ in\ kg}$$

For example, if a participant who weighs 68.0 kg has an age-adjusted $\dot{V}O_2$max of 2.35 L·min⁻¹, then the relative $\dot{V}O_2$max is 2350 mL·min⁻¹ divided by body mass (BM); thus, the relative $\dot{V}O_2$max is 35 mL·kg⁻¹·min⁻¹.

Results and Discussion

The original norms of Åstrand were derived mainly from Swedish physical education students. The original norms had higher standards than the ones presented in Table 14.7, which are based on 450 healthy Americans, who mainly were tested on cycle ergometers (Preventive Medicine Center, Palo Alto, CA, and NAHI, Inglewood, CA).

Table 14.7 Norms for Evaluating Åstrand Cycle Test Performance

Age	Aerobic Fitness Categories					
	Very High	High	Good	Average	Fair	Low
	Maximal Oxygen Consumption ($mL \cdot kg^{-1} \cdot min^{-1}$)					
Men						
20–29	> 61	53–61	43–52	34–42	25–33	< 25
30–39	> 57	49–57	39–48	31–38	23–30	< 23
40–49	> 53	45–53	36–44	27–35	20–26	< 20
50–59	> 49	43–49	34–42	25–33	18–24	< 18
60–69	> 45	41–45	31–40	23–30	16–22	< 16
Women						
20–29	> 57	49–57	38–48	31–37	24–30	< 24
30–39	> 53	45–53	34–44	28–33	20–27	< 20
40–49	> 50	42–50	31–41	24–30	17–23	< 17
50–59	> 42	38–42	28–37	21–27	15–20	< 15
60–69	> 39	35–39	24–34	18–23	13–17	< 13

Source: Preventive Medicine Center, Palo Alto, CA: National Athletic Health Institute, Inglewood, CA.

It is also important to consider the mode of exercise for establishing the norms. For example, maximal (peak) oxygen consumptions elicited from treadmill tests are at least 5 % to 10 % greater than those elicited by cycle ergometry.[10,18]

References

1. American College of Sports Medicine. (1991). *Guidelines for exercise testing and prescription.* Philadelphia: Lea & Febiger.
2. American College of Sports Medicine. (2000). *ACSM's guidelines for exercise testing and prescription.* Philadelphia: Lippincott Williams & Wilkins.
3. Åstrand, I. (1960). Aerobic work capacity in men and women with special reference to age. *Acta Physiologica Scandinavica, 49* (Suppl. 169).
4. Åstrand, P.-O. (1988). *Work tests with the bicycle ergometer.* Varberg, Sweden: Monark Crescent AB.
5. Åstrand, P.-O., & Rodahl, K. (1977). *Textbook of work physiology.* San Francisco: McGraw-Hill.
6. Åstrand, P.-O., & Ryhming, I. (1954). A nomogram for calculation of aerobic capacity (physical fitness) from pulse rate during submaximal work. *Journal of Applied Physiology, 7,* 218–221.
7. Coast, J. R., & Welch, H. G. (1985). Linear increase in optimal pedalling rate with increased power output in cycle ergometry. *European Journal of Applied Physiology, 53,* 339–342.
8. DePasquale, N. P., Burch, G. E., & Philips, J. H. (1968). The second heart sound. *American Heart Journal, 76,* 419–431.
9. deVries, H. A. (1971). Prescription of exercise for older men from telemetered exercise heart rate data. *Geriatrics, 26,* 102–111.
10. deVries, H. A. (1994). *Physiology of exercise.* Dubuque, IA: Brown & Benchmark.
11. Dickson, T. B. (1985). Preventing overuse cycling injuries. *Physician and Sportsmedicine, 13*(10) 118–123.
12. Edgren, B., Marklund, G., Nordesjo, L., & Borg, G. (1976). The validity of four bicycle ergometer tests. *Medicine and Science in Sports, 8,* 179–185.
13. Edington, D. W., & Cunningham, L. (1975). *Biological awareness.* Englewood Cliffs, NJ: Prentice-Hall.
14. Faria, I. E., & Cavanagh, P. R. (1978). *The physiology and biomechanics of cycling.* New York: John Wiley & Sons.
15. Gledhill, N., & Jamnik, R. (1995). Determining power outputs for cycle ergometers with different sized flywheels. *Medicine and Science in Sports and Exercise, 27,* 134–135.
16. Golding, L. A., Myers, C. R., & Sinning, W. E. (1989). *Y's way to fitness: The complete guide to fitness testing and instruction.* Champaign, IL: Human Kinetics.
17. Hagberg, J. M., Mullin, J. P., Giese, M. D., & Spitznagel, E. (1981). Effect of pedaling rate on submaximal exercise responses of competitive cyclists. *Journal of Applied Physiology, 51,* 447–451.
18. Hermansen, L., & Saltin, B. (1969). Oxygen uptake during maximal treadmill and bicycle exercise. *Journal of Applied Physiology, 26,* 31–37.
19. Kasch, F. W. (1984). The validity of the Åstrand and Sjostrand submaximal tests. *The Physician and Sportsmedicine,* 47–51, 54.
20. Leger, L., & Thivierge, M. (1988). Heart rate monitors: Validity, stability, and functionality. *The Physician and Sportsmedicine, 16*(5), 143–151.
21. Lehmann, J. (1972). Auscultation of heart sounds. *American Journal of Nursing, 72,* 1242–1246.
22. Littmann, D. (1972). Stethoscope and auscultation. *American Journal of Nursing, 72,* 1238–1241.

23. Luisada, A. A., & Zalter, R. (1960). Phonocardiography. In American College of Chest Physicians (Eds.), *Clinical cardiopulmonary physiology* (pp. 75–83). New York: Grune and Stratton.

24. Mahar, M., Jackson, A. S., Ross, R. L., Pivarnik, J. M., & Pollock, M. L. (1985). Predictive accuracy of single and double stage submax treadmill work for estimating aerobic capacity. *Medicine and Science in Sports and Exercise, 17,* Abstract #4, 206–207.

25. Mathews, D. K., & Fox, E. L. (1976). *The physiological basis of physical education and athletics.* Philadelphia: W. B. Saunders.

26. McArdle, W. D., Katch, F. I., & Katch, V. L. (1991). *Exercise physiology: Energy, nutrition, and human performance.* Philadelphia: Lea & Febiger.

27. Noble, B. J. (1986). *Physiology of exercise and sport.* St. Louis: Times Mirror/Mosby.

28. Powell, B. (1982). Correction and prevention of bicycle saddle problems. *The Physician and Sportsmedicine, 10(10),* 60–64, 67.

29. Rappaport, M. B., & Sprague, H. B. (1941). Physiologic and physical laws that govern auscultation, and their clinical application. *American Heart Journal, 21,* 257–318.

30. Robergs, R. A., & Roberts, S. O. (1997). *Exercise physiology: Exercise, performance, and clinical applications.* St. Louis: Mosby.

31. Rowell, L. B., Taylor, H. L., & Wang, Y. (1964). Limitations to prediction of maximal oxygen intake. *Journal of Applied Physiology, 19,* 919–927.

32. Seifert, J. G. (1991). The comparison of physiological responses from cycling on friction-braked and electromagnetic ergometers. *Research Quarterly for Exercise and Sport, 62,* 115–117.

33. Shennum, P. L., & deVries, H. A. (1976). The effect of saddle height on oxygen consumption during bicycle ergometer work. *Medicine and Science in Sports, 8,* 119–121.

34. Shephard, R. J. (1970). Computer programs for solution of the Åstrand nomogram and the calculation of body surface area. *Journal of Sports Medicine and Physical Fitness, 10,* 206–210.

35. Shephard, R. J. (1972). *Alive man: The physiology of physical activity.* Springfield, IL: Charles C Thomas.

36. Swain, D. P., & Wilcox, J. P. (1992). Effect of cadence on the economy of uphill cycling. *Medicine and Science in Sports and Exercise, 24,* 1123–1127.

37. Swain, D. P., & Wright, R. L. (1997). Prediction of $\dot{V}O_2$ peak from submaximal cycle ergometry using 50 versus 80 rpm. *Medicine and Science in Sports and Exercise, 29,* 268–272.

38. Terry, J. W., Tolson, H., Johnson, D. J., & Jessup, G. T. (1977). A workload selection procedure for the Åstrand-Ryhming test. *Journal of Sports Medicine and Physical Fitness, 17,* 361.

39. Widrick, J. J., Freedson, P. S., & Hamill, J. (1992). Effect of internal work on the calculation of optimal pedaling rates. *Medicine and Science in Sports and Exercise, 24,* 376–382.

40. Williams, L. (1975). Reliability of predicting maximal oxygen intake using the Åstrand-Ryhming nomogram. *Research Quarterly, 46,* 12–16.

41. Wyndham, C. H., Strydom, N. B., Moritz, J. S., Morrison, J. F., Peter, J., & Potgieter, Z. U. (1959). Maximum oxygen intake and maximum heart rate during strenuous work. *Journal of Applied Physiology, 14,* 927–936.

Form 14.1

Practice of Heart Rate (HR) Auscultation, Timing, and Calculation

Name [ ] Date [ ] Time [ ] A.M. [ ] P.M. [ ]

Age [ ] y   Gender (M or W) [ ]   Ht [ ] cm   Wt [ ] kg   [ ] N   Tech. Initials [ ]

Meteorological Data

T [ ] °C (closest 0.1 °C)   RH % [ ] P_B [ ] mm Hg × 1.333 = [ ] hPa (mbar)

Stethoscopic Auscultation Quality

Tech. Initials   Apical   (check one at each site)   Base

Men	Excellent		Good	Fair	Poor		Excellent	Good	Fair	Poor
1.	[ ]	[ ]	[ ]	[ ]	[ ]		[ ]	[ ]	[ ]	[ ]
2.	[ ]	[ ]	[ ]	[ ]	[ ]		[ ]	[ ]	[ ]	[ ]

Technician's Initials:

Women			Apical				Base			
1.	[ ]	[ ]	[ ]	[ ]	[ ]		[ ]	[ ]	[ ]	[ ]
2.	[ ]	[ ]	[ ]	[ ]	[ ]		[ ]	[ ]	[ ]	[ ]

Timing Heartbeats and Calculating Heart Rate

Tech. Initials   Site (check one)

Men   1800/(30 b t) in s (closest 0.1 s) = HR (b·min^{-1})   Apical   Base

Men		1800 ÷ [ ] s	= [ ] b·min^{-1}	Apical	Base
1. [ ]		1800 ÷ [ ] s	= [ ] b·min^{-1}	[ ]	[ ]
2. [ ]		1800 ÷ [ ] s	= [ ] b·min^{-1}	[ ]	[ ]

Women					
1. [ ]		1800 ÷ [ ] s	= [ ] b·min^{-1}	[ ]	[ ]
2. [ ]		1800 ÷ [ ] s	= [ ] b·min^{-1}	[ ]	[ ]

Maximal Heart Rate Correction Factor (HRmax CF from Table 14.6): [ ]

Form 14.2

Individual Data for Åstrand Cycle Test

Name [   ] Date [   ] Time [   ] A.M. [   ] P.M. [   ]

Age [   ] y   Gender (M or W) [   ]   Ht [   ] cm   Wt [   ] kg   [   ] N   Tech. Initials [   ]

Meteorological Data

T [   ] °C (closest 0.1 °C)   RH % [   ] P_B [   ] mm Hg × 1.333 = [   ] hPa (mbar)

Individual Data for Åstrand Cycle Test

Bike Model [   ]   Seat-Post ht [   ]   Bike-Seated HR = 1800 ÷ [   ] (closest 0.1 s) = [   ] $b \cdot min^{-1}$

Target HR Range: < 30 y = 150–160 $b \cdot min^{-1}$ ≥ 30 y (see Table 14.2 or Eq. 14.7) [   ] – [   ] $b \cdot min^{-1}$

Initial Power: [   ] $kg \cdot m \cdot min^{-1}$; × 2; + 300 = $\dot{V}O_2SM$ [   ] $mL \cdot min^{-1}$; = [   ] $L \cdot min^{-1}$

[   ] W; × 12; + 300 = $\dot{V}O_2SM$ [   ] $mL \cdot min^{-1}$; = [   ] $L \cdot min^{-1}$

Time	Exercise HR (Eq. 14.6b)		
min:s	1800 ÷	30-b time (s)	= $b \cdot min^{-1}$
1:30–2:00	1800 ÷	_____	_____
2:30–3:00	1800 ÷	_____	_____
3:30–4:00	1800 ÷	_____	_____
4:30–5:00	1800 ÷	_____	_____
5:30–6:00	1800 ÷	_____	_____
6:30–7:00	1800 ÷	_____	_____
7:30–8:00	1800 ÷	_____	_____

[   ] W (circle one)
Adjusted Power if Warranted: [   ] $kg \cdot m \cdot min^{-1}$

Average of 5th and 6th min HR (if differ by < 6 $b \cdot min^{-1}$)

[   ] $b \cdot min^{-1}$

6th min HR (if 5th & 6th min differ between 6 and 10 $b \cdot min^{-1}$)

HR if 5th and 6th min HR differ by > 10 $b \cdot min^{-1}$ or if power adjustment was made.

Absolute $\dot{V}O_2max$ ($L \cdot min^{-1}$; $mL \cdot kg^{-1} \cdot min^{-1}$) for MEN (M) and WOMEN (W) using Equations 14.9 and 14.10, respectively:

$\dot{V}O_2SM$ [   ] $L \cdot min^{-1}$ × {[(220 – Age [   ] y) – 61 M] ÷ (HRsm [   ] $\genfrac{}{}{0pt}{}{- 72\ W}{- 61)}$}

= $\dot{V}O_2SM$ [   ] $L \cdot min^{-1}$ × ([   ] ÷ [   ])

= $\dot{V}O_2SM$ [   ] $L \cdot min^{-1}$ × [   ] = [   ] $L \cdot min^{-1}$; × 1000 = [   ] $mL \cdot min^{-1}$;

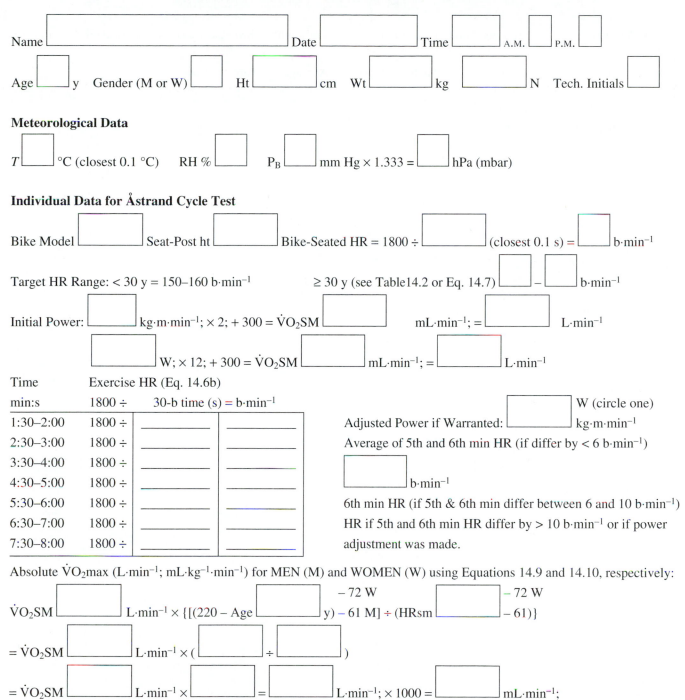

$\dot{V}O_2$max using table method for men (Table 14.4) and women (14.5) or Eq. 14.9:

$\dot{V}O_2$max ⬚ L·min^{-1} (from Table 14.5) × HRmax CF (from Form 14.1 or Table 14.6) ⬚

= ⬚ L·min^{-1} = ⬚ mL·min^{-1}; divided by body mass ⬚ kg = ⬚ mL·kg^{-1}·min^{-1}

Relative $\dot{V}O_2$max (mL·kg^{-1}·min^{-1}) = $\dot{V}O_2$max ⬚ mL·min^{-1} ÷ BM ⬚ kg = ⬚ mL·kg^{-1}·min^{-1}

Fitness Category (circle one): Very High   High   Good   Average   Fair   Low

Form 14.3

Group Data for Åstrand Cycle Test

M E N

Initials or I.D.	$\dot{V}O_2max$ (mL·kg⁻¹·min⁻¹)	Fitness Category
1.		
2.		
3.		
4.		
5.		
6.		
7.		
8.		
9.		
10.		
11.		
12.		
13.		
14.		
15.		
16.		
17.		
18.		
19.		
20.		
21.		
22.		
M		
Minimum		
Maximum		

W O M E N

Initials or I.D.	$\dot{V}O_2max$ (mL·kg⁻¹·min⁻¹)	Fitness Category
1.		
2.		
3.		
4.		
5.		
6.		
7.		
8.		
9.		
10.		
11.		
12.		
13.		
14.		
15.		
16.		
17.		
18.		
19.		
20.		
21.		
22.		
M		
Minimum		
Maximum		

MAXIMAL OXYGEN CONSUMPTION

A test of aerobic fitness that truly qualifies as a laboratory test is the Maximal Oxygen Consumption ($\dot{V}O_2$max) Test. Although this test may involve a substantial anaerobic contribution to metabolism at the terminal portion of the test, it is primarily an aerobic test.

Whereas the run/walk and cycle tests attempt to *predict* aerobic power as accurately as possible, the $\dot{V}O_2$max Test actually *measures* aerobic power. The run/walk tests, for example, predict maximal oxygen consumption based on the relationship between maximal oxygen consumption and time or distance of running or walking; some run/walk tests combine running or walking performance with heart rate. The step tests and cycle tests *estimate* the maximal oxygen consumption based on the relationship among heart rate, oxygen consumption, and power level. Because the $\dot{V}O_2$max Test directly measures oxygen consumption, it requires more expensive and sophisticated equipment than that required by field or field/lab tests.

In this chapter, the direct measurement of oxygen consumption is described for submaximal and maximal exercise. Special importance is given to the latter stages of the exercise protocol, because that is when the *maximal* oxygen consumption typically occurs.

Purpose of the Maximal Oxygen Consumption Test

The purpose of the Maximal Oxygen Consumption Test is to measure aerobic fitness. Aerobic fitness is synonymous with several other terms, such as *aerobic power, cardiovascular fitness, cardiovascular endurance, circulorespiratory endurance,* and *cardiorespiratory endurance.* Cardiovascular fitness, as estimated by $\dot{V}O_2$max, is inversely related to coronary heart disease and all-cause mortality in adult women.[11,38]

The Maximal Oxygen Consumption Test has received more recognition than any other exercise physiology laboratory test. Testimony to this is the fact that the purpose of many field and field/lab tests is to predict maximal oxygen consumption—the variable that often has been used synonymously with aerobic fitness.[57,71,78] Traditionally, no other single laboratory test has been used as frequently to indicate a person's aptitude for success in events calling upon maximal efforts longer than 2 min. In addition, combined with some anaerobic tests, it helps indicate success for events lasting 1 min to 2 min. In conjunction with measures of efficiency (economy), ventilatory threshold/breakpoint, glycogen storage, acclimatization, and fractional utilization of maximal oxygen consumption, the $\dot{V}O_2$max Test is also an important indicator of success for all-out events lasting between 20 min and 4 h.[70]

Also, the Maximal Oxygen Consumption Test provides insight into the cardiorespiratory system. For example, the clinical severity of disease decreases with an increase in functional aerobic fitness.[16] Thus, the Maximal Oxygen Consumption Test has been used to assess not only mixed aerobic-anaerobic fitness, short aerobic fitness, and long aerobic fitness, but also the abilities of the cardiovascular and respiratory systems to transport and diffuse oxygen.

Physiological Rationale

The ability to consume oxygen is important for the metabolic function of body cells. Cellular activity is dependent upon oxygen because the cell derives its energy from adenosine triphosphate (ATP). Aerobic metabolism produces large volumes of ATP via the oxidative pathway. This pathway reflects the ability of the muscles' mitochondria to synthesize the phosphagen ATP.

The maximal consumption of oxygen is dependent not only upon the cells' ability to extract and use oxygen but also upon the ability of the cardiovascular and respiratory systems to transport this oxygen to the cells. Cardiovascularly, the transport of oxygen is represented by the cardiac output, the amount of blood pumped by a heart ventricle per minute. Thus, a greater maximal cardiac output leads to a greater maximal oxygen consumption under normal conditions. The respiratory system's transport of oxygen is represented by ventilation, which is measured as liters of air per minute. A greater ventilation capacity usually is associated with a greater maximal oxygen consumption. It now appears that respiratory muscle work during heavy maximal exercise affects exercise performance by decreasing leg blood flow.[42]

The highest oxygen value achieved during the $\dot{V}O_2$max Test represents the maximal oxygen consumption. This peak is most likely to occur at the final minute of the progressive exercise test. Because peak oxygen consumption varies with the mode of exercise and performer symptoms, the term **peak oxygen consumption** denotes the highest oxygen consumption for a specific type of exercise, and the term **maximal oxygen consumption** denotes the single highest oxygen consumption elicited among the different modes of exercise.[12] For example, peak oxygen consumption values are similar for treadmill and step tests for most people, but they are about 5 % to 10 % higher on a treadmill than on a cycle ergometer.[43] For trained cyclists, however, similar results may be achieved on bicycle and treadmill ergometry. Another example is the $\dot{V}O_2$ peak elicited by arm ergometry, which is 63 % of that elicited by the treadmill.[8] Thus, the term *peak* should be used to denote the highest oxygen consumption value achieved for a particular mode of exercise, and the term *maximal* should be used for the highest value achieved among all the modes, which is usually treadmill ergometry. The performer's symptom-limited peak $\dot{V}O_2$ is the highest value achieved before abnormal symptoms dictated the halt of the test rather than physiological limits. In general, the peak oxygen consumption relates to the muscle mass involved in the ergometric task and reflects the performer's specific training.

Method

The methods and procedures for the administration of oxygen consumption (metabolic) testing may seem complicated, especially for first-year exercise physiology students. However, it is certainly possible for novices to gain an appreciation and understanding of maximal oxygen consumption testing simply by observing the performer and by monitoring the instruments during the exercise test. The methods include a description of the equipment, the exercise protocol, the procedures, and the calculations. A description of the accuracy of the $\dot{V}O_2$max Test is in Box 15.1.

Equipment

Until the 1970s, the equipment used for measuring oxygen consumption consisted of several instruments purchased from separate manufacturers. The investigator then would interface the individual instruments so that online testing could be accomplished, or the investigator would collect the exhaled air in special bags for post-test analysis of oxygen and carbon dioxide concentrations and ventilation volumes. Today a variety of manufacturers combine the individual components into a single package. These interfaced consoles often include a computer to make all the calculations for deriving the metabolic and respiratory values (Ametec™; Consentius Technologies™). Improved and consolidated instrumentation has led to portable and breath-by-breath capabilities in measuring oxygen consumption (Cosmed™; Sensor Medics™).

The equipment for Maximal Oxygen Consumption Tests may be categorized into three areas: (1) ergometers, (2) respiratory equipment and metabolic equipment, and (3) auxiliaries.

Ergometers

It is best to use the type of ergometer that simulates the type of movement for which the performer has been training. For

---

BOX 15.1　Accuracy of the $\dot{V}O_2$max Test

The accuracy of the Maximal Oxygen Consumption Test is maximized by achieving the traditional criteria of the max test, such as (1) the plateau of the oxygen consumption despite an increase of power level, (2) the attainment of respiratory exchange ratios > 1.0, (3) the plateau of heart rate, (4) high blood lactates, and (5) the exhaustion of the performer.

Validity

The validity of any exercise test is partly dependent upon the exercise modality and the specific fitness of the performer. Although not supported by all physiologists,[27,60] most investigators and reviewers [3, 57, 71, 78] have supported the maximal oxygen consumption value as the best single physiological indicator of a person's capacity for endurance-activities dependent upon the cardiorespiratory system. High maximal oxygen consumptions, when expressed relative to body mass ($mL \cdot kg^{-1} \cdot min^{-1}$), are associated with successful running performance in events lasting more than a couple min. For example, correlations of .90 and .91 have been reported between $\dot{V}O_2$max and 12 min distance.[25,37] However, a lower correlation of −.74 was reported between $\dot{V}O_2$max and 1.5 mile time.[53]

Reliability

The test-retest reliability of maximal oxygen consumption tests is high—about .95[61,78] to .99.[16] The intraclass correlation coefficient is .93 and the day-to-day variability is < 5 % or ≈ 2 $mL \cdot kg^{-1} \cdot min^{-1}$.[67] The standard error *(SE)* of the $\dot{V}O_2$max Test may range from a low of about 2.5 %[78] to a high of about 5 % to 6 %[49] of the mean score for an average person; it may extend up to about 8 % in aerobically trained males.[21] Thus, an individual would be expected to vary by about 2 to 4 $mL \cdot kg^{-1} \cdot min^{-1}$, even when tested weeks apart.[16,55,78] For example, if a person's maximal oxygen consumption is truly 40 $mL \cdot kg^{-1} \cdot min^{-1}$, then repeated tests with an *SE* of 5 % would be expected to vary between 38.0 and 42.0 $mL \cdot kg^{-1} \cdot min^{-1}$ [calculated as: 40 $mL \cdot kg^{-1} \cdot min^{-1}$ ± (5 % × 40)]. The $\dot{V}O_2$max is highly consistent even over four months, having an average coefficient of variation [*(SD/M)* × 100] of about 4.3 %.[86]

---

example, runners should be tested on treadmills, cyclists on cycle ergometers, rowers on rowing ergometers, wheelchair athletes on wheelchair or arm ergometers, cross-country skiers on ski ergometers, and swimmers in swim flumes, on swim benches, or in a pool while tethered to weighted pulleys. Another consideration is the norms by which the performer will be evaluated. The Maximal Oxygen Consumption Test should be performed on the same ergometer as that which was used by those performers whose scores generated the norms. A practical consideration is the cost and ancillary objectives of the test. For example, a step bench is inexpensive but is not a specific mode for a swimmer. A cycle ergometer facilitates the measurement of blood pressure by clinicians but is not specific for walkers and joggers.

The treadmill (TM) has two basic units of measure: (1) speed and (2) slope or grade (Table 15.1). Maximal

Table 15.1 Conversions for Speed and Slope for Treadmill Ergometry

Speed (Based upon 1 mph = 1.609 km·h⁻¹ = 26.8 m·min⁻¹)

mph	km·h⁻¹	m·min⁻¹	mph	km·h⁻¹	m·min⁻¹
1.7	2.74	45.6	8.5	13.68	228.0
2.0	3.22	53.6	9.0	14.48	241.4
2.5	4.02	66.7	9.5	15.29	254.8
3.0	4.83	80.4	10.0	16.09	268.2
3.5	5.63	94.0	10.5	16.89	281.6
4.0	6.44	107.2	11.0	17.70	295.0
4.5	7.24	121.0	11.5	18.50	308.5
5.0	8.04	134.1	12.0	19.31	322.0
5.5	8.85	148.0	12.5	20.11	335.3
6.0	9.65	161.0	13.0	20.92	348.7
6.5	10.46	174.3	13.5	21.72	362.1
7.0	11.26	188.8	14.0	22.53	375.5
7.5	12.07	201.2	14.5	23.33	389.0
8.0	12.87	215.0	15.0	24.13	402.3

Slopea

Degree (°)	Grade (%)	Degree (°)	Grade (%)
1	1.75	6	10.49
2	3.49	7	12.24
3	5.24	8	13.99
4	6.99	9	15.74
5	8.74	10	17.49

Note: aFor each degree increase in slope, the percent grade increases by ≈ 1.75 % units.

speeds (mph or mi·h⁻¹; km/h or km·h⁻¹) may vary with different treadmills from 12 mph (19.3 km·h⁻¹) to 15 mph (24 km·h⁻¹) to 25 mph (40.2 km·h⁻¹). The maximal slopes or grades of laboratory treadmills are about 25 %, but some can reach 40 % grade (≈ 22°). Table 15.1 provides the equivalent speeds in the American and metric systems, along with the slopes in degrees and percent grade. The calibration of treadmills is described in Box 15.2.

Respiratory and Metabolic/Gas Equipment (Figure 15.1)

The pieces of equipment that aid in the measurement of the volume of air breathed by the performer are (1) a noseclip, (2) a mouthpiece, (3) an air volume meter, (4) a respiratory valve, and (5) ventilatory hoses. The pieces of equipment that promote the measurement of the metabolic gases are (1) an oxygen analyzer, (2) a carbon dioxide analyzer, (3) a mixing chamber, and (4) a drying tube. A description of the calibrations for metabolic equipment is presented in Box 15.3.

Respiratory Equipment
A **noseclip** prevents the inhalation and exhalation of air through the nose. Otherwise, if air is breathed through the nose, it is unaccounted for at the air volume meter.

A **rubber mouthpiece** attaches to the respiratory valve and is similar to a scuba mouthpiece. The flanges of the mouthpiece prevent the leakage of air around the performer's mouth, while the protruding tabs allow gripping the piece with the teeth.

An **air volume meter** of some sort (electronic pneumotachometer, turbine flow, tissot spirometer, or mechanical bellows) is used to measure the volume of air inspired or expired per minute ($\dot{V}_I$ or $\dot{V}_E$). The recorded unit of measure is liters per minute (L·min⁻¹). Either the inspiratory or expiratory volume, or both, are measured by the air volume meter. When measuring inspired air, the inspiratory air flows from the inlet of the air volume meter to its outlet and on toward the respiratory valve via the ventilatory hose (Figure 15.1). Contrarily, when measuring expired air volume, the expiratory air flows from the respiratory valve outlet to the inlet of the air volume meter.

A **respiratory valve** (Figure 15.2) is a two-way valve that prevents inspired air from returning to the port where it entered. The inspired air comes into the inlet side of the respiratory valve but cannot return out the same inlet during expiration. The expired air is directed to the outlet on the other side of the respiratory valve.

Ventilatory hoses are internally smooth (noncorrugated), flexible tubes that conduct air to or from the air volume meter and mixing chamber. Sometimes metal clamps secure the hose endings to the respiratory valve and volume meter.

Metabolic/Gas Equipment The metabolic/gas equipment directs, dries, and analyzes the performer's expired air as it passes from the ventilatory tube at the outlet of the respiratory valve and through the mixing chamber to the respective gas analyzers.

Many electronic **oxygen analyzers** use paramagnetic or galvanic fuel cell principles to determine the fractional (or percentage) concentration of oxygen in the expired air (F_EO_2). Most metabolic analyzers are designed to be most accurate between oxygen concentrations of 15 % to 21 %. Many electronic **carbon dioxide analyzers** use an infrared principle to determine the fractional (F) concentration (or %) of carbon dioxide in the expired air (F_ECO_2). Mass spectrometers can measure both carbon dioxide and oxygen concentrations. Nitrogen analyzers are not necessary for measuring oxygen consumption because nitrogen concentration can be calculated as the balance from the other two gas measures.

The samples of gas can be directed to and from a mixing chamber, or they can be sampled after being collected in small rubber bags (aliquots) or large collection bags (meteorological; Douglas bag). The **mixing chamber,** usually a 4 L to 10 L box or cylinder made of clear plexiglass, allows the expired air to be uniformly distributed due to its internal bevels. Air samples then pass into the gas analyzers via small tubes for online analysis.

A **drying tube** consists of a small (≈ 4 in. × 0.5 in.) container holding a suitable drying agent, or desiccant (e.g., calcium sulfate), and filter that prevent damp (saturated) and dusty air from entering the analyzers. Although not universally used, the drying tube prolongs the life of the analyzers and eliminates the need to correct mathematically for the

Both the speed and slope of a treadmill (TM) should be calibrated annually. Instructions for TM calibration are usually in the manufacturer's instruction manual and other sources.[22,40]

Speed Calibration

1. If the length of the TM belt is not given in the manufacturer's instruction manual, then measure the belt length as follows:
   a. Mark (#1) the exposed belt with a piece of easily visible tape at the front of the TM (but not on the curved surface).
   b. Place a chalk or pen mark at a second point (mark #2) at the rear flat portion of the TM belt.
   c. Using a meter-stick or metric tape, measure the distance between marks #1 and #2 to the nearest 0.1 cm; record the value (e.g., 153.2 cm; 1.532 m).
   d. Expose another belt portion by pushing it backward with your foot, but stop it when the #1 mark is at the back of the TM.
   e. Make mark #3 at the front flat portion of the TM belt.
   f. Measure the distance from the tape mark (#1) now at the back of the belt to mark #3; record the value (e.g., 144.3 cm).
   g. Again move the belt; then stop it when the original rear chalk or pen mark (#2) is visible at a flat portion at the front of the TM belt.
   h. Measure the distance between mark #3 and mark #2; record the value (e.g., 141.0 cm; 1.410).
   i. Add the three values; the total is the length of the belt (e.g., 438.5 cm, or 4.385 m).
2. Measure the number of revolutions as follows if the TM has no automatic counter:
   a. Start the treadmill and set the speed control to a slow speed (e.g., 4.0 km·h⁻¹; km/h).
   b. Mark a fixed point outside the TM belt (e.g., the inside edge at the rear of the TM where the belt descends or disappears).
   c. Start a stopwatch the instant that the tape mark (#1) passes the fixed mark; remove other tapes.
   d. Count the number of belt revolutions by counting the number of times the belt mark passes the fixed point.
   e. Stop the watch at a complete (whole) revolution that is closest to 60 s; record the number of revolutions.
   f. Record the time to closest tenth of a second (e.g., 59.6).
3. Convert the revolutions to revolutions per minute (rpm) by using Equation 1:

$$\text{rpm} = \text{revolutions (\#)} \div (t \text{ in s} / 60 \text{ s})$$ Eq. 1

Sample calculation: If revolutions = <u>17</u> and time = <u>59.6</u> s
then rpm = 17 ÷ 59.6 / 60;
= 17 ÷ 0.99;
= 17.17

4. The distance (D) covered in 1 min is calculated according to Equation 2:

$$\text{D·min}^{-1} = \text{rpm} \times \text{belt length in m}$$ Eq. 2

Using the prior example, then D·min⁻¹ = 17.17 × 4.385 m = 75.30 m·min⁻¹, which is faster than the expected 66.7 m·min⁻¹ (Table 15.1).
5. The distance in m·h⁻¹ is calculated by multiplying the m·min⁻¹ by 60:

$$75.30 \times 60 = 4518 \text{ m·h}^{-1}$$

6. The distance in km·h⁻¹ = 4.518, which is faster than the expected 4.0 km·h⁻¹ (Table 15.1).
7. The distance in mph = 4.518 km·h⁻¹ ÷ 1.609 = 2.80 mph, which is faster than the expected 2.50 mph (Table 15.1).
8. The treadmill controller's zero set screw must be adjusted until the speed reads the same as the controller's gauge.

Slope Calibration

Zero

1. Run the treadmill at a slow speed while the elevation setting is at 0 % or 0°.
2. Stop the treadmill.
3. Place a carpenter's level on the TM belt.
4. Check the bubble on the level to make sure it is centered.
5. If it is not centered, then run and stop the TM repeatedly while changing the slope setting until the carpenter's level indicates zero slope.
6. Once the TM is level, change the slope indicator to zero by making an adjustment at a small screw sometimes found on the meter's face.

Range

1. Place the treadmill to a given percent slope (e.g., 20 %).
2. Measure a fixed distance on the floor parallel and at the edge of the treadmill (e.g., 20 in.).
3. Measure the perpendicular height of the treadmill at the low part of the parallel distance (e.g., 15 in.).
4. Measure the perpendicular height of the treadmill at the high part of the parallel distance (e.g., 19 in.).
5. Calculate the percent slope according to Equation 3:

$$\% \text{ slope} = [(\text{Highest ht} - \text{lowest ht}) \div \text{parallel distance}] \times 100$$ Eq. 3

E.g., 20 % = [(19 − 15) ÷ 20] × 100 = (4 ÷ 20) × 100
6. Adjust, if necessary, the potentiometer on the control-meter to the appropriate percent slope (e.g., 20 %).

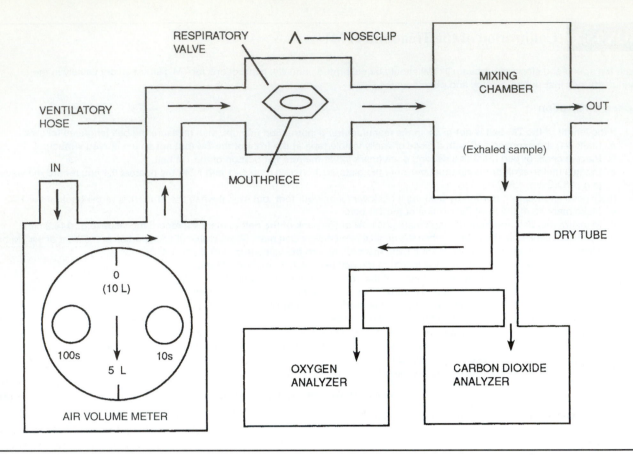

Figure 15.1 Schematic depiction of the airflow circuit for measuring the inspiratory volume of air ($\dot{V}_I$) and the expired fractional concentrations of oxygen (F_EO_2) and carbon dioxide (F_ECO_2). The air volume meter has three dials—the big circle representing 0 L to 10 L, the two smaller circles representing 10 L to 100 L and 100 L to 1000 L, respectively.

BOX 15.3 Calibration of Metabolic Instruments

Calibration can be performed by the instructor or lab assistants prior to the test. The gold standards of gas calibration are based on the measurement of oxygen and carbon dioxide from one of three methods: (1) Scholander technique[73]; (2) Haldane technique; and (3) mass spectrometry. The former two methods require inexpensive apparatuses that measure volumes of oxygen and carbon dioxide after each has been absorbed by respective chemical reagents.[24] These two methods are gradually giving way to the more rapid mass spectrometry method.

    Some commercial metabolic instruments (e.g., Sensor Medics MMC4400) have autocalibration devices using gas tanks with 24 % and 12 % oxygen, as well as 8 % and 0 % carbon dioxide.[59]

    It is not unusual to calibrate the analyzers against standardized gas tanks of known concentrations before each test. Ideally, a three-point calibration is recommended,[46] whereby certified calibrated gases at the zero are at 0 %, with the high span for carbon dioxide and oxygen at 6 % and 18 % fractional concentrations, respectively, and the midranges at 3 % and 15 %, respectively.

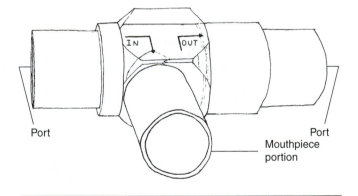

Figure 15.2 A two-way, non-rebreathing respiratory valve prevents air from exiting the same port that it entered.

percentage of water vapor in the gas samples. Because the airflow through the drying tube is slower than normal, a delay in the circuit of about 15 s,[79] or up to 30 s, should be accounted for when analyzing the data. Computerized metabolic consoles automatically correct for such delays.

Auxiliaries

The need for auxiliary equipment is dependent upon the type of basic equipment available to the investigator. For example, some computerized metabolic consoles also contain gauges for monitoring temperature and pressure. To measure oxygen consumption, a laboratory needs auxiliary equipment for such purposes as (1) monitoring the environment; (2) measuring the participant's stature and body mass; (3) providing comfort to the participant; (4) calibrating instruments and gases; (5) timing; (6) recording; and (7) protecting the instruments.

Various **meteorological gauges** for measuring environmental air temperature, barometric pressure, and relative humidity are necessary to correct for temperature, pressure, and saturation of the observed inspiratory and/or expiratory air volumes.

Either a **balance-beam** or **electronic scale** may be used to measure the participant's stature and body mass just prior to the test. These techniques were described in Chapter 3.

A **respiratory valve support** may consist of a hanging support from an overhead rail or ceiling or from a commercially available waist-harness. Without such a support, the performer has trouble keeping the valve in the mouth, especially during treadmill exercise. Some valves permit **saliva collectors** to be attached.

Calibrative auxiliaries include such items as gas cylinders and air volume syringes. The cylinders should contain certified precise CO_2, O_2, and N_2 gases; substantiation of such gases can be made with a Scholander apparatus.[73] The 3 L to 5 L air volume syringes (Figure 15.3) insert a precise volume of air into the air volume meter, pneumotach, or metabolic instrument.[5]

A **laboratory timer,** easily visible to all technicians, is used for timing various events such as the exercise protocol and air/gas recordings. Timers are described in Chapter 9—"Anaerobic Cycling."

A **ventilation recorder** is an optional auxiliary instrument. Some are capable of graphing inspirations and expirations, thus enabling the calculation of such respiratory parameters as ventilatory volume, frequency, and tidal volume. Of these three variables, only ventilatory volume is essential for the calculation of oxygen consumption. If the air volume meter has no electrical output by which to record the volume electronically, then the technician must simply record the values indicated by the pointers on the air volume meter (review Figure 15.1).

Exercise Protocol

The Maximal Oxygen Consumption Test usually requires the performer to exercise to exhaustion, although it need not

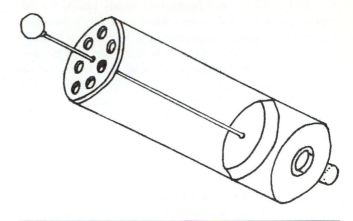

Figure 15.3   A 3 L syringe helps calibrate the ventilation volume measured by an air volume meter.

be quite so stressful as long as the other traditional criteria are met. The exercise may be performed on various modalities, such as (a) step bench, (b) cycle ergometer, (c) treadmill, (d) swim flume, (e) wheelchair ergometer, (f) rowing ergometer, (g) skiing ergometer, and others. The test protocol, which consists of the prescription for time spent at each power level, is often a continuous and progressive type that eventually exceeds the aerobic power of the exerciser. Thus, the test includes submaximal, maximal, and supramaximal exercise relative to $\dot{V}O_2max$. The supramaximal portion contributes highly to the performer's exhaustion.

Several protocols may be used to elicit peak or maximal oxygen consumption.[3] Some of these are described in Chapter 19 on the ECG Test, while two protocols are presented for the cycle ergometer and one for the treadmill, in this chapter.

Although it is possible to reach nearly the maximal oxygen consumption level in 1 min when performing an all-out 90 s cycling task,[75] the test (excluding warm-up) is seldom less than 5 min and often no longer than 9 min. Occasionally, it is as long as 20 min for aerobically fit individuals starting at low stages, or if a longer time for monitoring the electrocardiogram is desired, or if mechanical efficiency is being measured simultaneously. Some investigators recommend a continuous protocol that brings performers to their limit of tolerance in about 10 min ± 2 min.[18] Continuous protocols have no active or passive recovery intervals between exercise test stages.

Cycling Protocols

Prior to the test, the estimated $\dot{V}O_2max$ of the performer from previous field or field/lab predictive tests helps in determining the proper protocol. If no prior tests exist, then questioning the performer about training habits is helpful.

% $\dot{V}O_2max$ Protocol   One recommended protocol is to start at 25 % to 40 % of the predicted $\dot{V}O_2max$ and then progress through the 1 min to 3 min stages by 10 % to 15 %

$\dot{V}O_2$max.[79] To achieve reasonable steady states, the one minute or two minute stages should use 10 % increases, whereas three minute stages use 15 % $\dot{V}O_2$max increases.

If no predictive $\dot{V}O_2$max is available, but the performer knows the highest power level that he or she can sustain for three or more minutes on a cycle ergometer, then Table 15.2 can be used to approximate the maximal oxygen consumption. The table gives MET values, multiples of resting metabolism, at various power levels during cycle ergometry for persons weighing between 50 kg and 100 kg. The approximate oxygen cost may be found by multiplying the MET value by 3.5 mL·kg⁻¹·min⁻¹. Once the $\dot{V}O_2$max value has been estimated, either the % $\dot{V}O_2$max protocol or a protocol from Table 15.3 may be used.

Table 15.3 Protocols The two cycle protocols presented in Table 15.3 are modifications of a former continuous protocol[52] and are based on the aerobic fitness status of the performer. They are for persons who are estimated to have maxi-

mal oxygen consumptions either above or below 3.0 L·min⁻¹. For persons with an estimated $\dot{V}O_2$max less than 3.0 L·min⁻¹, the initial power level is 100 W (600 kg·m·min⁻¹) and increases by 25 W for subsequent 2 min power intervals. A similar protocol is followed for persons with estimated $\dot{V}O_2$max levels greater than 3.0 L·min⁻¹, except that the initial power level is 175 W. For persons with suspected $\dot{V}O_2$max levels that are exceptionally high, the starting power level can be higher than 175 W in order to keep the duration of the test close to a 9 min maximum. For some elite cyclists who reach 450 W, the test duration would be 30 min if they started at 175 W. Often, the final power level of a performer cannot be sustained for an entire 2 min stage due to the performer's fatigue.

$\dot{V}O_2$max Criteria The performer is encouraged to exercise to exhaustion in order to assure that peak oxygen consumption has been achieved. Traditionally, researchers sought a leveling off or plateauing of oxygen consumption at the end of the test. A primary criterion for attainment of maximum is an increase in oxygen consumption no greater than 150 mL·min⁻¹ at a succeeding power level.[78] This means, for example, that, for a change in power level equivalent to 25 W (or 150 kg·m·min⁻¹) on the cycle ergometer, or a power level of 2.5 % grade change on the treadmill, the change in oxygen consumption should not exceed 150 mL·min⁻¹.[78] An expected increase for 25 W is 300 mL·min⁻¹ or 0.3 L·min⁻¹. Thus, the lower value of 150 mL indicates that the performer cannot meet the oxygen requirement. For treadmill protocols, the MET unit is helpful in determining the plateau criterion. Thus, if the next stage dictates a MET increase of 2.8 but the performer only increases by 0.6 MET, then surely the plateau criterion is achieved.[44] Thus, it is likely that performers truly reach peak oxygen consumptions when this criterion

Table 15.2 Conversion of Power to Energy Cost (MET) of Cycle Ergometry

Body Mass (kg)	Power (W)						
	50	75	100	125	150	175	200
				MET			
50	5.1	6.6	8.2	9.7	11.3	12.8	14.3
60	4.6	5.9	7.1	8.4	9.7	11.0	12.3
70	4.2	5.3	6.4	7.5	8.6	9.7	10.8
80	3.9	4.9	5.9	6.8	7.8	8.8	9.7
90	3.7	4.6	5.4	6.3	7.1	8.0	8.9
100	3.5	4.3	5.1	5.9	6.6	7.4	8.2

Note: Table derived from the following equation for leg ergometry: $\dot{V}O_2$ in mL·kg⁻¹·min⁻¹ ÷ 3.5, where $\dot{V}O_2$ = [(10.8 × W)/BM] + 7; W = watt; BM = body mass (kg).[3]

Table 15.3 Cycle Ergometer Protocols for $\dot{V}O_2$max Test

Time (min:s)	Power (W; N·m·min⁻¹; kg·m·min⁻¹)[a]					
	"Guesstimated" Maximal Oxygen Consumption (L·min⁻¹)					
	< 3.0 L·min⁻¹			≥ 3.0 L·min⁻¹		
Warm-up	W	N·m·min⁻¹	kg·m·min⁻¹	W	N·m·min⁻¹	kg·m·min⁻¹
0:00–5:00	75	4500	450	150	9000	900
"Rest" (0:00-2:00)	0–25	0–1500	0–150	25–50	1500–3000	150–300
Max Test						
0:00–2:00	100	6000	600	175	10 500	1050
2:00–4:00	125	7500	750	200	12 000	1200
4:00–6:00	150	9000	900	225	13 500	1350
6:00–8:00	175	10 500	1050	250	15 000	1500
8:00–10:00	200	12 000	1200	275	16 500	1650
10:00–12:00	225	13 500	1350	300	18 000	1800
12:00–14:00	250	15 000	1500	325	19 500	1950
Recovery						
0:00–3:00	50–75	3000–4500	300–450	125–150	7500–9000	750–900

Note: [a]For approximate oxygen cost of each power level up to 200 W, see Table 2.1 in Chapter 2 or calculate milliliters per minute as the product of body mass (kg), MET (Table 15.2), and 3.5.

is met. If oxygen consumptions at the last power level increase by more than 150 mL·min⁻¹, then it is more likely that they will reach a higher oxygen consumption if proceeding to a higher power level.[20]

However, some reviewers note that a significant percentage of persons, especially children, elderly, and low-fit persons, fail to reach an oxygen plateau as defined by this criterion.[46,78] If this primary criterion is not met, peak oxygen consumption may still have occurred if secondary criteria have been met. For example, the respiratory exchange ratio (RER) is another common indicator of $\dot{V}O_2$max achievement. Some investigators would expect a ratio greater than 1.0;[13,54,58,84] and some exercise physiologists recommend minimum ratios from 1.05[30] to 1.1[44] or 1.15.[3,6,72]

Other secondary criteria are (1) high blood lactates (e.g., > 8 mM);[3] (2) rate of perceived exertion (RPE) greater than 17[3] and 8 for the original category scale and the category-ratio scale, respectively; (3) the reaching of previously *measured* maximal heart rate; (4) heart rate fails to increase with further increase in exercise intensity;[3] and (5) exhaustion of the performer. Because of the large standard deviation in maximal heart rate between persons (±10–12 b·min⁻¹), the *predicted* maximal heart rate from such formulas as 220 minus age should not be used as a criterion. In summary, if the attainment of $\dot{V}O_2$max criteria is questionable, then the more apt term may be peak $\dot{V}O_2$ rather than maximal $\dot{V}O_2$. In a study designed specifically to examine $\dot{V}O_2$max criteria, the investigators concluded that "only the RER and blood lactate standards appear to be of general value."[32]

Pedal Revolutions per Minute (RPM)   Although economy or efficiency of cycling may vary with pedal rpm during submaximal exercise[23,33,41,64,65,74,77] it does not mean that rpm will necessarily alter the peak or maximal oxygen consumption.[68] Also, some suggest that cyclists stand on the pedals during the last moments of cycling in order to cause the cycling peak $\dot{V}O_2$ value to approximate more closely the treadmill peak $\dot{V}O_2$. However, this has not been confirmed.[2,39]

Treadmill (TM) Protocol

It appears that similar results are obtained with a variety of treadmill protocols (see Chapter 19, Table 19.2 and Figure 19.1), although some take less time than others.[34] One of the most popular treadmill tests is the Bruce Test, the earliest standard treadmill test.[55] Although it is often used for cardiovascular screening purposes,[17] it also is a common protocol for predicting[1,10,51] and directly measuring maximal oxygen consumption.[61]

The Bruce protocol (Table 15.4) consists of seven 3 min stages. Most performers should walk during the initial three stages in the first 9 min.[13] Although the initial stages are important for cardiovascular screening (e.g., ECG monitoring), they are sometimes deleted when the primary purpose is to measure maximal oxygen consumption;

in these cases, the initial stage for $\dot{V}O_2$max testing is dependent upon the fitness level of the performer. Table 15.4 also lists the approximate MET for each completed stage of the Bruce protocol.[3]

Treadmill Technique   A common question is "Is treadmill running the same as overground running"? A group of investigators reported no difference in the oxygen cost.[9] A person should never be standing on a stationary treadmill belt when it is placed in the On position. To enter and exit a moving belt of a treadmill, both sides of the hand-rails should be used. There are two common ways of stepping onto the moving belt of a treadmill. One way is to stand alongside the moving belt and then to lean over the belt while grasping both rails for support. Then one foot is placed onto the belt and allowed to coast briefly; that foot is then returned to its original position. This is repeated until the performer establishes a rhythm or pace. Once the performer feels secure about the pace, the other foot is placed on the belt while the upper body is still substantially supported by the handrails; finally, the performer releases the handrails. The other method is to straddle the moving belt and then proceed as in the previous method. The oxygen cost of treadmill running is reduced if the performer relies on the handrails.[15] Therefore, tables and equations relating $\dot{V}O_2$ to exercise stages are not valid when the performer uses the handrails. While on the treadmill, the performer should look straight ahead to prevent possible nausea from viewing the moving belt.

Procedures for the Maximal Oxygen Consumption Test

The initial steps for the $\dot{V}O_2$max Test consist of calibrating the metabolic instruments (review Box 15.3) and preparing the performer for exercise.

Table 15.4	Bruce Treadmill Protocol for the $\dot{V}O_2$max Test				
Time min:s	Bruce Stage	Speed mph	km/h	Slope %	MET
Walk					
0:00–3:00	1	1.7	2.7	10	5
3:00–6:00	2	2.5	4.0	12	7
Jog/Walk					
6:00–9:00	3	3.4	5.5	14	10
9:00–12:00	4	4.2	6.8	16	13
Run					
12:00–15:00	5	5.0	8.0	18	16
15:00–18:00	6	5.5	8.0	20	18
18:00–21:00	7	6.0	9.7	22	22
Recovery (Jog/Walk)					
0:00–2:00	2	2.5	4.0	12	7

Preparations

The **performer** should arrive for testing under similar conditions as those presented for performers of the Step Test. Thus, the performer should be refreshed, euhydrated, dressed in lightweight exercise clothes, and not under the influence of drugs, hunger, or fullness.

The technician assigned as the performer's **caretaker** should oversee the gathering of the basic data, such as stature, body mass, and age. The caretaker should also prepare the performer for the ergometer (e.g., adjust the seat post of the cycle ergometer) and adjust the respiratory valve. After the caretaker explains the exercise protocol, risks, benefits, and objectives of the Maximal Oxygen Consumption Test, the performer signs the Informed Consent or gives verbal consent if it is a classroom situation.

The technician assigned as the **meteorologist** is responsible for observing and recording the environmental temperature, barometric pressure, and relative humidity (see Chapter 2).

Procedures during the Exercise Test

After the initial steps, the exercise begins, and various technicians perform their specific duties at significant times in the exercise protocol (Form 15.1).

The initial stages of the exercise protocol (review Tables 15.3 and 15.4) are not critical for measuring maximal oxygen consumption, but they are important for submaximal measurements. They also serve as a warm-up, allow the technicians to become familiar with their roles, and possibly alert them to any technical or performer problems. The step-by-step procedures are as follows:

1. Start laboratory timer when performer begins the initial power level of the chosen protocol.
2. Record the fraction of expired oxygen (F_EO_2) every 15 s.
3. Record the fraction of expired carbon dioxide (F_ECO_2) every 15 s.
4. Record ventilation ($\dot{V}_E$ or $\dot{V}_I$) from the air volume meter every 60 s early in the test, but every 30 s as the performer nears the expected maximal level.
5. Change the power level at the appropriate time in the exercise protocol.
6. If using a treadmill, note when the performer switches from walking to running; record the first complete minute of running, which usually occurs between the 6th and 12th min of the Bruce protocol.
7. Because the valve restricts the speech of performers, periodically have them indicate their condition by a thumb-up ("I'm OK"), thumb-sideways ("I'm nearing the end"), or thumb-down ("I'm going to stop") signal, or use a Rate-of-Perceived-Exertion chart (review Chapter 12).
8. As the performer begins to lose coordination due to fatigue (e.g., lots of extraneous movements), encourage continuation to exhaustion.
9. Place a spotter near the performer.
10. When the performer reaches exhaustion, record the exact time of stopping the test.
11. If the treadmill is not the type that automatically decreases the slope and speed after pressing the STOP button, then restart it in order to provide a recovery period on the treadmill; ask the performer to walk in place on the platform alongside the treadmill belt, until the proper recovery speed of the treadmill is obtained; if there is no space alongside the treadmill, ask the performer to grasp the siderails for support while continuing to jog/walk as the technician decreases the slope and speed of the treadmill. If using a cycle ergometer, quickly adjust to the proper recovery level and ask the performer to resume pedalling.
12. Remove the noseclip and respiratory valve from the performer.
13. Calculate the maximal oxygen consumption.

Calculation of Maximal Oxygen Consumption

Computerized instruments instantly provide the metabolic and ventilatory results. Their monitors and printers also graph the variables over time (Figure 15.4). However, students are less likely to understand the complexities, concepts, and principles behind the calculations unless they manually perform them. The equations used to calculate $\dot{V}O_2max$ can look rather intimidating. Some of this might be lessened by first trying to grasp the concepts surrounding the calculation.

Concepts

Several concepts can help us to understand the calculation of maximal oxygen consumption. One concept (Eq. 15.1) presents oxygen consumption ($\dot{V}O_2$) as the product of **true oxygen** (true O_2) and ventilation ($\dot{V}_I$ or $\dot{V}_E$). The true O_2 represents the oxygen percentage extracted from the ventilation or, stated differently, the amount of oxygen (mL) consumed for every 100 mL of air inspired or expired. Ventilation is the volume of air expired ($\dot{V}_E$) or inspired ($\dot{V}_I$) during each minute ($L \cdot min^{-1}$) of the test.

$$\dot{V}O_2 \ (L \cdot min^{-1}) = \text{true } O_2 \ \% \times \dot{V}_E \qquad \text{Eq. 15.1}$$

where:

$$\text{true } O_2 \ \% \ = \ \frac{1 - F_EO_2 - F_ECO_2}{0.7904} \times (0.2093 - 0.162)$$

The **ventilation** concept leads to the calculation of oxygen consumption by subtracting the amount of oxygen in the expired air from the volume of the oxygen in inspired air (Eq. 15.2). The fraction of oxygen in inspired air (F_IO_2) and expired air (F_EO_2) is usually expressed as a percentage or a decimal (e.g., 20.93 % or 0.2093), rather than as a fraction (20.93/100). The direct application of this concept requires the measurement of both the inspired and expired volumes but eliminates the need to measure carbon dioxide.

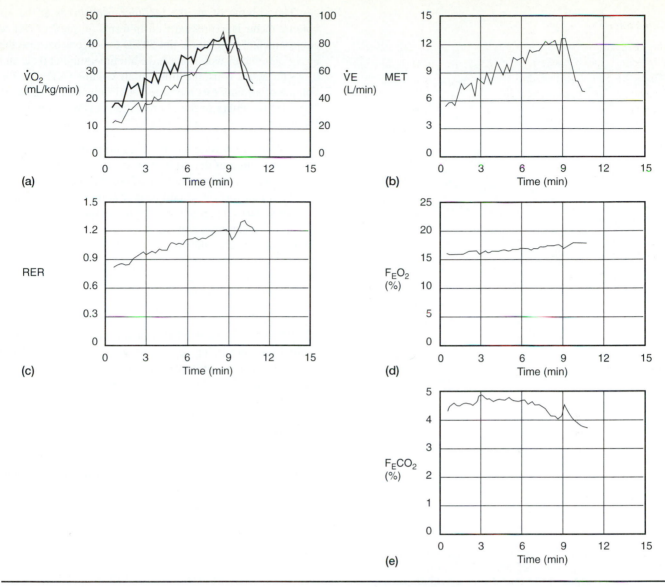

Figure 15.4 This sample of a graphic display from a computerized automated metabolic instrument shows the (a) relative oxygen consumption ($\dot{V}O_2$; mL·kg^{-1}·min^{-1}; bold line) and ventilation ($\dot{V}_E$; L·min^{-1}; light line); (b) MET; (c) respiratory exchange ratio (RER); (d) fractional concentration of expired oxygen (F_EO_2; %); and (e) fractional concentration of carbon dioxide (F_ECO_2; %). Courtesy of Parvo Medic™, Consentius Technologies, Sandy, UT.

$$\dot{V}O_2 \, (\text{L·min}^{-1}) = (\dot{V}_I \times F_IO_2) - (\dot{V}_E \times F_EO_2) \quad \text{Eq. 15.2}$$

The **carbon dioxide** concept incorporates some of the factors that led to Equations 15.1 and 15.2. As with the true O_2 concept, it considers the fraction of carbon dioxide in the expired air (F_ECO_2) as a result of its metabolic production. As with the ventilation concept, the carbon dioxide concept includes the volume of inspired air ($\dot{V}_I$) and the fractional concentration of inspired (0.2093) and expired oxygen. This may be presented in Equation 15.3 as[81]

$$\dot{V}O_2 (\text{L·min}^{-1}) \quad \text{Eq. 15.3}$$
$$= \dot{V}_I \times \left[\frac{[0.2093 \times (1 - F_ECO_2) - F_EO_2]}{1 - F_EO_2 - F_ECO_2} \right]$$

Application of the Calculation Concepts

In order to make the necessary calculations, of course, the values of the components on the right side of the equation must be known. Two components required for all of the conceptual equations are ventilatory volume and fractional concentration of expired oxygen. Two of the equations require the value for the fractional concentration of carbon dioxide in the expired air.

Calculation of the Ventilatory Volume ($\dot{V}_E$ or $\dot{V}_I$)

A nomogram (Figure 15.5) facilitates the calculation of oxygen consumption via the true O_2 concept. However, after inserting the nomogram's true O_2 value into Equation 15.1, the second part of the equation—ventilatory volume—must be

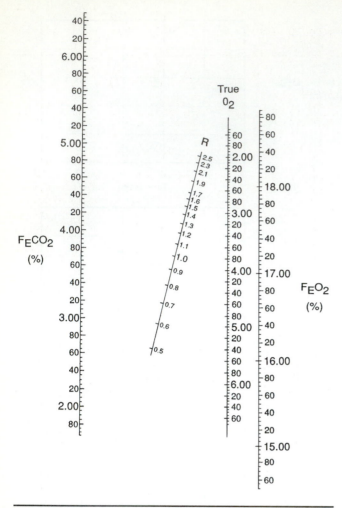

Figure 15.5 Nomogram for determination of R and true O_2 from the fractional concentrations of expired oxygen (F_EO_2) and carbon dioxide (F_ECO_2). Both the true O_2 and R may be found simultaneously by placing a straight-edge at the F_ECO_2 and F_EO_2 points of the outside vertical lines and then reading the R and true O_2 values on the inside lines. From Figure 1 on p. 134 of Dill, D. B., & Folling, A. (1928). Studies in muscular activity. II. A nomographic description as published in *Journal of Physiology, 66* and in Consolazio et al., 1963, p. 10. Copyright © 1963 The Physiological Society, Oxford.[31]

corrected for the effects of temperature (*T*), barometric pressure (P_B; mm Hg), saturation (S), and dryness (D). By convention, all ventilatory volumes used to express a *metabolic* amount (such as oxygen consumption) should be presented in *standard* terms.[24] The term *standard (S)* is used to refer to a dry (D) gas (e.g., oxygen) that is of a universally designated temperature (0 °C; 273 K) and pressure (760 mm Hg[a]; sea level). Thus, metabolic gases are expressed as STPD volumes.

---

[a]Although hectopascal is the International System's recognized unit of measure for environmental pressure, I am using millimeter of mercury (mm Hg) units because of the prevalence of the latter on mercury barometers and computerized instruments.

The volume of air the technician observes at the air volume meter is expressed first in terms of ambient (A) or environmental conditions, not STPD conditions because the air volume meter would not have a temperature at 0 °C and 0 % saturation. Thus, the ambient air volume (ATPS) is the volume of air under its measured environmental conditions. The specific letters in the abbreviation ATPS represent the following:

A = Ambient (environmental; laboratory; air meter)
T = Temperature of the expired or inspired air (°C); it is based on the thermometer reading at a specific site within the airflow circuit near or at the air meter. Some computerized systems use the midpoint between 37 °C and room air temperature.
P = Barometric pressure (P_B; mm Hg) in the laboratory.
S = Saturation; wet expiratory air; air in a wet spirometer is always 100 % saturated; the vapor pressure ($P-H_2O$; mm Hg) of inspiratory air is dependent upon relative humidity (RH) and temperature.

When the air is saturated, which is always the case with expired air from living organisms, it has a greater volume than when it is dry. Because scientific convention requires that all metabolic volumes be expressed in standard (thus, dry and freezing—0 °C) conditions, the volume must be converted to the smaller STPD volume. This universal volume then can be compared with other STPD volumes derived from tests undertaken at different meteorological conditions.

Correction Factors (cf) The ATPS volume may be converted to STPD by simply locating the correction factor (cf) in Table 15.5[19,56,66] or by calculating STPDcf by multiplying the correction factors for standard (S) air temperature (STcf) and air pressure dry (SPDcf) as in Equation 15.4.

$$STPDcf = STcf \times SPDcf \qquad Eq.\ 15.4$$

where:

$$STcf = \frac{273\ K}{273\ K + T_A}$$

$$SPDcf = \frac{P_B - P\text{-}H_2O\ at\ T_A}{760}$$

When the appropriate constant values for temperature (273 °K) and barometric pressure (760 mm Hg) are inserted into Equation 15.4 along with the measured values, the former equation now appears as Equation 15.5.

$$STPDcf = \frac{273\ K}{273\ K + T_A} \times \frac{P_B - P\text{-}H_2O\ at\ T_A}{760} \qquad Eq.\ 15.5$$

Although using Equation 15.5 is more complicated than using Table 15.5, once it is programmed into a calculator or computer the STPDcf is easily derived.

The kelvin scale is used for the **temperature** correction because of its absolute zero property—that is, no minus val-

Table 15.5 Correction Factors for Reducing ATPS Expiratory Volume (100% Saturated) to STPD (0 °C; 760 mm Hg) Volume

P_B mm Hg / T (°C)	16	17	18	19	20	21	22	23	24	25	26	27	28
740	0.900	.896	.892	.887	.883	.878	.874	.869	.864	.860	.855	.850	.845
742	.903	.898	.894	.890	.885	.881	.876	.871	.867	.862	.857	.852	.847
744	.906	.901	.897	.892	.888	.883	.878	.874	.869	.864	.859	.855	.850
746	.908	.903	.899	.895	.890	.886	.881	.876	.872	.867	.862	.857	.852
748	.910	.906	.901	.897	.892	.888	.883	.879	.874	.869	.864	.860	.854
750	.913	.908	.904	.900	.895	.890	.886	.881	.876	.872	.867	.862	.857
752	.915	.911	.906	.902	.897	.893	.888	.883	.879	.874	.869	.864	.859
754	.918	.913	.909	.904	.900	.895	.891	.886	.881	.876	.872	.867	.862
756	.920	.916	.911	.907	.902	.898	.893	.888	.883	.879	.874	.869	.864
758	.923	.918	.914	.909	.905	.900	.896	.891	.886	.881	.876	.872	.866
760	.925	.921	.916	.912	.907	.902	.898	.893	.888	.883	.879	.874	.869
762	.928	.923	.919	.914	.910	.905	.900	.896	.891	.886	.881	.876	.871
764	.930	.926	.921	.916	.912	.907	.903	.898	.893	.889	.884	.879	.874

Note: Slight differences occur among tables and equations due to rounding of temperatures and water vapor pressures.

ues. The STPD correction factor will never be a number greater than 1.0 at typical laboratory conditions because both the temperature and pressure parts of Equation 15.4 produce a fraction that, in turn, results in a ratio (correction factor) less than 1.0. Thus, the standard volume will always be less than the ambient volume under normal laboratory conditions. For example, under normal laboratory conditions, the temperature and humidity (P-H$_2$O) will be greater than 0 °C and 0 mm Hg (dry), respectively. When the STPDcf is known, the standard air volume can be found by multiplying the ATPS air volume by the STPD correction factor according to Equation 15.6.

$$\dot{V}_E \text{ or } \dot{V}_I \text{ (STPD)} = \text{STPDcf} \times \dot{V}_E \text{ or } \dot{V}_I \text{ (ATPS)} \quad \text{Eq. 15.6}$$

where:

$$\dot{V}_E \text{ or } \dot{V}_I \text{ (ATPS)} = \text{the measured volume of air (L·min}^{-1})$$

Air becomes saturated and warmed (or cooled if the ambient air temperature is > 37 °C) by being exposed to the lungs. The air in the lungs is 37 °C and 100 % saturated. This corresponds to a **water vapor pressure** of 47 mm Hg (P-H$_2$O). As the air is expelled under normal laboratory conditions, however, the air is condensed and cooled from a typical mouth temperature of about 33 °C to approximately 31 °C and 28 °C at the respiratory valve and unheated pneumotach or air volume meter, respectively.[50] This lower temperature decreases the amount of water vapor pressure in the expired air. The farther the thermometer is from the performer's mouth, the lower the exhaled air temperature, and consequently the P-H$_2$O, under normal laboratory conditions. Table 15.6 provides estimates of P-H$_2$O at various ambient temperatures; as the temperature increases at 100 % RH, the P-H$_2$O increases.

Inspired volumes rarely are 100 % saturated and thus do not exert water vapor pressures as high as those presented in Table 15.6.[20,62,82,83] By measuring the relative humidity (RH)

Table 15.6 Water Vapor Pressure (P-H$_2$O) at 100% Saturation at Given Temperatures (T)

°C	K	P-H$_2$O mm Hg	°C	K	P-H$_2$O mm Hg
20	293	18	31	304	34
21	294	19	32	305	36
22	295	20	33	306	38
23	296	21	34	307	40
24	297	22	35	308	42
25	298	24	36	309	45
26	299	25	37	310	47
27	300	27	38	311	50
28	301	28	39	312	52
29	302	30	40	313	55
30	303	32			

with a hygrometer or sling psychrometer, the pressure of water vapor (P-H$_2$O) for any given temperature may be found by using Equation 15.7 in conjunction with Table 15.6.

$$\text{P-H}_2\text{O (mm Hg)} = \text{RH \%} \times \text{P-H}_2\text{O at 100 \% RH} \quad \text{Eq. 15.7}$$

For example, Table 15.6 shows that an ambient temperature of 25 °C is equivalent to a water vapor pressure of 24 mm Hg. Because this table value represents 100 % saturation (RH), it must be corrected to the observed ambient relative humidity (e.g., 60 % RH) by using Equation 15.7. Thus, the water vapor pressure becomes 0.60 × 24 mm Hg = 14.4 mm Hg.

Minute (min) Volumes If the performer stops exercising before 30 s of air has been measured during the last starting minute of exercise, then only the preceding minute's volume should be used to calculate $\dot{V}O_2$max. If the performer stops between 30 s and 60 s, then the appropriate arithmetical

| Table 15.7 | Fractions (%) of Inspired (F_I) and Expired (F_E) Gases | |

Gas	Fractional Concentrations	
	Inspired	Expired at Exercise
Oxygen (O_2)	20.93	14.5–18.5
Carbon dioxide (CO_2)	0.03–0.04	2.5–5.5
Nitrogen (N_2)	79.03–79.04[a]	78.5–82.5

Note: [a]The nitrogen fraction includes rare gases such as argon.

adjustment should be made to account for a minute's worth of ventilation (e.g., double the volume based on 30 s value or multiply by 1.33 if based on 45 s value).

At rest, or during submaximal exercise when the respiratory exchange ratio (R) is less than 1.0, the inspired air volume is greater than the expired air volume. But during near maximal and maximal exercise when the R is greater than 1.0, then the expired air volume is greater than the inspired air volume. When R = 1.0 the two volumes are equal.

Fractions of Inspired and Expired Gases

One must know the fractional concentration of three gases in order to calculate oxygen consumption. The major gases are oxygen, carbon dioxide, and nitrogen (Table 15.7). All other gases (e.g., helium and argon) are either inert or insignificant for calculating oxygen consumption. An inert gas does not enter into biological metabolism. One of the three major components of the environmental air, nitrogen, is an inert gas.

The fractional concentrations of the expired gases (F_EO_2 or F_ECO_2) are expressed as percentages or decimals. Expired nitrogen concentration (dry) may be calculated from Equation 15.8.[29]

$$F_EN_2 = 1.0 - F_EO_2 - F_ECO_2 \qquad \text{Eq. 15.8}$$

Expired concentrations of oxygen and carbon dioxide are dependent upon the intensity of exercise. Expected fractional concentrations of expired gases in exercising persons may range according to those illustrated in Figure 15.4 or listed in Table 15.7. For example, if the F_EO_2 is 16 % (0.16) and the F_ECO_2 is 5.0 % (0.05), then, by substitution, Equation 15.8 becomes

$$F_EN_2 = 1.0 - 0.16 - 0.05 = 0.79$$

The exact amount of oxygen extracted from the volume of air ($\dot{V}_E$ or $\dot{V}_I$) cannot be calculated directly by multiplying this minute volume (L·min^{-1}) by the fractional concentration of oxygen unless the respiratory exchange ratio is equal to 1.0. This is because the volume of oxygen consumed is dependent not only upon the fractional concentration of the expired oxygen but also upon the fractional concentration of expired carbon dioxide. Consequently, when F_ECO_2 is included in the calculation of oxygen consumption, the term used to represent the true amount of oxygen extracted is called the true O_2. The true O_2 can be calculated from Equation 15.1 or from the nomogram in Figure 15.5.

Respiratory Exchange Ratio

True O_2 is dependent upon the ratio of carbon dioxide produced to oxygen consumed. The $\dot{V}CO_2$:$\dot{V}O_2$ ratio is called the respiratory exchange ratio (R), although it has sometimes been referred to as the respiratory quotient (RQ). However, R should be reserved for respiratory purposes while RQ should be used for nutritional or dietary considerations.

As exercise intensifies, the R value increases due to the release of greater quantities of carbon dioxide from the buffering of lactic acid. The R may change from a typical resting value of 0.83[35] to typical maximal exercise values between 1.0 and 1.25; values at supramaximal exercise may reach as high as 1.3 and, during recovery, lower than 0.7.[47] The R is often used as a criterion to indicate the achievement of true maximal oxygen consumption. When the R is 1.0, it means that the production of carbon dioxide ($\dot{V}CO_2$) is equivalent to the consumption of oxygen ($\dot{V}O_2$). The respiratory exchange ratio is calculated either from a nomogram (Figure 15.5) using the F_EO_2 and F_ECO_2 values or from the STPD volumes of carbon dioxide and oxygen (Eq. 15.9).

$$R = \dot{V}CO_2 / \dot{V}O_2 \qquad \text{Eq. 15.9}$$

For example, if the volume of carbon dioxide produced is 3.5 L·min^{-1} and the consumption of oxygen is 3.5 L·min^{-1}, then the respiratory exchange ratio is calculated as follows:

$$R = 3.5 \div 3.5 = 1.0$$

Although the *percent* of carbon dioxide is necessary to calculate oxygen consumption, it is not necessary to know the *volume* of carbon dioxide to calcute $\dot{V}O_2$. Its volume may be calculated easily from Equation 15.10.

$$\dot{V}CO_2 \, (\text{L·min}^{-1})\text{STPD} = \dot{V}_E \times (F_ECO_2 - F_ICO_2) \quad \text{Eq. 15.10}$$

For example, if expired ventilation STPD is 100 L·min^{-1} and F_ECO_2 is 5.0 % and F_ICO_2 is .03 %, then

$$\dot{V}CO_2 = 100 \times (5.0 \% - 0.03 \%)$$
$$= 100 \times 4.97 \% = 4.97 \text{ L·min}^{-1}$$

After calculating the volume of carbon dioxide produced by using Equation 15.10, the respiratory exchange ratio may be calculated from Equation 15.9 as soon as the volume of oxygen consumed is known, or simply from the nomogram (Figure 15.5) when the F_ECO_2 and F_EO_2 are known. For example, if the $\dot{V}CO_2$ is 4.97 and the $\dot{V}O_2$ is 4.93, then solving for Equation 15.9 is as follows:

$$R = \dot{V}CO_2 / \dot{V}O_2 = 4.97 \div 4.93 = 1.01$$

Interaction of Ventilatory Volume and Gas Concentrations

The volumes of inspired and expired air differ from each other at rest and throughout most stages of exercise intensity. Because maximal oxygen consumption can be measured using either the inspired and expired volumes alone or together, all three methods are explained here. The inspired or expired[29,85] air volumes may be calculated from the known value of the other by using Equations 15.11 and 15.12, respectively.

$$\dot{V}_I = \dot{V}_E \times (F_E N_2 \div F_I N_2)$$
$$= \dot{V}_E \times [(1.0 - F_E O_2 - F_E CO_2) \div 0.7904] \quad \text{Eq. 15.11}$$

where:

$$F_I N_2 = 79.04\ \%$$
$$\dot{V}_E = \dot{V}_I \times (F_I N_2 / F_E N_2)$$
$$= \dot{V}_I \times (0.79 / F_E N_2) \quad \text{Eq. 15.12}$$

Expired Air Volume   The concentrations of the inspired gases are essentially constant. Thus, when using expired ventilation to calculate oxygen consumption, Equation 15.13 may be used.

$$\dot{V}O_2 = \dot{V}_E \times \left[(F_E N_2 / F_I N_2) \times (F_I O_2 - F_E O_2) \right]$$
$$= \dot{V}_E \times \left[\frac{(1.0 - F_E O_2 - F_E CO_2)}{0.79} \times (0.209 - F_E O_2) \right]$$

$$\text{Eq. 15.13}$$

Both Expired and Inspired Air Volumes   If both volumes of inspired and expired air were measured, then carbon dioxide need not be measured or calculated;[80] thus, oxygen consumption is calculated according to the conceptual Equation 15.2[54] presented earlier as

$$\dot{V}O_2 = (\dot{V}_I \times F_I O_2) - (\dot{V}_E \times F_E O_2)$$

where:

$$F_I O_2 = 20.93\ \% \ (0.2093)$$

Inspired Air Volume   If only the inspired volume is measured, oxygen consumption can be calculated from Equation 15.14[54] or simply by converting the $\dot{V}_I$ to $\dot{V}_E$ by Equation 15.12 and then using the nomogram (Figure 15.5) to find true O_2 % or by using Equation 15.13.

$$\dot{V}O_2 = \dot{V}_I \times \left[F_I O_2 - \left(\frac{F_I N_2}{F_E N_2} \times F_I O_2 \right) \right]$$
$$\text{Eq. 15.14}$$

Calculating Relative Maximal Oxygen Consumption

When other factors are equal, larger persons (especially those with larger muscle mass) will have higher maximal oxygen consumptions. It is often appropriate to convert the absolute value of liters per minute to milliliters per minute (Eq. 15.15); this is then divided by body mass (BM) in order to derive the *relative* value, which is expressed in units of $mL \cdot kg^{-1} \cdot min^{-1}$ (Eq. 15.16). Sometimes the absolute value is divided by the lean body mass if the latter is known.

$$\dot{V}O_2 max\ (mL \cdot min^{-1}) = 1000 \times L \cdot min^{-1} \quad \text{Eq. 15.15}$$

$$\text{relative } \dot{V}O_2 max\ (mL \cdot kg^{-1} \cdot min^{-1}) \quad \text{Eq. 15.16}$$
$$= (mL \cdot min^{-1}) \div kg\ BM$$

For example, if a person weighing 65 kg has a maximal oxygen consumption of 4.0 $L \cdot min^{-1}$, then the following calculations would give the relative maximal oxygen consumption:

$$mL \cdot min^{-1} = 1000 \times 4.0\ L \cdot min^{-1} = 4000$$

$$mL \cdot kg^{-1} \cdot min^{-1} = 4000\ mL \cdot kg^{-1} \cdot min^{-1} \div 65\ kg = 61.5$$

Calculating MET Values

MET is the term used to denote the multiple of the resting oxygen consumption. Ideally, the directly measured resting oxygen consumption should be used instead of the generic "3.5." The generic maximal MET (METmax) is calculated from Equation 15.17 by simply dividing the relative maximal oxygen consumption by the assumed resting value of 3.5 $mL \cdot kg^{-1} \cdot min^{-1}$.[3]

$$\text{METmax} = \text{relative } \dot{V}O_2 max \div 3.5 \quad \text{Eq. 15.17}$$

Thus, using the relative maximal oxygen consumption from the previous example, the calculation appears as

$$\text{METmax} = 61.5\ mL \cdot kg^{-1} \cdot min^{-1} \div 3.5 = 17.6$$

Although the example used the maximal $\dot{V}O_2$ to obtain the maximal MET, any of the submaximal $\dot{V}O_2$ can be used to derive the submaximal MET values.

Ventilatory Threshold/Breakpoint ("Anaerobic Threshold")

The approximate ventilatory breakpoint occurs at the lowest point of a line, just before it rises, on a graph describing the relationship between ventilation and oxygen consumption ($\dot{V}_E$ vs. $\dot{V}O_2$). It is sometimes referred to as the "anaerobic threshold,"[82] but not without controversy. Although computer programs can select the ventilatory breakpoint by plotting the change in linearity between $\dot{V}O_2$ and $\dot{V}_E$, it can be estimated by plotting the points on a graph and noting the point where the line changes slope.

Summary of the Calculation of Maximal Oxygen Consumption

Although the numerous equations presented appear to be quite formidable, the tables and nomogram simplify the calculation of oxygen consumption. The summarized steps and examples for calculating $\dot{V}O_2 max$ with and without the nomogram and using inspired or expired ventilatory volumes are presented.

Nomogram Method When Measuring Expired Air Volume

1. Record the correction factors (cf) for STPD volumes by
    a. consulting Table 15.5 or

b. calculating STPDcf from Eq. 15.5 in conjunction with Table 15.6 (P-H_2O vs. T).

2. Convert the volume of air ($\dot{V}_E$) from ATPS to STPD by using Equation 15.6.

3. Determine the R and true O_2 values by placing a straight-edge on the two vertical lines denoting fractions of expired gases and reading the answers on the diagonal R line and vertical true O_2 line of the nomogram (Figure 15.5).

4. Insert the values found in Steps #2 ($\dot{V}_E$ STPD) and #3 (true O_2) into Equation 15.1.
   For example, if $\dot{V}_E$ is 100 L·min^{-1} and true O_2 is 4.0 %, then

   $$\dot{V}O_2 = \dot{V}_E \text{ STPD} \times \text{true } O_2$$

   $$= 100 \text{ L·min}^{-1} \text{ (STPD)} \times 4.0 \text{ % (or 0.04)}$$

   $$= 4.0 \text{ L·min}^{-1}$$

5. Convert L·min^{-1} to mL·min^{-1} by multiplying L·min^{-1} by 1000 (Equation 15.15).

6. Convert mL·min^{-1} to relative $\dot{V}O_2$max (mL·kg^{-1}·min^{-1}) by dividing mL·min^{-1} by body mass (Equation 15.16).

7. Calculate MET value by dividing mL·kg^{-1}·min^{-1} by 3.5 (Equation 15.17).

Example of Nomogram Method
When Measuring Expired Air Volume

```
Given Conditions:

Performer's body mass: 70 kg
V̇E ATPS = 100 L·min⁻¹
Saturation (RH) = 100 %
T = 25.0 °C
PB = 751 mm Hg
FEO₂ = 16.20 %; FECO₂ = 5.00 %
```

1. Convert the volume of expired air from ATPS to STPD (Equation 15.5):

   $$\dot{V}_E \text{ STPD} = 100 \text{ L·min}^{-1} \text{ ATPS} \times \text{STPDcf}$$

   $$= 100 \times [273 / (273 + 25)] \times [(751 - 24) / 760]$$

   $$= 100 \times (273 / 298) \times (727 / 760)$$

   $$= 100 \times (0.916 \times 0.956)$$

   $$= 100 \times 0.876^b \text{ (slightly > 0.873 from Table 15.5)}$$

   $$= 87.6 \text{ L·min}^{-1} \text{ STPD}$$

2. The R and true O_2 values from the nomogram (Figure 15.5) are

   R = 1.08 (but not needed for the $\dot{V}O_2$ max calculation)

   True O_2 = 4.65 % (0.0465)

---

[b]Agrees with table in Wasserman et al., 1994, p. 469.[82]

3. The volume of oxygen consumed (STPD) calculated from Equation 15.1 is

   $$\dot{V}O_2\text{STPD} = 87.6 \text{ L·min}^{-1} \times 0.0465$$

   $$= 4.073 \text{ L·min}^{-1}$$

4. The value of 4.073 L·min^{-1} converted to mL·min^{-1} is

   $$4.073 \text{ L·min}^{-1} \times 1000 = 4073 \text{ mL·min}^{-1}$$

5. The relative value is

   $$4073 \div 70 \text{ kg} = 58.2 \text{ mL·kg}^{-1}\text{·min}^{-1}$$

6. The generic MET value is

   $$58.2 \div 3.5 \text{ mL·kg}^{-1}\text{·min}^{-1} = 16.6$$

Nomogram Method When Measuring Inspired Air Volume

1. Convert the volume of inspired air from ATPS to STPD by using Table 15.6 (P-H_2O vs. T) and Equation 15.7 (RH %), along with Equations 15.5 (STPD) and 15.6.

2. Convert the STPD inspired volume to an expired volume by using Equation 15.12.

3. Then follow the same Steps #2 through #5 as used for expired air.

Example of Nomogram Method
When Measuring Inspired Air Volume

```
Given Conditions:

Performer's body mass: 70 kg
V̇IATPS = 100 L·min⁻¹
Saturation (RH) = 40 %
T = 25.0 °C
PB = 751 mm Hg
FEO₂ = 16.50 %; FECO₂ = 4.50 %
```

1. The volume of inspired air is converted from ATPS to STPD:

   $$\dot{V}_I\text{STPD} = 100 \text{ L·min}^{-1} \times \text{STPDcf}$$

   a. Find P-H_2O at 100 % RH (Table 15.6) and convert to 40 % RH:

   P-H_2O (mm Hg at 40 % RH) = 40 % RH × 24 (Table 15.6)

   $$= 9.6 \text{ mm Hg or rounded off to 10 mm Hg}$$

   b. Now the pressure and temperature are inserted into Equation 15.5:

   $$\dot{V}_I \text{ STPDcf} = \frac{273 \text{ K}}{273 \text{ K} + 25 \text{ °C}} \times \frac{751 - 10}{760}$$

   $$= (273 / 298) \times (741 / 760)$$

   $$= 0.916 \times 0.975 = 0.893$$

c. Thus,

$$\dot{V}_I \text{ STPD} = 100 \text{ L·min}^{-1} \times 0.893$$

$$= 89.3 \text{ L·min}^{-1}$$

2. Convert the $\dot{V}_I$ STPD value to $\dot{V}_E$ STPD by using Equation 15.12

$$\dot{V}_E \text{ STPD} = 89.3 \times [0.79 \div (1.0 - 0.1650 - 0.0450)]$$

$$= 89.3 \times (0.79 \div 0.79)$$

$$= 89.3 \times 1.0$$

$$= 89.3 \text{ L·min}^{-1}$$

3. Now follow same Steps #2 through #6 as for expired volume.

4. Obtain the R and true O_2 values from the nomogram (Figure 15.5):

$$R = 1.0 \text{ (but not needed for the } \dot{V}O_2\text{max calculation)}$$

True O_2 = 4.50 % (when R = 1.0, the F_EO_2 %
= true O_2 %, and $\dot{V}_I = \dot{V}_E$)

5. The volume of oxygen consumed (STPD) found from Equation 15.1 is

$$\dot{V}O_2\text{STPD} = 89.3 \text{ L·min}^{-1} \times 0.0450$$

$$= 4.019 \text{ L·min}^{-1}$$

6. The value of 4.019 L·min^{-1} converted to mL·min^{-1} is

$$4.019 \text{ L·min}^{-1} \times 1000 = 4019 \text{ mL·min}^{-1}$$

7. The relative value is

$$4019 \div 70 \text{ kg} = 57.4 \text{ mL·kg}^{-1}\text{·min}^{-1}$$

8. The generic MET value is

$$57.4 \div 3.5 \text{ mL·kg}^{-1}\text{·min}^{-1} = 16.4$$

Non-Nomogram Method When Measuring Expired Air Volume

1. Same as Step #1 for nomogram method when measuring expired air: Convert the volume of expired air to STPD from Table 15.5, or use Equations 15.5 and 15.6 in conjunction with Table 15.6.
2. Find oxygen consumption (L·min^{-1}) using Equation 15.13.
3. Follow same Steps #4 through #6 as nomogram method when expired air was measured: Convert the L·min^{-1} value to mL·min^{-1} by multiplying the L·min^{-1} by 1000 (Equation 15.15).
4. Find the relative $\dot{V}O_2$max by dividing the mL·min^{-1} value by the body mass (kg) of the performer (Eq. 15.16).
5. Find the generic MET value by dividing mL·kg^{-1}·min^{-1} by 3.5 (Eq. 15.17).

Example of Non-Nomogram Method
When Measuring Expired Air Volume

Given Conditions:

Same as for nomogram method for expired air volume:
70 kg; 100 L·min^{-1}; 25 °C; 100 % saturation; 751 mm Hg;
F_EO_2 = 16.20 %; F_ECO_2 = 5.00 %

1. Same as Step #1 for nomogram method when measuring expired air: The volume of expired air is converted from ATPS to STPD:

$$\dot{V}_E \text{ STPD} = 100 \text{ L·min}^{-1} \text{ ATPS} \times \text{STPDcf}$$

$$= 100 \text{ L·min}^{-1} \text{ ATPS} \times 0.876 \text{ (or 0.873)}$$

$$= 87.6 \text{ L·min}^{-1}$$

2. Find $\dot{V}O_2$max by inserting the appropriate conditions into Eq. 15.13:

$$\dot{V}O_2 = 87.6 \times \frac{1 - 0.1620 - 0.0500}{0.7904} \times (0.2093 - 0.1620)$$

$$= 87.6 \times [(0.788 / 0.7904) \times (0.0473)]$$

$$= 87.6 \times (0.997 \times 0.0473)$$

$$= 87.6 \times 0.0472$$

$$= 4.134 \text{ L·min}^{-1} \text{ (slight difference from nomogram method [4.073] due to imprecise reading of nomogram and rounding off)}$$

3. The value of 4.134 L·min^{-1} converted to mL·min^{-1} is (Eq. 15.15)

$$4.134 \text{ L·min}^{-1} \times 1000 = 4134 \text{ mL·min}^{-1}$$

4. The relative $\dot{V}O_2$max is (Eq. 15.16)

$$4134 \div 70 \text{ kg} = 59.1 \text{ mL·kg}^{-1}\text{·min}^{-1}$$

5. The generic METmax value is (Eq. 15.17)

$$59.1 \text{ mL·kg}^{-1}\text{·min}^{-1} \div 3.5 = 16.9$$

Non-Nomogram Method When Measuring Inspired Volume

1. Same as nomogram method for inspired air: Convert the volume of inspired air from ATPS to STPD by using Table 15.6 (P-H_2O vs. *T*) in conjunction with Equation 15.7 (RH %), along with Equations 15.5 ($\dot{V}_I$) and 15.6 (STPD).
2. Calculate $\dot{V}O_2$ by inserting the inspired STPD volume into Equation 15.3.
3. Follow the same last three steps as for the other methods:
   a. Convert L·min^{-1} to mL·min^{-1} by multiplying L·min^{-1} by 1000 (Eq. 15.15).

b. Find the relative $\dot{V}O_2$max by dividing mL·min^{-1} by body mass (Eq. 15.16).

c. Find generic MET value by dividing mL·kg^{-1}·min^{-1} by 3.5 (Eq. 15.17).

Example of Non-Nomogram Method When Measuring Inspired Air Volume

Given Conditions:

Same as for nomogram inspired air volume:
70 kg; V_I ATPS = 100 L·min^{-1}; RH = 40 %; T = 25.0 °C; P_B = 751 mm Hg; F_EO_2 = 16.50 %; F_ECO_2 = 4.50 %

1. Follow the same Step #1 as the nomogram method measuring the inspired air to convert 100 L·min^{-1} ATPS to 89.3 STPD.

2. Insert appropriate values into Equation 15.3:

$$\dot{V}O_2 (L\cdot min^{-1})$$

$$= 89.3 \times \left\{ \frac{[0.2093 \times (1 - 0.045) - 0.165]}{1 - 0.1650 - 0.0450} \right\}$$

$$= 89.3 \times \{[(0.2093 \times 0.955) - 0.1650] / 0.79\}$$

$$= 89.3 \times [(0.1999 - 0.1650) / 0.79]$$

$$= 89.3 \times 0.0349 / 0.79$$

$$= 89.3 \times 0.0442$$

$$= 3.947 \text{ L·min}^{-1} \text{ (slight difference from nomogram method)}$$

or (a) change $\dot{V}_I$ to $\dot{V}_E$ (Eq. 15.12) and (b) solve for $\dot{V}O_2$ with $\dot{V}_E$ (Eq. 15.13)

a. $\dot{V}_E = 89.3 \text{ L·min}^{-1} \times \dfrac{0.79}{1 - 0.1650 - 0.0450}$

$$= 89.3 \text{ L·min}^{-1} \times (0.79 / 0.79)$$

$$= 89.3 \text{ L·min}^{-1} \text{ (when R = 1.0, then } \dot{V}_I = \dot{V}_E)$$

b. Follow Step #2 of *expired* non-nomogram method:

$$\dot{V}O_2 = 89.3 \times$$

$$\left[\left(\frac{1 - 0.1650 - 0.0450}{0.790} \right) \times (0.2093 - 0.1650) \right]$$

$$= 89.3 \times [(0.79 / 0.790) \times (0.2093 - 0.165)]$$

$$= 89.3 \times (1.0 \times 0.0443)$$

$$= 89.3 \times 0.0443$$

$$= 3.956 \text{ L·min}^{-1} \text{ (slight difference from first method due to rounding off)}$$

3. Convert L·min^{-1} to mL·min (Eq. 15.15):

$$1000 \times 3.956 = 3956 \text{ mL·min}^{-1}$$

4. Relative $\dot{V}O_2$max (Eq. 15.16):

$$\dot{V}O_2\text{max (mL·kg}^{-1}\cdot\text{min}^{-1}) = 3956 \div 70 \text{ kg} = 56.5$$

5. Generic METmax (Eq. 15.17):

$$\text{METmax} = 56.5 \text{ mL·kg}^{-1}\cdot\text{min}^{-1} \div 3.5 = 16.1$$

Results and Discussion

Earlier investigators and reviewers[57,71,78] supported the maximal oxygen consumption as probably the best single physiological indicator of a person's capacity for maintaining endurance-type activity. This contrasts with one authority who questions the interpretation of maximal oxygen consumption[27] and with those who caution that other factors such as running economy[28] and the ability to use a high percent of the maximal oxygen consumption (fractional utilization)[26] and ventilatory threshold[81] also are important indicators of success in aerobic performance. For example, two investigators[53] reported a higher correlation ($r = -.86$) between fractional utilization of $\dot{V}O_2$max and 1.5 mi time than between $\dot{V}O_2$max and 1.5 mi time ($r = -.74$). A high relative $\dot{V}O_2$max reflects the ability to sustain a high percentage of $\dot{V}O_2$max during an aerobic activity. In fact, $\dot{V}O_2$max has been shown to be an ineffective discriminator of aerobic endurance time among persons with fairly similar maximal oxygen consumptions.[26]

In general, maximal oxygen consumption is higher in men than in women, in younger adults than in older adults, and in aerobically conditioned persons than in untrained persons.

$\dot{V}O_2$max on Treadmill Versus Cycling, Stepping, and Arm Ergometry

Typically, treadmill protocols elicit maximal oxygen consumptions that are from 5 % to 8 %,[30] or 10 %,[43] or 14 %,[45] or even up to 25 %[69] higher than $\dot{V}O_2$max elicited by cycle protocols.[c] The variability is dependent upon the specificity of training by the performer. Due to the "principle of the specificity of training," however, trained cyclists may achieve similar values on treadmill and cycle protocols. Maximal oxygen consumption values during certain step-test protocols appear to compare favorably ($r = .95$) with those during treadmill protocols.[48] Arm ergometry produces about 20 % to 30 % lower $\dot{V}O_2$max values than treadmill ergometry.[36] Again, this would depend on specificity of training and, in this case, arm strength.

---

[c] D. B. Dill ("father" of exercise physiology in the United States) had 20 % higher maximal oxygen consumptions on his treadmill tests than on his cycle tests.[45]

Norms for $\dot{V}O_2max$

Cycling Norms

Some popular norm tables were derived mainly by performers using cycle ergometers.[4,7,14] Therefore, in order to make valid comparisons, the values of performers tested on treadmills should be adjusted downward by $\approx 10\%$ depending upon the performer's training status and leg strength.

Generic Norms

Adjustments for treadmill testing are not necessary if using the norms (Figures 15.6 through 15.9) compiled from 62 studies of apparently healthy but untrained men and women ages 6 y to 75 y from the United States, Canada, and seven European countries.[76] The norms are based on directly measured maximal oxygen consumption tests from treadmill, cycle, and stepping ergometry. They are similar to the norms published in *ACSM's Guidelines* (2000)[3] based upon the Aerobics Research Institute's Balke treadmill tests.

The graphic norms show that the **absolute $\dot{V}O_2max$ ($L \cdot min^{-1}$)** increases in male youths from about 1.0 $L \cdot min^{-1}$ at age 6 y to over 3.0 $L \cdot min^{-1}$ at age 18 y (Figure 15.7). The men then decline to about 1.5 $L \cdot min^{-1}$ by age 75 y. The females follow a similar trend by increasing initially from about 0.8 $L \cdot min^{-1}$ at age 6 y to about 2.2 at age 18 y, then by decreasing to about 1.0 $L \cdot min^{-1}$ by age 75 y (Figure 15.9).

Relative $\dot{V}O_2max$ ($mL \cdot kg^{-1} \cdot min^{-1}$) shows smaller differences between the sexes and not nearly as great an increase during youth than that of absolute maximal oxygen consumption. The relative $\dot{V}O_2max$ decreases in males (Figure 15.6) from about 50 $mL \cdot kg^{-1} \cdot min^{-1}$ during late adolescence to about 25 $mL \cdot kg^{-1} \cdot min^{-1}$ in 75-year-old persons; females decrease from about 40 $mL \cdot kg^{-1} \cdot min^{-1}$ in early adolescence to about 17 "mL's" at age 75 y.

The seven **fitness categories** depicted in Figures 15.6 through 15.9 represent the following percentages of the sample population based on the means and standard deviations:

Very poor and excellent = 3 % each
Poor and very good = 8 % each
Fair and good = 22 % each
Average = 34 %

For example, Figure 15.6 shows that an excellent rating is warranted for all adult males age 26 y if their relative maximal oxygen consumption is 60 $mL \cdot kg^{-1} \cdot min^{-1}$. Figure 15.8

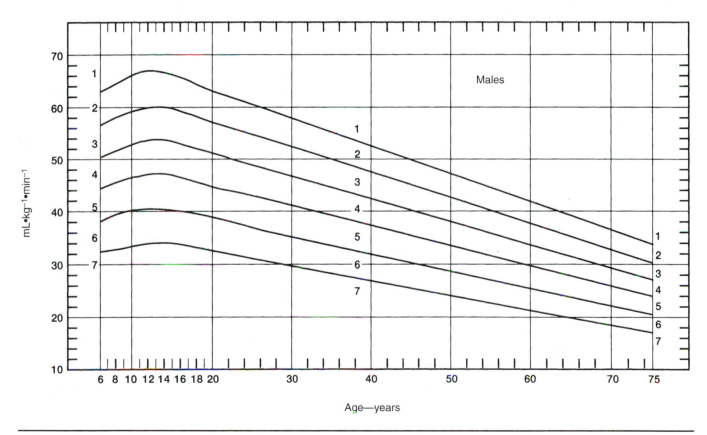

Figure 15.6 The relative maximal oxygen consumption ($mL \cdot kg^{-1} \cdot min^{-1}$) in **males** aged 6 y to 75 y. 1 = excellent; 2 = very good; 3 = good; 4 = average; 5 = fair; 6 = poor; 7 = very poor. From E. Shvartz and R. C. Reibold, "Aerobic Fitness Norms for Males and Females. . . ," in *Aviation Space, and Environmental Medicine, 61,* 3–11, 1990. Copyright © Aerospace Medical Association, Alexandria, VA.[76]

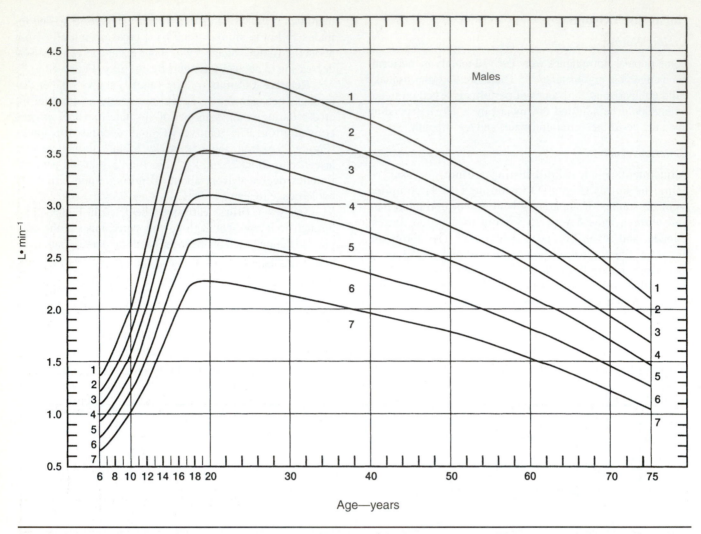

Figure 15.7 The absolute maximal oxygen consumption (L·min⁻¹) in **males** aged 6 y to 75 y. 1 = excellent; 2 = very good; 3 = good; 4 = average; 5 = fair; 6 = poor; 7 = very poor. From E. Shvartz and R. C. Reibold, "Aerobic Fitness Norms for Males and Females. . . ," in *Aviation Space, and Environmental Medicine, 61,* 3–11, 1990. Copyright © Aerospace Medical Association, Alexandria, VA.[76]

shows that women at age 26 y obtain an excellent rating if reaching 50 mL·kg⁻¹·min⁻¹.

Direct measurements of maximal oxygen consumption in large numbers of older adults is rare. Table 15.8, however, includes norms from nearly 300 men and women between the ages of 55 y and 86 y.[63] The linear decrease in relative maximal oxygen consumption was 0.31 mL·kg⁻¹·min⁻¹·y⁻¹ in men and 0.25 mL·kg⁻¹·min⁻¹·y⁻¹ in women. The investigators stated that their men needed at least a $\dot{V}O_2$max of 17.7 mL·kg⁻¹·min⁻¹ and their women at least 15.4 mL·kg⁻¹·min⁻¹ to cope with the daily activities of independent living.

Comparison of Predicted and Direct $\dot{V}O_2$max The results of the Maximal Oxygen Consumption Test can be compared with those from previous predictive tests (Form 15.6). It would be interesting to see which predictive test came the closest to predicting the actual $\dot{V}O_2$max for those students who performed the direct test. Conclusions would be tentative if only a few students performed the direct test.

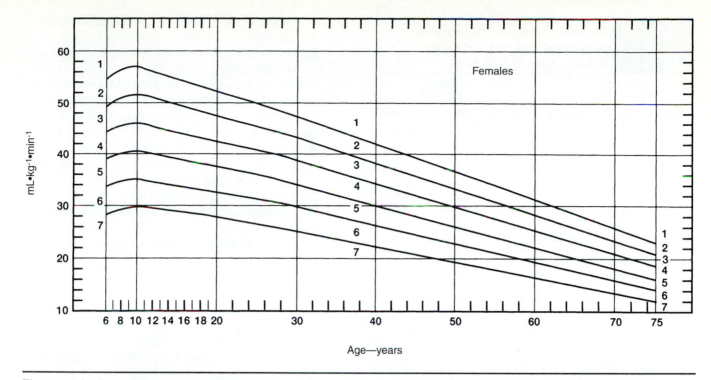

Figure 15.8 The relative maximal oxygen consumption ($mL \cdot kg^{-1} \cdot min^{-1}$) in **females** aged 6 y to 75 y. 1 = excellent; 2 = very good; 3 = good; 4 = average; 5 = fair; 6 = poor; 7 = very poor. From E. Shvartz and R. C. Reibold, "Aerobic Fitness Norms for Males and Females. . . ," in *Aviation Space, and Environmental Medicine, 61,* 3–11, 1990. Copyright © Aerospace Medical Association, Alexandria, VA.[76]

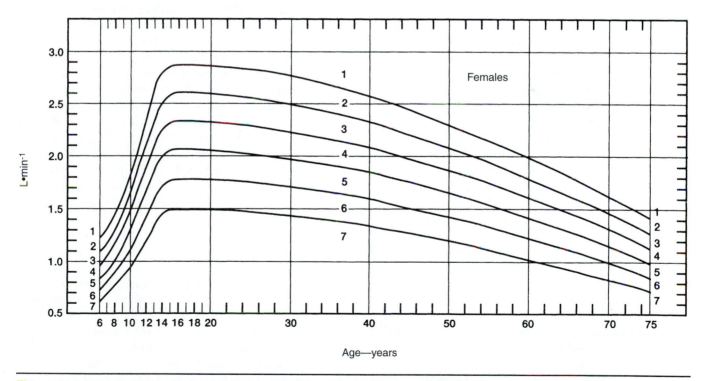

Figure 15.9 The absolute maximal oxygen consumption ($L \cdot min^{-1}$) in **females** aged 6 y to 75 y. 1 = excellent; 2 = very good; 3 = good; 4 = average; 5 = fair; 6 = poor; 7 = very poor. From E. Shvartz and R. C. Reibold, "Aerobic Fitness Norms for Males and Females. . . ," in *Aviation Space, and Environmental Medicine, 61,* 3–11, 1990. Copyright © Aerospace Medical Association, Alexandria, VA.[76]

Table 15.8 Maximal Oxygen Consumption of Noninstitutionalized Older Adults, Ages 55 y to 86 y

Age y	$\dot{V}O_2max$ mL·kg⁻¹·min⁻¹ Men	Women	Age y	$\dot{V}O_2max$ mL·kg⁻¹·min⁻¹ Men	Women
55	27.18	22.88	71	22.22	18.88
56	26.87	22.63	72	21.91	18.63
57	26.56	22.38	73	21.60	18.38
58	26.25	22.13	74	21.29	18.13
59	25.94	21.88	75	20.98	17.88
60	25.63	21.63	76	20.67	17.63
61	25.32	21.38	77	20.36	17.38
62	25.01	21.13	78	20.05	17.13
63	24.70	20.88	79	19.74	16.88
64	24.39	20.63	80	19.43	16.63
65	24.08	20.38	81	19.12	16.38
66	23.77	20.13	82	18.81	16.13
67	23.46	19.88	83	18.19	15.88
68	23.15	19.63	84	18.19	15.63
69	22.84	19.38	85	17.88	15.38
70	22.53	19.13	86	17.57	15.13

Table derived from linear regressions of Paterson, D. H., Cunningham, D. A., Koval, J. J., & St. Croix, C. M. (1999). Aerobic fitness in a population of independently living men and women aged 55–86 years. *Medicine and Science in Sports and Exercise, 31,* 1813–1820.[3]
Note: Linear regression equations: Men—$\dot{V}O_2max$ (mL·kg⁻¹·min⁻¹) = $(-0.31 \times age) + 44.23$ (SEE = 4.45); Women—$\dot{V}O_2max = (-0.25 \times age) + 36.63$ (SEE = 3.42).

References

1. Alexander, J. F., Liang, M. T. C., Stull, G. A., Serfass, R. C., Wolfe, D. R., & Ewing, J. L. (1984). A comparison of the Bruce and Liang equations for predicting $\dot{V}O_2max$ in young adult males. *Research Quarterly for Exercise and Sport, 55,* 383–387.

2. Allen, T. E., Hatcher, P. G., Lewis, J. B., Adams, F. S., & Brown, P. M. (1988). Standing and seated bicycle ergometry for elicitation of maximum oxygen uptake in women. *Medicine and Science in Sports and Exercise, 20* (Suppl.), Abstract #100, S17.

3. American College of Sports Medicine. 2000. *ACSM's guidelines for exercise testing and prescription.* Philadelphia: Lippincott Williams & Wilkins.

4. American Heart Association Committee on Exercise. (1972). *Exercise testing and training in apparently healthy individuals: A handbook for physicians.* New York: Author.

5. American Thoracic Society. (1987). Standardization of spirometry—1987 update. *American Review of Respiratory Diseases, 136,* 1285–1298.

6. Andersen, K. L., Shephard, R. J., Denolin, H., Varnauskas, E., & Masironi, R. (Eds.). (1971). *Fundamentals of exercise testing.* Geneva, Switzerland: World Health Organization.

7. Åstrand, P.-O., & Ryhming, I. (1954). A nomogram for calculation of aerobic capacity (physical fitness) from pulse rate during submaximal work. *Journal of Applied Physiology, 7,* 218–221.

8. Bar-Or, O., & Zwiren, L. D. (1975). Maximal oxygen consumption test during exercise—Reliability and validity. *Journal of Applied Physiology, 38,* 424–426.

9. Bassett, D. R., Giese, M. D., Nagle, F. J., Ward, A., Raab, D. M., & Balke, B. (1985). Aerobic requirements of overground versus treadmill running. *Medicine and Science in Sports and Exercise, 17,* 477–481.

10. Baumgartner, T. A., & Jackson, A. S. (1987). *Measurement for evaluation in physical education and exercise science.* Dubuque, IA: Wm. C. Brown.

11. Blair, S. N., Kohl, H. W., Paffenbarger, R. S., Clark, D. G., Cooper, K. H., & Gibbons, L. W. (1989). Physical fitness and all-cause mortality. *JAMA, 262,* 2395–2401.

12. Brooks, G. A., & Fahey, T. D. (1984). *Exercise physiology: Human bioenergetics and its application.* New York: John Wiley & Sons.

13. Brooks, G. A., & Fahey, T. D. (1987). *Fundamentals of human performance.* New York: Macmillan.

14. Bruce, R. A. (1972). Multi-stage treadmill test of submaximal and maximal exercise. In American Heart Association's Committee on Exercise (Ed.), *Exercise testing and training of apparently healthy individuals: A handbook for physicians* (pp. 32–34). New York: American Heart Association.

15. Bruce, R. A. (1974). Methods of exercise testing. *The American Journal of Cardiology, 33,* 715–720.

16. Bruce, R. A., Kusumi, F., & Hosmer, D. (1973). Maximal oxygen intake and nomographic assessment of functional impairment in cardiovascular disease. *American Heart Journal, 85,* 546–562.

17. Bruce, R. A., & McDonough, J. R. (1969). Stress testing in screening for cardiovascular disease. *Bulletin of New York Academy of Medicine, 45,* 1288.

18. Buchfuhrer, M. J., Hansen, J. E., Robinson, T. E., Sue, D. Y., Wasserman, K., & Whipp, B. J. (1983). Optimizing the exercise protocol for cardiopulmonary assessment. *Journal of Applied Physiology, 55,* 1558–1564.

19. Carpenter, T. M. (1948). *Tables, factors, and formulas for computing respiratory exchange and biological transformations of energy.* 4th (ed.). Publication 303C. Washington, DC: Carnegie Institute of Washington.

20. Clarke, D. H. (1975). *Exercise physiology.* Englewood Cliffs, NJ: Prentice-Hall.

21. Clear, M. S., & Frisch, F. (1984). Intra-individual biological variability in maximum aerobic power of trained and untrained individuals. *International Journal of Sportsmedicine, 5,* (Abstract) 162.

22. Coast, J. R., Crouse, S. F., & Jessup, G. (1995). *Exercise physiology videolabs.* Dubuque, IA: Brown & Benchmark.

23. Coast, J. R., & Welch, H. G. (1985). Linear increase in optimal pedal rate with increased power output in ergometry. *European Journal of Applied Physiology, 53,* 339–342.

24. Consolazio, C. F., Johnson, R. E., & Pecora, L. J. (1963). *Physiological measurements of metabolic functions in man.* New York: McGraw-Hill.

25. Cooper, K. H. (1968). Testing and developing cardiovascular fitness within the United States Air Force. *Journal of Occupational Medicine, 10,* 636–639.

26. Costill, D. L., Thomason, H., & Roberts, E. (1973). Fractional utilization of the aerobic capacity during distance running. *Medicine and Science in Sports and Exercise, 5,* 248–252.

27. Cureton, T. K. (1973). Interpretation of the oxygen intake test—What is it? *American Corrective Therapy Journal, 27,* 17–23.

28. Daniels, J. T. (1985). A physiologist's view of running economy. *Medicine and Science in Sports and Exercise, 17,* 332–338.

29. Davis, J. A., Caiozzo, V. J., Lamarra, N., Ellis, J. F., Vandagriff, R., Prietto, C. A., & McMaster, W. C. (1983). Does the gas exchange anaerobic threshold occur at a fixed blood lactate concentration of 2 or 4 mM? *International Journal of Sports Medicine, 4,* 89–93.

30. deVries, H. A. (1986). *Physiology of exercise for physical education and athletics.* Dubuque, IA: Wm. C. Brown.

31. Dill, D. B., & Folling, A. (1928). Studies in muscular activity. II. A nomographic description of expired air. *Journal of Physiology, 66,* 133.

32. Duncan, G. E., Howley, E. T., & Johnson, B. N. (1997). Applicability of $\dot{V}O_2$max criteria: Discontinuous versus continuous protocols. *Medicine and Science in Sports and Exercise, 29,* 273–278.

33. Eckermann, P., & Millahn, H. P. (1967). Der einfluss der drehzahl auf die herzfrequenz und die sauerstoffaufnahme bei konstanter leistung am fahrradergometer. *Int. Z. Angew. Physiol. Arbeitsphysiol, 23,* 340–344.

34. Falls, H. B., & Humphrey, D. H. (1973). A comparison of methods for eliciting maximum oxygen uptake from college women during treadmill walking. *Medicine and Science in Sports, 5,* 239–241.

35. Foss, M. L., & Keteyian, S. J. (1998). *Fox's physiological basis for exercise and sport.* Boston: WCB McGraw-Hill.

36. Franklin, B. A. (1985). Exercise testing, training and arm ergometry. *Sports Medicine, 2,* 100–119.

37. Getchell, L. H., Kirkendall, D., & Robbins, G. (1977). Prediction of maximal oxygen uptake in young adult women joggers. *Research Quarterly, 48,* 61–67.

38. Gibbons, L. W., Blair, S. N., Cooper, K. H., & Smith, M. (1983). Association between coronary heart disease risk factors and physical fitness in healthy adult women. *Circulation, 67,* 977–983.

39. Goffredo, M. A., Rich, G. Y., & Holland, G. J. (1983). The influence of treadmill, sitting, and standing bicycle ergometry upon maximal oxygen uptake and anaerobic threshold. *International Journal of Sports Medicine, 4* (Abstract) 136.

40. Grantham, W. C., & Howley, E. T. (1993). Facility design, equipment selection, and calibration. In American College of Sports Medicine (Ed.), *ACSM's resource manual for guidelines for exercise testing and prescription* (pp. 539–550). Philadelphia: Lea & Febiger.

41. Hagberg, J. M., Mullin, J. P., Giese, M. D., & Spitznagel, E. (1981). Effect of pedaling rate on submaximal exercise responses of competitive cyclists. *Journal of Applied Physiology, 51,* 447–451.

42. Harms, C. A., & Dempsey, J. A. (1999). Cardiovascular consequences of exercise hyperpnea. In J. O. Holloszy (Ed.), *Exercise and sport sciences reviews* (pp. 37–62). Philadelphia: Lippincott Williams & Wilkins.

43. Hermansen, L., & Saltin, B. (1969). Oxygen uptake during maximal treadmill and bicycle exercise. *Journal of Applied Physiology, 26,* 31–37.

44. Holly, R. G. (1993). Fundamentals of cardiorespiratory exercise testing. In American College of Sports Medicine (Ed.), *Resource manual for guidelines for exercise testing and prescription* (pp. 247–257) Philadelphia: Lea & Febiger.

45. Horvath, S. M., & Yousef, M. K. (1981). *Environmental physiology: Aging, heat and altitude.* New York: Elsevier/North-Holland.

46. Howley, E. T., Bassett, D. R., & Welch, H. G. (1995). Criteria for maximal oxygen uptake: Review and commentary. *Medicine and Science in Sports and Exercise, 27,* 1292–1301.

47. Issekutz, B., & Rodahl, K. (1961). Respiratory quotient during exercise. *Journal of Applied Physiology, 16,* 606–610.

48. Kasch, F. W., Phillips, W. H., Ross, W. D., Carter, J. E. L., & Boyer, J. L. (1966). A comparison of maximal oxygen uptake by treadmill and step test procedures. *Journal of Applied Physiology, 21,* 1387–1388.

49. Katch, V. L., Sady, S. S., Freedson, P. (1982). Biological variability in maximum aerobic power. *Medicine and Science in Sports and Exercise, 14,* 21–25.

50. Kolkhorst, F. W., Toepfer, T. D., & Dolgener, F. A. (1995). Expired air temperature during steady-state running. *Medicine and Science in Sports and Exercise, 27,* 1621–1625.

51. Liang, M. T. C., Alexander, J. F., Stull, G. A., & Serfass, R. C. (1982). The use of the Bruce equation for predicting $\dot{V}O_2$max in healthy young men. *Medicine and Science in Sports and Exercise, 14,* Abstract #129.

52. Luft, V. C., Cardus, D., Lim, T. P. K., Anderson, E. C., & Howarth, J. L. (1963). Physical performance in relation to body size and composition. *Annals of N.Y. Academy of Science, 110,* 795–808.

53. Mayhew, J. L., & Andrew, J. (1975). Assessment of running performance in college males from aerobic capacity percentage utilization coefficients. *Journal of Sports Medicine and Physical Fitness, 15,* 342–346.

54. McArdle, W. D., Katch, F. I., & Katch, V. L. (1991). *Exercise physiology.* Philadelphia: Lea & Febiger.

55. McDonough, J. R., & Bruce, R. A. (1969). Maximal exercise testing in assessing cardiovascular function. *Journal of South Carolina Medical Association, 65* (Suppl.) 26–33.

56. Michael, E. D., Burke, E. J., & Avakian, E. V. (1979). *Laboratory experiments in exercise physiology.* Ithaca, NY: Mouvements.

57. Mitchell, J. H., Sproule, B. J., & Chapman, C. B. (1958). The physiological meaning of the maximal oxygen intake test. *Journal of Clinical Investigation, 37,* 538.

58. Myerson, M., Gutin, B., Warren, M. D., May, M. T., Contento, I., Lee, M., Pi-Sunyer, F. Y., Pierson, R. N., & Brooks-Gunn, J. (1988). Resting metabolic rate and energy balance in amenorrheic and eumenorrheic runners. *Medicine and Science in Sports and Exercise, 23,* 15–22.

59. Nieman, D. C., Berk, L. S., Simpson-Westerberg, M., Arabatzis, K., Youngberg, S., Tan, S. A., Lee, J. W., & Eby, W. C. (1989). Effects of long-endurance running on immune system parameters and lymphocyte function in experienced marathoners. *International Journal of Sports Medicine, 10,* 317–323.

60. Noakes, T. D. (1988). Implications of exercise testing for prediction of performance: A contemporary perspective. *Medicine and Science in Sports and Exercise, 20,* 319–330.

61. Noble, B. J. (1986). *Physiology of exercise and sport.* Santa Clara, CA: Times Mirror/Mosby College.

62. Norton, A. C. (1976). *Technical memorandum. Methodologies for metabolic measurements.* Schiller Park, IL: Beckman.

63. Paterson, D. H., Cunningham, D. A., Koval, J. J., & St. Croix, C. M. (1999). Aerobic fitness in a population of independently living men and women aged 55–86 years. *Medicine and Science in Sports and Exercise, 31,* 1813–1820.

64. Patterson, R. P., & Moreno, M. I. (1990). Bicycle pedalling forces as a function of pedalling rate and power output. *Medicine and Science in Sports and Exercise, 22,* 512–516.

65. Patterson, R. P., & Pearson, J. L. (1983). The influence of flywheel weight and pedalling frequency on the biomechanics and psychological responses to bicycle exercise. *Ergonomics, 26,* 659–668.

66. Peters, J. P., & Van Slyke, D. D. (1932). *Quantitative clinical chemistry. Vol. II (Methods).* Baltimore: Williams & Wilkins.

67. Pivarnic, J. M., Dwyer, M. C., & Lauderdale, M. A. (1996). The reliability of aerobic capacity ($\dot{V}O_2$max) testing in adolescent girls. *Research Quarterly for Exercise and Sport, 67,* 345–348.

68. Pivarnik, J. M., Montain, S. J., Graves, J. E., & Pollock, M. L. (1988). Effects of pedal speed during incremental cycle ergometer exercise. *Research Quarterly for Exercise and Sport, 59,* 73–77.

69. Pollock, M. L., Wilmore, J. H., & Fox, S. M. (1984). *Exercise in health and disease: Evaluation and prescription for prevention and rehabilitation.* Philadelphia: W. B. Saunders.

70. Powers, S. K., & Howley, E. T. (1990). *Exercise physiology.* Dubuque, IA: Wm. C. Brown.

71. Robinson, S. (1938). Experimental studies of physical fitness in relation to age. *Arbetsphysiologia, 10,* 251–323.

72. Rogers, M. A., Yamamoto, C., Hagberg, J. M., Martin, W. H., Ehsani, A. A., & Holloszy, J. O. (1988). Effect of six days of exercise training on responses to maximal and submaximal exercise in middle-aged men. *Medicine and Science in Sports and Exercise, 20,* 260–264.

73. Scholander, P. F. (1947). Analyzer for accurate estimations of respiratory gases in one-half cubic centimeter samples. *Journal of Biological Chemistry, 167,* 235–250.

74. Seabury, J. J., Adams, W. C., & Ramey, M. R. (1977). Influence of pedalling rate and power output on energy expenditure during bicycle ergometry. *Ergonomics, 20,* 491–498.

75. Serresse, O., Lortie, G., Bouchard, C., & Boulay, M. R. (1988). Estimation of the contribution of the various energy systems during maximal work of short duration. *International Journal of Sports Medicine, 9,* 456–460.

76. Shvartz, E., & Reibold, R. C. (1990). Aerobic fitness norms for males and females aged 6 to 75 years: A review. *Aviation, Space, and Environmental Medicine, 61,* 3–11.

77. Tanaka, H., Bassett, D. R., Swensen, T. C., & Sampredo, R. M. (1993). Aerobic and anaerobic power characteristics of competitive cyclists in the United States Cycling Federation. *International Journal of Sports Medicine, 14,* 334–338.

78. Taylor, H. L., Buskirk, E., & Henschel, A. (1955). Maximal oxygen intake as an objective measure of cardiorespiratory performance. *Journal of Applied Physiology, 8,* 73–80.

79. Thoden, J. S. (1991). Testing aerobic power. In J. D. MacDougall, H. A. Wenger, & H. J. Green (Eds.), *Physiological testing of the high performance athlete* (pp. 107–173). Champaign, IL: Human Kinetics.

80. Thomson, J. M., & Garvie, K. J. (1981). A laboratory method for determination of anaerobic energy expenditure during sprinting. *Canadian Journal of Applied Sport Science, 6,* 21–26.

81. Vago, P., Mercier, J., Ramonatxo, M., & Prefant, C. (1987). Is ventilatory anaerobic threshold a good index of endurance capacity? *International Journal of Sports Medicine, 8,* 190–195.

82. Wasserman, K., Hansen, J. E., Sue, D. Y., Whipp, B. J., & Casaburi, R. (1994). *Principles of exercise testing and interpretation.* Philadelphia: Lea & Febiger.

83. Weast, R. C. (Ed.). (1967). *Handbook of chemistry and physics,* 54th (ed.). Cleveland, OH: The Chemical Rubber Co.

84. Wilmore, J. H., & Costill, D. L. (1974). Semiautomated systems approach to the assessment of oxygen uptake during exercise. *Journal of Applied Physiology, 36,* 618–620.

85. Wilmore, J. H., & Norton, A. C. (1974). *The heart and lungs at work.* Schiller Park, IL: Beckman Instruments.

86. Wyndham, C. H., Strydom, N. B., Maritz, J. S., Morrison, J. F., Peter, J., & Potgieter, Z. U. (1959). Maximum oxygen intake and maximum heart rate during strenuous work. *Journal of Applied Physiology, 14,* 927–936.

Form 15.1

Assignments for $\dot{V}O_2max$ Testing

Assignment	Name
1. Calibrator	_____
2. Performer	_____
3. Performer's caretaker	_____
4. Basic data recorder	_____
5. Meteorologist	_____
6. Oxygen recorder	_____
7. Carbon dioxide recorder	_____
8. Air volume recorder	_____
9. Protocol controller	_____
10. Starter/timer	_____

Form 15.2

F_EO_2 (%) and F_ECO_2 (%)[a]

Time	F_EO_2	F_ECO_2	Time	F_EO_2	F_ECO_2	Time	F_EO_2	F_ECO_2
1:15			6:15			11:15		
1:30			6:30			11:30		
1:45			6:45			11:45		
2:00			7:00			12:00		
M			M			M		
2:15			7:15			12:15		
2:30			7:30			12:30		
2:45			7:45			12:45		
3:00			8:00			13:00		
M			M			M		
3:15			8:15			13:15		
3:30			8:30			13:30		
3:45			8:45			13:45		
4:00			9:00			14:00		
M			M			M		
4:15			9:15			14:15		
4:30			9:30			14:30		
4:45			9:45			14:45		
5:00			10:00			15:00		
M			M			M		
5:15			10:15			15:15		
5:30			10:30			15:30		
5:45			10:45			15:45		
6:00			11:00			16:00		
M			M			M		

[a]An adjustment of 15 s to 30 s may be necessary due to the delay through the mixing chamber and the drying tube of the analyzers; unaccounting for the delay would produce an error in O_2 of less than 2 %.[29]

Form 15.3

Ventilation ($\dot{V}_E$ or $\dot{V}_I$ ATPS, STPD)

Time min:s	Air Volume Meter Reading	$\dot{V}_E$ or $\dot{V}_I$ ATPS L·min⁻¹	STPDcf = [ ]	Ventilation STPD ($\dot{V}_E$ or $\dot{V}_I$) L·min⁻¹ (check one) $\dot{V}_E$ _____ $\dot{V}_I$ _____
0:00				
1:00		0– 1 =	× cf =	
2:00		1– 2 =	× cf =	
3:00		2– 3 =	× cf =	
4:00		3– 4 =	× cf =	
5:00		4– 5 =	× cf =	
6:00		5– 6 =	× cf =	
7:00		6– 7 =	× cf =	
8:00		7– 8 =	× cf =	
9:00		8– 9 =	× cf =	
10:00		9–10 =	× cf =	
11:00		10–11 =	× cf =	
12:00		11–12 =	× cf =	
13:00		12–13 =	× cf =	
14:00		13–14 =	× cf =	
15:00		14–15 =	× cf =	
16:00		15–16 =	× cf =	

Calculation of the final minute's ventilation if the participant lasts as long or longer than 30 s of that final "minute":
Projected final minute's $\dot{V}_E$ or $\dot{V}_I$ = (60 s ÷ t) × Partial minute's $\dot{V}_E$ or $\dot{V}_I$

$\dot{V}_E$ or $\dot{V}_I$ = (60 s ÷ [   ] s) × [   ] L

= [   ] × [   ] L = [   ] L·min⁻¹

Form 15.4

Maximal Oxygen Consumption ($\dot{V}O_2$max)

Name ☐ Date ☐ Time ☐ A.M. ☐ P.M. ☐

Age ☐ y   Gender (M or W) ☐   Ht ☐ cm   Wt ☐ kg   ☐ N   Tech. Initials ☐

Meteorological Data

T ☐ °C (closest 0.1 °C)   RH % ☐ P_B ☐ mm Hg × 1.333 = ☐ hPa

Mode: TM ☐   Cycle ☐   Seat Ht ☐   Other ☐   Time to Exhaustion ☐ min:s

Time	Power or Stage[a]	F_EO_2 (%)	F_ECO_2 (%)	$\dot{V}_E$ or $\dot{V}_I$ STPD	True O_2 (%)	R	$\dot{V}O_2$ L·min^{-1}	$\dot{V}O_2$ mL·kg^{-1}·min^{-1}
0–1								
1–2								
2–3								
3–4								
4–5								
5–6								
6–7								
7–8								
8–9								
9–10								
10–11								
11–12								
12–13								
13–14								
14–15								
15–16								

[a]*Note:* The first complete whole min of running occurred between _____ min.

Form 15.5

Calculations for $\dot{V}O_2$max Test Using Nomogram and Expired Air Volume

1. Convert $\dot{V}_E$ ATPS to $\dot{V}_E$ STPD:

   a. Get STPDcf from Table 15.5 or Eq. 5 by calculation using Table 15.6.

   STPDcf (Table 15.5) = [＿＿＿] or STPDcf (Eq. 15.5 and Table 15.6) = [＿＿＿]

   $$\text{STPDcf (Eq. 15.5 and Table 15.6)} = \frac{273\ K}{273\ K + T_A \boxed{}\ °C} \times \frac{P_B\text{-}H_2O \text{ at } T_A \boxed{}\ °C \text{ (Table 15.6)}}{760}$$

   $$= (273\ K / \boxed{}\ K) \times (\boxed{}\ mm\ Hg/760)$$

   $$= \boxed{} \times \boxed{} = \boxed{}\ cf$$

   b. Get $\dot{V}_E$ STPD (L/min) (from Eq. 15.6).

   $$\dot{V}_E \text{ STPD (L/min)} = \dot{V}_E \text{ ATPS} \boxed{}\ L/min \times cf \boxed{} = \boxed{}\ L/min$$

2. Determine the R and true O_2 values from the nomogram in Figure 15.5.

   R from Fig. 15.5 = [＿＿＿]   True O_2 from Fig. 15.5 = [＿＿＿] %

3. Get $\dot{V}O_2$max from Equation 15.1.

   $$\dot{V}O_2 \text{ (L/min)} = \dot{V}_E \text{ STPD} \boxed{}\ L/min \times \text{true } O_2 \boxed{}\ \%$$

   $$= \boxed{}\ L/min$$

4. Get $\dot{V}O_2$ in units of mL/min from Equation 15.15.

   $$\dot{V}O_2 \text{ (mL/min)} = \boxed{}\ L/min \times 1000 = \boxed{}\ mL/min$$

5. Get relative maximal oxygen consumption from Equation 15.16.

   $$\dot{V}O_2 \text{ mL/(kg} \times min) = \boxed{}\ mL/min \text{ divided by body mass } \boxed{}\ kg$$

   $$= \boxed{}\ mL/(kg \times min) \text{ or } mL{\cdot}kg^{-1}{\cdot}min^{-1}$$

6. Get METmax from Equation 15.17.

   $$\text{METmax} = \boxed{}\ mL/(kg \times min) \text{ divided by } 3.5\ mL/(kg \times min) = \boxed{}\ MET$$

Form 15.6

Comparisons between Predictive and Direct Aerobic Tests

Maximal Oxygen Consumption (mL·kg^{-1}·min^{-1})
Name of Test
Predictive Tests

Initials	Run/Walk	Step	Cycle	Measured $\dot{V}O_2max$
1.				
2.				
3.				
4.				
5.				
6.				
7.				
8.				
9.				
10.				
11.				
12.				
13.				
14.				
15.				
16.				
17.				
18.				
19.				
20.				
21.				
M				

Cardiovascular tests often have clinical implications. The emphasis in *Exercise Physiology Laboratory Manual* is on testing apparently healthy persons. However, certain clinical criteria are explained as a cautionary measure due to the uncertainty of knowing a healthy person from a person with cardiovascular disease until the person is in the process of being tested. It would not be pedagogically sound to forbid teachers and students from administering cardiovascular tests just on the basis that there *might* be a person with unknown cardiovascular disease among the so-called apparently healthy persons. The uncertainty associated with the term *apparently healthy* also lends uncertainty to the required qualifications of kinesiology laboratory technicians.

In their Clinical Competence Statement, the American College of Cardiology (ACC) and the American Heart Association (AHA) states three conditions for a physician's presence or availability during exercise testing.[1] The first condition requires that a physician be able to observe any patient with any of the following:

• Seven- to ten-day history of acute coronary syndrome
• Severe left ventricular dysfunction

• Severe valvular stenosis (narrow heart valves)
• Complex arrhythmia (abnormal heart rhythm)

The second condition of the ACC/AHA statement recognizes that some patients may be tested while the physician is close enough in the facility to respond to an emergency. The third condition requires the physician to be reached by phone or page. The statement encourages nonphysicians who test patients (no comment on apparently healthy persons) to be certified by such organizations as the American College of Sports Medicine.

The American College of Sports Medicine provides risk criteria to assure the testing of only healthy persons.[2] The ACSM has three categories of risks—low, moderate, and high. Low-risk persons are men less than 45 y of age and women less than 55 y of age who are asymptomatic and have no more than one risk factor. Moderate-risk persons are either ≥ 45 y for men and ≥ 55 y for women or those who have two or more risk factors. High-risk persons have one or more symptoms or known cardiovascular, pulmonary, or metabolic disease.

References

1. American College of Cardiology and American Heart Association. (2000). American College of Cardiology/American Heart Association clinical competence statement on stress testing. *Circulation, 102,* 1726.
2. American College of Sports Medicine. (2000). *ACSM's guidelines for exercise prescription.* Philadelphia: Lippincott Williams & Wilkins.

RESTING BLOOD PRESSURE

Numerous researchers have reported an inverse (negative) relationship between physical activity or fitness and morbidity (disease rate) or mortality (death rate), not only from coronary heart disease[4,5,11,32,39,41,44] but from all causes.[5,6] Thus, physical activity and fitness are associated with a reduced risk of cardiovascular disease (CVD), as well as reduced deaths from CVD and all causes. In light of such evidence it seems prudent that the student of exercise physiology be knowledgeable about cardiovascular tests.

Blood pressure measurement is one of the most common clinical tests. It is recommended that all persons over 3 y of age check their blood pressure annually.[45,46]

Because blood pressure screening or monitoring is such an important part of many physical fitness clinics, the technique of measuring blood pressure should be learned by many types of allied health personnel. Dr. H. K. Hellerstein, a renowned cardiologist, speaking as a member of the American Medical Association's Committee on Exercise, said, "Certainly every physical educator should know how to take blood pressure and record it."[20] Additionally, every physical educator should know how to interpret blood pressure.

Purpose of Blood Pressure Measurement

Millions of Americans are hypertensive, with more men than women, until older adulthood, and more blacks than whites classified as hypertensive. *Primary hypertension* means that the cause of hypertension is not known; *secondary hypertension* means that it is caused by known endocrine or structural disorders.[1] Although the cause of hypertension (high blood pressure) in at least 90 % of adults is unknown, it is associated with a high risk for future cardiovascular morbidity and mortality.[15] Hypertensive persons are more likely to accelerate atherosclerosis (hardening of arteries) that may cause vascular occlusions and ruptures about 20 y earlier than in normotensives.[27] If there were obvious symptoms (e.g., pain, nausea) associated with high blood pressure, there would be less need to measure the actual pressure. However, high blood pressure may not be noticed outwardly until a fatal or near-fatal heart attack or stroke occurs. Thus, the primary clinical purpose of measuring blood pressure is to determine the potential risk of cardiovascular disease; if the pressure is high, then appropriate medications or lifestyle changes are recommended. Periodic monitoring of the blood pressure is done in order to check the efficacy of such recommendations.

Another purpose of measuring resting blood pressure is to establish a baseline by which to compare the effect of exercise on blood pressure. Thus, the effects of different types, intensities, or durations of exercise may be compared by noting their effects upon the baseline value. For example, blood pressure comparisons may be made between (1) static versus dynamic exercise, (2) different intensities of muscle actions (e.g., 30 % vs. 80 % maximal forces), and (3) short versus long durations of exercise.

Physiological Rationale

High blood pressure is unhealthy; blood pressure, per se, is not unhealthy. Without blood pressure there would be no blood flow. Blood pressure is primarily dependent upon the volume of blood and the resistance of the blood vessels. The blood pressure that is commonly measured is that of the arteries. Thus, blood pressure may be defined for laboratory purposes as the force of blood distending the *arterial* walls. Typically, the brachial artery is sampled because of convenience and its position at heart level. The brachial artery (Figure 16.1) is a continuation of the axillary artery and extends medially alongside the humerus; it gradually moves centrally as it nears the antecubital fossa (anterior crease of the elbow), where it divides into the radial and ulnar arteries.[22]

Korotkoff Sounds

The determination of blood pressure in the typical laboratory setting is based upon the sounds made by the vibrations from the vascular walls. These sounds are referred to as Korotkoff sounds (named after their discoverer in 1905) (Figure 16.2). In brief, when there is no blood flow (as when a tourniquet is applied), there will be no vibrations and thus no sound. Paradoxically, when there is completely nonobstructed flow of the blood, there is also no vibration and thus no sound; this is due to the streamlined flow of the blood. When blood flow is restricted by the application of a tourniquet or by any kind of pressure, and then gradually released, there will be a bolus of blood escaping at the peak point of blood pressure coinciding with left ventricular contraction (systole). This bolus of blood will cause vascular vibrations which result in a faint sound (phase 1); this is **systolic pressure.** As the restriction or pressure continues to be released, more blood escapes, causing even greater vibration and louder sounds. Phases 2

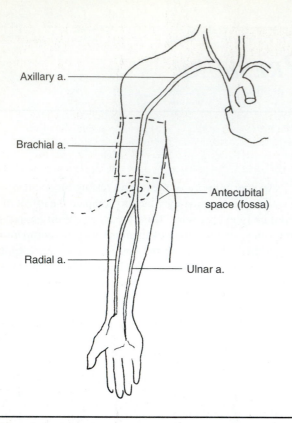

Figure 16.1 An internal view of the brachial artery and its origins and branches; the dotted diaphragm of the stethoscope is at the antecubital fossa (a. = artery).

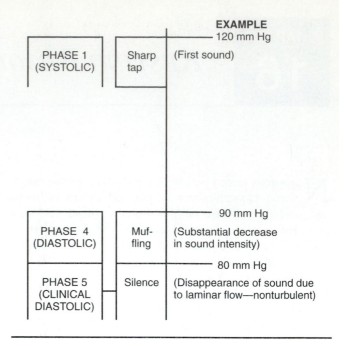

Figure 16.2 The three major phases of Korotkoff sounds when systolic pressure (first phase) is 120 mm Hg and diastolic pressures (fourth and fifth phases) are 90 and 80 mm Hg, respectively. Phase 2 (swishing sound) and phase 3 (crisp and intense) are not shown.

and 3 are not commonly used in recording blood pressures and, therefore, have been deleted in Figure 16.2. More blood escapes as the cuff pressure continues to decrease. However, after phase 3, as the blood flow becomes more streamlined due to less compression, there is a reduction of vibrations, causing a muffling sound (phase 4). The fourth phase is sometimes difficult to distinguish. The American Heart Association describes it as ". . . a distinct, abrupt, muffling of sound (usually of a soft, blowing quality) . . .".[15] Identifying phase 4 is more difficult than identifying phase 5.[14] When blood flow is completely streamlined (laminar flow), there is a disappearance of sound (phase 5). The disappearance denotes **diastolic pressure,** the lowest pressure that exists in the arteries. However, the fourth phase is closer to the actual invasive diastolic pressure; hence, it is sometimes referred to as the true diastolic pressure. The fifth phase is often referred to as the clinical diastolic pressure because it is the reference for normative classification.

The Task Force on Blood Pressure Control in Children[45,46] recommends that both the point of muffling (phase 4) and the point of disappearance (phase 5) of the sound be recorded when taking blood pressure in children. Because of the frequency of these occurring simultaneously or of the fifth phase's not occurring at all in children, the Task Force and the American Heart Association use the fourth phase to interpret children's norms and the fifth

phase for all persons above 12 y of age. Occasionally, phase 4 should be used for adults whose sounds remain very faint to near zero levels.[48] Usually, the fourth phase is significantly higher than the fifth phase by about 5 mm of mercury (Hg).[10] Rarely do true diastolic pressures reach less than 40 mm Hg.[12] Thus, for any person whose sounds can be heard below this level, it seems logical to use the fourth phase instead of the fifth phase as the true diastolic pressure. Exercise technicians are encouraged to practice recording the fourth phase in all persons because of the fourth phase's importance during exercise (Chapter 17).

Pulse Pressure and Mean Pressure

Pulse pressure (PP) is the difference between systolic and diastolic pressures. High pulse pressures—that is, large differences between SP and DP—may indicate increased risk of heart attack (myocardial infarction).[35] Pulse pressure reflects the vascular compliance (distensibility) in large arteries. Pulse pressure is used to calculate mean blood pressure (MBP).

MBP is based upon the actual pressure that the arteries would sustain if blood flow were not pulsating. Because arterial blood pressure under resting conditions is at systolic level only about one-twentieth of the time during a cardiac cycle, mean pressure is always closer to diastolic pressure than it is to systolic pressure. Resting MBP is usually estimated as one-third the distance between fifth-phase diastolic pressure and systolic pressure[43] (Eq. 16.1), or, similarly, by multiplying the difference between SP and DP—that is, PP, by 0.33[51] (Eq. 16.2). MBP is typically between 90 mm Hg and 100 mm Hg at rest.

$$MBP = (PP/3) + DP \qquad \text{Eq. 16.1}$$

where:

PP = pulse pressure; SP – DP

Example: MBP (mm Hg) = $\dfrac{130 - 80}{3} + 80$

$$= (50 / 3) + 80$$
$$= 17 + 80$$
$$= 97 \text{ mm Hg}$$

or:

$$MBP = (0.33 \times PP) + DP \qquad \text{Eq. 16.2}$$

Example: MBP (mm Hg) = $[0.33 \times (130 - 80)] + 80$

$$= (0.33 \times 50) + 80$$
$$= 17 + 80$$
$$= 97 \text{ mm Hg}$$

Method

The accuracy of blood pressure measurements is described in Box 16.1. Many types of instruments exist for measuring blood pressure. The original instrument in 1733, water in a glass tube, was used to measure the blood pressure of a horse.[3] Due to water's light weight (lower density) in comparison with mercury—the liquid now being used—a ladder was needed to enable the investigator to read the water column, which had risen about 10 ft. Mercury, being nearly 14 times heavier than water, enables the measurement of blood pressure with a glass tube, which can be about one-fourteenth the length of the original water-filled glass tubes. If we still used water to measure human blood pressure, the tube would have to be a minimum of six feet tall, and the column of water would oscillate by more than one foot with each heartbeat.[21]

The International System's unit of measure for pressure is the hectopascal. However, due to the traditional use of mercury in blood pressure instrumentation, the unit of measure for blood pressure recordings is millimeters of mercury (mm Hg; Hg = hydrargyrum; g = j sound). Regardless of the type of blood pressure method or instrument, the unit of measure remains mm Hg. The graduations on the sphygmomanometer gauge are in 2 mm divisions and extend to 300 mm Hg.

The methods of blood pressure measurement may be divided into two categories—invasive and noninvasive. The *invasive* method is the more valid of the two methods and is usually reserved for clinical settings or precise research investigations. A thin teflon tube, called an endhole catheter or cannula, is connected on one end to a pressure transducer. The sensor end of the catheter is inserted into

---

<table>
<tr><td style="background:black;color:white;">BOX 16.1</td><td>**Accuracy of Blood Pressure Measurements**</td></tr>
</table>

Validity

The cuff method of measuring systolic and fifth-phase diastolic blood pressure is usually lower than the more accurate invasive method of measuring blood pressure by about 10 mm Hg (8 %) and 5 mm Hg (6 %), respectively; the fourth phase, however, is not significantly different from the invasive measurement of diastolic pressure.[43] Thus, the fourth phase appears to be the most valid indicator of diastolic pressure, although the fifth phase is commonly used for calculating mean pressures during a resting body state.

Reliability

The ability of the human ear to hear sounds is dependent upon the frequency (Hz) and decibels (dB) of the sounds. Unfortunately, Korotkoff sounds are neither of high frequency nor high decibel—both being less than the optimal hearing of the human ear.[33] Acceptable reliability coefficients can be obtained for the test-retest values of systolic (r = .89) and diastolic (r = .83) blood pressures.[a] The diastolic values of the fifth phase may be more repeatable than those of the fourth phase due to greater difficulty in determining muffling points of fourth phases versus disappearance points of fifth phases. In fact, one investigator encourages the use of the fifth phase for this reason, although it may not be hemodynamically justified for all persons.[29]

[a]Adams, G. M. (1968). Blood pressure reliability in the elderly. Unpublished raw data.

---

the brachial artery or ascending aorta while the transducer end is connected to a recorder. Although the invasive method is accurate for mean and diastolic pressures in the ascending aorta,[16] it is expensive, elaborate, and traumatic, compared with the noninvasive method.

Two major methods are used to measure *noninvasive blood pressure*—cuff manometry and ultrasound Doppler. The cuff manometry method uses an instrument called a sphygmomanometer (*sphygmo* = pulse; pronounced sfig-mo-ma-nóm-a-ter); it is more easily referred to as a manometer. Both aneroid and mercury methods of manometry require a cuff with an air bladder; thus, the method is sometimes referred to as the cuff method (Figure 16.3). Although aneroid manometers are not favored over mercury manometers,[1,24] if the aneroids are calibrated routinely (Box 16.2), they are acceptable. Validated electronic devices can be used also, but finger sphygmomanometers are not recommended.[24] The aneroid manometers use a metal bellows device that drives tiny gears that move the dial's pointers. Commercial electronic automated blood pressure instruments have not been endorsed by the American Heart Association, partly because of the difficulty in checking their accuracy and their infrequent use by health personnel. The safety and performance requirements of nonautomated[42] and automated[49]

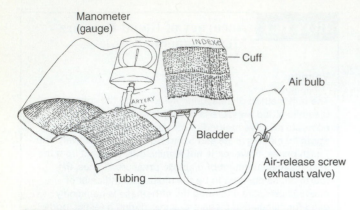

Manometer (gauge)

Cuff

Air bulb

Bladder

Air-release screw (exhaust valve)

Tubing

ARTERY

INDEX

Figure 16.3 The main parts of an aneroid sphygmomanometer are the gauge, tubing, cuff, bladder, air bulb, and air-release screw.

sphygmomanometers have been reported by the American Standards Institute.

Mercury and aneroid sphygmomanometers require a stethoscope to auscultate the Korotkoff sounds; when this is done, the noninvasive method may be referred to as the **auscultatory method.** Surprisingly, experienced participants can sense their blood pressure fairly accurately while the technician or clinician is auscultating it.[13] Ambulatory blood pressure monitors can be programmed to take readings every 5 min to 120 min throughout a 24 h period. The pressures can be analyzed after being downloaded on a computer.[13]

Procedures

Certain preparations, such as calibration and participant orientation, should be made in order to facilitate blood pressure measurement. **Calibration** of aneroid manometers, using a mercury manometer, should be done at six-month[24,27] to annual[28,46] intervals (Box 16.2).

Participant orientation includes such preparatory rules that were suggested for the stepping test (Chapter 13) and cycling test (Chapter 14). Whereas those tests prescribed abstaining from smoking and caffeine for 3 h prior to testing, the Joint National Committee on Detection, Evaluation, and Treatment of High Blood Pressure prescribes only a 30 min abstention.[24] The participant should relax for at least five minutes in a comfortable environment prior to the blood pressure measurement.[15,24] Also, sleeveless shirts/blouses or loose-fitting sleeves are recommended attire; if the sleeve appears to fit tightly around the person's arm when the sleeve is rolled up, the shirt or sweater should be removed. The cuff and stethoscope should not be placed over cloth. Most of the following procedures for measuring blood pressure are the recommendations of the Joint National Committee on Detection, Evaluation, and Treatment of High Blood Pressure (1997).[24]

BOX 16.2	Calibration of Aneroid Sphygmomanometer

Assumption: The method of calibrating the aneroid sphygmomanometers assumes that the mercury sphygmomanometer is accurate. A good sphygmomanometer will not shift its indicating pointer or mercury column when the air-release screw is closed.

Zero

Most pointers on the dials of the aneroid sphygmomanometers are designed to rest at the zero when no air has been inserted into the bladder. However, some aneroid sphygmomanometers are not designed to return to the zero. Thus, the return of the indicator to zero is not an infallible criterion for accuracy in all aneroid manometers. Those that are designed to rest at zero should be returned to the manufacturer if they do not do so.

Range

Equipment: (1) Mercury sphygmomanometer; (2) a "Y" connector; the Y section joining the binaurals of some stethoscopes may be used; (3) a short (about 4 in.) piece of surgical tubing; (4) (optional) a can or bottle that approximates the circumference of a person's upper arm.

Configuration: (1) Wrap the cuff around the can or bottle; (2) connect the tube of the cuff's bladder to one end of the "Y" connector; (3) connect the tube of the mercury sphygmomanometer to another end of the Y; and (4) connect the tube of the air bulb to the third end of the Y connector (Figure 16.4).

Procedure: (1) Inflate the cuff's bladder until the aneroid dial reads 40 mm Hg; (2) read the dial on the mercury sphygmomanometer; (3) record actual mercury reading; (4) deflate the bladder; (5) repeat the same procedure at increments of 20 mm Hg; (6) if necessary, devise a mathematical correction based upon the readings or return the aneroid to the manufacturer if values disagree.

Procedural Steps

1. The participant should sit comfortably in a chair with a backrest for at least 5 min. The arm bared is at heart level and resting on the armrest of a chair or on a table (Figure 16.5).
2. The manometer should be clearly visible to the technician; mercury gauges should read so that the meniscus (top of mercury) is at eye level.
3. For persons with suspected small or large arm circumferences, the technician measures the circumference of the participant's upper arm.
   a. The appropriate cuff size is selected based on the arm circumference guidelines in Table 16.1.
   b. Some cuffs have index lines that indicate if the cuff is too small or too large (Figure 16.6). In general the *bladder* should wrap around at least 80 % of the arm.

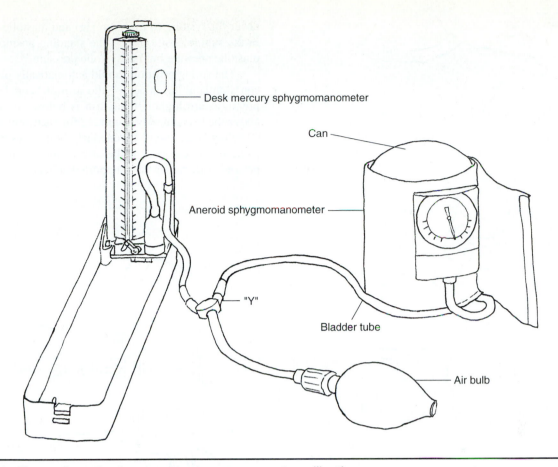

Figure 16.4   The configuration for aneroid sphygmomanometer calibration.

4. The technician snugly places the blood pressure cuff so that the lower edge is approximately 2.5 cm (1 in.) above the antecubital space.[30]
   a. The center of the bladder should be over the brachial artery.
   b. Some cuffs have a mark to line-up with the brachial artery. To assure alignment, it may be helpful to palpate the brachial artery along the medial side of the antecubital space.[15]
5. The technician places the diaphragm, or bell, of the stethoscope firmly, but not tight enough to indent the skin, over the nonvisible brachial artery in the antecubital space.
6. After turning the air-release screw clockwise, the technician quickly inflates the cuff to any of the three following levels:
   a. 160 mm Hg
   b. 20 mm Hg above expected or known SP
   c. 20 mm Hg to 30 mm Hg above the disappearance of the palpated radial pulse[15]
7. The technician turns the air-release screw counterclockwise so that the cuff pressure decreases at a rate of about 2 mm Hg to 3 mm Hg per second.[24]
8. The technician listens carefully and mentally notes the first Korotkoff sound of two consecutive beats—systolic pressure (first phase)—then fourth phase

(muffling)—then fifth phase (disappearance)—at the nearest 2 mm mark on the manometer, respectively.
9. The technician continues listening for 10 mm Hg to 20 mm Hg below the last sound heard to confirm disappearance.
10. The technician rapidly deflates the cuff.
11. The technician records the values in even numbers according to the accepted format: e.g., systolic/fourth phase DP/fifth phase DP. Thus, a hypothetical recording would appear as 128/92/86 mm Hg.
12. The technician notes the presence or absence of auscultatory gaps and/or irregular pulse rhythm.
13. The technician repeats the measurement after 2 min, then averages the two readings unless they differ by more than 5 mm Hg—in which case, additional readings are made.[24,27] If more than two readings are necessary, the technician averages them all.
14. The technician uses the first and fifth phases to classify persons according to Tables 16.2 and 16.4.

Comments on Blood Pressure Procedures

Body and Arm Position

There is no *practical* difference in blood pressure measured in the seated position versus that measured in the supine position. However, *statistically*, slightly higher values occur for systolic (6 to 7 mm Hg) and diastolic (1 mm Hg) in the supine position.[31,47] The standing position increases diastolic pressure but not systolic pressure.[18]

The sitting position should automatically place the person's antecubital space of the arm at heart level. Blood pressures are higher if the arm is below the heart versus above the heart (nearly 1 mm Hg for each centimeter above or below heart level). Erroneously higher systolic and diastolic pressures occur if the arm is allowed to hang at the person's side rather than supported at heart level.[47]

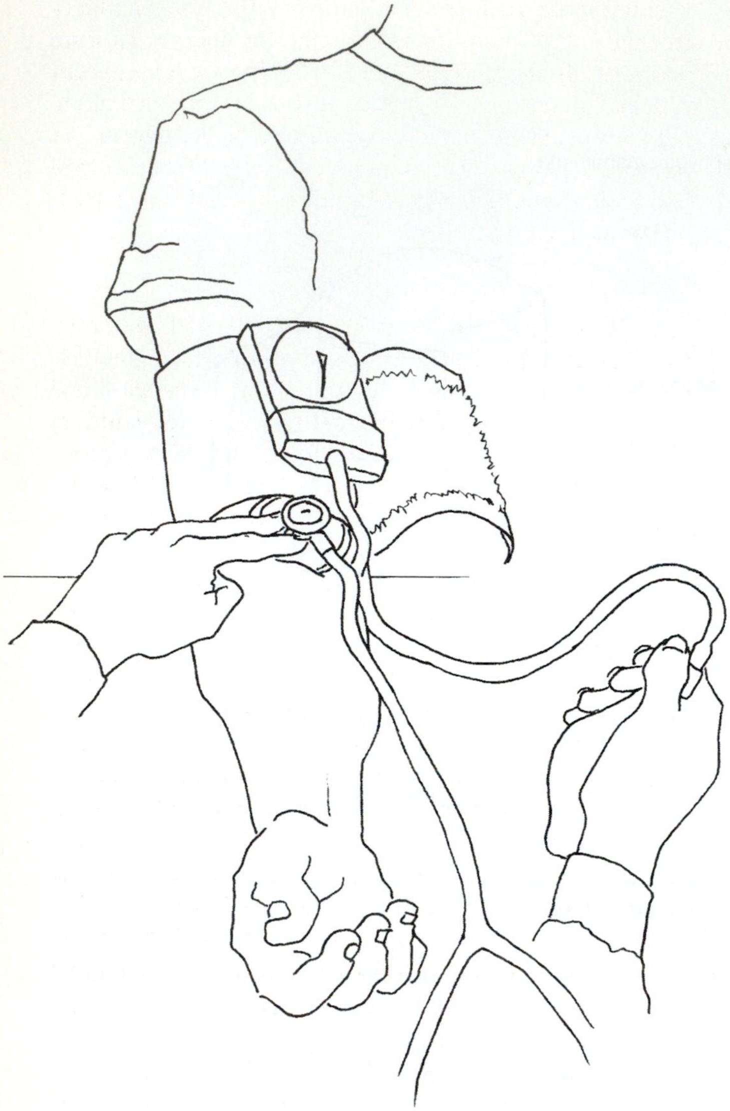

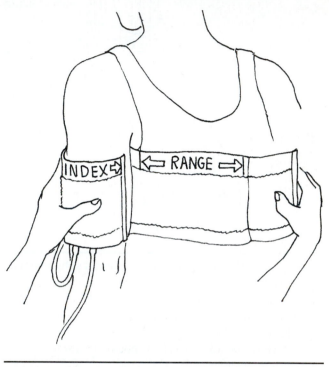

Figure 16.5 The bottom border of the cuff is placed about 1 in., or 2.5 cm, above the antecubital space and diaphragm of the stethoscope.

Figure 16.6 The cuff's index and range lines determine the appropriate cuff size for some sphygmomanometers.

Table 16.1	Guidelines for Type of Blood Pressure Cuff According to Limb Circumference (cir.)

Limb Size (cm)	Type of Cuff[a]	Bladder Size (cm)	
Upper Arm Cir.		Length	Width
32–42	Large adult	33 or 42	15
24–32	Adult (standard)	24	12.5
18–24	Child	21.5	10
	(3 y to 12 y)	18	8
Thigh Cir.			
42–50	Thigh	37	18.5

Note: [a]Other types of cuffs are newborn and infant.

Table 16.2	Blood Pressure (mm Hg) Criteria for Various Categories and Follow-Up Recommendations

Category	Criteria (mm Hg)		
	Systolic	Diastolic (5th phase)	Follow-Up
Optimal	< 120	< 80	Recheck in 2 y
High normal	130–139	85–89	Recheck in 1 y
Hypertension			
Stage 1	140–159	90–99	Confirm within 2 mo
Stage 2	160–179	100–109	Evaluate or refer to care within 1 mo
Stage 3	≥ 180	≥ 110	Evaluate or refer to care immediately or within 1 wk depending on clinical situation

Source: Joint National Committee on Detection, Evaluation, and Treatment of High Blood Pressure. (1997). The sixth report of the Joint National Committee on Detection, Evaluation, and Treatment of High Blood Pressure (JNC VI). NIH Publication No. 98-4080.

For best exposure of the antecubital position, it helps to have the person's palm upward with the thumb-side rotated outwardly (the anatomical position) and to have the arm nearly straight while resting on a platform (e.g., table). This provides the best contact with the brachial artery. The antecubital space should be left clear for the stethoscope's diaphragm.[7]

Various authorities recommend that the right arm be chosen for the blood pressure measurement.[8,46] This is partly because of the remote possibility that the genetic anomaly of coarctation (abnormal narrowing) between the aorta and subclavian artery will cause an elevated blood pressure. If the pressure in the right arm is normal, it is likely to be normal everywhere. However, higher right-arm values were not confirmed by some investigators,[10,17] nor did the investigators in the famous epidemiological study in Framingham, Massachusetts, measure blood pressure in the right arm.[25] In older patients, one group of investigators found that the systolic pressure in the right arm was not more than a few millimeters higher than in the left arm and that the diastolic pressure was virtually the same in both arms.[19] The American Heart Association recommends that both arms be measured at the initial examination and the arm with the higher pressure be measured in subsequent examinations.[15] Another consideration should be the comfort and convenience of both the technician and the participant.

Cuff Size

Special cuff sizes are available for small or large arms. Cuffs that are too small will overestimate blood pressure, whereas cuffs that are too large will underestimate blood pressure. The average overestimation by narrow cuffs is about 9 mm Hg and 5 mm Hg for SP and DP, respectively.[36] The ideal cuff size is when the cuff is 20 % wider than the diameter of the arm and bladder length is 80 % of arm circumference.[24]

Some cuff manufacturers print a criterion index line by which to determine proper cuff size (review Figure 16.6). For example, the cuff is placed so that the vertical arrow printed on the cuff is over the brachial artery. After the cuff encircles the arm, the index line should fall within the two horizontal range lines, otherwise, the cuff is too small. These index lines can vary considerably among manufacturers. Thus, lab personnel are encouraged to mark a line on the interior surface of the cuff at a distance of 32 cm from the standard cuff's left border.[36] Table 16.1 provided the proper guidelines for cuff size. Either the larger or smaller cuff may be used for overlapping values found in that table. A distended, bulging, or balooning bladder is a sign that something is wrong with the manometer.

Controlling the Manometer and Stethoscope

No air spaces should be allowed between the skin and the diaphragm of the stethoscope. By not pressing heavily on

---

Table 16.3 Age Prevalence Rates for Hypertension

	Percent
Total Adult Population[a]	25 to 33
Age-Specific Estimates[b]	
18 y to 29 y	4
30 y to 39 y	11
40 y to 49 y	21
50 y to 59 y	44
60 y to 69 y	54
70 y to 79 y	64
80+ y	65

Sources: [a]Joint National Committee on Detection, Evaluation, and Treatment of High Blood Pressure. (1993). The fifth report of the Joint National Committee on Detection, Evaluation, and Treatment of High Blood Pressure (JNCV). *Archives of Internal Medicine, 153,* 154–183. [b]National High Blood Pressure Education Program Working Group. (1993). Report on primary prevention of hypertension. *Archives of Internal Medicine, 153,* 186–208.

Table 16.4 Percentile Norms for Blood Pressure in Active Men and Women, Ages 20 y to 39 y

	Men				Women			
	Systolic		Diastolic		Systolic		Diastolic	
	Age (y)				Age (y)			
%ile	20–29	30–39	20–29	30–39	20–29	30–39	20–29	30–39
99th	94	96	60	60	90	90	56	60
90	110	108	70	70	99	100	63	65
80	112	110	72	74	101	104	68	70
70	118	116	78	78	106	110	70	70
60	120	120	80	80	110	110	72	74
50	121	120	80	80	112	114	75	76
40	128	124	80	81	118	118	78	80
30	130	130	84	85	120	120	80	80
20	136	132	88	90	122	122	80	82
10	140	140	90	92	130	130	82	90
1st	158	168	110	110	141	160	90	110
n	367	1615			118	301		

Source: Data from Pollock, M. L., Wilmore, J. H., & Fox, S. M. et al., *Health and Fitness Through Physical Activity,* 1978. Copyright © 1978 John Wiley & Sons, Inc., New York, NY.

the bell or diaphragm, the technician can avoid turbulent blood flow induced by the diaphragm. Turbulence can lower the diastolic pressure reading but is unlikely to distort systolic.[34] The technician should clear the cuff bladder's tubing away from the diaphragm because when they touch each other it sounds much like the Korotkoff sounds.

The technician should place the air bulb deep in the palm of the hand so that the thumb and index finger control the air-release screw. Although an effective method for knowing when to stop inflating the cuff is by palpating the person's radial artery, it can be an awkward procedure. The technician has to take one hand off the stethoscope's diaphragm while palpating the pulse. Often, technicians decrease the pressure too fast. Low systolic and high diastolic readings may occur when the rate of deflation is too fast.[15] Very slow deflation rates should be avoided in order to prevent prolonged discomfort, apprehensiveness, and fidgeting in the participant, all of which may increase the individual's blood pressure. If the person requires a repeated measurement for any reason, the pressure cuff should remain deflated for about 2 min between determinations.[24] This will allow the blood in the venous circulation to return to normal.[15]

The meniscus level (the peak of the "hump") at the top of the column of mercury is the measuring point when using **mercury** manometers. The indicating pointer is used for the **aneroid** gauge. If using the mercury manometer, the observer's eyes should be level with the meniscus in order to avoid parallax (angle distortion). When reading the aneroid dial, the observer's eyes should be directly in front of the gauge. Inexperienced technicians have a tendency to record pressures in deca-rounded numbers, such as 130/80/70.

Results and Discussion

The interpretation of blood pressure is based upon the criteria that have been established by various professional medical groups. These criteria are established from large-scale studies that indicate the norms for that particular population and/or subpopulation, such as, African Americans, males, females, and children.

Blood pressure criteria are based upon the contribution of blood pressure to the risk of death from cardiovascular disease—heart attacks, strokes, and congestive heart failure—and kidney damage, blindness, and dimentia.[24] The authoritative study groups on blood pressure such as the American Heart Association,[2] the Task Force on Blood Pressure,[45,46] the Joint National Committee,[24] and National High Blood Pressure Program[38] indicate that the criteria for systolic hypertension and diastolic hypertension are equally important. However, the Joint National Committee indicates that systolic pressure in older adults is a superior predictor of cardiovascular events.[24] Because blood pressure may be affected by nonpathological (nondisease) factors, such as emotions, it is recommended that no one be

classified as hypertensive on the basis of only one day's measurements. A person should be classified as hypertensive only when measurements taken on two separate visits are over the established hypertension criteria.[24]

Hypertension   The classification criteria listed in Table 16.2 are based on the Korotkoff sounds of the first and fifth phases. The criterion of 140/90 mm Hg is the recognized criterion for hypertension.[24,50] All that is necessary to meet the criterion is for either systolic or diastolic pressure to reach the respective value, not necessarily both of them. When only one of the pressures exceeds the criterion it is often referred to as *isolated* systolic (or diastolic) hypertension. Various authorities have suggested a category of high normal for younger persons with systolic pressure between 130 and 139 mm Hg, and diastolic pressure between 85 and 89 mm Hg.[24,26,45] The persons in the high normal category of Table 16.2 have an increased risk for future hypertension and target organ damage despite their seemingly benign blood pressures of 130–139/85–89 mm Hg.[24] Subdivisions of the hypertension category are Stages I, II, and III. Age prevalence percentages are presented in Table 16.3.[23,38]

Average BP   The average pressures of over 5000 men, ages 20 y to 60+ y, who were tested at a fitness clinic were 125/82 mm Hg.[40] These values are probably less than in a random sample because they are men who have been tested at a fitness clinic, presumably with the intention of planning to exercise or to evaluate their existing exercise programs. The women's averages (119/78 mm Hg) are from the same investigators and include 914 active women the same ages as the men—that is, between 20 y and 60+ y.

Optimal BP   Although the Joint National Committee[24] categorizes optimal as blood pressures < 120/< 80, the exact criteria for optimal SP and DP may not exist. For example, if the criteria were less than 120/80, then criteria would also have to consider the person's symptoms.[24] Thus, the lowest blood pressure may be the best as long as symptoms such as lightheadedness, dizziness, and/or faintness (syncope) are absent.

Hypotension   There are no increased risks for cardiovascular disease in hypotensive persons; in fact, lower pressures reduce the cardiovascular risk.[15] A hypotension criterion of 90 mm Hg is meant only for systolic pressure; there is no accepted criterion for diastolic pressure with respect to hypotension, although less than 60 mm Hg is unusual.[37] As with optimal blood pressure, hypotensive criteria really should be based upon symptoms. Thus, if an individual is experiencing dizziness, syncope, coldness, pallor, nausea, low urine output, and high arterial blood lactates when blood pressure decreases to a certain point, then that point should be the criterion for hypotension for that person.[9]

Norms are based on the average and standard deviation of blood pressures from a large population. Norms for active persons of both sexes between the ages of 20 y and 39 y are found in Table 16.4.[40] In general, women have lower blood pressures than men; younger persons have lower pressures than older persons.

The *mean blood pressure* of 507 healthy men and women at an average age of 35 y (± 13.2 y) was 85 mm Hg (± 9.0).[52] These persons were sedentary and included 166 Blacks among the Whites. Their blood pressures were taken with a calibrated automated device.

Lifestyle Modification of Hypertension Prevention

The Joint National Committee lists seven lifestyle changes that could prevent or control hypertension.[24]

* Lose weight if overweight.
* Limit alcohol to one drink per day.
* Increase aerobic activity to 30 + min most days of the week.
* Reduce sodium to < 2.4 g/d or NaCl to < 6 g/d.
* Maintain dietary potassium of ≈ 90 mmol/d.
* Maintain dietary calcium and magnesium.
* Stop smoking and reduce saturated fat and cholesterol.

References

1. American College of Sports Medicine. (2000). *ACSM's guidelines for exercise testing and prescription.* Philadelphia: Lippincott Williams & Wilkins.
2. American Heart Association. (1991). *1992 heart and stroke facts.* Dallas: Author.
3. Best, C. H., & Taylor, N. B. (1956). *The human body.* New York: Henry Holt & Co.
4. Blackburn, H., & Jacobs, D. R. (1988). Physical activity and the risk of coronary heart disease. *New England Journal of Medicine, 319,* 1217–1219.
5. Blair, S. N., Kampert, J. B., Kohl, H. W., Barlow, C. E., Paffenbarger, R. S., & Gibbons, L. W. (1996). Influences of cardiorespiratory fitness and other precursors on cardiovascular disease and all-cause mortality in men and women. *JAMA: The Journal of the American Medical Association, 276,*(3), 205–210.
6. Blair, S. N., Kohl, H. W., Paffenbarger, R. S., Clark, D. G., Cooper, K. H., & Gibbons, L. W. (1989). Physical fitness and all-cause mortality. A prospective study of healthy men and women. *Journal of the American Medical Association, 262,* 2395–2401.
7. Boyer, J. (1976). Exercise and hypertension. *The Physician and Sportsmedicine, 4*(12) 35–49.
8. Burch, G. E. (1976). *Consultations in hypertension: A clinical symposium.* Rochester, NY: Pennwalt Prescription Products.
9. daLuz, P. L., Weil, M. H., Liu, V. Y., & Shubin, H. (1974). Plasma volume prior to and following volume loading during shock complicating acute myocardial infarction. *Circulation, 49,* 98–105.
10. Das, B. C., & Mukherjee, B. N. (1963). Variation in systolic and diastolic pressure with changes in age and weight. *Gerontologia, 8,* 92–104.
11. Ekelund, L.-G., Haskell, W. L., Johnson, J. L., Whaley, F. S., Criqui, M. H., & Sheps, D. S. (1988). Physical fitness as a predictor of cardiovascular mortality in asymptomatic North American men. The Lipid Research Clinics' mortality follow-up study. *New England Journal of Medicine, 319,* 1379–1384.
12. Engler, R. L. (1977). Historical and physical findings in patients with aortic valve disease. *The Western Journal of Medicine, 126,* 463–467.
13. Estes, S. B. (1977, May). Putting the cuff on hypertensive patients. *Patient Care,* p. 25.
14. Freis, E. D., & Sappington, R. F. (1968). Dynamic reactions produced by deflating a blood pressure cuff. *Circulation, 38,* 1085–1096.
15. Frohlich, E. D., Grim, C., Labarthe, D. R., Maxwell, M. H., Perloff, D., & Weidman, W. H. (1987). *Recommendations for human blood pressure determination by sphygmomanometers: Report of a special task force appointed by the steering committee, American Heart Association.* Dallas: National Center, American Heart Association.
16. Griffen, S. E., Robergs, R. A., & Heyward, V. H. (1977). Blood pressure measurement during exercise: A review. *Medicine and Science in Sports and Exercise, 29,* 149–159.
17. Harrison, E. G., Foth, G. M., & Hines, E. A. (1960). Bilateral indirect and direct arterial pressures. *Circulation, 22,* 419–436.
18. Hasegawa, M., & Rodbard, S. (1979). Effect of posture on arterial pressures, timing of the arterial sounds, and pulse wave velocities in the extremities. *Cardiology, 64,* 122–132.
19. Hashimoto, F., Hunt, W. C., & Hardy, L. (1984). Differences between right and left arm blood pressures in the elderly. *Western Journal of Medicine, 141,* 189–192.
20. Hellerstein, H. K. (1976). Exercise and hypertension. *The Physician and Sportsmedicine, 4*(12) 35–49.
21. Hill, A. V. (1927). *Living machinery.* New York: Harcourt, Brace, & Co.
22. Jackson, C. M. (Ed.). (1923). *Morris' human anatomy.* Philadelphia: P. Blakiston's Son & Co.
23. Joint National Committee on Detection, Evaluation, and Treatment of High Blood Pressure. (1993). The fifth report of the Joint National Committee on Detection, Evaluation, and Treatment of High Blood Pressure (JNC V). *Archives of Internal Medicine, 153,* 154–183.

24. Joint National Committee on Detection, Evaluation, and Treatment of High Blood Pressure. (1997). The sixth report of the Joint National Committee on Detection, Evaluation, and Treatment of High Blood Pressure (JNC VI). NIH Publication No. 98-4080. Bethesda, MD.

25. Kannel, W. B., Philip, A. W., McGee, D. L., Dawber, T. R., McNamara, P., & Castelli, W. P. (1981). Systolic blood pressure, arterial rigidity, and risk of stroke. *Journal of the American Medical Association, 245,* 1225–1229.

26. Kaplan, N. M. (1976). Diagnosis and testing of the hypertensive patient. In G. Burch (Ed.), *Consultations in hypertension: A clinical symposium* (pp. 6–11). New York: Pennwalt Prescription Products.

27. Kaplan, N. M. (1983). Hypertension. In N. Kaplan & J. Stannler (Eds.), *Prevention of coronary heart disease. Practical management of risk factors.* Philadelphia: W. B. Saunders.

28. Kaplan, N. M., Deveraux, R. B., Miller, H. S. (1994). Systemic hypertension. *Medicine and Science in Sports and Exercise, 26*(10), S268–S270.

29. King, G. E. (1969). Taking the blood pressure. *Journal of the American Medical Association, 209,* 1902–1904.

30. Kirkendall, W. M., Burton, A. C., Epstein, F. H., & Freis, E. D. (1967). Recommendations for human blood pressure determination by sphygmomanometry. *Circulation, 36,* 980.

31. Lategola, M. T., & Busby, D. E. (1975). Differences between seated and recumbent resting measurements of auscultative blood pressure. *Aviation, Space, & Environmental Medicine, 46,* 1027–1029.

32. Leon, A. S., Connett, J., Jacobs, D. R., & Rauramaa, R. (1987). Leisure time physical activity levels and risk of coronary heart disease and death: The multiple risk factor intervention trial. *Journal of the American Medical Association, 258,* 2388–2395.

33. Lightfoot, J. T., Tuller, B., & Williams, D. F. (1996). Ambient noise interferes with auscultatory blood pressure measurement during exercise. *Medicine and Science in Sports and Exercise, 28,* 502–508.

34. Londe, S., & Klitzner, T. S. (1984). Auscultatory blood pressure measurement—Effect of pressure on the head of the stethoscope. *Western Journal of Medicine, 141,* 193–195.

35. Madhavan, S., Ooi, W. L., Cohen, H., & Alderman, M. H. (1994). Relation of pulse pressure reduction to the incidence of myocardial infarction. *Hypertension, 24,* 368.

36. Manning, D. M., Kuchirka, C., & Kaminski, J. (1983). Miscuffing: Inappropriate blood pressure cuff application. *Circulation, 68,* 763–766.

37. Milnor, W. R. (1968). Normal circulatory function. In V. B. Mountcastle (Ed.), *Medical physiology I* (pp. 118–133). St. Louis: Mosby.

38. National High Blood Pressure Education Program Working Group. (1993). Report on primary prevention of hypertension. *Archives of Internal Medicine, 153,* 186–208.

39. Peters, R. K., Cady, L. D., Bischoff, D. P., Bernstein, L., & Pike, M. C. (1983). Physical fitness and subsequent myocardial infarction in healthy workers. *Journal of the American Medical Association, 249,* 3052–3056.

40. Pollock, M. L., Wilmore, J. H., & Fox, S. M. (1978). *Health and fitness through physical activity.* Santa Barbara, CA: John Wiley & Sons.

41. Powell, K. E., Thompson, P. D., Caspersen, C. J., & Kendrick, J. S. (1987). Physical activity and the incidence of coronary heart disease. *Annual Review of Public Health, 8,* 253–287.

42. Prisant, L. M., Alpert, B. S., Robbins, C. B., Berson, A. S., Hayes, M., Cohen, M. L., & Sheps, S. G. (1995). American national standard for nonautomated sphygmomanometers. Summary report. *American Journal of Hypertension, 8,* 210–213.

43. Robinson, T. E., Sue, D. Y., Huszczuk, A., Weiler-Ravell, D., & Hansen, J. E. (1988). Intra-arterial and cuff blood pressure responses during incremental cycle ergometry. *Medicine and Science in Sports and Exercise, 20,* 142–149.

44. Slattery, M. L., Jacobs, D. R., & Nichaman, M. Z. (1989). Leisure time physical activity and coronary heart disease death: The U.S. railroad study. *Circulation, 79,* 304–311.

45. Task Force on Blood Pressure Control in Children. (1977). Report of the task force on blood pressure control in children. *Pediatrics 59* (Suppl.), 797–820.

46. Task Force on Blood Pressure Control in Children. (1987). Report of the task force on blood pressure control in children. *Pediatrics, 79,* 1–25.

47. Webster, J., Newnham, D., Petrie, J. C., & Lovell, H. G. (1984). Influence of arm position on measurement of blood pressure. *British Medical Journal, 288,* 1574–1575.

48. Walther, R. J., Tifft, C. P. (1985). High blood pressure in the competitive athlete: Guidelines and recommendations. *The Physician and Sportsmedicine, 13*(3) 93–114.

49. White, W. B., Berson, A. S., Robbins, C., Jamieson, M. J., Prisant, L. M., & Roccella, S. G. (1993). National standard for measurement of resting and ambulatory pressures with automated sphygmomanometers. *Hypertension, 21,* 504–509.

50. WHO/ISH. (1983). Guidelines for the treatment of mild hypertension. Memorandum from a WHO/ISH meeting. *Hypertension, 5,* 394–397.

51. Wilmore, J. H., & Costill, D. L. (1994). *Physiology of sport and exercise.* Champaign, IL: Human Kinetics.

52. Wilmore, J. H., Stanforth, P. R., Gagnon, J., Rice, T., Mandel, S., Leon, A. S., Rao, D. C., Skinner, J. S., & Bouchard, C. (2001). Heart rate and blood pressure changes with endurance training: The HERITAGE Family Study. *Medicine and Science in Sports and Exercise, 33,* 107–116.

Form 16.1

Individual Data for Resting Blood Pressure

Name [＿＿＿＿＿＿＿＿＿＿] Date [＿＿＿＿] Time [＿＿] A.M. [＿] P.M. [＿]

Age [＿] y   Gender (M or W) [＿]   Ht [＿＿] cm   Wt [＿＿] kg   [＿＿] N   Tech. Initials [＿]

Meteorological Data

Temperature (T) [＿＿] °C   RH [＿＿] % P_B [＿＿] mm Hg

Blood Pressure Data

Arm circumference [＿] cm   Cuff type: Large adult [＿] Adult [＿] Child

Body position: Seated [＿]   Supine [＿]   Standing [＿]   Arm: Rt [＿] Left [＿]

Auscultatory Method of Sphygmomanometry

Aneroid: (Rt. arm)   **(Left arm)**   **Mercury: (Rt. arm)**   **(Left arm)**

1st	4th	5th		1st	4th	5th		1st	4th	5th		1st	4th	5th	
[＿]	/ [＿]	/ [＿] mm Hg;		[＿]	/ [＿]	/ [＿] mm Hg;		[＿]	/ [＿]	/ [＿] mm Hg;		[＿]	/ [＿]	/ [＿] mm Hg	

Additional measurement
If first two differ > 5mm Hg:

1st	4th	5th		1st	4th	5th		1st	4th	5th	
[＿]	/ [＿]	/ [＿] mm Hg;		[＿]	/ [＿]	/ [＿] mm Hg;		[＿]	/ [＿]	/ [＿] mm Hg	

Average of two
or more measurements:

1st	4th	5th		1st	4th	5th		1st	4th	5th	
[＿]	/ [＿]	/ [＿] mm Hg;		[＿]	/ [＿]	/ [＿] mm Hg;		[＿]	/ [＿]	/ [＿] mm Hg	

Auscultatory gap: [＿] Yes [＿] No   Irregular pulse: [＿] Yes [＿] No   %tile [＿] Table 16.4

PP = SP [1st ＿] – DP [5th ＿] = [＿] mm Hg (use highest average of arms)

MBP = [(SP [1st ＿] – DP [5th ＿])/3] + DP [5th ＿] mm Hg

      SP – DP (or PP)

= ([＿])/3 + DP [5th ＿]

   (SP – DP)/3

= [＿] + DP [5th ＿] = [＿] mm Hg

Form 16.2

Group Data for Resting (Sitting) Blood Pressure (mm Hg)

Initials	Systolic	Diastolic 4th	Diastolic 5th	Initials	Systolic	Diastolic 4th	Diastolic 5th
MEN				WOMEN			
1.				1.			
2.				2.			
3.				3.			
4.				4.			
5.				5.			
6.				6.			
7.				7.			
8.				8.			
9.				9.			
10.				10.			
11.				11.			
12.				12.			
13.				13.			
14.				14.			
15.				15.			
16.				16.			
17.				17.			
18.				18.			
19.				19.			
20.				20.			
M				M			
Minimum				Minimum			
Maximum				Maximum			

EXERCISE BLOOD PRESSURE

It is just as important to measure blood pressure at exercise as it is to measure heart rate. If only heart rate is measured, blood pressure is neglected as a contributor to the total power output of the heart. The consideration of both heart rate and blood pressure provides a better estimate of myocardial oxygen consumption than heart rate alone, and the calculation of the rate-pressure product provides an indication of the heart's power output.[10,37]

The measurement of systolic pressure during progressive exercise may provide input toward diagnosing heart disease[56] and may reveal potential problems in those persons who show exaggerated increases in exercise blood pressure despite being normotensive under a resting state.[18,35,36] Conversely, decreases in systolic blood pressure, despite increases in exercise intensity, may be clinically significant if accompanied by cardiac ischemia or pectoris angina (chest pain).[2]

The pulse pressure—the difference between systolic and diastolic pressure—provides the basis for calculating mean pressure at exercise (Figure 17.1). Last, the measurement of blood pressure during recovery from exercise may lead to the prevention of syncope (fainting) in the performer.

Physiological Rationale

Numerous factors may affect blood pressure at exercise. These include characteristics of the performers, such as their age, muscle mass, fitness level, and smoking status. Also, the type of exercise may affect blood pressure.[57] For example, weight lifting in five 22- to 28-year-old body builders increased intra-arterial blood pressure during leg presses to 355 mm Hg over 281 mm Hg.[11] This is higher than in rhythmical aerobic exercise, such as cycling or walking. Differences are found even among types of aerobic exercise; cycling, for example, elicits higher blood pressures than treadmill exercise.[31,48] Additionally, the exercise protocol itself may affect the rate of increase and absolute levels of blood pressure during exercise.

Blood pressure is mainly a function of cardiac output and peripheral resistance. The increase in blood pressure during exercise is due to the increased cardiac output. Despite a decrease in peripheral resistance due to dilation of muscle arterioles, the large increase in cardiac output more than makes up for the decreased peripheral resistance.

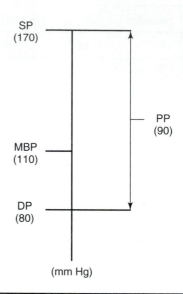

Figure 17.1 Mean blood pressure (MBP) is one-third of pulse pressure (PP) plus diastolic pressure (DP). For example, a blood pressure during exercise of 170/80/80 mm Hg produces a pulse pressure of 90 mm Hg and a mean pressure of 110 mm Hg.

Blood Pressure During Aerobic Exercise

Systolic pressure is expected to increase rather linearly,[3,54] and diastolic pressure changes very little, if at all, during progressive aerobic exercise (Figure 17.2)[9,13,16] when measured by noninvasive sphygmomanometry.

As mentioned in Chapter 16, mean blood pressure (MBP) is calculated from pulse pressure (PP). The traditional equation is recommended, although one group of investigators concluded that it may be more valid to use one-half the distance between cuff-determined fifth-phase diastolic pressure and systolic pressure, as the mean pressure.[54]

The traditional mean pressure as one-third the distance between systolic and diastolic pressure appears to be justified until further research confirms otherwise.

The Power Output of the Heart

The heart is affected by both its rate of pumping (b·min⁻¹) and the force or resistance (mm Hg) it has to pump against. This power output of the heart is often referred to as either the **double product** or the **rate-pressure product (RPP)** because of the multiplication of the two factors,

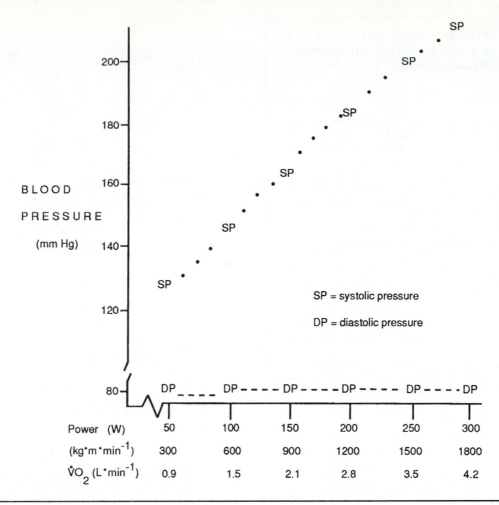

Figure 17.2 Relationship between systolic and fifth-phase diastolic blood pressures versus exercise intensity in a typical 70 kg man.

heart rate (HR) and systolic pressure (SP). The RPP, as calculated from Equation 17.1, is not meant to reflect differences in stroke volumes between individuals but is an accurate reflection of the myocardial oxygen requirement.[2,20,40] The product of HR and SP is divided by 100 in order to reduce the value to a convenient unit[53] and to agree closely with the oxygen consumption (mL·min⁻¹) of the heart. The *rate* of myocardial fiber shortening, an important factor in the contractility of the heart, is not included in the derived RPP.[24]

$$RPP = (HR \times SP) \div 100 \qquad \text{Eq. 17.1}$$

where:

HR = heart rate (b·min⁻¹)

SP = systolic pressure (mm Hg)

For example, if the heart rate is 150 b·min⁻¹ and systolic pressure is 200 mm Hg during exercise, then the RPP may be calculated as

$$(150 \times 200) \div 100 = 30\,000 \div 100 = 300$$

Method

The measurement of blood pressure during exercise is one of the most common measurements in an exercise laboratory. However, the technique is one of the most difficult to master, requiring many trials before the technician becomes confident. Although standards exist for measuring *resting* blood pressure, no such standards exist for *exercise* blood pressure.[25]

As expected, there are many similarities between the measurement of blood pressure at rest and at exercise. The differences include minor adjustments to the blood pressure technique and a more intense concentration on the fourth phase (muffling). During exercise it is not unusual for the vibrations to be heard even near zero levels[43] due to enhanced vasodilation at exercise.[22] Thus, the fifth phase is not a valid indicator of diastolic pressure during exercise tests in some people. For this reason, the American Heart Association recommends the recording of the fourth phase for exercise testing.[23] See Box 17.1 for a discussion on the accuracy of exercise blood pressure measurements.

BOX 17.1 Accuracy and Calibration of Exercise Blood Pressure Measurements

Validity

The ability to measure exercise blood pressure accurately is complicated by the noise of the equipment and movement of the performer. Although the indirect noninvasive measurement of **systolic pressure** has been reported to be satisfactory,[47] it appears that the noninvasive cuff method of measuring systolic pressure underestimates the invasive direct measure of systolic pressure anywhere from 8 mm Hg[30,45] up to 11 mm Hg[54] or 15 mm Hg[30] during aerobic exercise.

One group of investigators[54] found that the intra-arterial **diastolic pressures** exceeded the noninvasive fourth and fifth phases for diastolic pressure by 5 mm Hg and 13 mm Hg, respectively. This supports the use of the indirectly measured fourth phase as the most valid diastolic pressure during exercise. Their correlations between intra-arterial pressures and cuff pressures were .95 and .84 for systolic and diastolic (fourth phase) pressures, respectively. However, the fourth phase is not as clearly distinguishable as the fifth phase.

One group of reviewers recommended manual or automated sphygmomanometry to measure systolic pressure if the goal is to estimate the rate-pressure product.[25]

Reliability

Although various investigators have not supported high reliabilities in automated blood pressure methods,[4,5,41,50] including the measurement of diastolic blood pressure during recovery,[36] some have concluded that a few automated devices are a suitable alternative to human auscultatory methods.[25,42]

Calibration of Automated Blood Pressure Instruments

Automated blood pressure instruments are more widely accepted for research if they have been calibrated. For example, the heralded HERITAGE Family Study investigators use an automated device (Colin-STBP-780™, San Antonio, TX) after calibrating it with a mercury manometer and verifying the readings by listening with headphones. They calibrate it at mercury manometer pressures of 0, 50, 100, 150, and 200 mm Hg.[59]

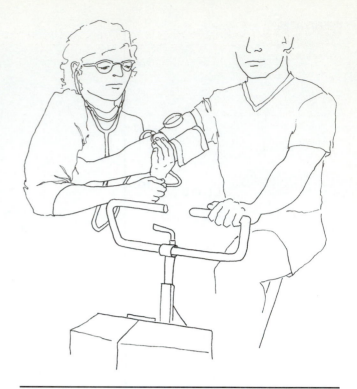

Figure 17.3 An appropriate position for the technician and performer while blood pressure is being measured at pre-exercise or during exercise.

so that the tubing runs along the back of the upper arm rather than the front, especially during treadmill exercise.

Contraindicative Blood Pressure

Another consideration in measuring blood pressure at exercise is whether to perform the exercise test in the first place. The term *contraindicative* means that for some people "the risks of exercise testing outweigh the potential benefits."[2] For example, the risk is greater than the benefit of exercise testing for someone who has just had a heart attack or someone with uncontrolled erratic heart rhythm accompanied by disturbing symptoms. Some authorities suggest that exercise testing is contraindicated if systolic is greater than 180 mm Hg or diastolic greater than 100 mm Hg.[51] The American College of Sports Medicine (2000) takes a more liberal view by having no **absolute** contraindication criteria for blood pressure but providing **relative** contraindicative criteria. This means that, if resting systolic pressures are greater than 200 mm Hg or diastolic pressures are greater than 110 mm Hg, then the risk-benefit ratio must be evaluated before exercise testing.[2]

Relative Contraindicative Blood Pressure	
SP > 200 mm Hg	DP > 110 mm Hg

If the performer tenses the arm while the technician is taking the blood pressure, it will cause large oscillations in the aneroid pointer or the mercury column. Presumably, this is due to the changes in upper arm circumference as the muscles contract and relax. Thus, it is very important to promote muscle relaxation of the performer's arm (Figure 17.3). Also, it is important to clear the antecubital space for the placement of the stethoscope's diaphragm. Sometimes the cuff will slide toward the elbow during exercise, or the bladder's rubber tubes will interfere with the antecubital space. Some researchers advise placing the cuff

Table 17.1 Cycling Protocols for Exercise Blood Pressure

Pre-exercise

Seated on cycle ergometer

	Exercise[a]		
	Low-Power	**Moderate-Power**	**High-Power**
$\dot{V}O_2$max (L·min⁻¹) history	< 2.1	2.1–2.9	> 2.9
Time	**Power Prescription (W)**		
0:00–3:00	50	75	100
3:00–6:00	100	125	150
6:00–9:00	150	175	200
	Recovery		
9:00–12:00 Cooldown on ergometer	25	50	75
11:00–14:00	Seated in chair		

Note: Treadmill protocols are in Chapters 15 and 19. [a]The three columns of exercise protocols represent three different fitness levels based on a person's maximal oxygen consumption.

Protocol for Exercise Blood Pressure

Three multistage cycling protocols are presented in Table 17.1. Technicians usually find it easier to measure blood pressure when performers cycle than when they walk or run on a treadmill. In order to prescribe an appropriate exercise protocol, consideration should be given to the performer's fitness level. The prescription can be based upon prior tests of aerobic or physical power on the prospective performer. An exercise interval of 3 min should assure a steady state at each stage.[43] The exercise period starts at 50, 75, or 100 W (300, 450, or 600 kg·m·min⁻¹), depending upon the fitness level of the performer. Power levels are increased by 50 W after each 3 min interval. Until the technician gains considerable confidence, repeated measures should be taken throughout the test; only the pressures measured at the last 30 s of each power level, however, need to be recorded.

In order to calculate the rate pressure product (RPP), the heart rate must be measured by either another technician with a stethoscope or by heart-rate monitor.

Summary of Procedures

The major differences in the technique for measuring blood pressure at exercise versus that at rest are the following: (a) the technician must support the exerciser's arm; (b) greater listening concentration is required due to the noise of the ergometer; and (c) the muffling point (fourth phase) is used sometimes as the primary indicator of diastolic pressure at exercise.[54,58] The procedural steps for measuring blood pressure are as follows.

Pre-Exercise

1. Obtain baseline blood pressures by measuring first-, fourth-, and fifth-phase pressures while the performer is resting on the cycle ergometer (or standing on the treadmill if it is the chosen mode).

a. With the cuff around the performer's arm, place that arm between your elbow and the side of your body (Figure 17.3).
b. Instruct the performer to relax the arm as much as possible.
c. While taking the pressure, maintain the performer's arm in an extended position.
d. Especially for treadmill exercise, tape or strap the stethoscope's diaphragm and the BP cuff to the performer's arm; you may need to remove the air bulb intermittently.

Exercise

2. Use Step #1 procedures for taking blood pressure during exercise, but allow cuff pressure to fall faster at about 5 to 6 mm Hg per second.[49]
3. Follow the exercise protocol for cycle ergometry (Table 17.1 or any of the Treadmill protocols in Chapters 15 and 19).
4. Record the blood pressure that was taken during the last 30 s of each exercise stage. Remeasure immediately if systolic pressure has decreased from prior stage's reading.
5. Take auscultatory or telemetered heart rate during these times in order to calculate rate-pressure product.

Recovery

6. Measure blood pressure during the last 30 s of each minute of the cooldown period while the performer pedals at 25 W, 50 W, or 75 W.
7. Measure blood pressure during the last 30 s of each minute during the recovery period while the performer is seated in a chair. Continue monitoring until blood pressure stabilizes.

Graph

8. Graph blood pressures (mean pressure optional) on Form 17.3.

Table 17.2 Comparative Blood Pressure Values at Submaximal Exercise, Maximal Exercise, and Recovery

	Systolic (mm Hg)	Diastolic (mm Hg)	
		4th Phase	5th Phase
Submaximal Exercise			
Cycling			
Normotense:	< 200	≈ ↑ from resting	↔ ≈ ↑ ≈ ↓ from resting
	10–18 per 50 W↑	7–11 per V̇O₂ L·min⁻¹↑	
	30 per V̇O₂ L·min⁻¹↑	≈ 5 per 50 W↑	
Hypotense:	↓ with P increase		
	↓ > 15 at given P		
Hypertense:	> normotense ↑		↑ > 10–15 from resting
Treadmill			
Normotense:	7–10 per MET↑	↑ < cycling ↑	
Hypertense:	> 20 per MET↑		
Maximal Exercise			≈ ↑ from resting
Normotense:			
General population	150–250		
Young adults:	150–250; 200		
Treadmill			
Active M (44 y)	190 ± 23		
Sedentary M (45 y)	185 ± 22		
Active W (42 y)	159 ± 19		
Sedentary W (48 y)	166 ± 23		
Hypertense:	220–230; ↑ > 96 from rest	95; ↑ > 15	
Hypotense:	↓ with P ↑; ↑ < 33 from rest to max		
Recovery	Return to pre-exercise level within 5 min to 8 min; possibly < pre-exercise up to 60 min to 90 min		

Note: ≈ = slight; ↑ = increase; ↔ = no change; ↓ = decrease; P = power level; M = men; W = women or watts.

Results and Discussion

Various criteria and expectations for exercise blood pressure are presented in Table 17.2 for comparative purposes. The table is organized into submaximal and maximal levels of exercise intensity, in addition to recovery from exercise.

Blood Pressure at Submaximal Aerobic Exercise

Even before exercise begins, persons anticipating the exercise test may have a systolic pressure about 10 mm Hg higher than their normal resting pressure.[14] Theoretically, **systolic pressure** is expected to increase somewhat linearly during aerobic cycling by approximately 10 mm Hg[44] or 15 mm Hg[3] for each 50 W (300 kg·m min⁻¹) increase in cycling power level. One group of investigators reported a rate of increase of 18 mm Hg per 50 W based on a 30 mm Hg increase per liter increase in oxygen consumption on less active persons monitored by intra-arterial catheter.[54]

During treadmill exercise, one might expect a 10 mm Hg (± 2) increase per MET increase.[2] It would be unusual for exercise heart rate to exceed systolic pressure in young adults. A hypertensive response in treadmill exercise may be indicated when systolic pressure increases at a rate greater than 20 mm Hg per MET,[19] or per 0.25 L·min⁻¹ oxygen consumption. If systolic pressure fails to increase at all with progressive exercise, or actually decreases, it may be a sign of coronary artery disease[56] or a high risk indication.[1,2,21]

More controversy exists regarding **diastolic pressure** changes than systolic pressure changes during exercise. Fifth-phase diastolic pressure usually decreases or stays the same in healthy persons.[2] Part of this controversy may be attributed to the method of measuring diastolic pressure. One group concluded that the noninvasive fifth-phase diastolic pressure decreases slightly from rest to heavy cycling by only 3 mm Hg, but the fourth-phase cuff pressure and intra-arterial diastolic pressure increases from rest through maximal cycling by about 7 to 11 mm Hg per liter of oxygen consumed.[54]

Some report decreases in fifth-phase diastolic pressure with progressive exercise in highly fit persons.[9,46] Others claim that a normal fifth-phase diastolic pressure response to exercise is one that does not increase by more than 10 mm Hg[18] to 15 mm Hg.[56] During treadmill exercise, many healthy persons show slight increases in diastolic pressure of no more than 10 mm Hg during the first couple of minutes, followed by a progressive reduction into the peak exercise period.[12] Others report a slight decrease or no change in diastolic pressure in healthy men during treadmill exercise.[60]

The **mean blood pressures (MBP)** of healthy sedentary males and females (17 y to 29 y) were determined at 50 W and 60 % V̇O₂max, respectively. The 95 males averaged a MBP of 94 (± 9.1) mm Hg and 105 (± 9.9) mm Hg, respectively. The 134 females' MBP were 90 (± 9.7) mm Hg and 101 (± 12.0) mm Hg, respectively.[59]

Blood Pressure at Maximal Aerobic Exercise

Quite often it is impossible to get a technically reliable blood pressure measurement while the performer is exercising at or near maximal intensity. In these cases, the blood pressure should be taken immediately after exercise with

Table 17.3 Peak Systolic and Diastolic Blood Pressures of Apparently Healthy Men and Women during Maximal Treadmill Testing[a]

Age y	Men		Women	
	Systolic *M (SD)*	Diastolic *M (SD)*	Systolic *M (SD)*	Diastolic *M (SD)*
20–29	182 (21)	71 (12)	156 (20)	70 (12)
30–39	184 (20)	76 (12)	160 (22)	74 (11)
40–49	188 (21)	80 (12)	167 (23)	78 (11)
50–59	193 (23)	83 (12)	177 (24)	81 (12)
60–69	197 (24)	84 (12)	186 (24)	81 (13)
70–79	196 (27)	84 (13)	185 (25)	83 (10)

Note: [a]Bruce protocol in 7863 men and 2406 women during the years 1988 to 1992. Adapted with permission from Daida, H., Allison, T. G., Squires, R. W., Miller, T. D., & Gau, G. T. (1996). Peak exercise blood pressure stratified by age and gender in apparently healthy subjects. *Mayo Clinic Proceedings, 71,* 445–452.

precautions taken to avoid postural (orthostatic) syncope in the performer; usually, this would mean easy walking on the treadmill (or in place) or easy pedalling on the ergometer. The peak blood pressure may be slightly underestimated by waiting to take blood pressure immediately after exercise, rather than during exercise.[32]

Maximal systolic pressure can be quite variable, ranging from 150 mm Hg to 250 mm Hg in men and women,[9] with an average in a normal young adult about 182 mm Hg[15] up to 200 mm Hg.[28] This concurs with other investigators who reported a maximal systolic pressure of 194 (± 20) mm Hg for running on the treadmill.[17] Normotensive middle-aged persons reach maximal systolic pressures between 180 mm Hg and 190 mm Hg.[10] Table 17.3 provides the mean systolic and diastolic pressures at peak exercise during treadmill testing of males and females from 18 y to 79 y of age. Men's pressures were higher than women's pressures and were positively related to age.[15] If systolic blood pressure exceeds 240 mm Hg, it may indicate a susceptibility for developing resting hypertension.[38]

Sometimes during an exercise test, the blood pressure reaches a level that calls for termination of the test. A systolic pressure greater than 260 mm Hg is a **general** indication by ACSM for stopping the test in a low-risk person.[2] Ruptures have occurred in the blood vessels of experimental animals when systolic pressures were between 260 and 280 mm Hg.[29] Others suggest caution and consider it a hypertensive response if the systolic pressure exceeds 220 mm Hg.[8,12] Some consider the exercise response as hypertensive if the systolic pressure increases by more than 96 mm Hg from the resting level, and as hypotensive if the systolic pressure does not increase more than 33 mm Hg at maximal exercise.[52]

Caution may be prudent when the performer's exercise **diastolic pressure** reaches 95 mm Hg.[8] However, the ACSM's indication for halting the test for low-risk adults is when DP exceeds 115 mm Hg.[2]

STOP Test!*	
SP > 260 mm Hg	DP > 115 mm Hg

*The ACSM criteria for stopping a test performed by a high-risk person under a clinical setting are ≥ 250 mm Hg and ≥ 110 mm Hg.[2]

Typical **mean** arterial pressures at maximal exercise are approximately 130 mm Hg, but may reach as high as 155 mm Hg.[9] A large group (*n* = 95) of 17- to 29-year-old males' MBP averaged 122 mm Hg at maximal cycling exercise. The average MBP for the females (*n* = 134) of the same age was 117 mm Hg.[59]

Blood Pressure during Recovery from Aerobic Exercise

Blood pressure often returns to the pre-exercise level within 5 min to 8 min after the cessation of moderate exercise.[34,44,55] It is not unusual for systolic pressure to drop slightly lower than the pre-exercise systolic pressure[6,27,28,39] and remain lower for several hours.[2] For example, from the 5th to the 60th,[38] or up to the 90th min[6] of recovery from treadmill walking, systolic blood pressure was slightly lower (8 to 12 mm Hg) than it was preceding exercise, possibly due to endorphin-like (opioid) effects.[7]

Usually, diastolic pressure during recovery remains similar to pre-exercise. The return of blood pressure to resting levels is affected by the type, intensity, and duration of the original exercise in addition to the type of recovery. For example, it requires more than 3 min for blood pressure to return to normal after heavy cycling exercise (85 % $\dot{V}O_2$max) if the cyclist recovers with unloaded pedaling at a slow rate.[54] However, if the performer were to stand upright immediately after the same exercise, it is quite possible that blood pressure would drop rapidly and drastically. Venous pooling of blood in the legs would reduce the blood flow to the brain and possibly lead to syncope. Post-exercise hypotensive symptoms are most likely after bouts of exercise lasting 30 min or more. Recovery hypotension is due to various factors besides venous pooling, such as cessation of muscle pump during passive recovery, loss of plasma volume due to sweating, reduced venous return, and reduced vasoconstriction.[26]

Rate-Pressure Product (RPP)

The mean resting rate pressure product in 1623 healthy men and women ranging from 20 y to 70 y of age was 75 ± 17.5 mm Hg. At maximal exercise of the Bruce treadmill protocol, the RPP averaged 328 ± 44.6.[33] The assumed myocardial oxygen consumption ($\dot{V}O_2$myo) at maximal exercise more than quadrupled the resting $\dot{V}O_2$myo. The men's maximal RPP was higher than the women's maximal RPP. Rate-pressure products at maximal exercise in active men and active women of a wide age range were 341 ± 55 and 281 ± 37 respectively.[10]

References

1. American Association of Cardiovascular and Pulmonary Rehabilitation. (1999). *Guidelines for cardiac rehabilitation and secondary prevention programs.* Champaign, IL: Human Kinetics.

2. American College of Sports Medicine. (2000). *ACSM's guidelines for exercise testing and prescription.* Philadelphia: Lippincott Williams & Wilkins.

3. Andersen, K. L., Shephard, R. J., Denolin, H., Varnauskas, E., & Masironi, R. (1971). *Fundamentals of exercise testing.* Geneva, Switzerland: World Health Organization.

4. Barker, W. F., Hediger, M. L., Katz, S. H., & Bowers, E. J. (1984). Concurrent validity studies of blood pressure instrumentation. *Hypertension, 6,* 85–91.

5. Becque, M. D., Katch, V., Marks, C., & Dyer, R. (1993). Reliability within subject variability of VE, $\dot{V}O_2$, heart rate and blood pressure during submaximum cycle ergometry. *International Journal of Sports Medicine, 14,* 220–223.

6. Bennett, T., Wilcox, R. G., & MacDonald, I. A. (1984). Postexercise reduction of blood pressure in hypertensive men is not due to an acute impairment of baroreflex function. *Clinical Science, 67,* 97–103.

7. Boone, J. B., Levine, M., Flynn, M. G., Przza, F. Y., Kubitz, E. R., & Andres, F. F. (1992). Opioid receptor modulation of postexercise hypotension. *Medicine and Science in Sports and Exercise, 24,* 1108–1113.

8. Boyer, J. (1976). Exercise and hypertension. *The Physician and Sportsmedicine, 4*(12) 35–49.

9. Brooks, G. A., & Fahey, T. D. (1984). *Exercise physiology: Human bioenergetics and its application.* New York: John Wiley & Sons.

10. Bruce, R. A. (1977). Current concepts in cardiology: Exercise testing for evaluation of ventricular function. *New England Journal of Medicine, 296,* 671–675.

11. Carswell, H. (1984). Brief reports. Headaches: A weighty problem for lifters? *The Physician and Sportsmedicine, 12*(7), 23.

12. Chung, E. K. (1983). *Exercise electrocardiography— A practical approach.* Baltimore: Waverly Press.

13. Clarke, D. H. (1975). *Exercise physiology.* Englewood Cliffs, NJ: Prentice-Hall.

14. Cooper, C. B. (2000). Blood pressure measurement, hypertension and endurance exercise. *ACSM's Health and Fitness Journal, 4,* 32–33.

15. Daida, H., Allison, T. G., Squires, R.W., Miller, T. D., & Gau, G. T. (1996). Peak exercise blood pressure stratified by age and gender in apparently healthy subjects. *Mayo Clinic Proceedings, 71,* 445–452.

16. deVries, H. A. (1986). *Physiology of exercise for physical education and athletics.* Dubuque, IA: Wm. C. Brown.

17. Dishman, R. K., Patton, R. W., Smith, J., Weinberg, R., & Jackson, A. (1987). Using perceived exertion to prescribe and monitor exercise training heart rate. *International Journal of Sports Medicine, 8,* 208–213.

18. Dlin, R. A., Hanne, N., Silverberg, D. S., & Bar-Or, O. (1983). Follow-up of normotensive men with exaggerated blood pressure response to exercise. *American Heart Journal, 106,* 316–320.

19. Dressendorfer, R. H. (1980, July). *ACSM workshop manual,* p. 110.

20. Edington, D. W., & Cunningham, L. (1975). *Biological awareness.* Englewood Cliffs, NJ: Prentice-Hall.

21. Fletcher, G. F., Balady, G., Froelicher, V. F., Hartley, L. H., Haskell, W. L., & Pollock, M. L. (1995). Exercise standards: A statement for health care professionals from the American Heart Association. *Circulation, 91,* 580–615.

22. Frohlich, E. D., Grim, C., Labarthe, D. R., Maxwell, M. H., Perloff, D., & Weidman, W. H. (1987). *Recommendations for human blood pressure determination by sphygmomanometers: Report of a special task force appointed by the steering committee, American Heart Association.* Dallas: National Center, American Heart Association.

23. Frohlich, E. D., Grim, C., Labarthe, D. R., Maxwell, M. H., Perloff, D., & Weidman, W. H. (1988). Recommendations for human blood pressure determination by sphygmomanometers: Report of a special task force appointed by the steering committee. *Hypertension, 11,* 210A–222A.

24. Gianelly, R. E., Goldman, R. H., Treister, B., & Harrison, D. C. (1967). Propranolol in patients with angina pectoris. *Annals of Internal Medicine, 67,* 1216–1224.

25. Griffin, S. A., Robergs, R. A., & Heyward, V. H. (1997). Blood pressure measurement during exercise: A review. *Medicine and Science in Sports and Exercise, 29,* 149–159.

26. Halliwill, J. R. (2001). Mechanisms and clinical implications of post-exercise hypotension in humans. *Exercise and Sport Sciences Reviews, 29,* 65–70.

27. Hannum, S. M., & Kasch, F. W. (1981). Acute postexercise blood pressure response of hypertensive and normotensive men. *Scandinavian Journal of Sport Science, 3,* 11–15.

28. Hayberg, J. M., Montain, S. J., & Martin, W. H. (1987). Blood pressure and hemodynamic responses after exercise in older hypertensives. *Journal of Applied Physiology, 63,* 270–276.

29. Hellerstein, H. K. (1976). Exercise tests inadequate for cardiac patients. *The Physician and Sportsmedicine, 4*(8) 58–62.

30. Henschel, A., De la Vega, F., & Taylor, H. L. (1954). Simultaneous direct and indirect blood pressure measurements in man at rest and work. *Journal of Applied Physiology, 6,* 506–512.

31. Hermansen, L., Ekblom, B., & Saltin, B. (1970). Cardiac output during submaximal and maximal treadmill and bicycle exercise. *Journal of Applied Physiology, 29,* 82–86.

32. Hollingsworth, V., Bendick, P., & Franklin, B. (1988). Validity of postexercise arm ergometer blood pressures? *Medicine and Science in Sports and Exercise, 20* (Suppl. 2), Abstract #435, S73.

33. Hui, S. C., Jackson, A. S., & Wier, L. T. (2000). Development of normative values for resting and exercise rate pressure product. *Medicine and Science in Sports and Exercise, 32,* 1520–1527.

34. Hyman, A. S. (1971). Cardiorespiratory endurance. In ACSM (Eds.), *Encyclopedia of sport sciences and medicine* (pp. 1067–1070). New York: Macmillan.

35. Jette, M., Landry, F., Sidney, K., & Blumchen, G. (1988). Exaggerated blood pressure response to exercise in the detection of hypertension. *Journal of Cardiopulmonary Rehabilitation, 8,* 171–177.

36. Jette, M., Landry, F., Tiemann, B., & Blumchen, G. (1991). Ambulatory blood pressure and Holter monitoring during tennis play. *Canadian Journal of Sport Science, 16,* 40–44.

37. Jorgensen, C. R. (1972). Physical training and myocardial function. *New England Journal of Medicine, 287,* 104–105.

38. Kaplan, N. M., Deveraux, R. B., & Miller, H. S. (1994). Systemic hypertension. *Medicine and Science in Sports and Exercise, 26*(10), S268–S270.

39. Kaufman, F. L., Hughson, R. L., & Schaman, J. P. (1987). Effect of exercise on recovery blood pressure in normotensive and hypertensive subjects. *Medicine and Science in Sports and Exercise, 19,* 17–20.

40. Kitamura, K., Jorgensen, C. R., Gobel, F. L., Taylor, H. L., & Wang, Y. (1972). Hemodynamic correlates of myocardial oxygen consumption during upright exercise. *Journal of Applied Physiology, 32,* 516–522.

41. LaBarthe, D. R. (1976). New instruments for measuring blood pressure. *Drugs, 11* (Suppl. I), 48–51.

42. Lightfoot, J. T., Tankersley, C., Rowe, S. A., Freed, A. N., & Fortney, S. M. (1989). Automated blood pressure measurements during exercise. *Medicine and Science in Sports and Exercise 21,* 698–707.

43. Lightfoot, J. T., Tuller, B., & Williams, D. F. (1996). Ambient noise interferes with auscultatory blood pressure measurement during exercise. *Medicine and Science in Sports and Exercise, 28,* 502–508.

44. Michael, E. D., Burke, E. J., & Avakian, E. V. (1979). *Laboratory experiments in exercise physiology.* Ithaca, NY: Mouvement.

45. Morehouse L. E., & Miller, A. T. (1976). *Physiology of exercise.* St. Louis: Mosby.

46. Nagle, F. J. (1975, May). *Conducting the progressive exercise test.* Symposium at the 22nd Annual American College of Sports Medicine Convention, New Orleans.

47. Nagle, F. J., Naughton, J., & Balke, B. (1966). Comparison of direct and indirect blood pressure with pressure-flow dynamics during exercise. *Journal of Applied Physiology, 21,* 317–320.

48. Niederberger, M., Bruce, R., Kusumi, F., & Whitkanack, S. (1974). Disparities in ventilatory and circulatory responses to bicycle and treadmill exercise. *British Heart Journal, 36,* 377–382.

49. Nieman, D. C. (1995). *Fitness and sports medicine: A health-related approach.* Palo Alto, CA: Bull.

50. O'Brien, E., Fitzgerald, D., & O'Malley, K. (1985). Blood pressure measurement: Current practice and future trends. *British Medical Journal, 290,* 729–733.

51. Pollock, M. L., Wilmore, J. H., & Fox, S. M. (1978). *Health and fitness through physical activity.* Santa Barbara, CA: John Wiley & Sons.

52. Pyfer, H. R., Mead, W. F., Frederick, R. C., & Doane, B. L. (1976). Exercise rehabilitation in coronary heart disease: Community group programs. *Archives of Physical Medicine and Rehabilitation, 57,* 335–342.

53. Robinson, B. F. (1967). Relation of heart rate and systolic blood pressure to the onset of pain in angina pectoris. *Circulation, 35,* 1073–1083.

54. Robinson, T. E., Sue, D. Y., Huszczuk, A., Weiler-Ravell, D., & Hansen, J. E. (1988). Intra-arterial and cuff blood pressure responses during incremental cycle ergometry. *Medicine and Science in Sports and Exercise, 20,* 142–149.

55. Ruddell, H., Berg, K., Todd, G. L., McKinney, M. E., Buell, T. C., & Eliot, R. S. (1985). Cardiovascular reactivity and blood chemical changes during exercise. *Journal of Sports Medicine, 25,* 111–119.

56. Sheps, D. S., Ernst, J. C., Briese, F. W., & Myerburg, R. J. (1979). Exercise-induced increase in diastolic pressure: Indicator of severe coronary artery disease. *The American Journal of Cardiology, 43,* 708–712.

57. Tuxen, D. V., Sutton, J., Upton, A., Sexton, A., McDougal, D., & Sale, D. (1983). Brainstem injury following maximal weight lifting attempts. *Medicine and Science in Sports and Exercise, 15* (Abstract), 158.

58. Walther, R. J., & Tifft, C. P. (1985). High blood pressure in the competitive athlete: Guidelines and recommendations. *The Physician and Sportsmedicine, 13*(3) 93–114.

59. Wilmore, J. H., Stanforth, P. R., Gagnon, J., Rice, T., Mandel, S., Leon, A. S., Rao, D. C., Skinner, J. S., & Bouchard, C. (2001). Heart rate and blood pressure changes with endurance training: The HERITAGE Family Study. *Medicine and Science in Sports and Exercise, 33,* 107–116.

60. Wolthius, R. A., Froelicker, V. F., Fischer, J., & Triehwasser, J. H. (1977). The response of healthy men to treadmill exercise. *Circulation, 55,* 153–157.

Form 17.1

Individual Data for Exercise Blood Pressure

Name _____ Date _____ Time _____ A.M. _____ P.M. _____

Age _____ y   Gender (M or W) _____   Ht _____ cm   Wt _____ kg   Tech. Initials _____

Meteorological Data

T _____ °C (closest 0.1 °C)   RH % _____ P_B _____ mm Hg × 1.333 = _____ hPa

Mode (check): Cycle _____   Other _____   Cycle Model _____   Seat Ht _____

Prior Test Score(s): $\dot{V}O_2$max _____ L·min⁻¹ _____ L·min⁻¹   Predicted (P) or Direct (D) $\dot{V}O_2$max (check) _____ P _____ D

Time	Power W	Systolic Pressure (SP)	Diastolic Pressure 4th Phase (DP-4th)	Diastolic Pressure 5th Phase (DP-5th)	Pulse Pressure (PP)	Heart Rate (HR)	Rate-Pressure Product (RPP)
Pre-exercise (on bike)	___	___	___	___	___	___	___
Exercise							
2:30–3:00	___	___	___	___	___	___	___
5:30–6:00	___	___	___	___	___	___	___
8:30–9:00	___	___	___	___	___	___	___
Recovery: Cooldown							
9:30–10:00	___	___	___	___	___	___	___
10:30–11:00	___	___	___	___	___	___	___
11:30–12:00	___	___	___	___	___	___	___
Chair Recovery							
12:30–13:00	___	___	___	___	___	___	___
13:30–14:00	___	___	___	___	___	___	___
14:30–15:00	___	___	___	___	___	___	___

Mean Blood Pressure (MBP)

Body State	Time	Pulse Pressure (PP)	PP ÷ 3	+ DP	= MBP
Pre-exercise		_____	_____	+ _____	= _____
Peak Exercise	8:30–9:00	_____	_____	+ _____	= _____
Recovery	11:30–12:00	_____	_____	+ _____	= _____
Recovery	14:30–15:00	_____	_____	+ _____	= _____

Form 17.2

Group Data for Exercise Blood Pressure

Power (W)	50			75			100			125			150			175			200		

Blood Pressure (mm Hg; 1st, 4th, and 5th phases)

Initials	1st	4th	5th	1st	4th	5th	1st	4th	5th	1st	4th	5th	1st	4th	5th	1st	4th	5th	1st	4th	5th
1.																					
2.																					
3.																					
4.																					
5.																					
6.																					
7.																					
8.																					
9.																					
10.																					
11.																					
12.																					
13.																					
14.																					
15.																					
16.																					
17.																					
18.																					
19.																					
20.																					
M																					
Minimum																					
Maximum																					

Form 17.3

Graph of Blood Pressure (BP) Before, During, and After Cycling

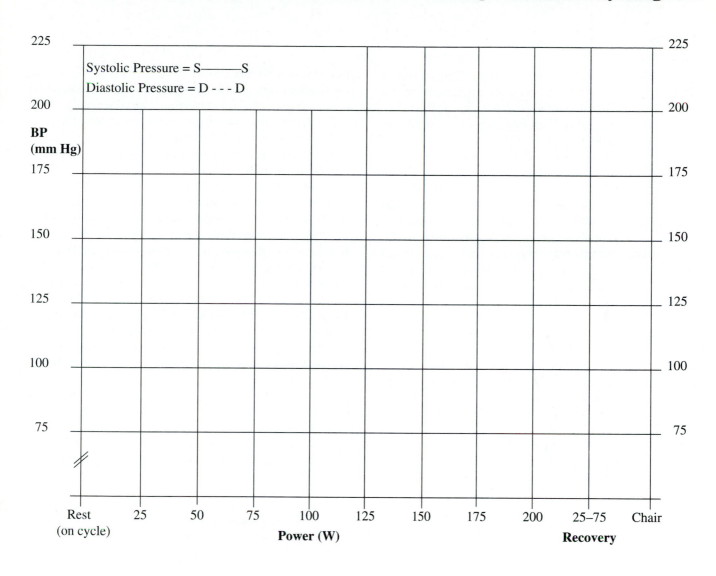

Systolic Pressure = S———S
Diastolic Pressure = D - - - D

BP (mm Hg)

Power (W)

Rest (on cycle)   25   50   75   100   125   150   175   200   25–75   Chair

Recovery

The diagnosis of the electrocardiogram (ECG) is one of the most important and accurate evaluations of the quantity and quality of heartbeats. Although 4 million electrocardiograms may have been interpreted by computer in the United States in 1975, that still leaves 76 million that were interpreted by the human brain.[10] An Englishman was the first (1887) to record electrical current from the human body's surface,[1,3] but it was a Dutchman, Willem Einthoven, who received the Nobel Prize in 1924 for his 1901 "elektrokardiograph" (EKG) because of his more sophisticated instrument and his publications on electrocardiography.[5] Although the electrocardiogram is widely known as a clinical test, it has been used numerous times by physiologists and kinesiologists to quantify accurately resting and exercise heart rates.

Physiological Rationale

The rationale for the ECG is based upon the heart's generation of an electrical current, which is then transferred to the skin through the body's salty fluid medium. The voltage from an ordinary flashlight battery is about 1500 times greater than the skin's voltage.[11] Voltage is an electromotive force that causes a current to flow between two points (electrodes). The electrodes (leads), which are placed on the skin, transfer this current from the skin to the electrocardiograph (the machine), where it is then recorded on special graph paper (electrocardiogram). Generally, when the current moves from the negative electrode to the positive electrode an upright deflection (positive wave) occurs on the graph paper. When the current moves from the positive electrode to the relatively negative electrode, a downward deflection or negative wave is recorded. When there is no movement of the current or when it is moving perpendicular to the two electrodes, the tracing is termed isoelectric; this means that there is neither a positive nor a negative deflection, thus remaining at baseline (Figure 18.1).[17]

The descriptions of the basic ECG waves and segments are presented in Table 18.1 and Figure 18.2. Einthoven arbitrarily assigned alphabetical letters to the waves of the ECG, starting with the middle of the alphabet to avoid confusion with the designations for vitamins.

To interpret the electrocardiogram, one must first understand the meaning of the graph paper when the electrocardiograph runs at standard operating speed (25 mm·s⁻¹). A magnified section of ECG paper is presented in Figure 18.3. The bold vertical lines divide the graph into 5 mm time lines, each representing 0.2 s. The thin vertical lines between the bold lines represent 1 mm or 0.04 s. The crisscrossing horizontal lines represent voltages; the divisions

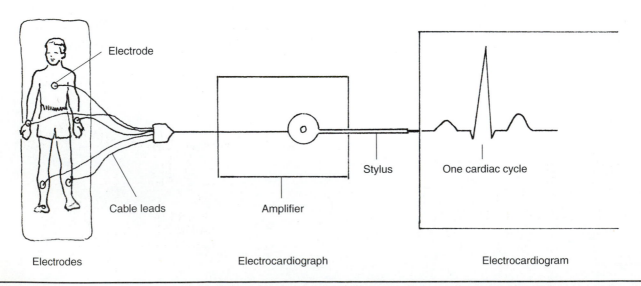

Electrode

Cable leads

Electrodes

Amplifier

Electrocardiograph

Stylus

One cardiac cycle

Electrocardiogram

Figure 18.1 Interfacing the heart with the ECG: The electrical currents from the heart are amplified by the electrocardiograph and recorded as the electrocardiogram. Only one of the six chest electrodes is shown.

between the horizontal bold lines represent 5 mm or 0.5 mv. The thin horizontal lines between the bold lines divide the graph into 1 mm or 0.1 mv sections.

Method

The technician should work calmly and unhurriedly; this will promote relaxation of the participant and provide an adequate rest period prior to the recording. While attaching the electrodes, the technician should set the person at ease by a calm, informal, yet professional manner. The technician need not interpret the tracing during testing unless an exercise ECG test immediately follows. In general, save interpretation for a later time when it can be studied more carefully.

Lead Nomenclature, Sites, and Skin Preparation

Leads may be classified anatomically into six limb (extremity) leads and six chest (precordial) leads. Also, they may be classified electronically, as bipolar standard (limb) leads or unipolar (augmented and chest) leads, based upon the electrocardiograph's mathematical manipulation of difference in voltage between two electrodes.

Bipolar Standard Leads (I, II, and III)

Bipolar leads represent the difference in electric potential between two sites and are recorded in the frontal plane (anterior surface of thorax). Thus, they depict direction and size of wave from right to left. The negative electrode is placed on the right arm (RA; medial wrist). The positive electrodes are on the left arm (LA; medial wrist) and left leg (LL; medial lower leg just above ankle) for leads I and II, respectively. The left arm is relatively negative to the positive left leg in lead III. The electrocardiograph mathematically makes leads I plus III equal to lead II. The ground electrode is placed on the right leg (RL; medially just above ankle). Table 18.2 summarizes the standard lead configuration.

Table 18.1	Basic ECG Waves, Complexes, Intervals, and Segments

Waves

P: The small, dome-shaped positive wave that represents the stimulus for atrial contraction; depolarization; atrial activation

Q: A little negative wave that initiates depolarization, the stimulus for contraction, of the ventricles

R: The large, triangular-shaped positive wave of ventricular depolarization; sometimes referred to as the "R spike"

S: The negative wave of ventricular depolarization

T: A medium-sized, dome-shaped positive wave representing repolarization of the ventricles; the stimulus for the ventricles to relax

Complex

QRS: The three waves of ventricular depolarization; the beginning of the Q-wave to the end of the S-wave

Intervals—Include Wave(s) and Segment(s)

Q-T: Ventricular systole; the beginning of the Q wave to the end of the T wave

Segment—Excludes Waves

ST: Horizontal line representing the early phase of ventricular repolarization; normally it is isoelectric, meaning that it is at baseline; the end of the S wave to the beginning of the T wave; sensitive to ischemia (below normal coronary blood flow)

PR: The end of the P wave to the beginning of the Q wave; technically, this segment should be called the P-Q segment

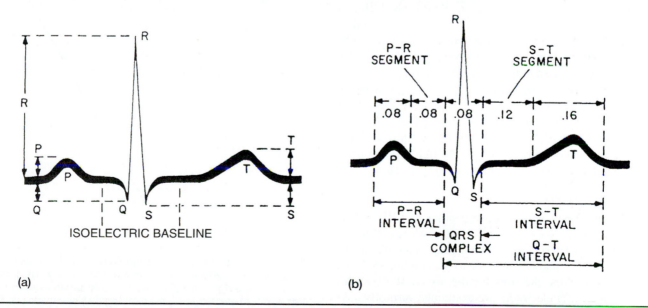

(a)   (b)

Figure 18.2 The basic waves and segments with their criteria for measuring (a) wave voltage amplitudes (mV) and (b) interval or segment durations (s).

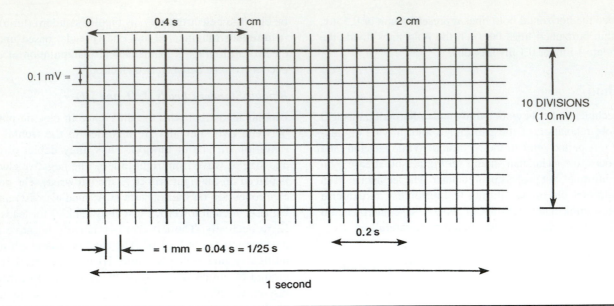

Figure 18.3 This magnified section of typical ECG paper shows the 1 mm squares whereby the horizontal distance represents 0.04 s and the vertical distance represents 0.1 mV.

Table 18.2	Standard Limb Lead Configuration and Sites		
Lead	**Site**	**Electrode Abbreviation**	**Electrode Color**
I	Right (−) and left (+) arms	RA - LA	RA = white
			LA = black
II	Right arm (−) and left leg (+)	RA - LL	LL = red
			RL = green
III	Left arm (−) and left leg (+)	LA - LL	Chest = brown
Ground	Right leg	RL; G	

Augmented Extremity Leads (aVR, aVL, and aVF)

The electrocardiograph makes three more leads by finding a central point of the three bipolar standard leads (I, II, and III), then comparing it to each of these three electrodes. This produces the unipolar augmented (a) leads aVR, aVL, and aVF. All modern electrocardiographs automatically record unipolar augmented leads. The term *augmented* means that the amplitude of the waves is 50 % greater than an older technique would produce. These three added limb leads essentially augment the three standard leads by connecting the standard leads to a common central lead and then viewing the positive current to the right (aVR) or left (aVL) shoulder or to the left leg (aVF)[5] (Figure 18.4).

Chest Leads (V₁–V₆)

The difference between the central point of I, II, and III versus each of the six chest leads produces leads V_1 to V_6. These are often referred to as the unipolar precordial leads; the six leads are named from V_1 to V_6. Figure 18.5 and Table 18.3 describe the sites for the six chest electrodes (V_{1-6} leads). Chest electrodes are positioned vertically relative to intercostal spaces (between ribs) and horizontally according to the sternum, clavicle, and axilla (armpit). The

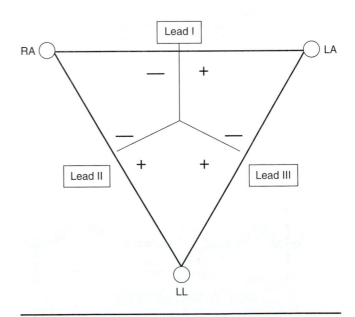

Figure 18.4 The Einthoven triangle diagrammatically illustrates the current flow of bipolar standard leads. For example, the right arm (RA) electrode is negative (−) to the left arm (LA) electrode (+) and left leg (LL) electrode (+). The intersection of the perpendiculars from each lead's axis theoretically represents the center of electrical activity.

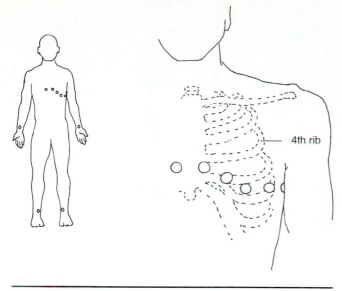

Figure 18.5 The typical electrode placement for the 12-lead system for resting ECG is shown on the left. The six chest electrodes are shown in more detail on the right.

4th rib

Table 18.3	Sites for Chest Precordial Electrodes
Chest Lead	**Anatomical Site**
V₁	4th intercostal space at *right* sternal margin
V₂	4th intercostal space at *left* sternal margin
V₃	Midpoint between V₂ and V₄
V₄	5th intercostal space at midclavicular line
V₅	Same horizontal level as V₄ at left anterior axillary line
V₆	Same horizontal level as V₄ and V₅ at left midaxillary line

technician locates the chest electrode positions by firmly palpating the person's chest along the vertical border of the sternum. The chest leads depict the direction and size of the electrical wave moving from front of the heart to the back (posterior).

Electrode Site Preparation

The inner surfaces of the wrists and ankles are preferred for leads I, II, and III because of the relative absence of hair. The electrode site is wiped with an alcohol pad; light rubbing will help remove dry skin, dirt, and/or oil, which all act as insulators to current and thus are poor conductors of electricity.

Electrocardiograph Procedures

The procedures for electrocardiograph calibration are presented in Box 18.1. Einthoven's original 1901 electrocardiograph required five people to operate and was so large that it occupied two rooms. A person's hands and left foot were placed into three buckets of a salt solution serving as electrodes. Since 1901, many types of electrocardiographs have been manufactured. Although electrocardiograph procedures may differ with different brands, the following procedures apply to most single-channel (one-lead-at-a-time) electrocardiographs. A multichannel ECG tracing is depicted in Figure 18.6.

1. Turn on *power switch*. Only a few seconds of warm-up is required due to the solid-state nature of electrocardiographs.
2. Turn lever of *amplifier* to On only after the person is connected to all limb (extremity; RA, LA, LL, and G) leads. Turning the amplifier on prior to these attachments will cause the stylus to swing wildly and possibly damage it.
3. *Print* the participant's name and the date on the ECG paper or input "patient" data into computer.
4. *Record* by shifting the Run lever or button to 25 so the paper will move at a speed of 25 mm/s; some machines can go 10 mm/s to 50 mm/s but the standard speed is 25 mm/s.
5. *Center* the ECG tracing with the Stylus Position control knob.
6. *Darken or lighten* the ECG tracing on old machines by adjusting the Stylus Heat screw with a screwdriver or strong fingernail.
7. *Standardize* the recording by pressing the Calibration-STD button. After the technician gains experience, the standardization process may be recorded while taking the actual ECG recordings of each lead. The standard deflection is placed between the T and P waves of two different cardiac cycles (see 10 mm deflection boxes at far right of Figure 18.6).
8. *Record* the 12 leads by rotating the Lead Selector knob; record for approximately 2.5 s to 5 s at each lead except for lead II (the standard lead), which should be recorded for 12 s; lead II can then be used to calculate resting heart rate.
9. Calculate an accurate resting heart rate by counting or measuring with a ruler the number of vertical 1 mm

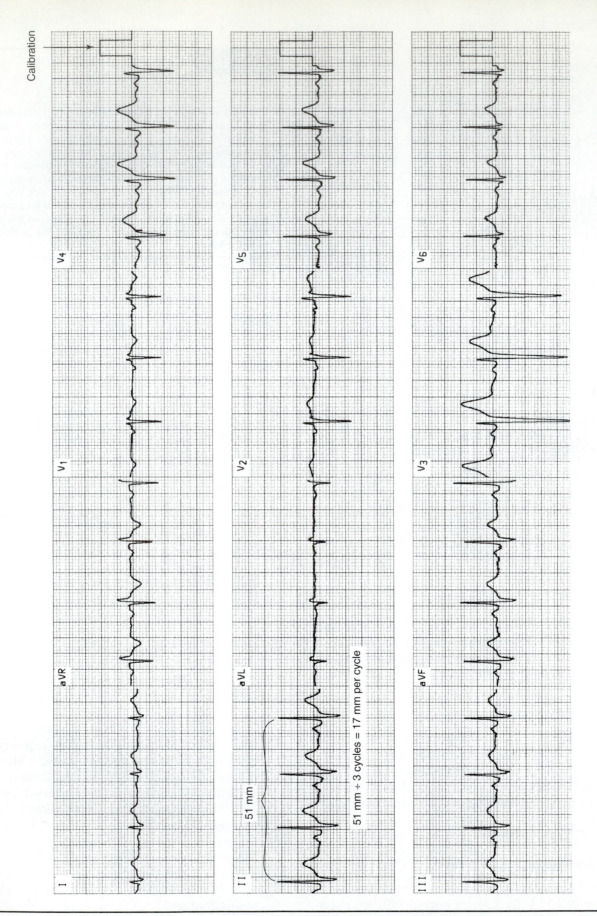

Figure 18.6 A multichannel ECG tracing. Some recorders present aV leads before standard I, II, and III leads. Lead II shows an average cycle length as 17 mm. This equates to a heart rate of 88 b·min⁻¹ (Eq. 18.1).

Table 18.4 Criteria for Normal in the Resting ECG

Component		Criteria		
HR	60–100 b·min⁻¹; Regular sinus rhythm			
Waves	Amplitude (mV)		Polarity (+, –, or isoelectric)	Duration (s)
P	< 2–3		+: I, II, aVF, V_{2-6}	< 0.11
Q			–: I–III, aVR, V_{5-6}	≤ 0.03
QRS (R)[a]	< 30 in II and V_5[b]		+: 2 of 3 std leads	0.05–0.12
	> 5 sum: I–III			
	> 5: $V_{1\ \&\ 6}$			
	> 7: $V_{2\ \&\ 5}$			
	> 9: $V_{3\ \&\ 4}$			
T	< 5: I–III		+: I, II; –: aVR; variable in III	
	< 10: V_{1-6} -leads		+: V_{3-6} (not notched)	
QRS axis	– 30° to + 110°			
Interval	Amplitude		Polarity	Duration
P-R (Q)			Isoelectric	0.12–0.20
Q-T			Mixed interval (+, –, iso)	0.30–0.43
Segment				
ST	0.0 relative to		Isoelectric (T-P or P-Q)	
			+: often $V_2 - V_4$ (elevated)	

Note: [a]axis = –30° to +90°. [b]QRS voltage should consider fitness training history—highly active persons tend toward high R spikes due to ventricular hypertrophy.
Source: Data from Goldman, M. J. (1967). *Principles of clinical electrocardiography,* Los Altos, CA: Lange Medical Publications.

lines between two R spikes. Or you may average the distance between more than two cardiac cycles. The 1 mm or 0.04 s vertical lines represent a minute rate of 1500 mm/min. For example, if the number of millimeters from the peak of one R wave (spike) to the next cardiac cycle's R peak is 17 mm, then heart rate may be calculated from Equation 18.1 as follows, as in lead II of Figure 18.6:[6]

$$HR\ (b\ /\ min) = 1500 \div \text{R-R mm} \qquad \text{Eq. 18.1}$$

$$= 1500 \div 17$$

$$= 88\ b\ /\ min\ \text{to closest whole beat}$$

where: 1500 = horizontal length in mm of a
   1 min section; 1500 mm·min⁻¹
   R-R = horizontal length (mm)
   of one cardiac cycle measured
   from peak of one R to the peak
   of the next R

10. Technician pays particular attention to rate, rhythm, and ST segment.
11. Remove electrodes and clean the application sites on the person.

Results and Discussion

The surgeon general and others have declared that daily moderate physical activity is protective against cardiovascular disease and all-cause mortality.[4,15] Clinical exercise physiologists often administer ECG tests to high-risk persons in the United States who may be following the advice of the surgeon general's *Physical Activity and Health report*[15] to initi-

Table 18.5 Clinical Types of Bradycardia

Bradycardia Type	Heart Rate
Mild	50–59
Moderate	40–49
Severe; pathologic	< 40

Source: Based on statements by Kammerling, J. M. (1988). Sinus node dysfunction. In D. P. Zipes & D. J. Rowlands (Eds.), *Progress in cardiology: Arrhythmias, Part II* (p. 210). Philadelphia: Lea & Febiger.

ate or increase their physical activity level. Three of the most basic variables encountered on an electrocardiogram are (1) heart rate, (2) heart rhythm, and (3) ST depression.

Heart Rate

Although the criteria for a normal resting ECG vary slightly with different investigators, those in Table 18.4[8] may serve as an appropriate guide. Persons with resting heart rates over 100 b·min⁻¹ are in a state of tachycardia, whereas those with resting heart rates less than 60 b·min⁻¹ are in bradycardia. Further divisions of bradycardia may be designated arbitrarily as depicted in Table 18.5.[9] Sinus bradycardia often does not indicate a clinically abnormal state. Table 18.5 indicates that rates between 40 b·min⁻¹ and 49 b·min⁻¹ are categorized as moderate bradycardia.[9,16] However, reports[9] of trained distance runners having heart rates of 43 (± 5 b·min⁻¹) during waking hours indicate a bradycardiac condition that is normal.

The seated heart rates for men and women from the ages of 18 y to over 65 y are presented in Table 18.6. Because heart rate is not known to differ with age in adult persons, I have reduced the original tables[7] to a single age

Table 18.6 Norms for Resting Heart Rate (HR) in Men and Women, Ages 18 y to 65+ y

Heart Rate Category	Heart Rates (b·min⁻¹)	
	Men	Women
Low	35–56	39–58
Moderately low	57–61	59–63
< Average	62–65	64–67
Average	66–71	68–72
> Average	72–75	73–77
Moderately high	76–81	78–83
High	82–103	84–104

Source: Based on data from Golding, L. A. (2000). *YMCA fitness testing and assessment manual.* Champaign, IL: Human Kinetics.

group. In general, the average man's heart rate (ranging from 66 to 71 b·min⁻¹) is slightly less than the average woman's (68 to 72 b·min⁻¹) heart rate. Although the original tables of the YMCA publication attach qualitative ("excellent," etc.) fitness categories to each heart-rate range, Table 18.6 simply provides nonqualitative categories such as "low," "average," and "high."

Heart Rhythm

When the rhythm of the heartbeats is irregular, it is referred to as arrhythmia. One author noted an arrhythmic criterion as a difference > 0.12 s (3 mm) between two adjacent cycle times (lengths).[14] Usually ventricular premature beats or contractions (VPB or VPC or PVC) are of greater concern than premature atrial (supraventricular) contractions (PAC). Usually, a VPB has no P wave.[2] One hierarchy of VPB severity ranges from an absence of severity if no VPB occur in one hour to a high severity if more than 30 VPB occur per hour. Also, the severity increases if the form of the VPB is multiform (varying shape), then repetitive couplets (e.g., bigeminy), then to ventricular tachycardia (> 3 consecutive VPB).[12]

ST Depression

The ST portion (Figure 18.2b) of the ECG is a segment that is often used to diagnose coronary heart disease. It is measured from the baseline (isoelectric), which can be defined as a "line connecting two consecutive P-Q junctions."[13] If the whole segment is more than 1 mm below the isoelectric line, it could indicate ischemic heart disease, depending upon other factors, such as angina and other ECG abnormalities. The final diagnosis should be made by a cardiologist.

References

1. Adrian, R. H., Channell, R. C., Cohen, L., & Noble, D. (1976, July). The Einthoven string galvanometer and the interpretation of the T-wave of the electrocardiogram. *Physiological Society,* pp. 67–70.

2. American College of Sports Medicine. (2000). *ACSM's guidelines for exercise testing and prescription.* Philadelphia: Lippincott Williams & Wilkins.

3. Besterman, E., & Creese, R. (1979). Waller—Pioneer of electrocardiography. *British Heart Journal, 42,* 61–64.

4. Blair, S. N., Kampert, J. B., Kohl, H. W., Barlow, C. E., Macera, C. A., Paffenbarger, R. S., & Gibbons, L. W. (1996). Influences of cardiorespiratory fitness and other precursors on cardiovascular disease and all-cause mortality in men and women. *JAMA, 276,* 205–210.

5. Brailey, A. G. (1978). Basic electrocardiography. In P. K. Wilson (Ed.), *Cardiac rehabilitation and adult fitness* (pp. 69–83).

6. Fisher, A. G., & Jensen, C. R. (1990). *The scientific basis of athletic conditioning.* Philadelphia: Lea & Febiger.

7. Golding, L. A. (2000). *YMCA fitness testing and assessment manual.* Champaign, IL: Human Kinetics.

8. Goldman, M. J. (1967). *Principles of clinical electrocardiography.* Los Altos, CA: Lange Medical Publications.

9. Kammerling, J. M. (1988). Sinus node dysfunction. In D. P. Zipes & D. J. Rowlands (Eds.), *Progress in cardiology* (pp. 205–230). Philadelphia: Lea & Febiger.

10. Laks, M. M., & Ginzton, L. (1979). Computerized ECG interpretation. *Practical Cardiology, 5,* 127–149.

11. Lemish, M. G. (1979, June). Trouble-free cardiac monitoring. *Emergency,* pp. 58–59.

12. Lown, B., & Wolf, M. (1971). Approaches to sudden death from coronary heart disease. *Circulation, 44,* 130–142.

13. Mason, R. E., Likar, I., Biern, R. O., & Ross, R. S. (1967). Multiple-lead exercise electrocardiography. *Circulation, 336,* 517–525.

14. Nieman, D. C. (1995). *Fitness and sports medicine: A health-related approach.* Palo Alto, CA: Bull.

15. United States Surgeon General's Office. (1996). *Physical activity and health: A report of the Surgeon General Executive Summary.* Washington, DC: U.S. Government Printing Office.

16. Viitasalo, M. T., Kala, R., & Eisalo, A. (1982). Ambulatory electrocardiographic recording in endurance athletes. *British Heart Journal, 47,* 213.

17. Winsor, T. (1968). The electrocardiogram in myocardial infarction. *Clinical Symposia, 20.*

Form 18.1

Resting ECG

Name [   ] Date [   ] Time [   ] A.M. [   ] P.M. [   ]

Age [   ] y   Gender (M or W) [   ]   Ht [   ] cm   Wt [   ] kg   Tech. Initials [   ]

Meteorological Data

Temperature (T) [   ] °C   RH [   ] % P_B [   ] mm Hg

HR = 1500 / R-R [   ] mm = [   ] b·min^{-1} Rhythm: Regular [   ] Irregular [   ]

Lead II or V$_5$ (circle one):

Wave	Amplitude (mv)	Polarity (+ or −)	Duration (s)	Comment
P				
Q				
R				
S				
T				
ST segment			x x x x x x x x x x x	
PR interval	x x x x x x x x x x x x	x x x x x x x x x x x x		
QT interval	x x x x x x x x x x x x	x x x x x x x x x x x x		

Mounting site for lead II and/or V$_5$ tracing:

EXERCISE ELECTROCARDIOGRAM

The Exercise ECG Test is often a part of the **stress** test. Less intimidating names are the **Graded Exercise Test (GXT)** and the **Exercise Tolerance Test (ETT)**. Also, these tests usually include the measurements of RPE, heart rate, and blood pressure. Sometimes, oxygen consumption is measured or predicted. The primary distinction of this test is the recording of the electrical conductivity of the heart—the **electrocardiogram (ECG).** The Exercise ECG Test has the advantage over some other evaluations of the cardiovascular system in that it is noninvasive, nonradiative, and relatively inexpensive.

There are at least three objectives in monitoring the electrocardiogram during the exercise test: (1) to assure the safety of the performer during exercise testing and training, (2) to measure accurate heart rates, and (3) to diagnose the performer or patient for cardiovascular disease.

The first two objectives—safety and accurate heart-rate recordings—may be accomplished by nonmedical personnel. However, the Exercise ECG may not be warranted for all asymptomatic—no cardiovascular disease (CVD) symptoms—and apparently healthy persons. The American College of Cardiology and the *American Heart Association Guidelines* state that the Exercise ECG Test is not warranted unless "healthy" people have two or more major risk factors—smoking, hypertension, hypercholesterolemia, and family history of CVD.[4] The American College of Sports Medicine does not consider an annual medical examination and the clinical Exercise ECG Test prerequisites if apparently healthy persons of any age at low or moderate risk perform only moderate exercise (≤ 60 % $\dot{V}O_2$max; 3 MET to 6 MET) during recreation or testing. The same holds true for vigorous exercise in low-risk persons.[7] Some believe that the exercise ECG is beneficial for all persons because it provides a baseline by which to compare their future Exercise ECG Tests.

The third objective—diagnosis of cardiovascular disease—is the primary responsibility of the physician, who may seek input from the allied health staff, which may include a clinical exercise physiologist and/or exercise technologist. Thus, the ECG Exercise Test often is an interdisciplinary test between medical and allied health personnel.[3] Although it is not within the role of an exercise laboratory technician to serve as a cardiologist, it is important for the technician to understand the basic concepts of electrocardiography and to recognize the most critical ECG abnormalities encountered in exercise testing.[37] For persons with

angina pectoris, the Exercise ECG Test is often the precursor test to one or more of the following tests: (1) angiography, which requires an X-ray-visible dye to be injected into the coronary arteries, (2) exercise scintigraphy, whereby radionuclide thallium allows the blood flow to be followed in the myocardium, (3) echocardiography, which provides views of the heart produced by ultrasound waves, and (4) calcium scanning of the arteries by electron-beam computed tomography. However, the Exercise ECG Test, using the exercise time, ST displacement, and angina index together can be as accurate as these sophisticated tests in predicting the risk of future cardiovascular events.[32]

Physiological Rationale

The exercise electrocardiogram is more apt to reveal latent (previously hidden) cardiovascular problems than the resting electrocardiogram.[25] For example, 10.2 % of 7023 normal resting ECG exams were deemed abnormal on maximal treadmill ECG tests.[20] Of those persons with known coronary heart disease, 30 % may not be revealed by resting ECG, but, if an exercise ECG is administered, 70 % of these will be revealed.[45]

Method

The Exercise ECG Test is usually preceded by a resting electrocardiogram in order to screen persons for whom exercise may be contraindicated and to enhance the interpretation of the exercise electrocardiogram. The Exercise ECG Test always includes measurements of heart rate and blood pressure periodically throughout the test. Often, a prediction of aerobic power ($\dot{V}O_2$max) is made on the basis of heart rate or exercise duration. Sometimes a scale for rating perceived exertion (RPE) is used to monitor the performer's perception of the exercise stress. Thus, the methodology of the Exercise ECG Test may be categorized into (a) exercise protocols; (b) the prediction of $\dot{V}O_2$; (c) the measurement of blood pressure, heart rate, and RPE; and (d) the ECG. See Box 19.1 for a discussion on the accuracy of the Exercise ECG and predictive $\dot{V}O_2$max Test.

Exercise Protocols

Although the first popular Exercise ECG Test used a step bench,[44] the most common protocols for these tests use either cycle ergometers or treadmills. The protocols for the Exercise ECG Test are usually continuous and progressive types. *Continuous,* as opposed to *intermittent,* is a term used to characterize a test in which the performer does not stop exercising until the end of the test. An intermittent, or noncontinuous, test has rest intervals between exercise bouts. *Progressive* simply means that the exercise intensity is graded—that is, the exercise bouts increase in intensity at periodic intervals.

Continuous-progressive protocols can be subdivided into two types based upon submaximal or maximal exercise. Submaximal tests often are targeted to a specified percent maximal heart-rate reserve (e.g., 85 % HRRmax) or to symptom-limited endpoints. If the performer is healthy and willing, however, it is preferable to perform a maximal test.

Cycling Protocols

In general, the continuous cycling protocols provide either 3 min or 4 min periods at each power level if the power increments are 50 W or greater. Less time (1 min or 2 min) permits reasonable steady-state heart rates if the power increments are 25 W or less[41] (Table 19.1). A suggested criterion for the achievement of steady-state heart rate is obtaining heart rates at each end of two consecutive minutes that are within 6 b·min^{-1} of each other.[7] Equation 19.1 enables the prediction of the gross steady-state oxygen cost for any given power (W) (*SEE* = 7 % mL·kg^{-1}·min^{-1}).[7]

$$\dot{V}O_2 \text{ (mL·kg}^{-1}\text{·min}^{-1}) = [(10.8 \times W) \div BM] + 7 \quad \text{Eq. 19.1}$$

Where:

> W = watts
>
> BM = body mass in kilograms
>
> 7 = sum of unloaded $\dot{V}O_2$ + resting $\dot{V}O_2$

A recovery period of 2 min to 4 min should be allotted for no-load or minimal-load cycling. The quality of the

---

Table 19.1 | **Sample of a Continuous-Progressive Protocol for Cycle Ergometry**

Time min	Force[a] N	W	Power[a] N·m·min^{-1}	Total Work kJ	Energy kcal·min^{-1}	Total Energy kcal
0–1	5	25;	1500	1.5	3.0	3.0
1–2	5	25;	1500	3.0	3.0	6.0
2–3	10	50;	3000	6.0	4.5	10.5
3–4	10	50;	3000	9.0	4.5	14.5
4–5	15	75;	4500	13.5	6.0	20.5
5–6	15	75;	4500	18.0	6.0	26.5
6–7	20	100;	6000	24.0	7.5	34.0
7–8	20	100;	6000	30.0	7.5	41.5
8–9	25	125;	7500	37.5	9.0	50.5
9–10	25	125;	7500	45.0	9.0	59.5
10–11	30	150;	9000	54.0	10.5	70.0
11–12	30	150;	9000	63.0	10.5	80.5
12–13	35	175;	10 500	73.5	12.0	92.5
13–14	35	175;	10 500	84.0	12.0	104.5
14–15	40	200;	12 000	96.0	14.0	118.5
15–16	40	200;	12 000	108.0	14.0	132.5
16–17	45	225;	13 500	121.5	16.0	148.5
17–18	45	225;	13 500	135.0	16.0	164.5
18–19	50	250;	15 000	150.0	17.5	182.0
19–20	50	250;	15 000	165.0	17.5	199.5

Note: [a]Force applicable for mechanically braked ergometers; power is based on 50 r·min^{-1} on Monark® ergometer.

Table 19.2 — The Oxygen Cost and MET for Various Stages of Four Treadmill Protocols

Treadmill Protocols							Mets
Balke-Ware	Ellestad		Bruce		Stanford		
Grade at 3.3 mph, 1 min stages	3/2/3 min stages		3 min stages		Grade at 3 mph, 3-min stages	Grade at 2 mph, 3-min stages	
	mph	gr	mph	gr			
26							19
25			5.5	20			
24	6	15	5.0	18			16
23							15
22							14
21	5	15					
20							
19			4.2	16			13
18					22.5		12
17							
16	5	10			20.0		11
15					17.5		10
14							
13			3.4	14	15.0		9
12							
11					12.5		8
10	4	10	2.5	12	10.0	17.5	7
9							
8					7.5	14	6
7							
6	1.7	10	1.7	10	5.0	10.5	5
5			1.7	5			
4					2.5	7	4
3			1.7	5	0.0	3.5	3
2			1.7	0			2
1							1

Adapted from Fig. 5-3 on pp. 92 and 93 of American College of Sports Medicine. (1995). *ACSM's guidelines for exercise testing and prescription.* © American College of Sports Medicine. Reprinted by permission.

electrocardiogram and the ease of measuring blood pressure is usually better during the cycling mode than during the treadmill mode of exercise.[7]

Treadmill Protocols

The treadmill ergometer is the most popular ergometer for ECG stress testing.[18,57] Table 19.2[6] and Figure 19.1[5] summarize several popular treadmill protocols. Table 19.3 and other summaries[6,7,15,46,53,58] of exercise protocols are available. The Bruce (also see Table 19.4) and Balke protocols are the most popular for exercise tests in apparently healthy persons.[56] The original **Bruce** Test lacked a good warm-up at Stage 1 for low-fit persons; however, the modified Bruce Test remedied this by providing a 0 % or 5 % slope instead of a 10 % slope at Stage 1.[48] The Balke and the Taylor protocols were designed originally for Maximal Oxygen Consumption Tests. The **Balke** protocol may be delimiting due to leg fatigue in some persons and is sometimes modified from 3.3 mph to 3.0 mph for women.[54] The **Ellestad** protocol has an endpoint at 95 % of age-predicted maximal heart rate.[26] As with the original Bruce Test, the first stage of the Ellestad Test may be too difficult for older or poorly fit persons. The **Naughton,**[50] or similar **Stanford,**[6] protocol is flexible and time efficient in that the first stage is chosen so that all persons can complete a minimum of 1.5 stages. For example, if the performers are likely to complete Stage 4, then they may begin at Stage 3. Protocols that increase intensities by small increments are best for less fit persons. The **Harbor** protocol increases the power continuously by a ramp method;[59] the uniform increase depends on the performer's fitness. The performer usually reaches $\dot{V}O_2$max in about 10 min. For all protocols, a recovery period of 4 min should be allotted for walking slowly at 0 % grade.

Prediction of $\dot{V}O_2$

The approximate **oxygen cost** and MET for each stage of various protocols is presented in Table 19.2[6] and again for the Bruce Test in Table 19.4.[5,16,17] The gross oxygen cost at steady state for any protocol can be predicted (SEE = 7 %), without actually measuring it, from ACSM equations for either walking (Eq. 19.2[a]) or running (Eq. 19.3[b]).[7]

$$\text{Walk: } \dot{V}O_2 \text{ (mL·kg}^{-1}\text{·min}^{-1}) = 3.5 + (0.1 \times S) + (S \times G \times 1.8) \qquad \text{Eq. 19.2}$$

[a]Appropriate for walking speeds of 50 m·min^{-1} (1.9 mph) to 100 m·min^{-1} (3.7 mph).
[b]Appropriate for jogging or running speeds over 80 m·min^{-1} (3 mph)— not if walking.

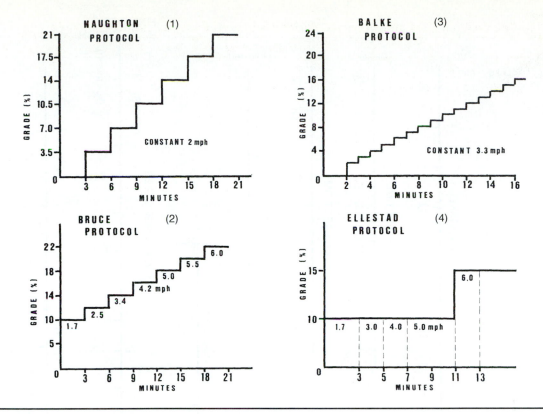

Figure 19.1 Four popular treadmill protocols: (1) Naughton, (2) Bruce, (3) Balke, and (4) Ellestad. From the American College of Sports Medicine, *Guidelines for Exercise Testing and Prescription,* 1986. Copyright © Lea & Febiger Publishers. Malvern, PA. Reprinted by permission.

Table 19.3   Summary of Four Common Treadmill Protocols

Protocol	Stages #	Speed Range mph	Speed Range m·min⁻¹	Grade Range %	Stage Time min/stage	Total Time minª
Bruce[b17]	7	1.7–6.0	46–161	10–22	3	21
Balke[8]	22	3.3	88	2–22	1	22
Naughton (original)[50]	13	1.0–2.0	27–54	0–22	2	30
Ellestad[26]	6	1.7–6.0	46–161	10; 15	2–3	13+

Note: ªOnly if performer can continue to the end of the protocol and starts at its beginning. ᵇBruce protocol for *clinical* testing may include two preliminary 3 min stages at 1.7 mph at 0 % and 5 % grade.

Table 19.4   Originalª Bruce Test Stages and Corresponding MET and Maximal Oxygen Consumption (mL·kg⁻¹·min⁻¹)

Stage	% grade	mph	km·h⁻¹	m·min⁻¹	MET	V̇O₂maxᵇ	Time (min)
1	10	1.7	2.7	45.6	5	17.5	3
2	12	2.5	4.0	72.4	7	24.5	6
3	14	3.4	5.5	91.1	10	35.0	9
4	16	4.2	6.8	112.6	13	45.5	12
5	18	5.0	8.0	134.0	16	56.0	15
6	20	5.5	8.8	147.4	19	66.5	18
7	22	6.0	9.7	160.8	22	77.0	21

Note: ªThe modified versions start at either 0 % or 5 % slope.[48] ᵇAssumes completion of given stage.

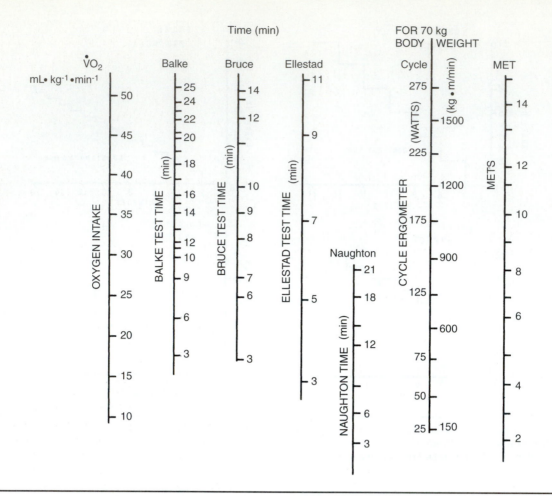

Figure 19.2 An estimate of metabolic cost is made by drawing a horizontal line from the time on a given exercise protocol to oxygen consumption or MET level. From the American College of Sports Medicine, *Guidelines for Exercise Testing and Prescription,* Fig. 2-4, p. 26, 1986. Copyright © Lea & Febiger Publishers. Malvern, PA. Reprinted by permission.

Run: $\dot{V}O_2$ (mL·kg^{-1}·min^{-1})   Eq. 19.3
$$= 3.5 + (0.2 \times S) + (S \times G \times 0.9)$$

where:

S = speed in meters per minute (m·min^{-1})

G = grade or slope as a fraction or decimal

3.5 = resting oxygen cost

For example, if a performer walks through Stage 2 of the Bruce Test at 2.5 mph (4.0 km·h^{-1}), or 67.0[c] m·min^{-1}, at 12 % slope, then the oxygen cost can be calculated according to Equation 19.2 as follows:

$$\dot{V}O_2 = 3.5 + (0.1 \times 67.0 \text{ m·min}^{-1}) + (67.0 \times 0.12 \times 1.8)$$

$$= 3.5 + 6.70 + 14.5$$

$$= 24.7 \text{ mL·kg}^{-1}\text{·min}^{-1}$$

The equivalent **MET** value may be calculated by dividing the oxygen cost by the generic one-MET value—3.5 mL·kg^{-1}·min^{-1} (Eq. 19.4).

$$\text{MET} = \dot{V}O_2 \div 3.5 \qquad \text{Eq. 19.4}$$

Therefore, the MET value of a performer walking at 67.0 m·min^{-1} on a 12 % grade is

$$\text{MET} = 24.7 \div 3.5 = 7.0 \text{ MET}$$

The **maximal oxygen consumption ($\dot{V}O_2$max)** for the Bruce test may be estimated from various regression equations, from Table 19.4, or from the nomogram in Figure 19.2[5] or by using the last complete stage of exercise.[7] Treadmill regression equations have been derived from the endurance times associated with the Bruce, Balke,[1,16,31] and Balke-modified protocols.[33] The regression equation for the Bruce test is selected based on its suitability for the performer—men or women,[16] or young men.[40]

Men: $\dot{V}O_2$max (mL·kg^{-1}·min^{-1})   Eq. 19.5
$$= (2.94 \times \text{min}) + 7.65$$

Women: $\dot{V}O_2$max $= (2.94 \times \text{min}) + 3.74$ Eq. 19.6

Young Men: $\dot{V}O_2$max $= (3.62 \times \text{min}) + 3.91$ Eq. 19.7

---

[c]1 mph = 26.8 m·min^{-1}.

where:

min = time to exhaustion in Bruce Test; decimal min

For example, if a woman completed Stage 2, a total time of 6 min, on the Bruce Test, then her $\dot{V}O_2$max based on Equation 19.6 is calculated as follows:

$$\dot{V}O_2max = (2.94 \times 6.0) + 3.74$$

$$= 17.64 + 3.7$$

$$= 21.34 \text{ mL} \cdot \text{kg}^{-1} \cdot \text{min}^{-1}$$

The advantage of using the ACSM steady-state equations for the terminal exercise stage to predict $\dot{V}O_2$max is that they can be applied to any protocol. However, the terminal stage's oxygen cost in a maximal test usually overestimates the performer's $\dot{V}O_2$max.[30] A more accurate prediction (*SEE* = 4.4 mL·kg^{-1}·min^{-1}) may be made if the ACSM value is corrected as follows in Equation 19.8:[30]

$$\dot{V}O_2max(\text{mL} \cdot \text{kg}^{-1} \cdot \text{min}^{-1}) \quad \text{Eq. 19.8}$$
$$= (0.869 \times \text{ACSM } \dot{V}O_2) - 0.07$$

For example, if a performer's ACSM oxygen cost at the terminal stage is calculated from Equation 19.3 as 40.05 mL·kg^{-1}·min^{-1}, then that person's $\dot{V}O_2$max calculated from Equation 19.8 is

$$\dot{V}O_2max(\text{mL} \cdot \text{kg}^{-1} \cdot \text{min}^{-1}) = (0.869 \times 40.08) - 0.07$$

$$= 34.82 - 0.07$$

$$= 34.75$$

The maximal oxygen consumption may also be estimated by consulting Table 19.4, which relates maximal oxygen consumption to the time to exhaustion on the Bruce Test. The nomogram in Figure 19.2 may be used for the Bruce Test and other protocols to predict maximal oxygen consumption and MET by drawing a horizontal line from the termination time (min) to $\dot{V}O_2$ and MET.[5]

Measurement of Blood Pressure, Heart Rate, and RPE

Blood Pressure

The American College of Sports Medicine recommends that blood pressure be measured with the performer in the supine, sitting, and standing positions prior to exercise.[7] Presumably, these measures are taken under relaxed conditions. Additional resting measures may be taken when the performer is prepared to exercise while seated on the cycle ergometer, standing on the treadmill, or in front of the step bench. These last measurements are referred to as the anticipatory or pre-exercise measures.

At exercise the blood pressure should be taken during the last minute of each stage or interval of the exercise protocol.[7] Usually, the technician starts pumping the sphygmomanometer's air bulb at the 30th s of the last minute of each stage. In recovery, it is taken immediately after exer-

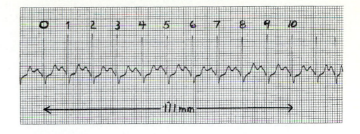

Figure 19.3 An actual ECG strip to calculate heart rate shows a length of 111 mm for 10 cycles, which translates to 0.444 s per cycle (0.004×111), thus 135 b·min^{-1} ($60 \text{ s} \div 0.444$).

cise and at 1 min to 2 min intervals for at least 5 min. The first few measurements of recovery blood pressure may be taken during *active* recovery (e.g., low-intensity cycling or walking slowly on the treadmill or in place), and subsequent measurements may be made while the person is *passive* (e.g., seated in a chair) until the pressure returns nearly to baseline.

Heart Rate

Calibrated **cardiotach** monitors can be useful to estimate the heart rate of the exerciser. Ideally, ECG simulators can be used to check the accuracy of the cardiotach.

Heart rate can be calculated from the **electrocardiogram** itself by taking the average distance for one cardiac cycle (one R-wave to the next R-wave) and dividing it into 1500. For example, 1500 divided by 9.0 mm results in a heart rate of 167 b·min^{-1} (sometimes abbreviated as b/min or bpm). By measuring the horizontal distance (mm) between 11 normal cardiac cycles (first to 11th R-spike), a more valid heart rate at exercise can be calculated from Equation 19.9.[35]

$$\text{HR (b·min}^{-1}) = 60 \text{ s} \div (0.1 \times 10 \text{ R-R mm} \times 0.04) \quad \text{Eq. 19.9}$$

where:

$$60 \text{ s} = 1 \text{ min}$$

$$10 \text{ R-R mm} = \text{distance of 10 cardiac cycles}$$

$$0.1 \times 10 \text{ R-R} = \text{average R-R interval; mm}$$

$$0.04 = \text{time (s) elapsing for each mm}$$

The equation may be simplified by multiplying the two constants, 0.1 and 0.04, and then using the product 0.004 to divide into 60 s. Thus, Equation 19.9 becomes

$$\text{HR (b·min}^{-1}) = 60 \text{ s} \div (0.004 \times 10 \text{ R-R mm}) \quad \text{Eq. 19.10}$$

For example, in Figure 19.3 the distance for 10 cardiac cycles (11 R spikes) during exercise is 111 mm. The following calculation provides an exercise heart rate of 135 b·min^{-1}:

$$\text{HR (b·min}^{-1}) = 60 \text{ s} \div (0.004 \times 111 \text{ mm})$$

$$= 60 \text{ s} \div 0.444$$

$$= 135 \text{ b·min}^{-1}$$

Another method of calculating heart rate uses the 3 s black marks at the top of some ECG paper. By multiplying the number of R-waves (to closest tenth of a cycle) in a 6 s interval by 10, the b·min⁻¹ is produced (Eq. 19.11).

$$b \cdot min^{-1} = \# \text{ of R-waves in 6 s} \times 10 \qquad \text{Eq. 19.11}$$

Also, the technician can make a rapid estimation of heart rate by memorizing the heart rate that is related to each **5 mm box.**[29] First, count the number of 5 mm boxes—indicated by bold vertical lines at every fifth vertical line (0.20 s)—from the first R-wave to the second. Then relate the number of boxes listed in Table 19.5 to the heart rate or simply divide the number of 5 mm boxes into 300. For example, the ECG in Figure 19.3 shows slightly over two boxes between R-waves. Therefore, the heart rate has to be between 150 b·min⁻¹ and 100 b·min⁻¹. The more exact rate is found by dividing 2.2 boxes into 300, thus 136 b·min⁻¹.

"Rulers" to measure heart rate are often provided free by electrocardiograph manufacturers and drug companies. The index line or arrow is placed on an R-spike; then the rate is read at the appointed cardiac cycle—usually three cycles for resting rates, and 10 cycles for exercise rates.

Table 19.5	Rapid Estimation of Heart Rate from the Number (#) of 5 mm Vertical Lines		
Boxes # from R-R	Length mm	Time s	Heart Rate b·min⁻¹
1	5	0.20	300
2	10	0.40	150
3	15	0.60	100
4	20	0.80	75
5	25	1.00	60

Rate of Perceived Exertion (RPE)

The reader may need to refresh the memory about RPE scales by referring back to Chapter 12. Prior to the Exercise ECG Test, the performer should be instructed as to the meaning of the RPE scale. The revised RPE scale with ratio properties may be more suitable for determining subjective symptoms associated with breathing, aches, and pains.[13] A large RPE poster should be prominently placed or held so that the exerciser has no trouble viewing the RPE scale. The tester should read aloud the instructions as printed in Chapter 12. Thumb signals may be necessary if the performer is using a respiratory valve. During the last 15 s of each stage, the tester asks the performer to indicate by pointing to the number on the poster (if respiratory valve) or saying the RPE number. The thumbs-up ("I'm OK"), sideways ("I'm tired"), down ("I'm quitting soon") signals can be used anytime during the test if the performer has the respiratory valve. The technician confirms the performer's RPE number by stating it aloud. Either the 6-to-20 or the category-ratio scale from 0-to-10 monitor the performer's stress. The authors of ACSM's guidelines state that the performers understand the 0 to 10 scale better than the 6 to 20 scale.[7] When performers indicate ratings between 18 and 19 ("very, very hard") and 9 to 10 ("extremely strong"; "strongest intensity") for either of the two scales, respectively, the testers will know that the performers are near exhaustion.[7]

The Electrocardiogram

The basic concept of exercise electrocardiography is depicted in Figure 19.4. The methods of electrocardiography are dependent upon the objectives of the test and the selected electrocardiograph and lead system.

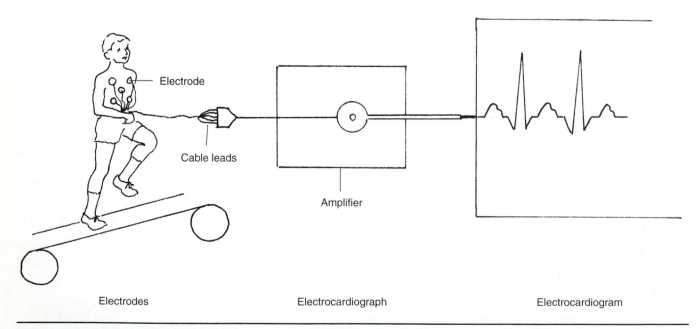

Figure 19.4 Interfacing the heart with the ECG. The electrical currents from the heart are transferred from the skin by the electrodes, amplified by the electrocardiograph, and then recorded as the electrocardiogram.

Electrocardiographic Equipment

Electrocardiograph and Monitor   The electrocardiograph is the recording machine, whereas the tracing is the electrocardiogram. Early technology used a single-channel ECG recorder with or without a monitor. Early monitors were the "bouncing-ball" type, which left only a readable trace for a fraction of a second; newer monitors enable persisting or "freezing" traces, and some can retrieve cycles from memory (Figure 19.5). Expensive electrocardiographs and monitors are available that display 3 to 12 channels nearly simultaneously instead of one (Chapter 18—Figure 18.6). They may include an ECG analysis system and an interface with the treadmill or ergometer for programming the protocol.

Leads and Cable   The lead/cable system for the Exercise ECG Test has improved tremendously since Einthoven's original system for resting electrocardiograms that required a person to maintain both hands and the left foot in three buckets of salt solution. The popular Master ECG Step Test from the 1930s to 1960s was a more portable system but still required the person to carry relatively thick and heavy cables while exercising. In fact, the system was so cumbersome that the person's movements made it impossible to take a readable recording during exercise; only after the exerciser stopped would the tracing be made. Today the electrodes and cables are very lightweight. Present electrodes come prepared with electrolyte solution and are disposable.

ECG Procedures

The procedures for administering the Exercise ECG Test are concerned with (1) safety, (2) application of the electrodes, and (3) ECG protocol.

Safety

Probably the most effective way to assure a safe Exercise ECG Test is to choose a healthy person to perform the test. The American College of Sports Medicine provides guidelines regarding who needs an exercise test before being cleared for exercise or who needs physician supervision dur-

ing the exercise test.[7] For **vigorous** (> 60 % $\dot{V}O_2$max) exercise, men ≥ 45 y of age and women ≥ 55 who have more than one risk factor for coronary artery disease (Table 19.6) need to be medically evaluated by a physician prior to exercise testing and be supervised by a physician during the exercise test.[7] Thus, both age and health-status criteria—such as being apparently healthy, or at higher risk, or diseased—are important considerations with respect to test supervision. For example, maximal treadmill tests of more than 24 000 men and women produced nearly 1100 abnormal exercise tests. Of these, men and women who were apparently healthy had lower abnormality rates than those at higher cardiovascular disease (CVD) risk and those with CVD. Second, the abnormal rate increased exponentially with age, regardless of health status.[38]

For **submaximal,** or **moderate,** (≤ 60 % $\dot{V}O_2$max) exercise testing, apparently healthy persons of any age may participate without prior medical examination or physician-supervised exercise test.[7,15] Hence, those persons without symptoms or disease or no more than one risk factor are free to partake in mild exercise tests.

The safety of the participant is partially dependent upon proper interpretation of the electrocardiogram. The risks associated with performing an Exercise ECG Test are often classified into morbidity and mortality—*morbidity* referring to injury or traumatic event and *mortality* referring to death. Bruce reported a morbidity rate of less than 0.1 % with no mortalities in more than 15 000 mainly coronary patients who performed the exercise test.[17] Also, morbidity and mortality rates of 2.4 and 1, respectively, per 10 000 tests occurred in a survey of 170 000 exercise tests.[55] These rates from physician-supervised tests do not differ from nonphysician-supervised tests, such as those supervised by exercise physiologists[37]—ideally, ACSM-certified exercise physiologists. Thus, with proper supervision, the exercise test is not very risky. Proper supervision also means that the ECG monitor should be observed at all times by at least one technician. Thus, it is important that the technician know how to interpret the ECG that is being viewed on the monitor or paper.

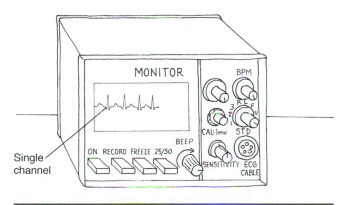

Figure 19.5   An example of an electrocardiograph with a single-channel display monitor.

Table 19.6	Cardiovascular Disease (CVD) Risk Factors	
Positive Risk Factor	**Criteria**	
Age	Men ≥ 45 y; women ≥ 55 y	
Family history	Premature CVD death or MI[a] in parents or siblings:	
	Men—before 55 y	
	Women—before 65 y	
Smoking	Current smoker	
High cholesterol	> 200 mg/dL (> 5.2 mmol/L)	
Diabetes	Insulin dependent (ID) > 30 y of age; non-ID > 35 y of age	
Very sedentary	Sitting nearly all day	

Adapted from Table 2-2, p. 18 of American College of Sports Medicine. (1995). *ACSM's guidelines for exercise testing and prescription.* © ACSM.; Indianapolis, IN 46206-1440.
Note: [a]MI = myocardial infarction (heart attack).

Table 19.7

Absolute and Relative Indications for Termination of an ECG Exercise Test

Absolute Indications for Stopping the Test

1. Acute MI or suspicion of myocardial infarction (MI)
2. Onset of moderate to severe angina (chest pain)
3. Drop in systolic blood pressure (SBP) with increasing power level accompanied by signs or symptoms or drop below standing resting SBP
4. Serious arrhythmias (e.g., second- or third-degree atrioventricular [AV] block, sustained ventricular tachycardia or increasing premature ventricular contractions [PVC], atrial fibrillation with fast ventricular response)
5. Signs of poor perfusion (blood flow), including pallor, cyanosis, or cold and clammy skin
6. Unusual or severe shortness of breath
7. Central nervous system symptoms, including ataxia (incoordination), vertigo (dizziness), visual or gait problems, or confusion
8. Technical inability to monitor the ECG
9. Performer's request

Relative Indications for Stopping the Test[a]

1. Pronounced ECG changes from baseline (> 2 mm of horizontal or downsloping ST-segment depression, or > 2 mm of ST-segment elevation; except in lead aVR)
2. Any chest pain that is increasing
3. Physical or verbal manifestations of severe fatigue or shortness of breath (dyspnea)
4. Wheezing
5. Leg cramps or intermittent claudication (grade 3 on 4-point scale)
6. Hypertensive response (SBP > 260 mm Hg; DBP > 115 mm Hg)
7. Less serious arrhythmias, such as supraventricular tachycardia
8. Exercise-induced bundle branch block that cannot be distinguished from ventricular tachycardia

From American College of Sports Medicine. (1995). *ACSM's guidelines for exercise testing and prescription*, 5th ed., p. 97, table 5-4, © 1995 American College of Sports Medicine.
Note: [a]A relative indication is one that may not call for immediate cessation but reevaluation "when sound clinical judgment supersedes the stated criteria."[7]

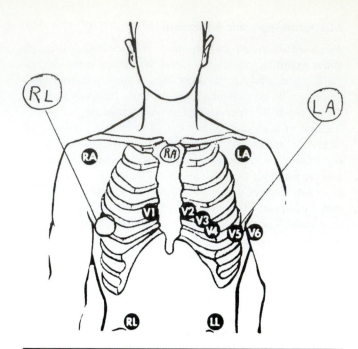

Figure 19.6 The Mason-Likar (blackened sites) and CM5 lead sites. The CM5 electrodes are the RA—placed at manubrium (M), LA—V₅ or chest (C), and RL—ground.

Also, the safety of the performer is enhanced if the technician and supervisor of the Exercise ECG Test are familiar with the criteria for stopping the test. It is not within the scope of this manual to explain all of the criteria listed by the American College of Sports Medicine,[6] but they are presented in Table 19.7 so that interested students will see the need to learn more about them by taking other courses or workshops. Some of the ECG variables that require in-depth study are (1) ectopic beats (e.g., premature ventricular contractions; PVC), (2) ST-depression, a common indicator of myocardial ischemia, and (3) conduction blocks.

Electrode Application

The procedures for applying electrodes can be simple or complex, depending upon the number of electrodes. A Mason-Likar modification[42] of the classic 12-lead (10 electrodes) resting electrocardiogram is often used for the clinical exercise test hookup.[7] However, the electrodes typically placed on the arms and legs in the resting ECG are placed instead on the upper torso when using the Mason-Likar configuration for the exercise test (Figures 19.4 and 19.6). The

right arm (RA; white) negative electrode avoids muscle mass just below (≈ 2 cm) the distal end of the clavicle at the infraclavicular fossa. The left arm (LA; black) positive electrode is placed similarly below the left clavicle. The left (LL; red) and right leg (RL; green) electrodes are placed just superior to the left and right anterior superior iliac spines, respectively, at the level of the navel[12] at the anterior axillary line.[43] Precordial unipolar chest leads are applied at the same sites as those for the resting ECG (Chapter 18).

For exercise tests of apparently healthy persons, a simple three-electrode lead system may be used that is somewhat similar to the V₅ unipolar and the CM5 bipolar lead systems[10,11,21,52] and Holland's[36] configurations. The RA electrode is placed on the person's manubrium, and the LA and RL electrodes are placed at the left V₅ and right side of the chest, respectively; the ECG selector switch is at lead 2. These less sensitive[5] but simpler and effective bipolar lead systems are often used in testing asymptomatic persons; it reduces the time and expense of electrode placement.

In order to avoid muscle and outside electrical interference (artifact), the skin of the person at each electrode site should be prepped before the electrode is applied. Three steps to prepping the skin are (1) scrubbing the site with alcohol, (2) shaving the skin with a razor if hairs are visible, and (3) abrading the skin lightly with fine-grain sandpaper, emery cloth, gauze, or an abrading pad. A final wiping of the skin with alcohol is sometimes performed. The alcohol swab, abrader, and razor must be discarded after their use on one person. First using a marking pen to mark each electrode site facilitates accurate site positioning and provides an indication of the extent of abrading. Inexpensive ohm meters reveal appropriate resistances.

The ECG Protocol

The technician records the ECG while the person is at rest, exercise, and recovery. The person's name, date, body position, and exercise stage should be labeled appropriately on the ECG strip.

Resting and/or Pre-exercise ECG   Ideally, a resting 12-lead ECG should be taken before administering the Exercise ECG Test. It should be required for persons who are at greater risk based on their medical history or risk factor analysis. Although some laboratories include a pre-exercise hyperventilation recording, some authorities do not recommend it because of reducing the tests specificity (i.e., the ability to detect true normals).[24] After taking the resting ECG, a pre-exercise recording should be taken while the performer is seated on the cycle or standing on the treadmill.

Exercise and Recovery ECG   During exercise and recovery, the ECG is monitored constantly, but a tracing may be recorded only at each stage of the test; more frequent recordings may be made if so indicated. The exercise recording usually is taken for the last 10 s to 15 s of each stage. A recording should be taken immediately after the last stage of exercise. A recording should be taken during active recovery at 1 min or 2 min, as well as at passive recovery at the 5th min of post-exercise. The participant should not be released from monitoring until at least 5 min and all subjective and physiological (e.g., ECG baseline) symptoms have stabilized at a reasonable level.

Results and Discussion

Persons performing the Exercise ECG Test can be evaluated according to their fitness and symptoms. The symptom, or variable, of special concern in this chapter is the ECG, which provides us with heart rate, ECG wave lengths, segments, and amplitudes. The interpretation of the performer's fitness can be made through a variety of sources, many found in the chapters on aerobic fitness in *Exercise Physiology Laboratory Manual*.

Heart Rate

A typical increase in heart rate during a progressive exercise test is about 10 b·min^{-1} ($\pm$ 2) for each MET increase. If the peak exercise heart rate is more than 20 b·min^{-1} lower than the age-predicted heart rate (220 – age), it is called chronotropic incompetence.[7] However, cautious interpretation of any criterion using predicted maximal heart rate is advised due to its high variability.[27] A heart rate at 1 min post-exercise that is only within 12 b·min^{-1} of peak exercise heart rate is a predictor of increased risk of mortality.[19]

Table 19.8	ECG Criteria for an Abnormal Exercise Test

1. Exercise-induced ST-depression or elevation of ≥ 1 mm relative to the Q-Q line, lasting ≥ 0.06 s[a] from the J-point
2. Ventricular tachycardia ("V-tach"; ≥ 3 consecutive PVC) or > 30 % frequency of PVC
3. Exercise-induced left or right bundle branch block (delayed and abnormal spread of excitation)
4. Sustained supraventricular tachycardia
5. R-on-T PVC
6. Exercise-induced second- or third-degree heart block
7. Post-exercise U-wave inversion (possible faulty repolarization of septum)
8. Inappropriate bradycardia (slow heart rate)

American College of Sports Medicine, *"Guidelines for Exercise Testing and Prescription,"* 1986, Lea and Febiger 200 Chesterfield Pkwy Malvern, PA 19355-9725. Reprinted by permission.
Note: [a]1995 ACSM "Guidelines"; 1986 "Guidelines" = 0.08 s.

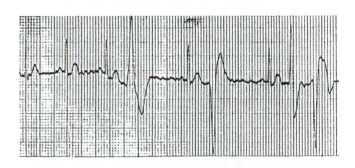

Figure 19.7   Premature ventricular contractions (depolarizations) of a multifocal nature. *Multifocal* means that the ectopic beats originate from more than one area (focus) of the heart.

ECG Interpretation

The Exercise ECG Test in epidemiological studies has demonstrated that asymptomatic men with abnormal tests have 10 to 15 times the risk of coronary artery disease than those with normal exercise tests.[22]

Table 19.8 presents ECG criteria for abnormality in exercise testing that have been endorsed by the American College of Sports Medicine,[5] whereas the following list provides the normal changes associated with exercise:[7]

1. Small changes in the shape and amplitude of the P wave
2. P wave moves closer to the T wave, forming before the T wave reaches baseline at high heart rates (Figure 19.3)
3. Q wave increase in amplitude
4. Slight decrease in R wave amplitude
5. Likely increase in T wave amplitude
6. Slightly shorter QRS duration
7. J point (end of ST) depression
8. Shorter Q-T interval

Arrhythmia

It is not abnormal for healthy persons to have an occasional "skipped" beat during the day.[49] Prevalence of these premature ventricular contractions (PVC; Figure 19.7) may vary

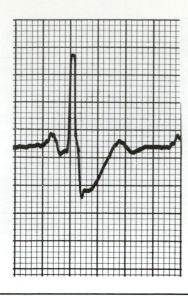

Figure 19.8 An example of severe ST-depression (6 mm to 7 mm) in an elderly man.

with the age of the population and the duration of the monitoring. Prevalency with 24 h monitoring of a young population is 50 %,[14] and about 5 % in only a 2 min monitoring of middle-aged men,[23] and nearly 3 % incidence in the typical time of a resting ECG recording.[51]

The chances of recording ECG abnormalities during exercise is greater than at rest.[39,47] During maximal exercise testing in normal men, the younger men averaged close to 30 % incidence of PVC, while the middle-aged men averaged close to 43 %.[28] Forty-four percent of normal men in another study experienced PVC during maximal exercise.[47] Older adults showed a prevalency of premature ventricular contractions of 16 % at rest and of 55 % during the combined exercise and recovery periods.[2]

S-T Segment

During ischemia, the affected myocardial fibers are slow in reestablishing normal polarity, thus changing the S-T segment[35] and, possibly, increasing the number of ectopic beats.[58] S-T segment depression in a true-positive test probably will not be evident unless a major coronary artery is 60 % occluded.[15] True-positive ST-depression, indicating myocardial ischemia, is best noted by the lateral leads, I, V_4, V_5, and V_6[24] with 1.0 mm of displacement continuing for 0.06 s (i.e., 60 ms).[6] The American Association of Cardiovascular and Pulmonary Rehabilitation[3] considers a moderate risk, especially in persons with cardiac symptoms, to be an exercise-induced ST-depression between 1 mm and 2 mm, whereas a higher risk is greater than 2 mm. Figure 19.8 shows a severe ST-depression of 6 mm to 7 mm. If clinically significant S-T segment depression occurs, especially accompanied by angina, then a follow-up thallium-imagery technique is sometimes advised to validate the positive stress ECG test.

References

1. Alexander, J. F., Liang, M. T. C., Stull, G. A., Serfass, R. C., Wolfe, D. R., & Ewing, J. L. (1984). A comparison of the Bruce and Liang equations for predicting $\dot{V}O_2$max in young adult males. *Research Quarterly for Exercise and Sport, 55,* 383–387.
2. Ambe, K. S., Adams, G. M., & de Vries, H. A. (1973). Exercising the aged. *Medicine and Science in Sports, 5* (Abstract), 63.
3. American Association of Cardiovascular and Pulmonary Rehabilitation. (1994). *Guidelines for cardiac rehabilitation programs.* Champaign, IL: Human Kinetics.
4. American College of Cardiology/American Heart Association Subcommittee on Exercise Testing. (1986). Guidelines for exercise testing: A report of the American College of Cardiology/American Heart Association Task Force on Assessment of Cardiovascular Procedures. *Journal of American College of Cardiology, 8,* 725–738.
5. American College of Sports Medicine. (1986 & 1991). *Guidelines for exercise testing and prescription.* Philadelphia: Lea & Febiger.
6. American College of Sports Medicine. (1995). *ACSM's guidelines for exercise testing and prescription.* Philadelphia: Williams & Wilkins.
7. American College of Sports Medicine. (2000). *ACSM's guidelines for exercise testing and prescription.* Philadelphia: Lippincott Williams & Wilkins.
8. Balke, B., & Ware, R. W. (1959). An experimental study of physical fitness of Air Force personnel. *U.S. Armed Forces Medical Journal, 10,* 675.
9. Baumgartner, T. A., & Jackson, A. S. (1988). *Measurement for evaluation in physical education and exercise science.* Dubuque, IA: Wm. C. Brown.
10. Blackburn, H. (1969). *Measurement in exercise electrocardiography.* Springfield, IL: Charles C Thomas.
11. Blackburn, H., Taylor, H. L., Vasquez, C. L., & Puchner, T. C. (1966). The electrocardiogram during exercise. *Circulation, 34,* 1034–1043.
12. Boone, T., & Zwiren, L. (1993). Surface anatomy for exercise programming. In ACSM (Ed.), *Resource manual for guidelines for exercise testing and prescription* (pp. 3–17). Philadelphia: Lea & Febiger.
13. Borg, G. A. V. (1982). Psychophysical bases of perceived exertion. *Medicine and Science in Sports and Exercise, 14,* 377–381.
14. Brodsky, M., Wu, D., Denes, P., Kanakis, C., & Rosen, K. (1977). Arrhythmias documented by 24-hour continuous electrocardiographic monitoring in 50 male medical students without apparent heart disease. *The American Journal of Cardiology, 39,* 390–395.
15. Brooks, G. A., & Fahey, T. D. (1987). *Fundamentals of human performance.* New York: Macmillan.

16. Bruce, R. A. (1972). Multi-stage treadmill test of submaximal and maximal exercise. In American Heart Association's Committee on Exercise (Ed.), *Exercise testing and training of apparently healthy individuals: A handbook for physicians* (pp. 32–34). New York: American Heart Association.

17. Bruce, R. A. (1974). Methods of exercise testing. *The American Journal of Cardiology, 33,* 715–720.

18. Chung, E. K. (1983). *Exercise electrocardiography: Practical approach.* Baltimore, MD: Williams & Wilkins.

19. Cole, C. R., Blackstone, E. H., Pashkow, F. J., Snader, C. E., & Lauer, M. S. (1999). Heart-rate recovery immediately after exercise as a predictor of mortality. *New England Journal of Medicine, 341,* 1351–1357.

20. Cooper, K. H. (1977). The treadmill re-examined. *American Heart Journal, 94,* 811–812.

21. Costill, D. L., Branam, G. E., Moore, J. C., Sparks, K., & Turner, C. (1974). Effects of physical training in men with coronary heart disease. *Medicine and Science in Sports, 6,* 95–100.

22. Council on Scientific Affairs. (1981). Indications and contraindications for exercise testing. *Journal of the American Medical Association, 246,* 1015–1018.

23. Crow, R. S., Pineas, R. J., Dias, V., Taylor, H. L., Jacobs, D., Blackburn, H. (1975). Ventricular premature beats in a population sample. *Circulation, 51,* (Suppl.), III-211–III-215.

24. Dubach, P., & Froelicher, V. F. (1991). Recent advances in exercise testing. *Journal of Cardiopulmonary Rehabilitation, 11,* 29–38.

25. Duda, M. (1984). Basketball coaches guard against cardiovascular stress. *The Physician and Sportsmedicine, 12,* 193–194.

26. Ellestad, M. H. (1980). *Stress testing. Principles and practice.* Philadelphia: F. A. Davis.

27. Engels, H.-J., Zhu, W., & Moffatt, R. J. (1998). An empirical evaluation of the prediction of maximal heart rate. *Research Quarterly for Exercise and Sport, 69,* 94–98.

28. Faris, J. V., McHenry, P. L., Jordan, J. W., & Morris, S. N. (1976). Prevalence and reproducibility of exercise-induced ventricular arrhythmias during maximal exercise testing in normal men. *The American Journal of Cardiology, 37,* 617–622.

29. Fisher, A. G., & Jensen, C. R. (1990). *The scientific basis of athletic conditioning.* Philadelphia: Lea & Febiger.

30. Foster, C., Crowe, A. J., Daines, E., Dumit, M., Green, M. A., Lettau, S., Thompson, N. N., & Weymier, J. (1996). Predicting functional capacity during treadmill testing independent of exercise protocol. *Medicine and Science in Sports and Exercise, 28,* 752–756.

31. Foster, C., Jackson, A. S., Pollock, M. L., Taylor, M. M., Hare, J., Sennett, S. M., Rod, J. L., Sarwar, M., & Schmidt, D. H. (1984). Generalized equations for predicting functional capacity from treadmill performance. *American Heart Journal, 107,* 1229–1234.

32. Franklin, B. A. (2000). Treadmill scores to diagnose heart disease and assess prognosis. *ACSM's Health and Fitness Journal, 4,* 29–31.

33. Frid, D. J., Ellefsen, K., Porcari, J., Ward, A., Ockene, I., & Rippe, J. (1988). Estimating $\dot{V}O_2$max from a modified Balke treadmill protocol: Validation in a young healthy population. *Medicine and Science in Sports and Exercise, 20* (Suppl.), Abstract #3, S1.

34. Ginder, J. (1984). *The Bruce vs. Cooper predictive tests for aerobic power in prospective fire fighters.* Unpublished master's project, California State University, Fullerton.

35. Goldman, M. J. (1967). *Principles of clinical electrocardiography.* Los Altos, CA: Lange Medical Publications.

36. Holland, G. J., Heng, M. K., & Weber, F. (1988). Conducting and interpreting exercise tests for asymptomatic adults. *Cardiovascular Reviews and Reports, 9,* 54–63.

37. Knight, J. A., Laubach, C. A., Butcher, R. J., & Menapace, F. J. (1995). Supervision of clinical exercise testing by exercise physiologists. *The American Journal of Cardiology, 75,* 390–391.

38. Kohl, H. W., Gibbons, L. W., Gordon, N. F., & Blair, S. N. (1990). An empirical evaluation of the ACSM guidelines for exercise testing. *Medicine and Science in Sports and Exercise, 22,* 533–539.

39. Kosowsky, B. D., Lown, B., Whiting, R., & Guiney, T. (1971). Occurrence of ventricular arrhythmias with exercise as compared to monitoring. *Circulation, 46,* 826–832.

40. Liang, M. T. C., Alexander, J. F., Stull, G. A., & Serfass, R. C. (1982). The use of the Bruce equation for predicting $\dot{V}O_2$max in healthy young men. *Medicine and Science in Sports and Exercise, 14* (Abstract), 129.

41. Luft, V. C., Cardus, D., Lim, T. P. K., Anderson, E. C., & Howarth, J. L. (1963). Physical performance in relation to body size and composition. *Annals of New York Academy of Science, 110,* 795–808.

42. Mason, R. E., & Likar, I. (1966). A new system of multiple-lead exercise electrocardiography. *American Heart Journal, 71,* 196.

43. Mason, R. E., Likar, I., Biern, R. D., & Ross, R. S. (1967). Multiple-lead exercise electrocardiography. *Circulation, 336,* 517–525.

44. Master, A. M., & Oppenheimer, E. J. (1929). A simple exercise tolerance test for circulatory efficiency with standard tables for normal individuals. *American Journal of Medical Sciences, 177,* 223–243.

45. McArdle, W. D., Katch, F. I., & Katch, V. L. (1991). *Exercise physiology: Energy, nutrition, and human performance.* Philadelphia: Lea & Febiger.

46. McArdle, W. D., Katch, F. I., & Katch, V. L. (1994). *Essentials of exercise physiology.* Philadelphia: Lea & Febiger.

47. McHenry, P. L., Morris, S. N., Kavalier, M., & Jordan, J. W. (1976). Comparative study of exercise-induced ventricular arrhythmia in normal subjects and patients with documented coronary artery disease. *The American Journal of Cardiology, 37,* 609–616.

48. McInnis, K. J., & Balady, G. J. (1994). Comparison of submaximal exercise responses using the Bruce vs. modified Bruce protocols. *Medicine and Science in Sports and Exercise, 26,* 103–107.

49. Misner, J. E., Bloomfield, D. K., & Smith, L. (1975). Periodicity of premature ventricular contractions (PVC) in healthy, active adults. *Medicine and Science in Sports, 7* (Abstract), 72.

50. Naughton, J. (1977). Stress electrocardiography in clinical electrocardiographic correlations. In J. C. Rios (Ed.), *Cardiovascular Clinics, 8,* 127–139. Philadelphia: F. A. Davis.

51. Okajuma, M., Scholmerich, P., & Simonson, E. (1960). Frequency of premature beats. *Minnesota Medicine, 43,* 751.

52. Phibbs, B. P., & Buckels, L. J. (1975). Comparative yield of ECG leads in multistage stress testing. *American Heart Journal, 90,* 275–276.

53. Pollock, M. L., Bohannon, R. L., Cooper, K. H., Ayres, J. J., Ward, A., White, S. R., & Linnerud, A. C. (1976). A comparative analysis of four protocols for maximal treadmill stress testing. *American Heart Journal, 92,* 39–46.

54. Pollock, M. L., Foster, C., Schmidt, D. H., Hellman, C., Linnerud, A. C., & Ward, A. (1982). Comparative analysis of physiological responses to three different maximal graded exercise test protocols in healthy women. *American Heart Journal, 103,* 363.

55. Rochmis, P., & Blackburn, H. (1971). Exercise tests: A survey of procedures, safety, and litigation experience in approximately 170,000 tests. *Journal of the American Medical Association, 217,* 1061–1066.

56. Stuart, R. J., & Ellestad, M. H. (1980). National survey of exercise stress testing facilities. *Chest, 77,* 94.

57. Thacker, S. B., & Berkelman, R. L. (1988). Public health surveillance in the United States. *Epidemiological Reviews, 10,* 164.

58. Wasserman, K., Hansen, J. E., Sue, D. Y., Whipp, B. J., & Casaburi, R. (1994). *Principles of exercise testing and interpretation.* Philadelphia: Lea & Febiger.

59. Whipp, B. J., Davis, J. A., Torres, F., & Wasserman, K. (1981). A test to determine parameters of aerobic function during exercise. *Journal of Applied Physiology, 50,* 217–221.

Form 19.1

Exercise ECG Test

Name [   ] Date [   ] Time [   ] A.M. [   ] P.M. [   ]

Age [   ] y Gender (M or W) [   ] Ht [   ] cm Wt [   ] kg Tech. Initials [   ]

Meteorological Data

T [   ] °C (closest 0.1 °C) RH % [   ] P_B [   ] mm Hg × 1.333 = [   ] hPa Fan: Yes [   ] No [   ]

Lead System: Mason-Likar [   ] CM5 [   ] Modified [   ]

Body State	1-R-R mm	Heart Rate (HR) 1500 ÷ R-R = b·min⁻¹	Blood Pressure (mm Hg) 1st Phase	4th	5th
Resting Supine					
Resting Sitting					
Resting Standing					
Bike Sitting or					
Treadmill Standing					

Exercise

Type of Test: Max [   ] Submax [   ] Target HR [   ] b·min⁻¹

Stage	Time[a] (W; % grade; mph; MET)	Power (P)	Heart Rate (b·min⁻¹)	Blood Pressure (mm Hg)	RPE	Arrhythmia (type; #)	ST-Depression (mV)
1	0:00–1:00						
	1:00–2:00						
2	2:00–3:00						
	3:00–4:00						
3	4:00–5:00						
	5:00–6:00						
4	6:00–7:00						
	7:00–8:00						
5	8:00–9:00						
	9:00–10:00						
6	10:00–11:00						
	11:00–12:00						
7	12:00–13:00						
	13:00–14:00						

Total Exercise Time _____ min _____ s; min + (s/60) = _____ decimal min

[a]Cycle protocol

Recovery Time	P or Position	HR	Blood Pressure	Arrhythmia	ST-Depression
0–30 s					
1:00					
3:00					
5:00					

PULMONARY TESTING

Chapter 20 *Resting Lung Volumes*
Chapter 21 *Exercise Ventilation*

The pulmonary (respiratory) tests presented in *Exercise Physiology Laboratory Manual* may be classified into two types—those performed under conditions of rest and those performed during exercise. The resting pulmonary tests presented in this laboratory manual are classified as laboratory tests but may also be classified as field/lab tests because some of the equipment is relatively inexpensive and portable, allowing simple techniques to test persons rather quickly.

Evaluation of pulmonary function is important for early diagnosis and management of pulmonary diseases, such as emphysema, chronic bronchitis, asthma, and pneumonia. The pulmonary tests essentially involve the determination of various lung volumes, airflow rates, and ventilatory volumes. The influence of environment, lifestyle, and age may be evaluated by periodically testing the lungs for deterioration or improvement.

The submaximal exercise test presented in Part 6 includes the measurement of (a) ventilation, (b) breathing frequency, and (c) tidal volume. Ventilatory equivalent, a combination variable that involves both the pulmonary and metabolic systems, is calculated from the exercise ventilation and the estimated oxygen consumption for a given exercise level. Ventilatory threshold also shows the interaction between these two systems.

RESTING LUNG VOLUMES

The measurement of lung volumes during rest enhances the interpretation of these volumes during exercise. The measurement of each of the four lung volumes demonstrates the physiology of respiration and tests for respiratory disease. For example, vital capacity, a composite of three lung volumes, has been used frequently for diagnosing lung disease.[30]

Physiologically, all four lung volumes are nonoverlapping divisions of the lungs at potentially different stages of breathing (Figure. 20.1). For example, the **inspiratory reserve volume (IRV)** is the volume of air that can be inspired maximally at the end of a normal inspiration. The volume of air in a normal breath is the **tidal volume (TV or V_T)**. The volume of air that can be expired maximally after a normal expiration is the **expiratory reserve volume (ERV)**. The **residual volume (RV)** is the volume of air remaining in the lungs after a maximal expiration. The **vital capacity (VC),** an overlapping volume, is a sum of three lung volumes (Eq. 20.1).

$$VC \text{ (mL or L)} = IRV + TV + ERV \qquad \text{Eq. 20.1}$$

VC (mL or L) = IRV + TV + ERV

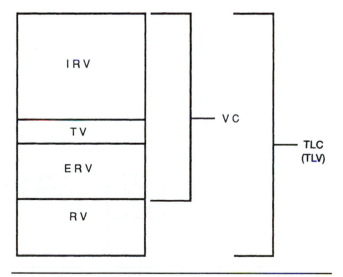

Figure 20.1 The four lung volumes (IRV, TV, ERV, RV) do not overlap as do the vital capacity (VC), and total lung volume (TLV) or capacity (TLC).

Vital Capacity and Forced Expiratory Volume

The vital capacity test is one of the oldest[17] and most common respiratory tests. The measurement of vital capacity (VC) simply requires that an individual blow as large a breath of air as possible into a spirometer. Thus, the person expels three of the four components of the total lung volume—the inspiratory reserve volume (IRV), the tidal volume (TV), and the expiratory reserve volume (ERV)—when performing the vital capacity test. It provides an indirect indication of the size of the lungs, although it is not a complete measure of the entire lung size because it does not account for residual volume. It is often measured in fitness and/or health clinics in order to assess the effects of smoking, disease, or environment or as a part of the hydrostatic weighing test for body composition. Restrictive lung diseases, such as fibrosis and pneumonia, and chest wall stiffness, or respiratory muscle weakness will reduce the vital capacity.

Large vital capacities have been associated with potentially high aerobic performances and breath-hold activities. In general, vital capacity relates to three uncontrolled characteristics: (1) age, (2) stature, and (3) gender. The older a person becomes, the less elastic (less compliant) become both the thoracic cage and respiratory muscles. The reduced expansion of the chest restricts lung expansion, which, along with reduced respiratory muscle strength, reduces vital capacity. The vital capacity is typically higher in taller people. This is basically a function of lung size, taller people having larger lungs. Chest circumference is not as closely related to lung size because chest muscle hypertrophy has little or nothing to do with lung size. Finally, with respect to gender, men have larger lungs than women, even when corrected for body size.

If the person is asked to exhale as fast as possible, the VC is termed more appropriately the Forced (or fast) Vital Capacity (FVC). If FVC is measured at various time intervals, such as at 1.0 s or 3.0 s, then these components of FVC are referred to as Forced Expiratory Volumes ($FEV_{1.0}$ or $_{3.0}$, respectively). Normally, VC and FVC are similar.[25] These timed volumes can be helpful in evaluating late-phase obstructive lung diseases, such as emphysema, bronchitis, and asthma. The only air volume that remains in the person's lungs after such a maximal effort is the residual volume, a volume that normally cannot be exhaled.

Method

The equipment and procedures for measuring the four lung volumes and vital capacity have many similarities. Depending upon the type of equipment, some of these measures can be taken sequentially without changing the instrumentation. Many of the procedures described here are those recommended by the American Thoracic Society's Committee on Proficiency Standards.[2] The accuracy of measuring vital capacity and residual volume is presented in Box 20.1.

Equipment for Measuring Vital Capacity and Timed Volumes

Spirometer is the name of an instrument for measuring lung volumes and ventilation. These may have a mechanical basis, an electronic basis, or a combination of both. Electronic instruments have transducers of various types: (1) pneumotach, (2) turbine, (3) variable orifice, (4) hot wire, and (5) ultrasonic.[25] These have the advantage over traditional mechanical-based spirometers by providing (1) visual displays on monitor and printout, (2) computerized calculations, and (3) direct comparison with computer-stored norms.

Vital capacity and timed volumes are measured easily with an automated electronic-mechanical spirometer such as the Vitalometer® (Warren E. Collins, Braintree, MA). Its features are similar to most other wet spirometers in that its container (body) is filled with distilled water.[a] A hollow tube runs through the middle and extends above the water level at one end and connects to an outside respiratory hose

containing a mouthpiece at the other end (Figure 20.2). A lightweight plastic bell with an open bottom is inside the body of the 9 L container. By enclosing the hollow tube, the bell will rise when a person exhales through the flexible external respiratory (ventilatory) hose. This causes the attached chain on a pulley to move the volume indicators (pointers) of the vitalometer. A *red* pointer on a circular scale indicates the vital capacity value. The *black* pointer indicates the designated *timed volumes* (0.5 s, 0.75 s, 1 s, 2 s, 3 s). A disadvantage of the vitalometer is that it fails to meet the American Thoracic Society's requirement of providing a digital or graphic recording.[2]

The vital capacity can be measured also with 9.0 L or 13.5 L spirometers (Figure 20.3), whose distinguishing features include the rotating drum (kymograph or ventilograph) and the container for carbon dioxide absorbent (e.g., barium hydroxide lime). The bell's counterbalanced chain passes over a pulley and is attached to a pen that records all respiratory movements on the spirogram (chart paper) of the kymograph. The kymograph or drum can rotate at slow (32 mm·min^{-1}), moderate (160 mm·min^{-1}), or fast (1920 mm·min^{-1}) speeds. A sample of an electronic spirometer with a pneumotach transducer is shown in Figure 20.4.

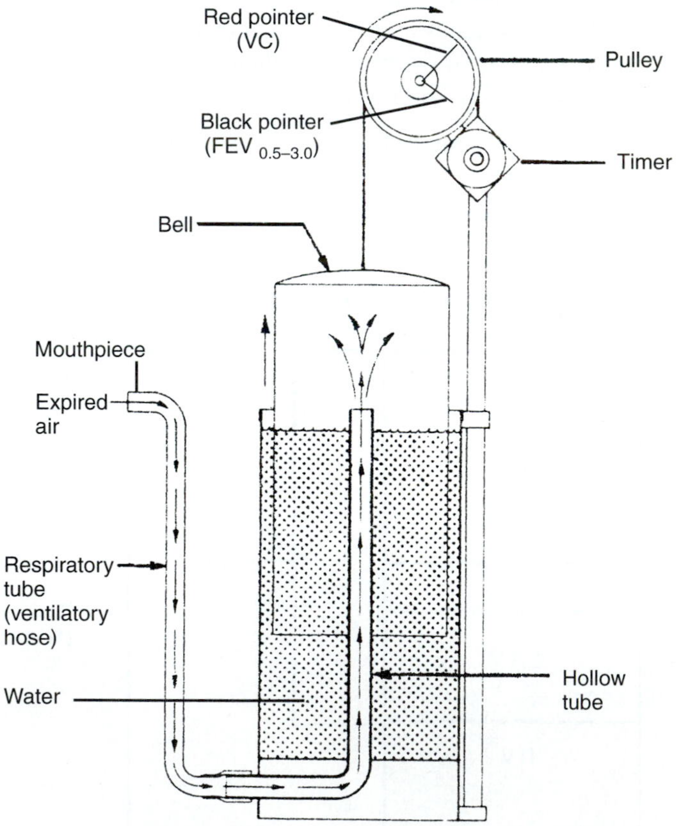

Figure 20.2 A schematic diagram of an automated wet spirometer (e.g., Vitalometer®), showing the upward movement of the bell as the person exhales through the respiratory tube into the water-filled container.

BOX 20.1 Accuracy of Lung Volume Tests

Vital Capacity

Reproducibility of the *best* vital capacity trial in a normal person should be within 50 mL to 100 mL over a period of a few days.[6] Vital capacity does not vary over 5 % from day to day,[15] or the second largest FVC does not vary over 5 % from the largest FVC during the same test.[2] The same criteria apply to FEV$_1$. The voluntary expulsion of air is affected by the cooperation of the participant. This can be a source of variation among persons or between trials of the same person.

Residual Volume

Residual volume may vary daily by about 5 % in either direction for healthy persons.[7] The standard error of measurement is about 100 mL based on a review of traditional methods[35] and about 125 mL when using a simplified method.[36] The oxygen dilution (simplified) method reliabilities range from $r = .96$[31] to .99,[36] with a validity coefficient of .92.[36]

---

[a]Distilled water prevents corrosion or lime development

Regardless of the instrument being used to measure vital capacity, the methods are similar. The pretest preparations should ensure that the equipment is ready for use and is properly sanitized and calibrated, in addition to ensuring that the participant is prepared.

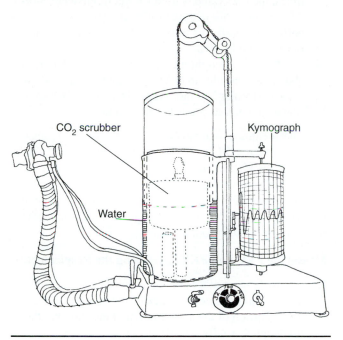

CO₂ scrubber

Kymograph

Water

Figure 20.3 A wet spirometer with the kymograph for recording lung volumes. It includes a two-way breathing valve and a container of CO_2 "scrubber."

Procedures for Measuring Lung Volumes

These procedures apply specifically to the measurement of vital capacity and forced expiratory volumes using the Vitalometer™ and Respirometer. However, most of the steps can be applied to all instruments. They also include detailed procedures for the simplified oxygen-dilution method of measuring residual volume. Brief comments are made regarding other methods of measuring residual volume, such as helium dilution and nitrogen washout.

Preparation for Vital Capacity and Timed Volumes

Some researchers are very strict regarding abstention from exercise within 12 h of pulmonary function testing.[10] This is partly because the vital capacity has been shown to be reduced temporarily after exercise.[21] However, 12 h may be overly restrictive because both vital capacity and $FEV_{1.0}$ may be decreased significantly at the 5th and 10th min but not at the 30th min after varying intensities of exercise.[28]

It is not unusual to measure lung volumes while the person is in the seated position. However, the standing position, which gives slightly greater volumes than sitting,[32] is recommended because the norms presented in this chapter are based on the standing position.[18,25,26]

Participants should wear noseclips if they are inexperienced in the vital capacity test or if the data are to be used for research. The technician should ask the person if it is possible to breathe with the mouth closed when wearing the

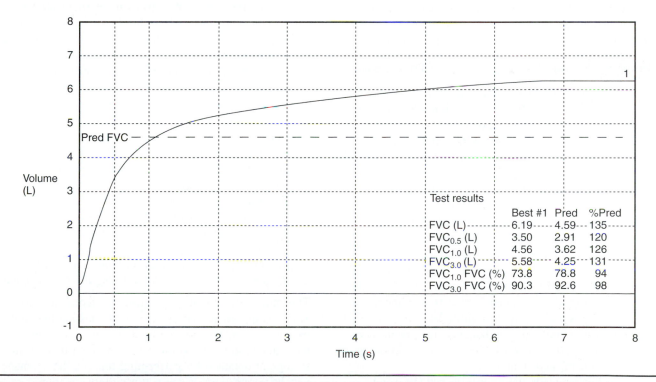

Figure 20.4 A computerized printout displays the forced vital capacity (FVC) and forced expiratory volumes (FEV$_{0.5 \text{ s to } 3.0 \text{ s}}$) of a 59-year-old man who is 175 cm (68.9 in.) tall and a lifetime nonsmoker. From the pneumotach-type instrument TrueMax 2400™ (Parvo Medics, Consentius Technologies, Sandy, UT).

Test results

	Best #1	Pred	%Pred
FVC (L)	6.19	4.59	135
FVC$_{0.5}$ (L)	3.50	2.91	120
FVC$_{1.0}$ (L)	4.56	3.62	126
FVC$_{3.0}$ (L)	5.58	4.25	131
FVC$_{1.0}$ FVC (%)	73.8	78.8	94
FVC$_{3.0}$ FVC (%)	90.3	92.6	98

noseclip. If the person can still breathe, the noseclip should be readjusted until he or she cannot breathe with the mouth closed. Valid tests of vital capacity in experienced persons are possible by simply having them pinch the nose with the fingers during the test. The technician, handling the mouthpiece with sterile gloves or a paper towel, inserts the cardboard disposable mouthpiece into the ventilatory hose.

In order to ensure that the participant knows exactly what to do, the technician and participant should rehearse the commands and practice the breathing maneuvers. The technician should demonstrate the maneuvers,[2] but need not use the spirometer. The participant can also practice the maneuver without actually exhaling into the mouthpiece. The calibration of respiratory instruments is presented in Box 20.2.

Measuring FVC and $FEV_{1.0-3.0}$ Using the Vitalometer

1. In preparation for the test, the bell of the vitalometer should be pushed to its lowest position. The indicator pointers—red and black—should be turned clockwise to the starting position (300 mL to 400 mL). The timing knob should be set at the 1.0 s position in order to measure $FEV_{1.0}$.
2. The performer holds the ventilatory tube at the junction of the mouthpiece and tube.
3. The performer inhales as deeply as possible (maximal inspiration) without inhaling *from* the respiratory tube.
4. At the point of maximal inspiration, the performer places the mouthpiece into the mouth and exhales as much air as possible and as fast as possible. The entire exhalation should last about 5 s[15] to 10 s,[2] although most persons will expire their entire VC within 4 s.[13,16] Technicians should give verbal encouragement, such as "Go," "All the way out," "Keep going," "Looking good," "Push," and "Gut it out!"
5. The technician reads and records the **red (VC)** and **black ($FEV_{1.0}$)** pointers to the closest 50 mL (or 0.05 L) (Figure 20.4).

6. The bell automatically returns nearly to the starting position after the performer removes his or her mouth from the breathing tube; if it does not, the technician should press gently down on the bell so that it does.
7. The technician and participant repeat the test three times; the *best* value is used for interpretive purposes.
8. After three trials with the timer at 1.0 s, the participant performs three trials at 3.0 s in order to measure the $FEV_{3.0}$.
9. The technician might mention that it is possible for the abdominal muscles to be slightly sore on the next day if the performer had more than six FVC trials.
10. The technician disposes the mouthpiece.

The breathing maneuver for measuring vital capacity when using the 9.0 L or 13.5 L respirometer is the same as that using the vitalometer. It may be more convenient, however, to measure vital capacity with the participant seated if the measurement is made sequentially from the other lung volume measurements. The techniques for making the measurement on the respirometer follow.

Measuring FVC and $FEV_{1.0-3.0}$ Using the Respirometer

1. The participant places the mouthpiece into the mouth.
2. The technician places the pen of the respirometer at the lower portion of the spirogram, making sure that there is enough space for the pen excursion for the expiratory capacity.
3. The technician switches the rotating drum to the slow speed (32 mm per min; 1 min between vertical lines).
4. After a few normal breaths by the participant, the technician requests him or her to perform the vital capacity maneuver that has been rehearsed—maximal inspiration followed by maximal expiration.
5. When the participant is nearly at the peak of the inspiratory capacity, the technician may opt to switch to the moderate (160 mm per min; 12 s between vertical lines) or fast (1920 mm/min; 1 s between vertical lines) speed.
6. The participant removes the mouthpiece and relaxes while the technician flushes the respirometer a few times (manually lifts and lowers the bell).
7. The test is repeated three times.
8. The technician calculates the vital capacity and the $FEV_{1.0}$ and $FEV_{3.0}$ from the spirogram.

Measuring Expiratory Reserve Volume, Tidal Volume, and Inspiratory Reserve-Volume Using the Respirometer

The measurement of lung volumes from the 9.0 L or 13.5 L respirometer can be done while testing the vital capacity. In fact, the tidal volume, expiratory reserve volume, and inspiratory volume may be measured from the spirogram obtained by performing the ventilatory maneuvers just prior to the VC test. It is simply a matter of calculating the respective volumes based upon the diagram presented in Figure 20.5.

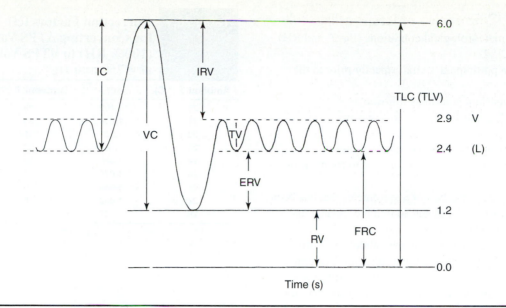

Figure 20.5 Spirogram of lung volumes and vital capacity (VC): TV = tidal volume, IRV = inspiratory reserve volume, ERV = expiratory reserve volume, RV = residual volume, IC = inspiratory capacity, FRC = functional residual capacity, TLC = total lung capacity or volume.

Measuring Residual Volume (RV) Using the Oxygen Dilution Method

The residual volume is the only lung volume that cannot be measured directly; it is also the most complicated and expensive method. Depending upon the chosen method and instrumentation, the reader may have to consult additional sources.[4,7,8,9,12,35,36]

Residual volume has been shown to increase temporarily after exercise.[14] It should not be measured for at least 30 min after exercise.[5]

Traditional methods to measure residual volume require expensive gas analyzers. The **nitrogen washout** method requires a nitrogen or oxygen analyzer, depending upon the use of the traditional or simplified version. The two **helium dilution methods** (multiple breath and single breath) require a helium analyzer, but neither is discussed here.

The rationale for using the nitrogen washout method of estimating residual volume is based upon the measurement of the functional residual capacity (FRC; see Figure 20.5). This is because residual volume cannot be measured directly but can be derived by subtracting the known expiratory reserve volume (ERV) from the FRC (Eq. 20.2).

$$RV \text{ (mL)} = FRC - ERV \qquad \text{Eq. 20.2}$$

The **simplified O_2 dilution** method eliminates the need for a nitrogen or helium analyzer but requires rapid-responding carbon dioxide and oxygen analyzers.[36] Fortunately, the analyzers are common in exercise physiology laboratories. A 5 L neoprene or rubber bag (anaesthesia bag) filled with oxygen is used to determine the extent of its dilution after having been breathed into by the participant.

The procedures for the oxygen dilution technique of reaching nitrogen equilibration by using only oxygen and carbon dioxide analyzers is conceptualized by Equation 20.3.

$$RV = \frac{\text{bag } \dot{V}O_2 \times N_2 \%}{79.8 - N_2 \%} \qquad \text{Eq. 20.3}$$

where:

$\dot{V}O_2$ = initial volume of oxygen in bag

$N_2 \%$ = $100 \% - (O_2 \% + CO_2 \%)$; represents the $N_2 \%$ in mixed air in the bag at the point of equilibrium

79.8 = given percentage of nitrogen by referenced researchers[36]

For example, if the initial volume of 100 % oxygen in the anaesthesia bag is 5 L and the post-breathing percentages of oxygen and carbon dioxide are 75 % and 5 %, respectively, then the calculation of residual volume is as follows:

$$RV(L) = \frac{5.0 \times (100 - 75 - 5)}{79.8 - (100 - 75 - 5)}$$

$$= \frac{5.0 \times 20}{79.8 - 20}$$

$$= \frac{100}{59.8} = 1.67 \text{ L}$$

Procedural Steps for Oxygen Dilution (Simplified) Method of RV Measurement

Several preparations are necessary before measuring the residual volume using the simplified method.

Preparatory steps

1. Record the meteorological conditions (P_B, T, and RH) onto Form 20.2.
2. Measure the participant's vital capacity prior to the RV test.
3. Set up the instrumentation as follows:
   a. attach a 5 L anesthesia bag to a two-way syringe stopcock,
   b. attach the other end of the bag to a three-way breathing valve that can be opened to room air or the bag,
   c. manually push the bell of a spirometer that has been filled with 100 % oxygen so that the oxygen flows into the bag,
   d. flush the bag with pure oxygen about three times,
   e. fill the bag with an accurately measured volume of oxygen that is 80 % to 90 % of the participant's vital capacity; measure the volume of oxygen, for example, by calculating the amount taken from the spirometer.

Testing Procedures

The technician and participant interaction occurs during the following procedures:

1. The participant, wearing a noseclip and in the sitting position, breathes normally via the mouthpiece attached to the three-way breathing valve opened to room air. However, if the main purpose of measuring RV is subsequently to measure body density by underwater weighing, then RV should be measured in the same position as the one in the water.
2. The technician instructs the participant to perform a maximal expiration after a normal breath.
3. At the end of the maximal expiration, the technician turns the three-way valve open to the 5 L bag of oxygen.
4. The technician instructs the participant to breathe deeply (but not depleting the oxygen volume in the bag) five to seven times at about one breath per 2 s.
5. Following the five to seven breaths, the technician instructs the participant to exhale to maximal expiration.
6. The technician turns the valve to close the 5 L bag, thus opening the valve to room air.
7. The technician asks the participant to breathe normally then removes the noseclip.
8. The participant removes his or her mouth from the mouthpiece.
9. The technician removes about 1 L of air from the bag; the remaining contents are analyzed using the carbon dioxide and oxygen analyzers.
10. A technician uses Equation 20.3 to find residual volume.
11. The technician repeats the procedure until readings are within 200 mL (a strict criterion may be 100 mL) of each other; the average of these is the participant's RV.

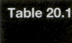

Table 20.1 Correction Factors (cf) for Converting ATPS Volumes (100 % RH) to BTPS Volumes at ≈ 760 mm Hg[a]

Ambient T (° C)	cf	Ambient T (° C)	cf
20	1.102	29	1.051
21	1.096	30	1.045
22	1.091	31	1.039
23	1.085	32	1.032
24	1.080	33	1.026
25	1.075	34	1.020
26	1.068	35	1.014
27	1.063	36	1.007
28	1.057	37	1.000

Note. [a] These cf approximate the cf provided by Equation 20.6. This is because the differences in laboratory pressures and sea level (760 mm Hg) are too small to make a significant difference.

12. The technician corrects the volume to BTPS using Equation 20.9 (or Eq. 20.8 and Table 20.1).
13. The total lung volume (TLV) or capacity (TLC) can be derived easily from a combination of lung volumes or capacities that are now known (Figure 20.5).

$$TLC = FRC + IC \qquad \text{Eq. 20.4}$$

where:

$$FRC = RV + ERV$$
$$IC = TV + IRV$$
$$TLC = RV + VC \qquad \text{Eq. 20.5}$$

Calculations and Corrections for Lung Volumes and Vital Capacity

Certain calculations are made in order to correct respiratory volumes to conventional units of measure. Additionally, simple calculations are necessary in some instances in order to allow for easier interpretation of the norms; an example of the latter is the conversion of the FEV values to a percentage of the VC value.

Correction of Lung Volumes to Conventional Volumes

The final recorded respiratory lung volumes are expressed in terms of BTPS, where the BT represents resting body temperature, the P represents the barometric pressure at the test site, and the S represents the saturation level of the air volume. However, the vital capacity value (liters or milliliters) that is read on the spirometer is in terms of ATPS. The ATPS abbreviation means that the volume of ambient (A) air is at laboratory pressure, at or near laboratory temperature, and is saturated. Some commercial metabolic systems use 31 °C. In other words, the air that is expired from the person's lungs decreases from the typical body temperature of 37 °C to 33 °C at the mouth exit[23] to that near the laboratory of spirometer temperature, usually

20 °C to 25 °C. The air remains saturated in a wet spirometer because of the water surrounding its bell. Even electronic spirometers sample exhaled air that is 100 % saturated. The barometric pressure is read from the laboratory barometer.

Volume Changes Due to Temperature Changes and Water Vapor

A correction must be made because of the temperature difference between the air in the lungs (body) and that of the air being measured in the ambient environment (spirometer). Air molecules expand at higher temperatures; thus, it is logical to expect the BTPS volumes to be higher than ATPS volumes (unless under unusually hot conditions whereby the ambient temperature is over 37 °C). The correction factors (cf) presented in Table 20.1 were derived from Equation 20.6, which accounts for both the expansion of gas and the increase of water vapor pressure at any given increase of temperature.

$$\text{BTPS cf} = \frac{273 \text{ K} + T_b \text{ °C}}{273 \text{ K} + T_A \text{ °C}} \qquad \text{Eq. 20.6}$$

$$\times \frac{P_B - \text{P-H}_2\text{O}_A}{P_B - \text{P-H}_2\text{O}_b}$$

where:

BTPS cf = the correction factor for respiratory volumes

T_b = body temperature (assumed to be 37 °C at rest)

T_A = ambient (environmental or spirometric) temperature

P_B = laboratory barometric pressure

$\text{P-H}_2\text{O}_A$ = vapor pressure of water at the T_A

$\text{P-H}_2\text{O}_b$ = vapor pressure of water at T_b (assumed, 47 torr)

Table 20.1 should serve all laboratory pressures because the differences are extremely small. The correction factors in Table 20.1 range from 1.0 (no correction) at 37 °C to about 1.1 at 20 °C. Hence, the BTPS volume would be 10 % (1.1 cf) larger than the ATPS volume only if the latter were measured at 20 °C. The correction factors are then used to multiply the ATPS volume in order to obtain the BTPS volume.[8]

The vapor pressure of water (P-H$_2$O) at 100 % saturation and at temperatures between 20 °C and 40 °C are listed in Table 20.2.

If a person's exhaled air is 25 °C at 100 % RH and the barometric pressure is 758 mm Hg, then by inserting the proper values into Equation 20.6 we could calculate the ATPS-to-BTPS correction factor as follows:

$$\text{BTPS cf} = \frac{273 \text{ K} + 37 \text{ °C}}{273 \text{ K} + 25 \text{ °C}}$$

Table 20.2 Water Vapor Pressure (P-H$_2$O) at 100 % Saturation at Given Temperatures (T)

T °C	T K	P-H$_2$O mm Hg	T °C	T K	P-H$_2$O mm Hg
20	293	18	31	304	34
21	294	19	32	305	36
22	295	20	33	306	38
23	296	21	34	307	40
24	297	22	35	308	42
25	298	24	36	309	45
26	299	25	37	310	47
27	300	27	38	311	50
28	301	28	39	312	52
29	302	30	40	313	55
30	303	32			

$$\times \frac{758 \text{ mm Hg} - 24 \text{ mm Hg}}{758 \text{ mm Hg} - 47 \text{ mm Hg}}$$

$$= \frac{310 \text{ K}}{298 \text{ K}} \times \frac{734 \text{ mm Hg}}{711 \text{ mm Hg}}$$

$$= 1.04 \times 1.03 = 1.07$$

We could have simply consulted Table 20.1 to obtain the same answer. Thus, by simply finding the respiratory correction factor (cf) and then multiplying the ATPS volume by that factor, one may calculate the BTPS volume (V_{BTPS}) (Eq. 20.7).

$$V_{BTPS} \text{ (L)} = \text{cf} \times V_{ATPS} \qquad \text{Eq. 20.7}$$

For example, if the vital capacity reads 5.40 L at an ambient temperature (T_A) of 22 °C, and pressure (P_B) of 758 mm Hg then by referring to Table 20.1 or by using Equation 20.6 the BTPS correction factor is 1.09. Then by using Equation 20.8 the following calculation determines the respiratory volume (V_{BTPS}):

$$V_{BTPS} \text{ (L)} = 1.09 \times 5.40 = 5.89 \text{ L}$$

The correction of the volume of air in the spirometer (V_{ATPS}) to the volume of air in the lungs (V_{BTPS}) can be summarized by Equation 20.8:

$$V_{BTPS} = V_{ATPS} \times \frac{310}{273 + T_A} \qquad \text{Eq. 20.8}$$

$$\times \frac{P_B - \text{P-H}_2\text{O}_A}{P_B - 47}$$

$$V_{BTPS} = V_{ATPS} \times \frac{310}{273 + 22} \times \frac{758 - 20}{758 - 47}$$

$$= V_{ATPS} \times \frac{310}{295} \times \frac{738}{711}$$

$$= 5.40 \times 1.0508 \times 1.0379$$

$$= 5.40 \times 1.091$$

$$= 5.89 \text{ L}$$

In summary, the BTPS volume reflects the actual environmental condition of the lungs, whereas the ATPS volume reflects the environmental condition at the test site.

Calculations to Facilitate the Interpretation of Scores

The observed vital capacity and forced expiratory volume can be interpreted more meaningfully if the expected (predicted; P) scores are known (Predicted VC or PVC and Predicted FEV or PFEV, respectively). It is also meaningful to know what percentage of the predicted score (% P) is represented by the observed vital capacity (VC_{obs}). Both the predicted and observed respiratory volumes should be presented in BTPS terms.

The predicted value of vital capacity may be approximated from the appropriate nomogram[25] for gender (Figure 20.6 for men; Figure 20.7 for women) or calculated from the regression equations (Equations 20.9 for men and 20.10 for women). These equations give values that are virtually identical to other equations published elsewhere.[1,22] The volumes may be multiplied by 0.85 for African Americans and Asians.[1] If the decimals are ignored in the equations, the answer will be in units of milliliters; thus, the equations will predict the vital capacity within 740 mL and 520 mL for two-thirds of the population at any given height (Ht) and age for men and women, respectively.[25,26]

Men: VC_{BTPS} (L) = 0.148 Ht (in.)   Eq. 20.9
[or 0.058 Ht (cm)] – 0.025 Age – 4.241

Women: VC_{BTPS} (L) = 0.115 Ht (in.)   Eq. 20.10
[or 0.045 Ht (cm)] – 0.024 Age – 2.852

For example, a 46-year-old man who is 69 in. (175.26 cm) tall would be expected to have a vital capacity of 4.8 L (4800 mL to closest 50 mL) based upon the following calculations:

$$VC_{BTPS} \text{ (L)} = (0.148 \times 69 \text{ in.}) - (.025 \times 46 \text{ y}) - 4.241$$

$$= 10.21 - 1.15 - 4.241 = 4.819 \text{ L}$$

$$\text{or using cm:} = (0.058 \times 175.26) - (0.025 \times 46)$$

$$- 4.241$$

$$= 10.17 - 1.15 - 4.241 = 4.779^{b}$$

Equation 20.11 is used to calculate the percent of predicted.

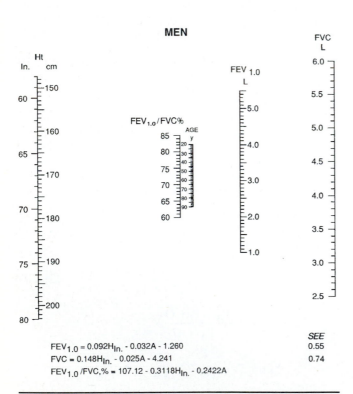

MEN

FEV$_{1.0}$ = 0.092H$_{In.}$ - 0.032A - 1.260   0.55
FVC = 0.148H$_{In.}$ - 0.025A - 4.241   0.74
FEV$_{1.0}$/FVC,% = 107.12 - 0.3118H$_{In.}$ - 0.2422A

Figure 20.6 Nomogram for predicting vital capacity (VC), Forced Expiratory Volume in 1.0 s (FEV$_1$) and FEV$_1$/FVC % (BTPS), in **men** between the ages of 20 y and 90 y. From J. F. Morris, "Spirometry in the Evaluation of Pulmonary Function," in *The Western Journal of Medicine, 125,* (2), fig. 2, p. 114, 1976. Copyright © 1976 California Medical Association.

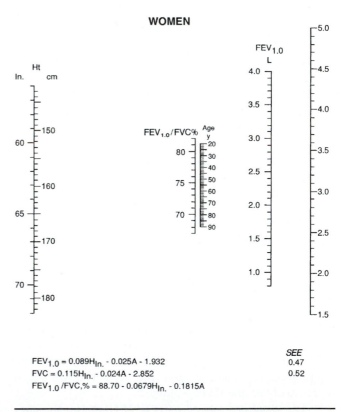

WOMEN

FEV$_{1.0}$ = 0.089H$_{In.}$ - 0.025A - 1.932   0.47
FVC = 0.115H$_{In.}$ - 0.024A - 2.852   0.52
FEV$_{1.0}$/FVC,% = 88.70 - 0.0679H$_{In.}$ - 0.1815A

Figure 20.7 Nomogram for predicting vital capacity (VC), forced expiratory volume in 1.0 s (FEV$_1$), and FEV$_1$/FVC % (BTPS) in **women** between 20 y and 90 y of age. From J. F. Morris, "Spirometry in the Evaluation of Pulmonary Function," in *The Western Journal of Medicine, 125,* (2), fig. 3, p. 115, 1976. Copyright © 1976 California Medical Association.

---

[b]Slight difference due to rounding.

$$\% \ P = (VC_{obs} / PVC) \times 100 \qquad \text{Eq. 20.11}$$

Thus, if the 46-year-old man in the previous example had an observed (obs) vital capacity of 6.00 L, then the percent predicted vital capacity (% VCP) would be calculated as follows:

$$\% \ PVC = (6.00 / 4.80) \times 100$$

$$= 1.25 \times 100$$

$$= 125 \ \%$$

The expected or predicted values for Forced Expiratory Volumes in 1.0 s for men and women are available from their respective nomograms in Figures 20.6 and 20.7 or from their predictive equations (Eq. 20.12 and 20.13). As with the prediction equation for vital capacity, the prediction equations for the forced expiratory volume in 1 s ($PFEV_1$) consider the gender, age, and height of the person.[25] The standard errors of the estimates are 0.55 L for men and 0.47 L for women.

Men: $PFEV_1$ (L) = 0.092 Ht (in.) − 0.032 Age − 1.260

$$\text{(cm use 0.036 Ht)} \qquad \text{Eq. 20.12}$$

Women: $PFEV_1$ (L) = 0.089 Ht (in.) − 0.025 Age − 1.932

$$\text{(cm use 0.035 Ht)} \qquad \text{Eq. 20.13}$$

For example, a 20-year-old woman who is 165.1 cm (65.0 in.) tall would have a predicted forced expiratory volume in 1 s ($PFEV_1$) of 3.346 L or 3350 mL to the closest 50 mL based upon the following metric calculation:

$$PFEV_1 = (0.035 \times 165.1 \text{ cm}) - (0.025 \times 20) - 1.932$$

$$= 5.778 - 0.5 - 1.932$$

$$= 3.346 \text{ L or } 3346 \text{ mL}$$

Results and Discussion

The focus of attention when discussing the results of the tests is on the interpretation of the test scores. The tests for the four lung volumes are of physiological significance and when interpreted in conjunction with vital capacity and FEV tests add a clinical significance. Although the norms are helpful for interpreting the results of a person's pulmonary test, serial test comparisons on a single person over a period of years can be even more helpful.[25]

Respiratory Lung Volumes

Some typical values for three respiratory volumes[7] have been converted to percentages of vital capacity and total lung volume in Table 20.3. As long as a person's respiratory values are normal, they are not good predictors of fitness or performance in a normal environment. This is especially true when such values are adjusted for body size, gender, and age. The approximated percentages for IRV, TV, and ERV are based on the assumption that the percentages do not vary with total lung volume. Absolute values for residual volume and total lung volume in a typical 20- to 30-year-old man and woman are presented also in Table 20.3. The man's values can also be deciphered from Figure 20.5. A slightly higher value for residual volumes in adult men (1300 mL) has been reported.[27]

Vital Capacity

More than 20 "norms" are commonly used by various laboratories.[2] The valid interpretation of vital capacity should consider the person's age, height, gender, and smoking status. The nomograms in Figures 20.6 and 20.7 are based on nearly 1000 nonsmoking men and women.[25,26] The nonsmoking normative values are equivalent to an improvement of lung function that represents a 10 y decrease in age,[24] compared with some traditional norms that included smokers.[17,18] This is attributed to destruction of the pulmonary tissues and consequent degrees of chronic obstructive pulmonary disease (COPD) in those persons with cigarette addiction. The investigators in the famous epidemiological heart study in Framingham, Mass., indicated that the vital capacity and the FEV_1 were associated with living capacity, thus suggesting that the lower the VC or FEV_1 %, the greater the risk of death.[3]

The vital capacities for a typical man and woman between the ages of 20 y and 30 y are 4.8 L (4800 mL) and 3.2 L (3200 mL), respectively (Table 20.3).[7] The highest vital capacity for a female measured in our laboratory was 5.98 L in a former swimmer who was predicted to be 3.99 based upon her age of 31 y and her height of 5.5 ft (167.6 cm). This observed value represented 150 % of her predicted value. One of the highest men's % PVC was 132 % by a 48-year-old who was predicted to have a VC of 4.77 L but had an observed VC of 6.32 L.

Table 20.3 Typical Respiratory Lung Volumes (% VC; % TLV mL) and Capacities (mL)

Lung Volume	% VC	% TLV	Absolute Volumes (mL)		Men	Women	Capacities		Men	Women
IRV	65	52	IRV		3100	1900	VC		4800	3200
TV	10	8	TV		400–500	350–450	IC		3600	2400
ERV	25	20	ERV		1200	900	FRC		2400	1800
RV		20	RV		1200	1000				
			TLV		6000	4200				

Table 20.4	Degrees of Restrictive or Obstructive Lung Disease Based upon VC, FEV_1, VC/PVC^b, $FEV_1/PFEV_1,^c$ and FEV_1/VC^c

Subjective Degree	Percentage
Normal	> 80
Mild; borderline[a]	65–80; 70–79
Moderate	50–64
Severe	35–49
Very severe	< 35

From J. F. Morris, "Spirometry in the Evaluation of Pulmonary Function," in *The Western Journal of Medicine, 125,* (2), Table 2, p. 116, 1976. Copyright © 1976 California Medical Association. *Note:* [a]Mahler's (1993) lower criterion for normal. [b]VC may be normal in some *obstructive* patients.[1] [c]FEV_1 may be normal, and FEV_1/FVC may be normal or increased in some *restrictive* patients.[1]

African American and Asian men and women have lower VC and FEV than White men and women, respectively.[1] A person's measured vital capacity (BTPS) should be a minimum of 80 % of the predicted value in order to be considered normal.[25] Percentages between 100 % and 120 % VC_{obs} would be considered good, and those above 120 % would be classified as high. The vital capacity and FEV_1 criteria for various degrees of ventilatory impairment—restrictive and obstructive—are presented in Table 20.4. Because the FEV_1/VC has been shown to decrease linearly through the course of chronic obstructive lung disease,[30] three of the table's variables are (1) the observed VC percent of predicted FVC, (2) the observed FEV_1 percent of predicted FEV_1, and (3) the observed FEV_1 percent of observed VC. Normal persons should be at least 80 % for all of the listed variables. The FEV should be 94 % during the first 2 s (FEV_2) and 97 % during the first 3 s (FEV_3).

A decrease in pre-exercise FEV_1 versus post-exercise FEV_1 of 10 % or greater following strenuous exercise might suggest exercise-induced bronchospasm.[19,20,29,33] This bronchospasm in most chronic asthmatics and many allergic persons is usually maximal between 5 min and 15 min after exercise.

References

1. American College of Sports Medicine. (2000). *ACSM's guidelines for exercise testing and prescription.* Philadelphia: Lippincott Williams & Wilkins.
2. American Thoracic Society. (1987). Standardization of spirometry—1987 update. *American Review of Respiratory Disease, 136,* 1285–1298.
3. Ashley, F., Kannel, W. B., Sorlie, P. D., & Masson, R. (1975). Pulmonary function: Relation to aging, cigarette habit, and mortality. *Annals of Internal Medicine, 82,* 736–745.
4. Brown, L. K., & Miller, A. (1987). In A. Miller (Ed.), *Pulmonary function tests* Orlando, FL: Grune & Stratton.
5. Buono, M. J., Constable, S. H., Morton, A. R., Rotkis, T. C., Stanforth, P. R., & Wilmore, J. H. (1981). The effect of an acute bout of exercise on selected pulmonary function measurements. *Medicine and Science in Sports and Exercise, 13,* 290–293.
6. Cissik, J. H., & Louden, J. A. (1979). Measurement precision of screening spirometry in normal adult men. *Cardiovascular Practice (CVP), 63,* 65–68.
7. Comroe, J. H., Forster, R. E., Dubois, A. B., Briscoe, W. A., & Carlsen, E. (1962). *The lung.* Chicago: Year Book Medical Publishers.
8. Consolazio, C. F., Johnson, R. E., & Pecora, L. J. (1963). *Physiological measurements of metabolic functions in man.* New York: McGraw-Hill.
9. Cooper, C. B. (1995). Determining the role of exercise in patients with chronic pulmonary disease. *Medicine and Science in Sports and Exercise, 27,* 147–157.
10. Cordain, L., Tucker, A., Moon, D., & Stager, J. M. (1990). Lung volumes and maximal respiratory pressures in collegiate swimmers and runners. *Research Quarterly for Exercise and Sport, 61,* 70–74.
11. Darling, R. C., Cournand, A., & Richards, D. W. (1940). Studies on the intrapulmonary mixture of gases. III. An open circuit method for measuring residual air. *Journal of Clinical Investigation, 19,* 609–618.
12. Enright, P. L., & Hyatt, R. E. (1987). *Office spirometry.* Philadelphia: Lea & Febiger.
13. Gaensler, E. A. (1951). Analysis of the ventilatory defect by timed capacity measurements. *The American Review of Tuberculosis, 64,* 256–278.
14. Girandola, R., Wiswell, R., Mohler, J., Romero, G., & Barnes, W. (1977). Effects of water immersion on lung volumes: Implications for body compositional analysis. *Journal of Applied Physiology, 43,* 276–279.
15. Goldman, A. L. (1979). Standardization of spirometry. *CVP, 7*(3) 35–39.
16. Hodgkin, J. E., Balchum, O. J., Kass, I., Glaser, E. M., Miller, W. F., Haas, A., Shaw, D. B., Kimbel, P., & Petty, T. L. (1975). Chronic obstructive airway diseases—Current concept in diagnosis and comprehensive care. *JAMA: The Journal of the American Medical Association, 232,* 1243.
17. Hutchinson, J. (1846). On capacity of lungs and on respiratory functions with view of establishing a precise and easy method of detecting disease by spirometer. *Tr. Med.-Chir. Society of London, 29,* 137.
18. Kory, R. C., Callahan, R., Boren, H. G., & Syner, J. C. (1961). The Veterans Administration-Army cooperative study of pulmonary function. *American Journal of Medicine, 30,* 243–258.
19. Kyle, J. M., Walker, R. B., Hanshaw, S. L., Leaman, J. R., & Frobase, J. K. (1992). Exercise-induced bronchospasms in the young athlete: Guidelines for routine screening and initial management. *Medicine and Science in Sports and Exercise, 24,* 856–859.

20. Mahler, D. A. (1993). Exercise-induced asthma. *Medicine and Science in Sports and Exercise, 25,* 554–561.

21. Maron, M., Hamilton, L., & Maksud, M. (1979). Alterations in pulmonary function consequent to competitive marathon running. *Medicine and Science in Sports and Exercise, 11,* 244–249.

22. Miller, A. (1986). *Pulmonary function tests in clinical and occupational lung disease.* Orlando, FL: Grune & Stratton.

23. Miller, M. R., & Pincock, A. C. (1986). Linearity and temperature control of the Fleisch pneumotachograph. *Journal of Applied Physiology, 60,* 710–715.

24. Mohler, S. R. (1981). Reasons for eliminating the "age 60" rule. *Aviation, Space, and Environmental Medicine, 52,* 445–454.

25. Morris, J. F. (1976). Spirometry in the evaluation of pulmonary function. *The Western Journal of Medicine, 125,* 110–118.

26. Morris, J. F., Koski, A., & Johnson, L. C. (1971). Spirometric standards for healthy nonsmoking adults. *American Review of Respiratory Disease, 103,* 57–68.

27. National Academy of Sciences. (1958). *Handbook of respiration.* Philadelphia: W. B. Saunders.

28. O'Krory, J. A., Loy, R. A., & Coast, J. R. (1992). Pulmonary function changes following exercise. *Medicine and Science in Sports and Exercise, 24,* 1359–1364.

29. Scoggin, C. (1985). Exercise-induced asthma. *Chest, 87* (Suppl.), 48S–49S.

30. Sobol, B. J., & Emirgil, C. (1977). Clinical significance of pulmonary function tests. *Chest, 72,* 81–85.

31. Thorland, W. G., Johnson, G. O., Cisar, C. J., & Housh, T. J. (1987). Estimation of minimal wrestling weight using measures of body build and body composition. *International Journal of Sports Medicine, 8,* 365–370.

32. Townsend, M. C. (1984). Spirometric forced expiratory volumes measured in the standing versus the sitting posture. *American Review of Respiratory Disease, 130,* 123–124.

33. Virant, F. S. (1992). Exercise-induced bronchospasm—Epidemiology, patho-physiology, and therapy. *Medicine and Science in Sports and Exercise, 24,* 851–855.

34. Wasserman, K., Hansen, J. E., Sue, D. Y., Whipp, B. J., & Casaburi, R. (1994). *Principles of exercise testing and interpretation.* Philadelphia: Lea & Febiger.

35. Wilmore, J. H. (1969). A simplified method for determination of residual lung volume. *Journal of Applied Physiology, 27,* 96–100.

36. Wilmore, J. H., Vodak, P. A., Parr, R. B., Girandola, R. N., & Billing, J. E. (1980). Further simplification of a method for determination of residual lung volume. *Medicine and Science in Sports and Exercise, 12,* 216–218.

Form 20.1

Individual Data for FVC, FEV$_{1.0}$ and $_{3.0}$ (Men)

Name ☐ Date ☐ Time ☐ A.M. ☐ P.M. ☐

Age ☐ y Gender M Ht ☐ cm Wt ☐ kg Tech. Initials ☐

Smoker: (check)

now _____

Meteorological Data

past _____

T ☐ °C (closest 0.1 °C)   RH % ☐ P_B ☐ mm Hg × 1.333 = ☐ hPa

never _____

Correction Factor (CF) ☐ (Table 20.1 or Eq. 20.6)   Body position ☐ sit ☐ stand

Forced Vital Capacity (ATPS)   Trial (circle highest): #1 ☐ mL   #2 ☐ mL   #3 ☐ mL

FVC (BTPS) = CF ☐ × VC (ATPS) ☐ (to closest 50 mL) = ☐ mL; ÷ 1000 = ☐ L

Predicted FVC (PVC)

PVC = (0.148 × ☐ in.) – (0.025 × ☐ y) – 4.241 = ☐ – ☐ – 4.241 = ☐ L

PVC (metric) = (0.058 × ☐ cm) – (0.025 × ☐ y) – 4.241 = ☐ – ☐ – 4.241 = ☐ L

%PVC

% PVC = (VC$_{obs}$BTPS ☐ L ÷ PVC ☐ L) × 100 = ☐ %

FEV$_{1.0}$ ATPS   Trial (circle highest): #1 ☐ mL   #2 ☐ mL   #3 ☐ mL

FEV$_1$BTPS = CF ☐ × FEV$_1$ ATPS ☐ mL = ☐ mL; ÷ 1000 = ☐ L

PFEV$_1$

PFEV$_1$ = (0.092 × ☐ in.) – (0.032 × ☐ y) – 1.260 = ☐ – ☐ – 1.260 = ☐ L

PFEV$_1$ (metric) = (0.036 × ☐ cm) – (0.032 × ☐ y) – 1.260 = ☐ – ☐ – 1.260 = ☐ L

%PFEV$_1$

%PFEV$_1$ = (FEV$_{1obs}$BTPS [　　　] ÷ PFEV$_1$ [　　　]) × 100 = [　　　] %

FEV$_{3.0}$ ATPS   Trial (circle highest): #1 [　　　] mL   #2 [　　　] mL   #3 [　　　] mL

FEV$_3$BTPS = CF [　　　] × [　　　] FEV$_3$ATPS = [　　　] mL; ÷ 1000 = [　　　] L

%FEV$_1$ of VC BTPS = (FEV$_1$ BTPS [　　　] mL ÷ VC BTPS [　　　] mL) × 100 = [　　　] %

%FEV$_3$ of VC BTPS = (FEV$_3$ BTPS [　　　] mL ÷ VC BTPS [　　　] mL) × 100 = [　　　] %

Form 20.2

Individual Data for FVC, FEV$_{1.0}$ and $_{3.0}$ (Women)

Name [   ] Date [   ] Time [   ] A.M. [   ] P.M. [   ]

Age [   ] y Gender [W] Ht [   ] cm Wt [   ] kg [   ] N Tech. Initials [   ]

Smoker: (check)

now _____

Meteorological Data

past _____

T [   ] °C (closest 0.1 °C) RH % [   ] P$_B$ [   ] mm Hg × 1.333 = [   ] hPa

never _____

Correction Factor (CF) [   ] (Table 20.1 or Eq. 20.6) Body position [   ] sit [   ] stand

Forced Vital Capacity (ATPS) Trial (circle highest): #1 [   ] mL #2 [   ] mL #3 [   ] mL

FVC (BTPS) = CF [   ] × VC (ATPS) [   ] (to closest 50 mL) = [   ] mL; ÷ 1000 = [   ] L

Predicted FVC (PVC)

PVC = (0.115 × [   ] in.) − (0.024 × [   ] y) − 2.852 = [   ] − [   ] − 2.852 = [   ] L

PVC (metric) = (0.045 × [   ] cm) − 0.024 × [   ] y − 2.852 = [   ] − [   ] − 2.852 = [   ] L

%PVC

% PVC = (VC$_{obs}$BTPS [   ] L ÷ PVC [   ] L) × 100 = [   ] %

FEV$_{1.0}$ ATPS Trial (circle highest): #1 [   ] mL #2 [   ] mL #3 [   ] mL

FEV$_1$BTPS = CF [   ] × FEV$_1$ ATPS [   ] mL = [   ] mL; ÷ 1000 = [   ] L

PFEV$_1$

PFEV$_1$ = (0.089 × [   ] in.) − (0.025 × [   ] y) − 1.932 = [   ] − [   ] − 1.932 = [   ] L

PFEV$_1$ (metric) = (0.035 × [   ] cm) − (0.025 × [   ] y) − 1.932 = [   ] − [   ] − 1.932 = [   ] L

%PFEV₁

$\text{\%PFEV}_1 = (\text{FEV}_{1\text{obs}}\text{BTPS}\ \boxed{} \div \text{PFEV}_1\ \boxed{}\ ) \times 100 = \boxed{}\ \%$

FEV₃.₀ ATPS   Trial (circle highest): #1 $\boxed{}$ mL   #2 $\boxed{}$ mL   #3 $\boxed{}$ mL

FEV₃BTPS $= \text{CF}\ \boxed{} \times \boxed{}\ \text{FEV}_3\text{ATPS} = \boxed{}\ \text{mL}; \div 1000 = \boxed{}\ \text{L}$

%FEV₁ of VC BTPS $= (\text{FEV}_1\ \text{BTPS}\ \boxed{}\ \text{mL} \div \text{VC BTPS}\ \boxed{}\ \text{mL}) \times 100 = \boxed{}\ \%$

%FEV₃ of VC BTPS $= (\text{FEV}_3\ \text{BTPS}\ \boxed{}\ \text{mL} \div \text{VC BTPS}\ \boxed{}\ \text{mL}) \times 100 = \boxed{}\ \%$

Form 20.3

Individual Data for Residual Volume

Name ☐ Date ☐ Time ☐ A.M. ☐ P.M. ☐

Age ☐ y Gender (M or W) ☐ Ht ☐ cm Wt ☐ kg ☐ N Tech. Initials ☐

Meteorological Data

T ☐ °C (closest 0.1 °C)   RH % ☐ P_B ☐ mm Hg × 1.333 = ☐ hPa

Body position: Sit ☐   Stand ☐   Other ☐

P_B ☐ mm Hg   Correction Factor (cf) ☐ (Table 20.1 or Eq. 20.6)   VC ☐ L (BTPS)

80 % × VC = ☐ L; 90 % × VC = ☐ L   Initial $\dot{V}O_2$ (bag) ☐ L (between 80 % and 90 % VC)

Oxygen % in Bag	Carbon Dioxide % in Bag
Trial #1:	
Trial #2:	
Trial #3:	

$$RV\ (L) = \frac{\dot{V}O_2\ \boxed{}\ L \times [100\ \% - (O_2\ \boxed{}\ \% + CO_2\ \boxed{}\ \%)]}{79.8\ \% - [100\ \% - (O_2\ \boxed{}\ \% + CO_2\ \boxed{}\ \%)]}$$

$$= \frac{\boxed{}\ L \times \boxed{}\ \%}{79.8\% - \boxed{}\ \%}\ \begin{array}{c}\dot{V}O_2 \times [100\ \% - (O_2\ \% + CO_2\ \%)]\\ \rule{4cm}{0.4pt}\\ [100\ \% - (O_2\ \% + CO_2\ \%)]\end{array}$$

$$= \boxed{}\ L$$

$$\rule{5cm}{0.4pt} = \boxed{}\ L; \times 1000 = \boxed{}\ mL$$

☐

Form 20.4

Group Data for Lung Volumes, Vital Capacity, and FEV$_{1.0}$ and FEV$_{3.0}$

Initials

Volumes and Capacities (BTPS; mL)

Men	IRV	TV (V$_T$)	ERV	RV	VC	FEV$_1$	FEV$_3$
1.							
2.							
3.							
4.							
5.							
6.							
7.							
8.							
9.							
10.							
11.							
Mean							
Women	IRV	TV (V$_T$)	ERV	RV	VC	FEV$_1$	FEV$_3$
1.							
2.							
3.							
4.							
5.							
6.							
7.							
8.							
9.							
10.							
11.							
Mean							

EXERCISE VENTILATION

Justification for exercise testing is based on the nonlinear relationship between functional capacity and symptoms.[24] Thus, it is not unusual to find persons who function non-symptomatically under resting conditions but have debilitating symptoms under exercise conditions. When an Exercise Ventilation Test is combined with metabolic measures, such as oxygen consumption and carbon dioxide production, it is a very effective, inexpensive, and noninvasive method for diagnosing exercise intolerance.[40]

The purpose of the Exercise Ventilation Test is to examine the influence of exercise upon such dynamic parameters as (a) minute ventilation volume, (b) breathing frequency, (c) tidal volume, (d) ventilatory equivalent, and (e) ventilatory threshold. A secondary purpose is to relate a measurement at rest—maximal voluntary ventilation—to exercise ventilation.

Physiological Rationale

Measurable differences exist in exercise respiratory parameters between aerobically fit and unfit people. In brief, fit people are expected to have lower minute ventilations, breathing frequencies, and ventilatory equivalents at any given exercise intensity (power). The dynamics of the various respiratory parameters for both fit and unfit persons are the following: (a) a positive linear relationship between minute ventilation and power level except for the change in linearity at the ventilatory threshold, (b) a positive curvilinear relationship between both breathing frequency and tidal volume versus power level, and (c) a horizontal (non-changing) relationship between ventilatory equivalent and power levels below the ventilatory threshold. The kinetics of most ventilatory variables are similar to those of oxygen consumption, heart rate, and blood pressure. Thus, the time required to achieve steady state usually occurs within 2 min to 6 min, depending primarily upon the intensity of the power level.

Minute Ventilation ($\dot{V}_E$ or $\dot{V}_I$)

The amount of air inspired (I) or expired (E) in one minute is termed minute ventilation ($\dot{V}_E$ or $\dot{V}_I$; $L \cdot min^{-1}$). Typical minute ventilations at rest range from 5 $L \cdot min^{-1}$ to 10 $L \cdot min^{-1}$ and at exhaustive exercise from 70 $L \cdot min^{-1}$ to 125 $L \cdot min^{-1}$ with the lower ventilations in women. Minute ventilation increases linearly with increased exer-

cise intensity in order to rid the body of carbon dioxide and provide more oxygen. The increase in minute ventilation changes disproportionately at a point usually between 50 % and 75 % of maximal oxygen consumption,[35] with less fit persons closer to the 50 % value.

Breathing Frequency (f)

The number of breaths taken each minute is referred to as **breathing frequency** or **respiratory rate.** At rest, typical frequencies range from 10 to 20 breaths per minute ($br \cdot min^{-1}$), whereas at maximal exercise they typically range from 40 $br \cdot min^{-1}$ to 55 $br \cdot min^{-1}$. The disproportionate rise in breathing frequency with increased power levels is gradual at low and moderate power levels but rapid at high power levels.[34]

Tidal Volume (TV or V_T)

The volume of air inspired or expired with each breath is called the tidal volume (TV; V_T). It may be expressed either in milliliters or liters and sometimes as a percentage of the vital capacity. At rest, typical tidal volumes are about 350 mL to 500 mL (about 10 % VC), whereas at maximal aerobic exercise they may reach about 1600 mL and 2400 mL for the typical woman and man, respectively (about 50 % VC to 60 % VC). The curvilinear rise in tidal volume with increased power levels is opposite that of breathing frequency; there is a rapid increase in TV when progressing from low to moderate power levels and smaller increases from moderate to high power levels. The larger tidal volume is due to both greater inspirations and expirations, thus encroaching upon the resting inspiratory and expiratory reserve volumes.[31]

Ventilatory Equivalent (VE)

The ratio of ventilation to oxygen consumption is referred to as the oxygen ventilatory (or ventilation) equivalent (O_2 VE). The oxygen ventilatory equivalent in equation form is

$$O_2 \text{ VE} = (\dot{V}_E \text{ or } \dot{V}_I) \div \dot{V}O_2 \qquad \text{Eq. 21.1}$$

Typical oxygen ventilatory equivalents at rest are about 20 L to 25 L of air for each liter of oxygen consumed, thus 20:1 to 25:1 ratios. The O_2 VE remains relatively constant during subventilatory threshold (or subventilatory breakpoint) exercise. Usually, the O_2 VE exceeds 25:1 above the ventilatory threshold; it exceeds 30:1 at and above maximal oxygen consumption. The ventilatory equivalent for carbon dioxide (CO_2 VE) is often combined with O_2 VE to determine the ventilatory threshold.

Ventilatory Threshold (Tvent)

The Tvent (Figure 21.1) is an important index of the capacity for prolonged exercise.[2] Originally, the ventilatory threshold was termed the anaerobic threshold (T_{an}), which was used as an indirect, or noninvasive, estimate of the lactate threshold. The terms *lactate threshold* and *anaerobic threshold* describe "the point at which blood lactic acid rises systematically during graded exercise"[36] and originally was thought to represent the start of anaerobic metabolism during exercise. Various researchers and reviewers have quarreled with both the term—T_{an}—and the physiological rationale.[4,6] Other terms often used, and confused, are (1) *onset of blood lactate accumulation (OBLA);* (2) *ventilatory inflection point—or breakpoint—or threshold;* and (3) *critical lactate clearance point (CLCP).* The newer terms also recognize the nonlinear, or disproportionate, increase in blood lactate or ventilation compared with $\dot{V}O_2$ increase but do not attribute these to the *beginning* of anaerobiosis.[31,42] The CLCP reflects the power output during several bouts of prolonged exercise beyond the performer's ability to clear lactate and prevent it from contin-uously rising.[6] The traditional lactate threshold occurs at a lower oxygen consumption than OBLA and CLCP.

The *ventilatory threshold (Tvent)* or *breakpoint* appears at the nonlinear increase, or exponential rise, in ventilation. This hyperventilation is caused by the increase in carbon dioxide, which results from the buffering by bicarbonate of the hydrogen ions from lactic acid.[14,42] Usually the Tvent occurs at about 50 % to 60 % of maximal oxygen consumption in the typical person[6,7,17] but may vary from 40 % to 85 % of $\dot{V}O_2$max.[26]

An increase in breathing frequency is mainly responsible for the increase in ventilation when the exercise level is above the ventilatory threshold, whereas an increase in tidal volume is mainly responsible for increased ventilation when the exercise level is below the ventilatory threshold. The Tvent has practical implications because fatigue occurs sooner at power levels above the Tvent than below it,[39] and this is even more evident for the critical lactate clearance point when CLCP is measured during continuous prolonged exercise.[6]

Maximal Voluntary Ventilation

The maximal voluntary ventilation test (MVV), reflects the overall capacity of the lungs and respiratory muscles to pump air. Thus, it is an indicator of maximal minute ventilation ($\dot{V}_E$max) during exercise. However, $\dot{V}_E$max values are about

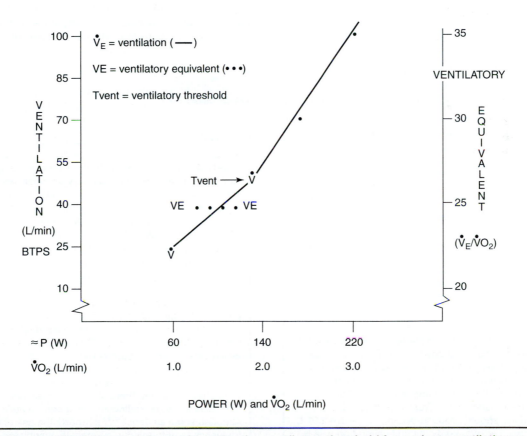

Figure 21.1 An example of the graph format for estimating ventilatory threshold from minute ventilation and oxygen ventilatory equivalent at exercise.

70 %[4] of MVV values. The maximum tolerable steady-state exercise ventilation is only about 64 % of the MVV.[19] This is due to the performer's ability to sustain voluntarily a maximal effort during a 12 s or 15 s MVV period[3] versus the longer, 1 min, period for exercise ventilation. Additionally, maximal exercise does not involuntarily stimulate maximal ventilations, and performers do not voluntarily force themselves to breathe faster and deeper at maximal exercise.

In respiratory patients at exercise, when the ventilation requirement exceeds 50 % of the MVV "the patient almost invariably complains of dyspnea (breathlessness)."[20] The correlation was –.49 between MVV and distance-run time in trained middle distance runners.[11]

The purpose of the MVV test is to measure the maximal amount of air that can be inspired (or expired) within a brief time period under resting conditions.

Maximal Voluntary Ventilation (MVV) Method

The methods for measuring MVV include the usual items of concern, such as equipment, calibration of equipment (Box 21.1), accuracy of the measurement (Box 21.2), and procedural steps. The calculations for MVV are made by the computer software, which uses the same equations that were presented in Chapter 20. In Chapter 20, however, we calculated all equations ourselves; this time the computer will do them.

Equipment

As mentioned in Chapter 20, pulmonary measurements can be made with mechanical (e.g., wet spirometers, bellows) instruments or electronic (e.g., pneumotach, turbine) instruments. The electronic ones usually attach to measurement modules that convert analog signals to digital signals so that computerized software can provide instantaneous calculations and monitored displays and printouts of the results in table and graph forms (Parvo Medics of Consentius Technologies, Sandy, UT; Physio-Dyne Instrument Corp., Quogue, NY; Quinton Instruments, Bothell, WA; SensorMedics Corp., Yorba Linda, CA).

A list of the items for the automated calibration and measurement of maximal voluntary ventilation usually includes the following: (1) 3 L or 7 L calibrating syringe; (2) noseclip; (3) mouthpiece; (4) two-way rebreathing valve; (5) ventilatory tubing; (6) disposable bacterial/viral filter; (7) pneumotach, turbine, or other type of electronic flowmeter; (8) software; (9) computer; and (10) printer.

A figure of a calibration syringe (3 L) was presented in Figure 15.3. The noseclip prevents air from entering and exiting from the nose—air that is not capable of being measured by the instruments. The mouthpieces for automated testing of MVV can be the same disposable cardboard ones used for testing lung volumes mentioned in Chapter 20 if the participant uses a *hand-held* pneumotach. However, for a more similar comparison to exercise ventilation and a more secure fitting into the mouth, I recommend using the rubber mouthpieces that fit onto respiratory rebreathing valves. These rubber mouthpieces are more expensive than the disposable cardboard ones and require washing and sterilizing after each test. A variety of sizes have flanges that fit between the gums and lips and two protruding tabs that the teeth grip (VacuMed,™ Ventura, CA). The two-way rebreathing respiratory valve's inlet port allows room air to enter the participant's mouth and then directs the exhaled air to the outlet port of the respiratory

---

BOX 21.1 Calibration

Ideally, the airflow meter should be calibrated prior to the test with a syringe that is, ideally, at least 3 L.[3] The technician should make sure that all connections are in proper order and are tightly sealed. In general, this means that the respiratory valve directs expiratory air to the airflow meter.

Be sure to place the pulmonary bacterial filter in front of the pneumotach to replicate the test setup. The computer will direct you to the flowmeter calibration option. Stroke the syringe four times to flush out any heated air. Then stroke three times each at five different speeds, starting slowly at ≈ 60 mL·min⁻¹ and increasing gradually with each set of three strokes to ≈ 600 mL·min⁻¹. The computer screen displays each stroke. The variance in readings should be < 0.1 L. Thus, a 3 L syringe should produce readings between 2.91 L and 3.09 L for each stroke. Verify the first calibration with a second calibration.

BOX 21.2 Accuracy of the MVV and Exercise Ventilation Tests

Dry airflow meters with bellows (e.g., Parkinson-Cowan) are not recommended for research studies that measure online high-flow rates. This means that pulmonary tests, such as vital capacity and forced expiratory volumes, and exercise ventilations should not utilize the bellows type of dry spirometer. The only precise way that they could be used for heavy exercise purposes is to collect the air in Douglas bags, meteorological balloons, or anesthetic bags and then pump the air at a slow rate of flow through the meter.

Pneumotachometers and turbines are accurate to ± 2 % or about ± 50 mL of air. Instruments that measure inspiratory air instead of expiratory air are accurate to ± 1.0 %. One guideline is to try obtaining MVV volumes that are reproducible within 5 % of each other.[22]

Oxygen and carbon dioxide analyzers are accurate to volume fractions of about 0.1 %. Probably the best that can be expected from the automated devices is an accuracy of ± 2 % for measuring oxygen consumption. Although knowing the oxygen consumption permits the determination of ventilatory threshold, there still may remain about 30 % of the cases where no deflection point can be deciphered.[9] Although some evidence[9, 23] supports the use of breathing frequency to determine accurately the ventilatory threshold, more confirmation is needed.

valve. For instruments that measure expiratory volumes, a transparent flexible tube connects the outlet port of the respiratory valve to the disposable bacterial/viral filter just in front of the pneumotach or other spirometry device. The ventilatory tubing requires washing and sterilization after each use. The pneumotach includes a pressure transducer and is the flowmeter of many automated systems. The computer and its software enable displays and printouts of the calculated results.

Procedural Steps for MVV

1. Turn on the system and allow 30 min for warm-up. Insert participant data and meteorological data into the computer.
2. Calibrate the flowmeter (Box 21.1).
3. If the performer's MVV is going to be compared to maximal ventilation during treadmill ergometry, then the MVV at rest is measured with the performer standing. If the performer is compared to cycle ergometry, then the resting MVV is measured with the performer sitting.
4. The performer breathes from a respiratory valve mouthpiece into the airflow meter.
5. After breathing normally for at least three consecutive breaths, the performer starts breathing as much air as possible. To maximize the MVV, the performer should approximate a breathing rate of at least one breath per s,

with tidal volumes about 50 % vital capacity; larger breaths may interfere with frequency of breathing, whereas faster breaths interfere with tidal volumes.

6. Immediately after the fast breathing starts, a technician clicks the computer screen (e.g., "Trial Run").
7. When the displayed tidal waves reach near the 20th s (sometimes 12th s or 15 s), a technician calls "STOP" and clicks "OK" on the computer. The performer breathes normally and removes the mouthpiece and noseclip.
8. Repeat the test two more times; use the best trial for data purposes.
9. Print and save the best test.
10. No calculations are necessary because the computer automatically converts 12 s of tidal waves to minute volumes and converts ATPS to BTPS (Figure 21.2).

Exercise Ventilation Method

The Exercise Ventilation Test demonstrates the effect of exercise upon such respiratory factors as ventilation, breathing frequency, tidal volume, ventilatory equivalent, and ventilatory threshold. The procedures and calculations are described here. The equipment is the same as for the MVV test with the addition of either a cycle ergometer or treadmill and gas analyzers. The analyzers enable the direct measurement of the oxygen and carbon dioxide ventilatory equivalents. They

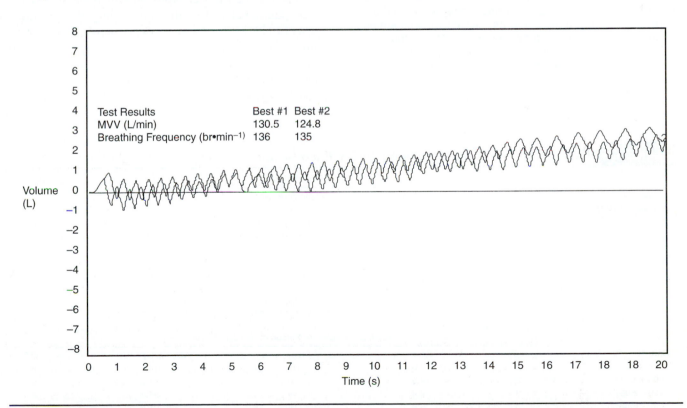

Test Results	Best #1	Best #2
MVV (L/min)	130.5	124.8
Breathing Frequency (br•min⁻¹)	136	135

Figure 21.2 The printed graph from an automated computerized measurement of a 45-year-old man, who is 162.5 cm tall, shows two superimposed trials of maximal voluntary ventilation (MVV). Although each trial lasted 20 s, only 12 s of each trial was used to calculate the projected MVV (L/min) and breathing frequency per minute. Courtesy of Parvo-Medic, Consentius Technologies, Sandy, UT.

also enhance the precision of the ventilatory threshold. For simplicity and conceptualization purposes, the oxygen ventilatory equivalent and ventilatory threshold can be estimated from basic power (W)-to-oxygen consumption conversions and breathing frequency, respectively. Figure 21.3 displays the typical configuration of an automated system for measuring expiratory air.

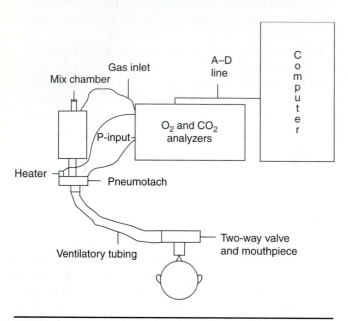

Figure 21.3 The interfaces (connections) between the participant's air and the computer are shown, in addition to the pressure (P) transducer line and heater of the pneumotach. Also shown is the analog to digital (A–D) converter line from the measurement module (analyzer console) to the computer.

Procedure

In addition to the actual conduction of the Exercise Ventilation Test, the technicians should be familiar with the proper preparations, such as calibration, meteorological data, and the exercise protocol.

The technician should record the **meteorological data** onto Form 21.1 and the computer screen. This is especially important for respiratory tests because of the influence of temperature, pressure, and saturation on air volumes. Conveniently, once the meteorological (environmental) data are into the computer, all conversions are made automatically.

As with most of the exercise tests described in this manual, the **performer** should abide by the standard guidelines prior to exercise testing. The performer should be fitted comfortably and securely with the noseclip and the respiratory valve.

The **exercise protocols** described in Table 21.1 are for cycle and treadmill ergometry, although other forms of ergometry may be used. The 4 min exercise bouts at each power level are designed to elicit steady-state conditions, especially for those power levels below the ventilatory threshold.[40] The protocols are not expected to elicit exhaustion. There are three exercise protocols for **cycle ergometry,** depending upon the low, moderate, or high fitness level of the performer. For example, those persons with $\dot{V}O_2$max values greater than 2.9 L·min^{-1} will use the high-power protocol, which has four 4 min stages starting at 100 W, then proceeding by 25 W increments to 175 W. The cycle recovery period returns to the initial stage of each protocol. The cycle protocols will approach maximal levels for persons who are only slightly above the fitness criterion of each protocol.

Table 21.1 **Exercise Protocols for Ventilation during Exercise and Recovery**

Fitness History	Cycle Exercise		
	Low-Power	Moderate-Power	High-Power
$\dot{V}O_2$max (L·min^{-1})	< 2.1	2.1–2.9	> 2.9
Time	Power Prescription (W)		
0:00–4:00	50	75	100
4:00–8:00	75	100	125
8:00–12:00	100	125	150
12:00–16:00	125	150	175
	Cycle Recovery		
16:00–20:00	50	75	100

Treadmill Exercise for Person of Average Fitness					
Time	mph	km·h^{-1}	Slope %	$\dot{V}O_2$ mL·kg^{-1}·min^{-1}	MET
0:00–4:00	3	4.8	0	10.5	3
4:00–8:00	3	4.8	5	17.5	5
8:00–12:00	3	4.8	10	24.5	7
12:00–16:00	3	4.8	15	31.5	9
			Treadmill Recovery		
16:00–20:00	3	4.8	0	11.55	3

The single treadmill protocol at the bottom of Table 21.1 is the Stanford protocol.[2] All four exercise stages, and the recovery stage, are at a speed of 4.8 km·h^{-1} (3.0 mph). The slope increases from 0 % at Stage 1 to 15 % at Stage 4. These 5 % increments at each stage cause a MET increase of 2 MET at each stage. Thus, the treadmill oxygen cost increases from 10.5 mL·kg^{-1}·min^{-1} (3 MET) at the first stage to 31.5 mL·kg^{-1}·min^{-1} (9 MET) at the fourth (final) exercise stage.

Conduction of the Test

For cycle ergometry, a technician starts the timer as soon as the performer reaches the appropriate pedal revolutions (50 rpm to 80 rpm for constant power ergometer) at the prescribed exercise level. For treadmill ergometry, the time starts when the performer is at the prescribed speed and slope and then releases the hands from the treadmill railings.

Many automated systems can be programmed to calculate minute ventilations by averaging single breaths, 15 s, 30 s, or 1 min volumes.

Calculations

The parameters of concern are minute ventilation, breathing frequency, tidal volume, ventilatory equivalent, and ventilatory threshold. As with the lung volumes measured under resting conditions (Chapter 20), the exercise ventilation volumes must be expressed in BTPS form. We will allow the computer of the automated system to make those conversions in this chapter. The computer will also convert oxygen consumption volumes to STPD. For a review of STPD, see Chapter 15. Our conceptualization of the computer's calculations is enhanced by examining some basic respiratory equations for ventilation, tidal volume, breathing frequency, ventilatory equivalents, and ventilatory threshold.

Interaction of Minute Ventilation, Tidal Volume (TV; V_T), and Breathing Frequency (f)

Equation 21.2 summarizes the interaction between the major ventilatory variables.

$$\dot{V}_E \text{ or } \dot{V}_I \text{ BTPS} = f \times \bar{V}_T \qquad \text{Eq. 21.2}$$

where:

$\dot{V}_E$ or $\dot{V}_I$ = minute ventilation expired or inspired in L·min^{-1} or mL·min^{-1}

f = frequency of breathing in breaths per minute (br·min^{-1})

$\bar{V}_T$ = tidal volume in liters or milliliters per breath (L·br^{-1}; mL·br^{-1})

For example, if breathing frequency is 30 br·min^{-1} and tidal volume is 2 L·br^{-1}, then

$$\dot{V}_E \text{ (L·min}^{-1}) = 30 \text{ br·min}^{-1} \times 2 \text{ L·br}^{-1} = 60 \text{ L·min}^{-1}$$

The average tidal volume could be determined by two methods if using an electronic recorder during the test. It would be possible to measure each tidal volume during the minute's interval and then get the average; however, even without the recorder it is much simpler to derive the $\bar{V}_T$ from Equation 21.2, which when transposed becomes Equation 21.3.

$$\bar{V}_T \text{ (L·br}^{-1}; \text{ mL·br}^{-1}) = (\dot{V}_E \text{ or } \dot{V}_I) \div f \qquad \text{Eq. 21.3}$$

For example, if minute ventilation equals 60 L·min^{-1} for the 12th min, and the frequency of breathing equals 30 br·min^{-1}, then the following calculation would provide the tidal volume:

$$\bar{V}_T \text{ (L·min}^{-1}; \text{ ml·br}^{-1}) = 60 \div 30$$

$$= 2 \text{ L·br}^{-1} \text{ or } 2000 \text{ mL·br}^{-1}$$

A meaningful calculation with respect to tidal volume is that which relates it to vital capacity. Equation 21.4 can be used to calculate the relative size of each breath:

$$\% \text{ VC} = (\bar{V}_T \div \text{VC}) \times 100 \qquad \text{Eq. 21.4}$$

For example, if tidal volume is 2000 mL·br^{-1} and vital capacity is 5000 mL, then the following calculation shows that the size of the tidal volume is 40 % VC:

$$\% \text{ VC} = (2000 \div 5000) \times 100$$

$$= 0.40 \times 100$$

$$= 40 \% \text{ VC}$$

Breathing frequency is calculated following the same principles as the calculation of tidal volume. If the minute ventilation and the mean tidal volume are known and Equation 21.2 is transposed, then Equation 21.5 enables the calculation of breathing frequency.

$$f \text{ (br·min}^{-1}) = V_E \div \bar{V}_T \qquad \text{Eq. 21.5}$$

For example, if minute ventilation is 60 L·min^{-1} and tidal volume is 2 L·br^{-1}, then

$$f \text{ (br·min}^{-1}) = 60 \text{ L·min}^{-1} \div 2 \text{ L·br}^{-1}$$

$$= 30$$

Oxygen Ventilatory Equivalent (O$_2$ VE)

An accurate measurement of the oxygen ventilatory equivalent requires the direct measurement of oxygen consumption and ventilation. However, estimates can be made by first equating the exercise power levels to oxygen consumption, then dividing the $\dot{V}O_2$ into the minute ventilation for each power level. To equate the power level of cycle ergometry with oxygen consumption, Table 21.2 or any of the Equations 21.6 to 21.9 may be used.

Table 21.2 **Expected Ranges for Oxygen Ventilatory Equivalent (O_2 VE), Frequency (f), Tidal Volume (TV), and Minute Ventilation ($\dot{V}_E$ or $\dot{V}_I$) during the Exercise Ventilation Test**

Power kg·m·min⁻¹	W	$\dot{V}O_2$ L·min⁻¹	$\dot{V}_E$ or $\dot{V}_I$ L·min⁻¹	f br·min⁻¹	TV mL·br⁻¹	VC %	O_2 VE Ratio
150	25	0.60	12–15	12–19	900–1400	20–35	20–25
300	50	0.90	15–23	13–20	1000–1500	20–40	20–25
450	75	1.20	24–32	15–21	1300–1700	25–45	20–25
600	100	1.50	32–39	17–23	1500–1900	30–50	21–26
750	125	1.80	40–49	20–25	1600–2000	35–55	22–27
900	150	2.10	48–59	23–30	1700–2100	35–55	23–28
1050	175	2.40	58–70	26–35	1800–2200	40–60	24–29
1200	200	2.80	70–84	30–40	1900–2300	40–60	25–30
Recovery (1st min)							
300	50	0.90	35–50	20–28	1400–2000	25–40	40–50

Note: It is possible to have values outside these ranges, depending upon fitness level and vital capacity.

$\dot{V}O_2$ (mL·min⁻¹) =

$$[P \text{ (in N·m·min}^{-1}) \times 0.2] + 300 \qquad \text{Eq. 21.6}$$

$$[P \text{ (in kg·m·min}^{-1}) \times 2] + 300 \qquad \text{Eq. 21.7}$$

$$[P \text{ (in W)} \times 12] + 300 \qquad \text{Eq. 21.8}$$

$$(10.8 \times W) + (7 \times BM) \qquad \text{Eq. 21.9[2]}$$

where: BM = body mass (kg)

Once the estimated oxygen consumption for the given power level is known, the oxygen ventilatory equivalent may be calculated from Equation 21.10.

$$O_2 \text{ VE} = (\dot{V}_I \text{ or } \dot{V}_E) \div \dot{V}O_2 \qquad \text{Eq. 21.10}$$

For example, Table 21.2 shows that the expected oxygen consumption for cycle ergometry at a power of 150 W is 2.1 L·min⁻¹. If the ventilation during the twelfth minute is 52.0 L·min⁻¹ BTPS, then the following calculation would provide an oxygen ventilatory equivalent of 24.8.

$$O_2 \text{ VE (ratio)} = 52.0 \text{ L·min}^{-1} \div 2.1 \text{ L·min}^{-1}$$

$$= 24.8$$

Thus, 24.8 L of air per minute was breathed by the performer for each liter of oxygen consumed while exercising at a steady-state power level of 150 W.

For the treadmill protocol, oxygen consumption in liters per minute or milliliters per minute may be estimated from the given mL·kg⁻¹·min⁻¹ values in Table 21.1 when used in conjunction with Equation 21.11.

$\dot{V}O_2$ (L·min⁻¹) =

$$\frac{MET \times 3.5 \text{ mL·kg}^{-1} \cdot \text{min}^{-1} \times BM \text{ in kg}}{1000} \qquad \text{Eq. 21.11}$$

For example, what would be the oxygen consumption (L·min⁻¹) if the mL·kg⁻¹·min⁻¹ value at the 12th min of the treadmill protocol (3 mph; 10 % slope) were 24.5 for a 70 kg person? By multiplying 24.5 by the body mass of the performer, 70 kg, the product is the amount of oxygen con-

sumed expressed in milliliters per minute—1715. This is converted to liters by dividing 1715 mL·min⁻¹ by 1000, resulting in an oxygen consumption of 1.72 L·min⁻¹.

Ventilation or oxygen consumption may be approximated if either of these two variables is known. This is because the expected range of ratios for the ventilatory equivalent is between 20 and 25 for submaximal exercise below the ventilatory threshold. For instance, if only oxygen consumption is measured, then ventilation may be estimated from Equation 21.12, which is a transposed form of Equation 21.1.

$$\dot{V}_E \text{ or } \dot{V}_I = \dot{V}O_2 \text{ (L·min}^{-1}) \times 20 \text{ to } 25 \qquad \text{Eq. 21.12}$$

For example, if the oxygen consumption is 3.0 L·min⁻¹, then the ventilation can be estimated as

$$\dot{V}_E \text{ or } \dot{V}_I = (20 \text{ to } 25) \times 3.0 \text{ L·min}^{-1}$$

$$= 60 \text{ L·min}^{-1} \text{ to } 75 \text{ L·min}^{-1}$$

Oxygen consumption may be calculated by using Equation 21.13[13] or by using Equation 21.14, which is also a transposition of Equation 21.1.

$$\dot{V}O_2 \text{ (L·min}^{-1}) = \dot{V}_E \text{ or } \dot{V}_I \times 0.04 \qquad \text{Eq. 21.13}$$

$$\dot{V}O_2 \text{ (L·min}^{-1}) = (\dot{V}_E \text{ or } \dot{V}_I) \div 25 \qquad \text{Eq. 21.14}$$

For example, if the minute ventilation is 60 L·min⁻¹, then the oxygen consumption can be estimated as follows:

$$\dot{V}O_2 \text{ (L·min}^{-1}) = 60 \text{ L·min}^{-1} \times 0.04$$

$$= 2.40 \text{ L·min}^{-1}$$

or

$$= 60 \text{ L·min}^{-1} \div 25$$

$$= 2.40 \text{ L·min}^{-1}$$

Ventilatory Threshold (Tvent; VT)

The Tvent (or VT) is at the point where the oxygen ventilatory equivalent increases without a similar increase in

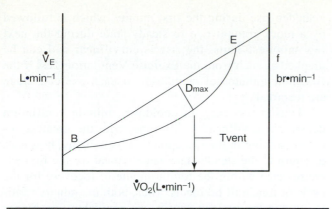

Figure 21.4 The Dmax method of determining the ventilatory threshold requires plotting ventilation ($\dot{V}_E$) or breathing frequency (vertical axis) with oxygen consumption (horizontal axis). Then the plotted points are connected with a smooth curved line, and the two endpoints (Beginning: B; Ending: E) of this line are connected with a straight line. Then a perpendicular line is drawn at the apparent maximal distance from the curved line and the straight line. The ventilatory threshold is where the Dmax line intersects the curved line.

the ventilation-to-carbon dioxide ratio (CO_2 VE) when oxygen consumption is plotted on the horizontal axis.[14,15] Ideally, examination of the $\dot{V}_E/CO_2$ relationship, and more data points for the $\dot{V}_E$ vs. $\dot{V}O_2$ relationship than the four produced by this exercise protocol, are recommended[41] for estimating the ventilatory threshold. Also, ideally, 15 s or 30 s data points, not just 1 min points, should be plotted in order to determine the change in slope or linearity between $\dot{V}CO_2$ and $\dot{V}O_2$.[28,37] Despite these limitations, Tvent can be approximated by using the graph developed from Form 21.3 (also see Figure 21.1). This is done by connecting the data points for ventilation at the four given exercise intensities and the four corresponding assumed oxygen consumptions of the protocol. The inflection point occurs where there is a disproportionate change of linearity (change in slope). This would represent the approximate ventilatory threshold.[36]

The Dmax method helps investigators in deciphering consistently the threshold from ventilation, breathing frequency, and carbon dioxide production.[9] It can also be used to decipher the lactate threshold if blood lactates are measured.[33] The term *Dmax* represents the maximal distance derived from the following computations or procedures (also see Figure 21.4):

1. Graphically plot ventilation and/or breathing frequency (vertical axis) with oxygen consumption (horizontal axis).
2. Connect the 15 s or 30 s points—usually forming a curved line.
3. Draw a straight line connecting the first plotted point to the last plotted point.
4. Draw a perpendicular line from the straight line to the curved line at the point appearing to produce the longest perpendicular line.

5. The ventilatory threshold is where the Dmax line intersects the curved line.[a]

It becomes apparent from the ventilatory equivalent and ventilatory threshold equations that there is a very close relationship between metabolism (oxygen consumption) and respiration (ventilation).

Results and Discussion

Maximal voluntary ventilation is lower in patients with obstructive and restrictive lung disease.[10] Maximal ventilation during exercise may be indicated by measuring the resting maximal voluntary ventilation (MVV). One investigator reported an average resting MVV of 189 L·min⁻¹, with the highest being 252 L·min⁻¹ in trained middle-distance runners.[11] Some norms use body surface area (m²) and age as a basis for predicting average MVV.[5] Other predictions of average MVV may use age and stature,[27] age alone,[32] and FEV.[21] High school boys average 146 L·min⁻¹ ($SD = 21$).[29] MVV decreases by about 25 % from ages in the 20 s to the 60 s.[8] Various methods of determining average values are presented as follows:

1. Use a nomogram[27] to predict the expected (normal) MVV based upon age, gender, and height, or use the prediction equation (21.15) for men only:[27]

   Men: MVV (L·min⁻¹) =   Eq. 21.15
   $(1.34 \times$ Ht in cm$) - (1.26 \times$ Age$)$

2. A prediction equation (Eq. 21.16) of MVV for men and women may be used by multiplying the Forced Expiratory Volume (FEV_1) by 40.[21]

   $$FEV_1 \times 40 = MVV \qquad \text{Eq. 21.16}$$

3. Tables are available that provide norms for adult men and women based upon body surface areas (BSA; Figure 21.5)[b] between 1.40 and 2.10 square meters (m²).[5] The regression equations for men (Eq. 21.17) and women (Eq. 21.18) were used to derive the nomograms.

   Men: MVV (L·min⁻¹) =   Eq. 21.17
   $(86.5 - 0.522$ Age$) \times$ m²

   Women: MVV (L·min⁻¹) =   Eq. 21.18
   $(71.3 - 0.474$ Age$) \times$ m²

4. Women's MVV may be predicted from age alone in Equation 21.19.[32]

   Women: MVV (L·min⁻¹) = $113 - 0.7$ Age   Eq. 21.19

---

[a]The original Dmax method[9] was modified in these procedures by not employing a third-order curvilinear regression to form the curved line of the plotted points.
[b]Dubois' classic BSA formula =[18] BSA (m²) = $0.202 \times$ (m^{0.425}$) \times$ H^{0.725}.

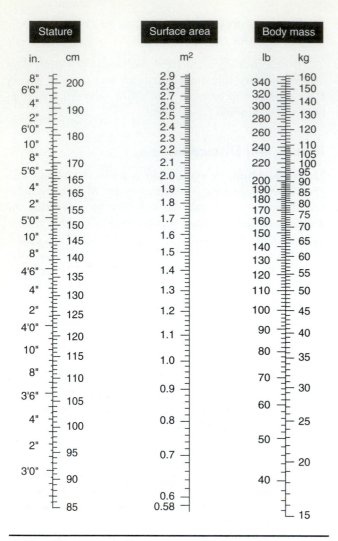

Figure 21.5 The body surface area (BSA) nomogram provides the BSA (m²) without making any calculations. Simply place a straight-edge or string on the stature (in. or cm) vertical line at the left side of the nomogram and pivot it to the body mass (lb or kg) vertical line at the far right. The intersecting point on the surface area (m²) vertical line gives the body surface area. For example, a person with a stature of 175 cm (69 in.) and body mass of 70 kg (154 lb) has a body surface area of 1.88 m². Nomogram is by the courtesy of Warren E. Collins, Braintree, MA.

Exercise ventilation may be evaluated by observing the kinetics of ventilation and the steady-state aspects of minute ventilation. The *kinetics of ventilation* refers to the nonsteady-state condition, whereby the ventilatory parameters are ascending to their plateaus at each exercise power level; *kinetics* may also refer to the ventilatory parameters descent to baseline during recovery from exercise.

Kinetics of Ventilation

The rise in ventilation at the onset of exercise is similar to the rise in heart rate and oxygen consumption; there is

a sudden rise during the first minute, which is followed by a more gradual rise to steady state during the next few minutes. Thus, the rise is curvilinear and can be graphed as such from the Exercise Ventilation Test if the first four minutes of ventilation at each exercise stage are recorded.

During recovery, or cooldown, minute ventilation decreases curvilinearly with time, with the greatest decrease ocuring in the first minute. It is unlikely, however, to return to the steady-state value typical for the first exercise stage within the fourth minute of recovery for the cycle or treadmill protocols. Thus, both the minute ventilation and the oxygen ventilatory equivalent are higher during early recovery of the cooldown period than during the same exercise power level at the start of the progressive exercise protocol.

Steady-State Ventilatory Values during Submaximal Exercise

Aerobically fit persons have lower ventilations, respiratory frequencies, and oxygen ventilatory equivalents for any given level of submaximal exercise than unfit people. With exercise training, persons with chronic airway obstruction reduce their ventilations and frequencies.[1] The approximate ranges for ventilation, breathing frequency, tidal volume, and ventilatory equivalent at given powers and oxygen consumptions were presented in Table 21.2.

Minute Ventilation and Oxygen Ventilatory Equivalent

At the higher power levels, or at some point between 50 % and 75 % maximal oxygen consumption, the minute ventilation would be expected to increase at an accelerated rate;[6] thus, the higher end of the ranges presented in Table 21.2 would be more appropriate for persons exercising at power levels above their ventilatory threshold. Aerobically unfit persons have higher ventilations at any given submaximal exercise intensity than fit persons.

The oxygen ventilatory equivalent is always lower than the carbon dioxide ventilatory equivalent when the respiratory exchange ratio is less than 1.0.[40] The O₂ VE is also lower in aerobically fit persons.

Tidal Volume and Breathing Frequency

The approximated tidal volumes in Table 21.2 are based upon typical vital capacities of 4.8 L and 3.2 L for men and women, respectively. Also, a somewhat linear relationship between tidal volume and oxygen consumption (or power) is assumed at the low and moderate exercise intensities (about 25 W to 150 W). As exercise intensity increases beyond the moderate levels, however, the greater ventilation requirement tends to be met by increased frequency, while the tidal volume tends to reach an asymptote (plateau).[40] The greater rate increase in frequency of breathing at high power levels is in contrast to its relatively slow increase at low and moderate levels of exercise.

Ventilatory Threshold

The Tvent may be closely related to a perceived exercise intensity of 12 to 15 on the 6–20 RPE scale. Semantically, this would equate to exercise intensities described as "somewhat heavy" to "heavy."[30] The sustained intensity of exercise for marathoners or 3 h cyclists coincides roughly with their oxygen consumption at the ventilatory threshold.[12] The higher along the oxygen consumption continuum that Tvent occurs, the faster will be the sustained exercise pace.

Maximal Exercise

Although the final stage of the exercise protocol used for this Exercise Ventilation Test may not stimulate maximal exercise ventilatory values in most performers, the discussion presented here can help interpret the ventilatory values produced by a maximal oxygen consumption test.

Maximal Minute Ventilation

Maximal breathing capacity is similar for treadmill and cycling ergometry.[40] Respiratory parameters are not limiting factors for maximal exercise capacity in the average healthy person. However, they do limit the maximal aerobic capacity of elite endurance athletes.[16,42] Even during maximal exercise, the performer could increase ventilation voluntarily if that were desired. Neither the average person nor the athlete is expected to have a maximal exercise ventilation that equals the minute ventilation derived from the 12 s maximal voluntary ventilation (MVV).

The breathing reserve may be expressed as the difference between the stationary MVV and the maximal exercise ventilation.[40] If a performer's $\dot{V}_E$ max is within 15 L·min^{-1} of the MVV, then that person may have a clinically significant ventilatory problem.[10] Thus, a normal person should have a ventilatory reserve of at least 15 L·min^{-1}. The ventilatory reserve ($\dot{V}$res) may be calculated from Equation 21.20.

$$\dot{V}res = MVV - \dot{V}_E \text{ or } \dot{V}_I \text{ max} \qquad \text{Eq. 21.20}$$

Another evaluative equation for ventilatory limitation uses the ratio of $\dot{V}_E$max to MVV (Eq. 21.21). Normally, the ratio should range from 0.5 to 0.7. A $\dot{V}_E$max: MVV ratio > 0.7 (same as a ventilatory reserve < 30 %) indicates a ventilatory limitation.[2]

$$\dot{V}_E \text{ ratio} = \dot{V}_E\text{max} \div MVV \qquad \text{Eq. 21.21}$$

Maximal Tidal Volume

In general, the maximal tidal volume at maximal exercise is 50 % to 55 % for men and 40 % to 45 % for women.[40] It can be expressed by Equation 21.22 as:[25]

$$\bar{V}_T \text{ max} = 0.74 \text{ VC} - 1.11 \qquad \text{Eq. 21.22}$$

Thus, the typical adult male with a vital capacity of 4.80 L would be expected to have a maximal tidal volume of about 2.44 L (2440 mL) to 2.64 L (2640 mL) or about 50 % to 55 % of the vital capacity; the typical female with a vital capacity of 3.20 L would be expected to have a maximal tidal volume of about 1.26 L (1260 mL) to 1.44 L (1440 mL) or 40 % to 45 % of the vital capacity. Probably, highly motivated exercisers would be able to achieve tidal volumes up to 60 % of their vital capacities at their exhaustive point of exercise.

Maximum breathing frequency in normal men between the ages of 34 y and 74 y is less than 50 br·min^{-1} in 95 % of these men at maximal exercise.[21,38]

References

1. Alison, J. A., Samios, R., & Anderson, S. D. (1981). Evaluation of exercise training in patients with chronic airway obstruction. *Journal of Physical Therapy, 61,* 1273–1277.
2. American College of Sports Medicine. (2000). *ACSM's guidelines for exercise testing and prescription.* Philadelphia: Lippincott Williams & Wilkins.
3. American Thoracic Society. (1995). Standardization of spirometry—1994 update. Official Statement of the American Thoracic Society, *American Journal of Respiratory Critical Care Medicine, 152,* 1107–1136.
4. Åstrand, P. O., & Rodahl, K. (1986). *Textbook of work physiology.* New York: McGraw-Hill.
5. Baldwin, E. D., Cournand, A., & Richards, D. W. (1948). Pulmonary insufficiency I, Physiologic classification, Clinical methods of analysis, Standard values in normal subjects. *Medicine, 27,* 243.
6. Brooks, G. A., Fahey, T. D., White, T. P., & Baldwin, K. M. (2000). *Exercise physiology: Human bioenergetics and its application.* (3rd ed.). Mountain View, CA: Mayfield.
7. Casaburi, R., Storer, T. W., Sullivan, C. S., & Wasserman, K. (1995). Evaluation of blood lactate elevation as an intensity criterion for exercise training. *Medicine and Science in Sports and Exercise, 27,* 852–862.
8. Chebotarev, D. F., Korkushka, D. V., & Ivanov, L. A. (1974). Mechanisms of hypoxemia in the elderly. *Journal of Gerontology, 29,* 393–400.
9. Cheng, B., Kuipers, H., Snyder, A.C., Keizer, H.A., Jeukendrup, A., & Hesseluk, M. (1992). A new approach for the determination of ventilatory and lactate thresholds. *International Journal of Sports Medicine, 13,* 518–522.
10. Cooper, C. B. (1995). Determining the role of exercise in patients with chronic pulmonary disease. *Medicine and Science in Sports and Exercise, 27,* 147–157.
11. Costill, D. L. (1971). Endurance running. In ACSM (Ed.), *Encyclopedia of sport science and medicine* (p. 338). New York: Macmillan.

12. Coyle, E. F. (1995). Integration of the physiological factors determining endurance performance ability. In J. O. Holloszy (Ed.), *Exercise and sport sciences Reviews 23* (pp. 25–63). Baltimore: Williams & Wilkins.

13. Datta, S. R., & Ramanathan, N. L. (1969). Energy expenditure in work predicted from heart rate and pulmonary ventilation. *Journal of Applied Physiology, 26,* 297–302.

14. Davis, J. A. (1985). Anaerobic threshold: Review of the concept and directions for future research. *Medicine and Science in Sports and Exercise, 17,* 6–18.

15. Davis, J. A., Frank, M. H., Whipp, B. J., & Wasserman, K. (1979). Anaerobic threshold alterations caused by endurance training in middle aged men. *Journal of Applied Physiology, 46,* 1039–1045.

16. Dempsey, J. A. (1986). Is the lung built for exercise? *Medicine and Science in Sports and Exercise, 18,* 143–155.

17. deVries, H. A. (1986). *Physiology of exercise in physical education and athletics.* Dubuque, IA: Wm. C. Brown.

18. Dubois, D., & Dubois, E. F. (1916). Clinical calorimetry: A formula to estimate the approximate surface area if height and weight be known. *Archives of Internal Medicine, 17,* 863.

19. Freedman, S. (1970). Sustained maximum voluntary ventilation. *Respiratory Physiology, 3,* 230–244.

20. Gaensler, E. A., & Wright, G. W. (1966). Evaluation of respiratory impairment. *Archives of Environmental Health, 12,* 146–189.

21. Hansen, J. E., Sue, D. Y., & Wasserman, K. (1984). Predicted values for clinical exercise testing. *American Review of Respiratory Disease, 12* (Suppl.), S49–S55.

22. Hill, N. S., Jacoby, C., & Farber, H. W. (1991). Effect of an endurance triathlon on pulmonary function. *Medicine and Science in Sports and Exercise, 23,* 1260–1264.

23. James, N. W., Adams, G. M., & Wilson, A. F. (1989). Determination of anaerobic threshold by ventilatory frequency. *International Journal of Sports Medicine, 10,* 192–196.

24. Jones, N. L. (1975). Exercise testing in pulmonary evaluation: Rationale, methods, and the normal respiratory response to exercise. *New England Journal of Medicine, 293,* 541–544.

25. Jones, N. L. (1984). Dyspnea in exercise. *Medicine and Science in Sports and Exercise, 16,* 14–19.

26. Jones, N. L., & Ehrsam, R. E. (1982). The anaerobic threshold. In R. Terjung (Ed.), *Exercise and sport sciences review* (pp. 49–83). New York: Franklin Institute Press.

27. Kory, R. C., Callahan, R., Boren, H. G., & Syner, J. C. (1961). The Veterans Administration–Army cooperative study of pulmonary function. *American Journal of Medicine, 30,* 243–258.

28. Lucia, A., Hoyos, J., Pérez, M., & Chicharro, J. L. (2000). Heart rate and performance parameters in elite cyclists: A longitudinal study. *Medicine and Science in Sports and Exercise, 32,* 1777–1782.

29. Pease, G. F. (1961). *Maximum breathing capacity in high school boys.* Unpublished master's thesis, San Diego State University, California.

30. Prusacyzk, W. K., Cureton, K. J., Graham, R. E., & Ray, C. A. (1992). Differential effects of dietary carbohydrate on RPE at the lactate and ventilatory thresholds. *Medicine and Science in Sports and Exercise, 24,* 568–575.

31. McArdle, W. D., Katch, F., & Katch, V. (1996). *Exercise physiology, energy, nutrition, and human performance.* Philadelphia: Williams & Wilkins.

32. Needham, C. D., Rogan, M. C., & McDonald, J. (1954). Normal standards for lung volumes, intrapulmonary gas-mixing and maximum breathing capacity. *Thorax, 9,* 313.

33. Nicholson, R. M., & Sleivert, G. G. (2001). Indices of lactate threshold and the relationship with 10-km running velocity. *Medicine and Science in Sports and Exercise, 33,* 339–342.

34. Origenes, M. M., Blank, S. E., & Schoene, R. B. (1993). Exercise ventilatory response to upright and aero-posture cycling. *Medicine and Science in Sports and Exercise, 25,* 608–612.

35. Powers, S. K., & Beadle, R. E. (1985). Onset of hyperventilation during incremental exercise: A brief review. *Research Quarterly for Exercise and Sport, 56,* 352–360.

36. Powers, S. K., & Howley, E. T. (2001). *Exercise physiology: Theory and application to fitness and performance.* (4th ed.). Boston: McGraw-Hill.

37. Schneider, D. A., Phillips, S. E., & Stoffolano, S. (1993). The simplified V-slope method of detecting the gas exchange threshold. *Medicine and Science in Sports and Exercise, 25,* 1180–1184.

38. Sue, D. Y., & Hansen, J. E. (1984). Normal values in adults during exercise testing. *Clinical Chest Medicine, 5,* 89–98.

39. Wasserman, K. (1986). Anaerobiasis, lactate and gas exchange during exercise: The issues. *Federation Proceedings, 45,* 2904–2909.

40. Wasserman, K., Hansen, J. E., Sue, D. Y., Whipp, B. J., & Casaburi, R. (1994). *Principles of exercise testing and interpretation.* Philadelphia: Lea & Febiger.

41. Wasserman, K., Whipp, B. J., Koyal, S. N., & Beaver, W. L. (1973). Anaerobic threshold and respiratory gas exchange during exercise. *Journal of Applied Physiology, 35,* 236–243.

42. Wilmore, J. H., & Costill, D. L. (1999). *Physiology of sport and exercise.* (2nd ed.). Champaign, IL: Human Kinetics.

Form 21.1

Individual Data for the Exercise Respiratory Test

Name [   ] Date [   ] Time [   ] A.M. [   ] P.M. [   ]

Age [   ] y Gender (M or W) [   ] Ht [   ] cm Wt [   ] kg [   ] N BSA [   ] m^2

Meteorological Data

Tech. Initials [   ] T [   ] °C (closest 0.1 °C) RH % [   ] P$_B$ [   ] mm Hg × 1.333 = [   ] hPa

VC BTPS [   ] L MVV [   ] L·min^{-1} BTPS $\dot{V}O_2$max [   ] L·min^{-1}

Ergometry Mode (check one): Cycle [   ] Treadmill [   ] Step [   ] Other [   ]

Time min	Power W; km·h^{-1}; %	MET	$\dot{V}$ATPS L·min^{-1}	$\dot{V}$BTPS L·min^{-1}	f br/min	TV mL/br	BTPS % VC	$\dot{V}O_2$ L·min^{-1}	O$_2$VE ratio
0:00–1:00									
1:00–2:00									
2:00–3:00									
3:00–4:00									
4:00–5:00									
5:00–6:00									
6:00–7:00									
7:00–8:00									
8:00–9:00									
9:00–10:00									
10:00–11:00									
11:00–12:00									
12:00–13:00									
13:00–14:00									
14:00–15:00									
15:00–16:00									
Recovery 16:00–17:00									
17:00–18:00									
18:00–19:00									
19:00–20:00									

Form 21.2

Graphic Analysis of Tidal Volume and Frequency

Tidal Volume (TV)

(mL·br⁻¹)

TV = TV --- TV --- TV

f = f . . . f . . . f

| | 3000 | | | | | | | | 50 |

BREATHING FREQUENCY (f)

(br·min⁻¹)

Cycle Power (W)	25	50	75	100	125	150	175	200
V̇O₂ (L·min⁻¹)	0.6	0.9	1.2	1.5	1.8	2.1	2.4	2.8
TM MET		3		5		7		9

Exercise Intensity

Form 21.3

Graphic Analysis of Ventilation and Ventilatory Equivalent

$\dot{V}_E = \dot{V}_E$ --- $\dot{V}_E$ --- $\dot{V}_E$
VE = VE. .VE. . .VE

Left axis (VENTILATION ($\dot{V}_E$) (L·min^{-1})): 90, 70, 50, 30, 10, 0

Right axis (OXYGEN VENTILATORY EQUIVALENT (O$_2$VE)): 35, 30, 25, 20, 15, 0

W:	25	50	75	100	125	150	175	200
L·min^{-1}:	0.6	0.9	1.2	1.5	1.8	2.1	2.4	2.8

Power (W) and $\dot{V}O_2$ (L·min^{-1})

Chapter 22 *Lower Trunk Flexibility*

Consideration of the range of joint motion is crucial in defining the term *flexibility*. Additionally, the measurement of range of motion may involve various types of movements in flexibility testing.

One meaningful definition of flexibility fitness is the optimal range of motion (ROM) permitted by connective and muscle tissue. This definition not only lends itself to quantifying flexibility in terms of distance or degree of ROM, but also includes the two main tissues influencing flexibility. Although neural tissue had been shown to contribute to resistance by eliciting an active contractile process,[49] it appears that this occurs only during fast stretching or if the slow stretching elicits pain.[14,22,48] Bone, histologically classified as a connective tissue,[23] can have incongruencies that also limit the range of motion.[59] The muscles' and tendons' extensibility allows them to stretch; their elasticity permits them to return from the stretched positions to their original lengths.[25] Extensibility without elasticity is plasticity, meaning that the tissues fail to return to their normal resting length. M. J. Alter's book[2] (1996) is an excellent resource for the anatomical and physiological basis of flexibility.[a]

Although the term *flexibility* is a popular one, it may be a misnomer because it implies that flexibility is concerned only with flexion. However, flexibility also consists of extension, abduction, adduction, and circumduction. Furthermore, flexion implies bending or folding of the tissue when, in fact, it is really a stretching or an elongation of the tissue. *Flexibility* has multiple definitions and can be organized into different categories. These definitions may include clarifications with respect to optimal range of motion and types of movement.

As an exercise physiologist, I appreciate the "optimal range of motion permitted by muscle and connective tissue" definition for flexibility fitness because it not only allows a means of quantifying flexibility (distance or degree) but also includes the tissues that are significant for flexibility. Thus, the two tissues involved in flexibility are

primarily the muscle and connective tissues. The term *optimal* implies that "too much" or "too little" flexibility may exist. Optimal is not encountered with respect to the other fitness components, such as strength, aerobic power, and anaerobic power. Thus, investigators did not suggest that a person could be too strong, too aerobically fit, too fast, or too powerful. In the case of flexibility, sometimes investigators do suggest that it may be undesirable to be too flexible. The desired amount of flexibility is dependent upon the performance goal. For example, the optimal flexibility of a football player is different from that of a gymnast. In fact, too much flexibility may result in such laxity (hypermobility) of the tissues that the football player may increase susceptibility to dislocations, subluxations, and sprains. On the other hand, too little flexibility (tightness) may increase the player's susceptibility to strains.[17,52] In the gymnast, hypermobility might permit certain maneuvers, but too much laxity in the spinal cord may cause lordotic vertebral problems.[47] Too much tightness in the swimmer may cause "swimmer's shoulder" or an impingement of the long head of the biceps and distal end of the supraspinatus,[21] but hypermobility can lead to subluxations.[56] Thus, either extreme of static flexibility (hypermobility and tightness) may increase the risk of musculoskeletal injuries.[38,40,59] For people who are content to perform daily movements successfully without undue pain, the term *functional range of motion* is applicable.

The types of flexibility are related to the types of movements performed. These movements are (1) slow-to-holding point; (2) fast-to-nonholding point; and (3) slow-assisted. These are measured usually with respect to movement range but sometimes they are measured in terms of dynamic flexibility—that is, the torque necessary to produce movement at a given joint. You may recall that torque represents the force at the lever arm in a radial movement. Dynamic flexibility may be measured by moving a body segment passively over a fixed range of movement. A strain gauge measures the torque necessary to overcome the joint resistance. Transducers convey the displacement and torque changes to an X-Y plot (a load-deformation loop or curve). Thus, dynamic flexibility reflects the stiffness accompanying a movement. The measurement of dynamic flexibility has practical importance because rarely do we move through the maximal range of motion, but we always need to overcome some joint resistance in all movements.

---

[a]All numbered references are found in the References of Chapter 22.

Slow-to-holding types of flexibility movements are usually referred to as static stretching maneuvers. They are often associated with Yoga-like positions. Thus, the body position is assumed gradually and then held for varying lengths of time. Static range of motion is a linear (cm) or angular (°) measurement.

Fast-to-nonholding types of flexibility movements are often referred to as "ballistic." Sometimes the term *dynamic* also is used but can be confused with torque dynamics. Thus, the body position is assumed quickly and not held. These types of flexibility exercises are associated with some popular calisthenics (e.g., twisting toe touchers).

Slow-assisted types of flexibility movements are achieved with the aid of another person, with heavy objects, or by pulling on an attached object. These are often done under the guidance of a therapist or trainer. Some weight machines are constructed so that they assist in stretching the individual prior to the execution of the movement.

In summary, *flexibility* is a term that is technically misleading but one that is popular and probably will remain for future generations. The range of motion (or movement) can be measured dynamically and statically, with the latter being approached slowly, quickly, or with assistance. Chapter 22 includes only lower trunk flexibility as a measure of static range of motion.

LOWER TRUNK FLEXIBILITY

Indirectly, the fitness component of flexibility was responsible for the formation of the President's Council on Physical Fitness and Sports (PCPFS). President Eisenhower formed this organization in the mid 1950s after his disenchantment with the fitness of our youth. He was stirred to action when investigators[42] reported American children from 6 y to 16 y of age compared poorly with European children. More than half of the American children had failed a fitness battery composed of six tests; this compared with less than one-tenth of the European children (Figure 22.1). Most of the American failures were due to poor flexibility, specifically the "floor-touch" (Kraus-Weber) test, which caused 44 % of the American children to fail.

Sit-and-Reach (SR) Test

Most Americans will suffer from low-back pain at least once in their lifetime. Although never documented by the Sit-and-Reach (SR) Test,[6,43] poor flexibility of low-back extensors and hamstrings has often been suggested to be associated with, or contribute to, muscular low-back pain.[6,37] In addition, poor hamstring flexibility may predispose injury to hamstrings.[63,67] Tests for these two muscle groups (lower back muscles and hamstring muscles) have received the most attention. For example, the Sit-and-Reach Test has

been incorporated as a health-related physical fitness item into such national fitness batteries as *AAHPERD Physical Best,*[5] the President's Council on Physical Fitness and Sports,[58] the Fitnessgram,[34] the AAHPERD Functional Fitness Assessment for Adults over 60 years,[10,54] and the American Alliance for Health, Physical Education, Recreation and Dance Health-Related Test.[3]

However, despite the positive claims supporting flexibility as a health-related fitness component, *hypermobility* in static flexibility tests does not appear to be associated with a reduced risk of injury.[59] Furthermore, the data are not convincing in connecting a reduced injury risk to a stretching regimen prior to exercise.[41,57,62] More studies are needed before definitive conclusions can be made—especially randomized prospective studies that include large numbers of participants and control groups. A variety of stretching regimens should be studied, and distinctions should be made between regimens that include warm-up with the stretching regimen. For the present, it appears that performers will continue to stretch prior to exercise based on nearly universal beliefs, their habitual routines, and their own intuitions regarding the safety of their musculoskeletal system during exercise. This is probably their most prudent course of action until evidence is strong enough to call for a modification of their present prior exercise regimen.

Method

Although some authorities would view the Sit-and-Reach (SR) Flexibility Test as a field test, it has some qualities that meet the criteria for a field/lab test. The SR Test requires close interaction between the technician and participant. Additionally, unless there are numerous measuring sticks or sit-and-reach boxes, it does not lend itself to simultaneous testing of many persons, as does a simple bendover toe-toucher field test.

Six methods of performing the Sit-and-Reach Test include modifications of the traditional one prescribed by the American Alliance for Health, Physical Education, Recreation and Dance.[3,4,5] The modifications are the YMCA,[19] Canadian,[16] Wall,[26,27,28,29] Back-Saver,[12] and V-sit[12] SR Tests (Table 22.1).

Although criterion tests of validity for the SR Tests retain the subjective characteristic of the performer's tolerance to discomfort, two criterion tests standout as the "gold standards." The MacRae and Wright (MW) Test is a criterion

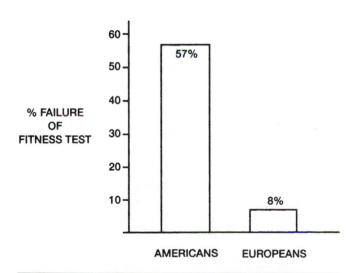

Figure 22.1 The fitness of American children in the 1950s based on a six-item fitness test was inferior to that of European children.

Table 22.1 Types of Sit-and-Reach Tests and Their Basic Characteristics

Type	Equipment	Heel Line (Index)	Hold (s)	Trials	Recorded
Traditional	Box: 12.75 in. high	23 cm; 9 in.	1–2	4[a]	4th
Canadian	Meter-stick and adjustable box—toe level	26 cm; ≈10 in.	2	2	Best
YMCA	Yardstick; tape; floor level	15 in.; 38 cm	≈ 2	3	Best
Wall SR	Traditional box with m/yd-stick or Acuflex 1™	0 cm; 0 in.	≥ 2	2 (3-phase stretch)	Average
V-sit	Meter-stick on floor	23 cm	1–2	4[a]	4th
Back-Saver	Box	23 cm	1–2	4 each leg[a]	4th

Note: [a]First three trials of traditional, V-sit, and Back-Saver SR Tests are practice trials.

BOX 22.1 Accuracy of Sit-and-Reach (SR) Tests

Validity

Flexibility testing is not wholly objective due to the variability in performers' tolerance at the limits of motion. Scientifically significant evidence to support the association between low-back pain and inflexibility is not clearly apparent.[53] Although SR tests are presumed to measure both lower back and hamstring flexibility, investigators conclude that the tests are more valid for hamstring than for back flexibility.[13,32,35,36,44,45,47] It is, secondarily, a test for the lower back, buttocks, and calf muscles. Specifically, the stretched muscles are the biceps femoris, semitendinosus, semimembranosus, erector spinae, gluteus maximus and medius, and gastrocnemius.

Many investigators agree that there is no such phenomenon as general flexibility.[6,24,30,31,33,50,61] In other words, one joint's range of motion cannot predict the range of motion of another joint. Few correlations between one body part and another exceed .40. Some exceptions are cited in a review of flexibility,[11] but a factor analytic study was quite convincing toward a specificity characteristic for flexibility.[24] It is reasonable that the relationship between the SR Test and the Standing Toe-Toucher Test is high ($r = .90$)[66] because these tests, essentially, are measuring the same muscle groups.

Not only is flexibility specific from one type of joint in the body to another type of joint in the body (e.g., legs vs. shoulders) but it is specific with respect to the same joint but on different sides of the body. For example, one shoulder is usually more flexible than the other shoulder.

The intraclass correlations ranged from .15 to .42 when the lower-back criterion was compared with the classic (Traditional) SR, Back-Saver, and V-sit SR Tests. The validity coefficients ranged from .39 to .58 when the same three SR Tests were compared with the hamstring criterion.[32]

Reliability

The test-retest reliability of the SR Test can be as high as .98[44] and is usually greater than .70, based upon the testing of more than 12 000 boys and girls 6 y to 18 y of age; the test-retest correlation over an 8 mo period in older persons (45 y to 75 y) was .83.[61] The test-retest reliability of the modified Wall SR Test for males and females tested on the same day ranges from .91 to .97.[29] The intraclass correlation coefficients of the traditional SR, V-sit, and Back-Saver Tests ranged between .89 and .98 in Asian adults.[32]

---

measure for lower back flexibility,[45] and the goniometrically measured straight-leg raise is a criterion measure for hamstring flexibility.[20] Other than the subjective aspect of these criteria tests, they meet all of the criteria to qualify as laboratory tests. Comments on the accuracy of the SR Tests are presented in Box 22.1.

Equipment

Table 22.1 presents the equipment for the six SR Tests, and Figure 22.2 shows other instruments for measuring range of motion. The test apparatus for the Traditional SR Test is a boxlike structure with a measuring scale on its upper surface labeled in 1 cm gradations. The 23rd cm (9 in.) line is exactly in line with the vertical plane of the participant's soles and heels, which are underneath the overhang and against the front edge of the box (Figures 22.3 and 22.4).

Procedures Common to and Distinct among All SR Tests

Certain procedures are the same for all six tests. Because flexion places strain on spinal ligaments, especially when performed ballistically,[1] and raises intradiscal pressures,[9,51,60] the participant should be "warm and loose" and perform the movement slowly. Although only the Canadian test prescribes a standard preparatory regimen, it seems that a standard prior exercise regimen of slow stretching and walking/jogging in place for five minutes would enhance the reliability and validity of the other tests also. It would also validate comparisons among SR tests.

The shoeless participants fully extend their legs, meaning that the back of the knees are against the floor, table, or bench. The hands are placed with palms down and one palm on top of the backhand of the other. The performer holds the final reach trial for at least a second or two.

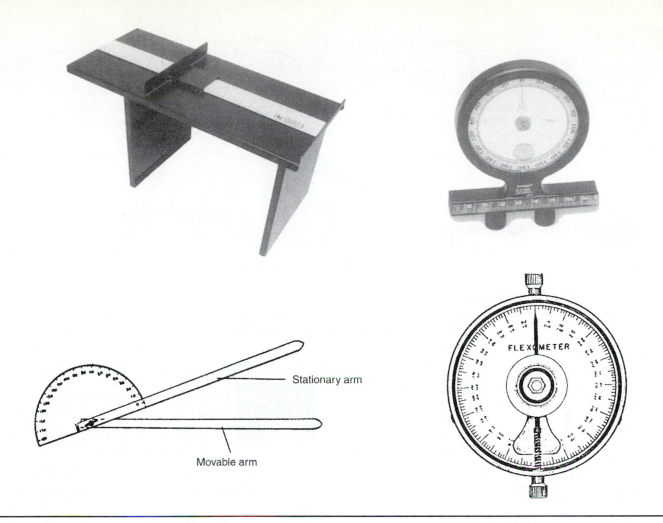

Figure 22.2 Some of the instruments used to measure range of motion. Top left: sit-and-reach box; top right: inclinometer; lower left: manual goniometer; lower right; Leighton Flexometer (courtesy of Lafayette Instruments, Lafayette, IN).

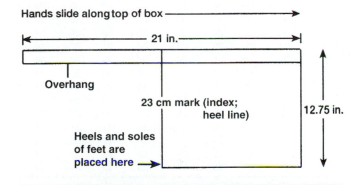

Figure 22.3 The Sit-and-Reach Test apparatus is boxlike with an overhang.

The tests are distinct in several ways. The most obvious is the initial body position—distance of the feet spread, a bent leg, hands on floor or on box. They may also vary in their choice of recorded trial—fourth, best, or average. Also, the index line (heel line) may vary—0 cm, 23 cm, 26 cm, and 38 cm. Other distinctions are presented in the specific procedures for each SR Test.

Specific Procedures for the SR Tests

Traditional SR Test

Figure 22.4 illustrates the proper technique to perform the traditional Sit-and-Reach Test. The sit-and-reach box should be braced against an object (e.g., wall) to prevent it from sliding away from the performer. Recognize that the index line (heel line) is at the 23 cm mark. Thus, any performer reaching beyond this line will have a recorded score greater than 23 cm. The procedural steps are as follows:

Performer

1. Perform a short bout (e.g., 5 min) of prior exercise.
2. Remove shoes.
3. Sit on the floor, bench, or table with feet against the testing apparatus (index; heel line).

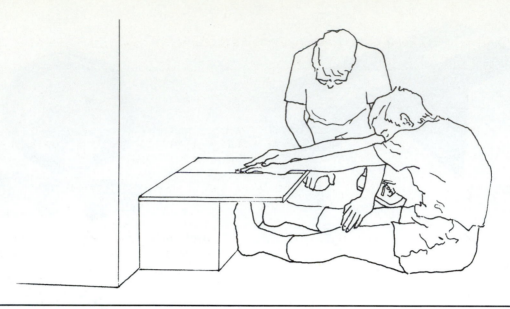

Figure 22.4 A participant performs the Sit-and-Reach Flexibility Test while the technician gently holds performer's knees.

4. Fully extend the legs, with the medial sides of the feet about 20 cm (≈ 8 in.) apart.

Technician

5. Hold one hand lightly against the performer's knees to ensure full leg extension.

Performer

6. Extend arms forward with the hands placed on top of each other, palms down.
7. Slowly bend forward along the measuring scale, not necessarily to the maximal on the first trial.
8. Repeat this forward stretch two more times.
9. Repeat the same stretch a fourth time, but now hold both hands at the maximal position for at least 1 s, but not necessarily beyond 2 s.

Technician

10. Observe and record the fourth (final) trial's score to the nearest centimeter.
11. Interpret the Traditional SR test value from Table 22.2.

Canadian SR Test[15,16]

Except for the specifically prescribed prior exercise regimen, the beginning steps of the Canadian SR Test are similar to those of the Traditional SR Test. The later steps include minor differences related to the height of the meter stick, separation of the performer's feet, the number of trials, and the recorded trial.

Performer

1. Performer executes the modified hurdle stretch (bent leg's sole of foot against inside of other leg), holding for 20 s, and repeated twice for each leg.

| Table 22.2 | **Percentile (%ile) Norms for the Traditional Sit-and-Reach Test for Men and Women, 18 y to 21 y of Age** |

	Sit-and-Reach (cm)[a]							
	Men				**Women**			
%ile	**18 y**	**19 y**	**20 y**	**21 y**	**18 y**	**19 y**	**20 y**	**21 y**
99	50	49	49	50	52	52	51	50
95	45	45	46	45	47	47	46	46
90	42	43	43	42	46	45	45	44
85	41	42	41	41	44	43	43	43
80	40	40	41	40	43	42	42	42
75	39	39	40	39	42	41	41	42
70	38	38	39	38	41	40	39	40
65	37	37	38	36	40	40	38	39
60	36	36	37	35	39	38	38	38
55	35	35	36	35	38	38	37	37
50	34	34	35	33	38	37	37	36
45	34	33	34	32	37	36	36	36
40	32	32	33	31	36	36	35	35
35	31	31	32	31	35	34	34	34
30	30	29	31	30	34	33	33	33
25	29	28	30	28	33	32	32	32
20	27	27	27	27	32	31	31	31
15	25	26	25	25	30	29	30	29
10	23	23	22	24	29	27	28	27
5	19	19	18	20	26	23	24	25

Reprinted from "Norms for College Students" with permission of the American Alliance for Health, Physical Education, Recreation and Dance, 1900 Association Dr., Reston, VA.
Note: [a]Index (heel line) is at 23 cm.

	%ile	15–19		20–29		30–39		40–49		50–59		60–69	
		M	W	M	W	M	W	M	W	M	W	M	W
High	81–100	38	42	39	40	37	40	34	37	34	38	32	34
> Ave	61–80	34–38	38–42	34–39	37–40	33–37	36–40	29–34	34–37	28–34	33–38	25–32	31–34
Ave	41–60	29–33	34–37	30–33	33–36	28–32	32–35	24–28	30–33	24–27	30–32	20–24	27–30
< Ave	21–40	24–28	29–33	25–29	28–32	23–27	27–31	18–23	25–29	16–23	25–29	15–19	23–26
Low	1–20	24	29	25	28	23	27	18	25	16	25	15	23

From Fitness and Lifestyle in Canada, Fitness and Lifestyle Research Institute, 1983. Fitness and Amateur Sport, Ottawa, Canada.
Note: [a]Index (heel line) is at 26 cm. Therefore, subtract 3 cm from the Canadian values if using the Traditional SR Test or V-sit Test.[6]

2. Performer removes shoes, sits on floor, table, or bench, and extends legs.
3. Performer places heels about 5 cm (≈ 2 in.) apart.

Technician

4. Technician places a meter stick at the performer's toe-level height or uses a height-adjustable box with meter stick attached.
5. The meter stick crosses the heel line (index) at the 26 cm (≈ 10 in.) mark.

Performer

6. Performer places hands on top of each other and slowly bends forward, running hands along meter stick, keeping head down.
7. Performer holds maximally extended position for 2 s.

Technician

8. Technician notes the distance of the reach to the closest centimeter. For example, if the performer reaches exactly to the index line at toe level, the score is recorded as 26 cm.

Performer

9. Performer repeats trial.

Technician

10. Technician records and interprets the best of the two trials using Form 22.1 and Table 22.3, respectively.

YMCA SR Test[19]

Except for the placement of the yardstick, index line, number of trials, and the recorded trial, most of the Y's procedures are the same as those of the Traditional SR Test.

The technician places a yard-/meter-stick on the floor, mat, table, or bench so that the zero end is toward the crotch. Because the yardstick is at a lower level than when it is on top of a 12 in. box, the reach scores may be about 1 in. or 2.5 cm lower than the reaches measured on the traditional box.[39] However, this deficit may be partly compensated by the plantar flexion permitted by this nonbox method.

1. Technician intersects the index line with a tape across the yardstick at 15 in. or 38 cm (equivalent to touching toes).

2. After warming up, the performer removes shoes; sits on floor, table, or bench; and extends legs, straddling yard-/meter-stick or measuring tape.
3. Performer abducts legs to separate heels by 10 in. to 12 in. (25 cm to 30 cm) and places heels perpendicular to and at the front edge of the index tape or mark. If the performer's heels slide over the tape, adjust heels accordingly.
4. Performer places hands on top of each other and slowly bends forward with head down, running hands along the top of the yard-/meter-stick. Technician gently holds participant's knees down.
5. Performer holds the extended position for about 2 s.
6. Technician notes the distance of the reach to the closest quarter or half inch. For example, if the performer reaches one-half inch past the index line, the score is recorded as 15.5 in. (39 cm).
7. Participant performs a second and third trial and can relax and flex legs between trials.
8. Technician records and interprets the best of the three trials using Form 22.1 and Table 22.4, respectively.

Wall SR Test[26,27,28,29]

This test has an added preliminary phase to the other SR Tests. This phase is performed against a wall in order to correct for any interindividual differences in appendage proportions, such as leg length versus trunk length.[8,27,28,64]

1. Performer executes a short bout (≈ 5 min) of prior exercise.
2. Performer removes shoes.
3. Performer sits on the floor, (or bench or table) with the back, hips, and head against a wall.
4. Performer places soles and heels of feet against the testing apparatus, which can be a commercial box (Acuflex 1™ in Figure 22.2) or the traditional box. The apparatus should be braced against the technician's feet or some object in order to prevent it from sliding away from the performer's feet.

Table 22.4   YMCA Sit-and-Reach Norms (in.) for Men (M) and Women (W), 18 y to 65+ y of Age[a]

Category	%ile	18 y to 25 y M	W	26 y to 35 y M	W	36 y to 45 y M	W	46 y to 55 y M	W	56 y to 65 y M	W	> 65 y M	W
Very high	100	26	27	25	26	24	25	23	24	21	23	20	22
	90	20	24	20	23	19	22	19	21	17	20	17	20
High	80	19	22	18	21	17	20	17	19	15	18	14	18
Above average	70	18	21	17	20	17	19	15	18	13	17	13	17
	60	17	20	16	19	15	17	14	17	13	16	11	16
Average	50	16	19	15	18	14	16	12	16	11	15	10	15
Below average	40	14	18	14	17	13	15	11	15	9	14	9	13
	30	13	17	12	16	11	14	10	14	9	13	8	12
Low	20	12	15	11	14	9	12	8	12	7	11	6	10
Very low	10	9	13	7	13	7	10	6	10	5	9	4	8
	0	2	8	2	8	1	6	1	4	1	3	0	2

Adapted from Golding, L. A. (1997). Flexibility, stretching, and flexibility testing: Recommendations for testing and standards. *ACSM's Health and Fitness Jounal, 1,* 17–20, 37–38.
Note: [a]Index (heel line) of the floor-level yardstick is at 15 in. (38 cm).

5. Performer fully extends the legs, with the feet about shoulder width (about 8 in. to 12 in. or 20 cm to 30 cm) apart. Technician does not need to hold the performer's knees but performer's legs remain extended.

6. Performer places one hand on top of the other as in the other tests.

7. The **starting (zero) position** is determined by:
   a. **Performer** reaching forward as far as possible along the measuring device without having the head and back leave the wall; however, the shoulders are permitted to hunch forward into a rounded position
   b. **Technician** recording the inch-mark to the closest 0.5 in. onto Form 22.1; using the Acuflex, simply slide the reach indicator to the person's finger tips and observe the score

8. After the recording or adjustment is made, the performer slowly reaches forward three times during a single maneuver along the device, with the third reach being held for 2 s or more.

9. Technician records the third phase of this reaching maneuver.

10. Technician records the actual back/hamstring flexibility value by subtracting the starting value from the end-reach value.

11. Performer executes another three-phase reach trial.

12. Technician records the second trial, then calculates and records the average flexibility value of the two trials.

13. Technician interprets the flexibility value by referring to Table 22.5.

V-Sit SR Test

The V-Sit SR Test is a modification of the Traditional SR Test. The only modifications are the removal of the box and a prescribed 30 cm separation of the heels, hence the V-sit position. All other procedures are the same, such as the following:

1. Performer executes a short bout of prior exercise.
2. Performer removes shoes.

Table 22.5   Percentiles (%ile) for the Wall Sit-and-Reach Test

%ile	≤ 35 y Men	Women	36 y to 49 y Men	Women	≥ 50 y Men	Women
	Flexibility Score (in.)[a]					
99	24.7	19.8	18.9	19.8	16.2	17.2
95	19.5	18.7	18.2	19.2	15.8	15.7
90	17.9	17.9	16.1	17.4	15.0	15.0
80	17.0	16.7	14.6	16.2	13.3	14.2
70	15.8	16.2	13.9	15.2	12.3	13.6
60	15.0	15.8	13.4	14.5	11.5	12.3
50	14.4	14.8	12.6	13.5	10.2	11.1
40	13.5	14.5	11.6	12.8	9.7	10.1
30	13.0	13.7	10.8	12.2	9.3	9.2
20	11.6	12.6	9.9	11.0	8.8	8.3
10	9.2	10.1	8.3	9.7	7.8	7.5
5	7.9	8.1	7.0	8.5	7.2	3.7
1	7.0	2.6	5.1	2.0	4.0	1.5

From *Principles and Laboratories for Physical Fitness and Wellness* (1991). Englewood, CO: Morton Publishing. Reprinted with permission.
Note: [a]The reference line is at zero inches.

3. Technician places meter stick's 23 cm line between the legs and at the heel line of performer.

4. Performer's legs are fully extended; technician gently holds knees to assure extension.

5. Performer's bottom hand and top hand of outstretched arms are directly aligned.

6. Performer slowly bends forward along the meter stick during three preparatory trials.

7. Performer makes a maximal stretch during the fourth trial.

8. Technician records the fourth trial to the nearest centimeter and interprets according to the same norms as the Traditional SR Test (Table 22.2).

Back-Saver SR Test[12]

Possible excessive posterior disc compression occurs when performing the maneuvers prescribed for the five previously discussed SR tests.[9] The Back-Saver SR Test was devised to reduce this compression when bending forward with *both* legs extended by prescribing forward bending with only *one* leg extended.[12] Unfortunately, some participants feel discomfort at the hip joint of the bent leg during the modified maneuver.[32] The Back-Saver SR Test is identical to the Traditional SR Test (with box) except for the four trials for each leg and the following modified body position:

- Floor-seated participant places the sole of the foot of a fully extended leg against the front and bottom edge of the sit-and-reach box.
- Participant bends the other leg so that the sole of the leg's foot is flat on the floor and about two or three inches ($\approx$ 5 cm to 7.5 cm) to the side of the extended knee of the other leg.
- Participant may have to move the bent leg to the side as the body moves forward along the box.

The technician records the fourth trial of the right leg and the left leg. The norms are the same as the Traditional SR Test (Table 22.2).

Specific Procedures for the Criterion Tests

The MacRae and Wright (MW) Test is a criterion measure for lower back flexibility,[45] and the goniometrically measured straight-leg raise is a criterion measure for hamstring flexibility.[20] The MW Test measures the maximal anterior flexion of the lower back and has a high validity coefficient ($r = .97$) with radiographically determined vertebral flexion.[45] The criterion test for hamstring flexibility uses a manual goniometer (review Figure 22.2). The test has a subjective endpoint whereby the technician and participant both sense tightness during the assisted straight-leg raise. Nevertheless, the reliability of this goniometric test is high.[7] The scores of all performers on the MW and goniometric criterion tests can then be correlated with one or more of the SR Tests as a validation check of lower back flexibility and hamstring flexibility, respectively.

Procedures for the MacRae-Wright (MW) Back Criterion Test[32,45,55]

1. Performer stands erect.
2. Technician locates the sacroiliac joint by palpation and marks it with a pen.
3. Technician measures and marks the points 5 cm below and 10 cm above the lumbosacral joint mark, thus producing a total distance of 15 cm between marks.
4. Performer sits with legs extended on the floor, mat, table, or bench.
5. Technician views the marks on performer's back while placing the tape measure on the low 5 cm mark.
6. As performer bends maximally forward, technician measures the distance from the lowest mark to the highest mark.
7. Technician subtracts the original position's 15 cm from the maximally stretched position's distance.

8. The procedure is repeated three times, with the average being recorded as the flexibility score.

Procedures for the Goniometric Hamstring Criterion Test

The goniometric test received its name because of the goniometer instrument but is often referred to as the straight-leg raise test. The raising of the leg is a passive maneuver on the performer's part because the technician lifts, and gently pushes against, the performer's leg. It may require two technicians—one to lift the performer's leg and another to make the goniometric measurement.

1. Technician aligns the axis of the goniometer with the axis of performer's hip joint.
2. Technician places the stationary arm of the manual goniometer (electronic goniometers, or "elgons," may be used) in line with the trunk and the mobile arm in line with the femur.
3. Technician holds performer's knee straight while moving that leg toward hip flexion.
4. When technician feels tightness (feedback from performer may help), the leg is held there while a reading to the closest degree is made from the angle produced by the stationary arm and mobile arm of the goniometer.
5. The average of three trials is used as the flexibility score.

Results and Discussion

Because extreme (hyper) mobility is not optimal, high flexibility scores are not classified as "excellent." A nonqualitative classification system ranging from low to high is used instead. It is apparent from the norm tables that women are more flexible than men. Asian adult women's scores were 4 cm to 13 cm higher than men's scores for the Traditional SR Test, the V-SR Test, and the Back-Saver SR Test.[32]

A remedial flexibility program is advised by AAHPERD if anyone falls below the 25th percentile (Table 22.2) in their traditional SR test. The 50th percentile is the average score. Standard scores (i.e., scores that are recommended) may be found in AAHPERD's *Physical Best* pamphlet.[5] The minimum standards for boys and girls on the Back-Saver Test are 20.3 cm (8 in.) and 25.4 cm (10 in.), respectively.[55]

Anthropometric factors may cause normal boys and girls between the ages of 10 y and 14 y to be unable to reach the 23 cm index mark in the Traditional Test.[3] This may be due to the preadolescent and adolescent growth spurt, which makes the legs disproportionately longer than the trunk. Except for the Wall Sit-and-Reach Test, other tests may favor persons with longer arms and/or trunk and disproportionately shorter legs.[27] However, the criterion MacRae-White Test showed that the other SR Tests are just as valid as the Wall Test.[32] This might be one of the reasons leading to higher scores in women than men—lower average leg length compared with their height.[65] Despite the bias attributed to disproportionate lengths, it appears that the nonwall SR Tests would be independent of total height.[8,61,64]

Norms for the Canadian SR Test in Table 22.3 are for a wider age range than those for the Traditional SR test in Table 22.2. The absolute values (cm) of the tests cannot be compared directly because the index points are different.

Equation 22.1 may be used to convert a floor measurement (e.g., YMCA SR Test) to a box test measurement (e.g., Traditional SR Test),[39] or simply add 0.7 in. (1.75 cm) to the floor score.[18]

$$\text{Box (in.)} = 5.86 + (\text{floor} \times 0.728) \qquad \text{Eq. 22.1}$$

Norms for the YMCA SR Test are presented in Table 22.4.[19] Flexibility scores from floor measuring sticks are lower than scores from boxes.[18,39]

The norms for the Wall SR Test are presented in Table 22.5.[26,29] The flexibility categories are based on the same percentile (%ile) categories as those for the Canadian SR Test. Thus, > 81st %ile is equivalent to the High category; 61–80 = > Ave.; 41–60 = Ave.; 21–40 = < Ave.; and < 20th %ile = Low.

References

1. Adams, M. A., & Hutton, W. C. (1983). The mechanical function of the lumbar apophyseal joints. *Spine, 8,* 327–330.

2. Alter, M. J. (1996). *Science of flexibility.* Champaign, IL: Human Kinetics.

3. American Alliance for Health, Physical Education, Recreation and Dance. (1980). *AAHPERD health related physical fitness test.* Reston, VA: Author.

4. American Alliance for Health, Physical Education, Recreation and Dance. (1985). *Norms for college students—The health related physical fitness test.* Reston, VA: Author.

5. American Alliance for Health, Physical Education, Recreation and Dance. (1988). *Physical best.* Reston, VA: Author.

6. American College of Sports Medicine. (2000). *ACSM's guidelines for exercise testing and prescription.* Philadelphia: Lippincott Williams & Wilkins.

7. Boone, D., Azen, S., Lin, G., Spence, C., Baron, C., & Lee, L. (1978). Reliability of goniometric measurements. *Physical Therapy, 58,* 1355–1360.

8. Broer, M. R., & Galles, N. R. G. (1958). Importance of relationship between various body measurements in performance of toe touch test. *Research Quarterly, 29,* 253–263.

9. Cailliet, R. (1988). *Low back pain syndrome* (4th ed.). Philadelphia: F. A. Davis.

10. Clark, B., Osness, W., Adrian, M., Hoeger, W. W. K., Raab, D., & Wiswell, R. (1989). Tests for fitness in older adults: AAHPERD Fitness Task Force. *Journal of Physical Education, Recreation and Dance, 60,* 66–71.

11. Clarke, H. H. (1975). Joint and body range of movement. *Physical Fitness Research Digest, 5,* 1–22.

12. Cooper Institute for Aerobics Research. (1992). *The Prudential FITNESSGRAM test administration manual.* Dallas, TX: Author.

13. Corbin, C. B., & Pangrazi, R. P. (1992). Are American children and youth fit? *Research Quarterly for Exercise and Sport, 63,* 96–106.

14. Davidoff, D. A. (1992). Skeletal muscle tone and the misunderstood stretch reflex. *Neurology, 42,* 951–963.

15. Fitness and Amateur Sport Canada. (1987). *Canadian Standardized Test of Fitness (CSTF) operations manual* (3rd ed.). Ottawa, Ontario: Canadian Association of Sport Sciences.

16. Fitness and Lifestyle Research Institute. (1983). *Fitness and lifestyle in Canada.* Ottawa, Canada: Fitness and Amateur Sport.

17. Gerber, S., & Marshall, J. (1974). Searching for loose and tight joints. *The Physician and Sportsmedicine, 2*(10) 50, 81–83.

18. Golding, L. A. (1997). Flexibility, stretching, and flexibility testing: Recommendations for testing and standards. *ACSM's Health and Fitness Journal, 1,* 17–20, 37–38.

19. Golding, L. A. (Ed.). (2000). *YMCA fitness testing and assessment manual* (4th ed.). Champaign, IL: Human Kinetics.

20. Goeken, L. N., & Holf, A. L. (1993). Instrumental straight-leg raising: Results in healthy subjects. *Archives of Physical Medicine and Rehabilitation, 74,* 194–203.

21. Greipp, J. F. (1985). Swimmer's shoulder: The influence of flexibility and weight training. *The Physician and Sportsmedicine, 13*(8), 92–98, 101–105.

22. Halbertsma, J. P. K., van Bolhuts, A. I., & Goeken, L. N. H. (1996). Sport stretching: Effect on passive muscle stiffness of short hamstrings. *Archives of Physical Medicine and Rehabilitation, 77,* 688–692.

23. Ham, A. W. (1969). *Histology.* Philadelphia: J. P. Lippincott.

24. Harris, M. L. (1969). A factor analytic study of flexibility. *Research Quarterly, 40,* 62–70.

25. Hinson, M. M. (1977). *Kinesiology.* Dubuque, IA: Wm. C. Brown.

26. Hoeger, W. W. K. (1989). *Lifetime physical fitness and wellness.* Englewood, CO: Morton.

27. Hoeger, W. W. K., & Hopkins, D. R. (1992). A comparison of the sit and reach and the modified sit and reach in the measurement of flexibility in women. *Research Quarterly for Exercise and Sport, 63,* 191–195.

28. Hoeger, W. W. K., Hopkins, D. R., Button, S., & Palmer, T. A. (1990). Comparing the sit and reach with the modified sit and reach in measuring flexibility in adolescents. *Pediatric Exercise Science, 2,* 156–162.

29. Hoeger, W. W. K., Hopkins, D. R., & Johnson, L. C. (1993). *The assessment of muscular flexibility.* Rockton, IL: Authors/Novel Products, Inc.

30. Holland, G. J. (1968). The physiology of flexibility. *Kinesiology Review, 49.* Cited by Clarke (1975).

31. Hubley, C. (1982). Testing flexibility. In D. McDougall, H. Wenger, & H. Green (Eds.), *Physiological testing of the elite athlete* (pp. 117–132). Ottawa, Canada: Canadian Association of Sport Sciences.

32. Hui, S. C., Yuen, P. Y., Morrow, J. R., & Jackson, A. W. (1999). Comparison of the criterion-related validity of sit-and-reach tests with and without limb length adjustment in Asian adults. *Research Quarterly for Exercise and Sport, 70,* 401–406.

33. Hupperich, F. L., & Sigerseth, P. O. (1950). The specificity of flexibility in girls. *Research Quarterly, 21,* 25–33.

34. Institute for Aerobics Research. (1988). *The Fitnessgram.* Dallas: Author.

35. Jackson, A. W., & Baker, A. A. (1986). The relationship of the sit and reach test to criterion measures of hamstring and back flexibility in young females. *Research Quarterly for Exercise and Sport, 57,* 183–186.

36. Jackson, A. W., & Langford, N. J. (1989). The criterion-related validity of the sit and reach test: Replication and extension of previous findings. *Research Quarterly for Exercise and Sport, 60,* 384–387.

37. Jackson A. W., Morrow, J. R., Brill, P. A., Kohl, H. W., Gordon, N. F., & Blair, S. N. (1998). Relations of sit-up and sit-and-reach test to lower back pain in adults. *The Journal of Orthopaedic and Sports Physical Therapy, 27,* 22–26.

38. Jones, B. H., & Knapik, J. J. (1999). Physical training and exercise-related injuries. *Sports Medicine, 27,* 111–125.

39. Jones, G. R., Boyce, R. W., Coolidge, W. A., & Hiatt, A. R. (1989). Comparison of two methods of sit and reach trunk flexion assessment. *Medicine and Science in Sports and Exercise, 21* (Suppl.), Abstract #691, S116.

40. Knapik, J. J., Jones, B. H., Bauman, C. L., & Harris, J. (1992). Strength, flexibility, and athletic injuries. *Sports Medicine, 14,* 277–288.

41. Knudson, D. (1999). Stretching during warm-up: Do we have enough evidence? *Journal of Health, Physical Education, Recreation and Dance, 70*(7), 27–27, 51.

42. Kraus, H., & Hirschland, R. P. (1954). Minimum muscular fitness tests in school children. *Research Quarterly, 125,* 178–188.

43. Kraus, H., & Raab, W. (1961). *Hypokinetic disease.* Springfield, IL: Charles C Thomas.

44. Liemohn, W., Sharpe, G. L., & Wasserman, J. F. (1994). Criterion related validity of the sit-and-reach test. *Journal of Strength and Conditioning Research, 8,* 91–94.

45. MacRae, I. F., & Wright, V. (1969). Measurement of back movement. *Annals of the Rheumatic Diseases, 28,* 584–589.

46. Martin, S. B., Jackson, A. W., Morrow, J. R., & Liemohn, W. P. (1998). The rationale for the sit and reach test revisited. *Measurement in Physical Education and Exercise Science, 2,* 85–92.

47. McAuley, E., Hudash, G., Shields, K., Albright, J. P., Garrick, J., Requa, R., & Wallace, R. K. (1988). Injuries in women's gymnastics. The state of the art. *American Journal of Sports Medicine, 16* (Suppl 1), S124–S131.

48. McHugh, M. P., Kremenic, I. J., Fox, M. B., & Gleim, G. W. (1998). The role of mechanical and neural restraints to joint range of motion during passive stretch. *Medicine and Science in Sports and Exercise, 30,* 928–932.

49. Moore, M. A., & Hutton, R. S. (1980). Electromyographic investigation of muscle stretching techniques. *Medicine and Science in Sports and Exercise, 12,* 322–329.

50. Munroe, R. A., & Romance, T. J. (1975). Use of the Leighton flexometer in the development of a short flexibility test battery. *American Corrective Therapy Journal, 29,* 22–29.

51. Nachemson, A. (1975). Towards a better understanding of low back pain: A review of the mechanics of the lumbar disc. *Rheumatic Rehabilitation, 14,* 129–143.

52. Nicholas, J. A. (1970). Injuries to knee ligaments. Relationship to tightness and looseness in football players. *The Journal of the American Medical Association, 212,* 2236–2239.

53. O'Connor, J. S., Hines, K., & Warner, C. A. (1996). Flexibility and injury incidence. *Medicine and Science in Sports and Exercise, 28*(5), Abstract #376, S63.

54. Osness, W. H., Adrian, M., Clark, B., Hoeger, W., Raab, D., & Wiswell, R. (1990). *Functional fitness assessment for adults over 60 years: A field-bond assessment.* Reston, VA: AAHPERD.

55. Patterson, P., Wiksten, D. L., Ray, L., Flanders, C., & Sanphy, D. (1996). The validity and reliability of the back saver sit-and-reach test in middle school girls and boys. *Research Quarterly for Exercise and Sport, 67,* 448–451.

56. Pfeiffer, R. P., & Mangus, B. C. (1998). *Concepts of athletic training.* Boston: Jones & Bartlett.

57. Pope, P. R., Herbert, R. D., Kirwan, J. D., & Graham B. J. (2000). A randomized trial of preexercise stretching for prevention of lower-limb injury. *Medicine and Science in Sports and Exercise, 32,* 271–277.

58. President's Council on Physical Fitness and Sports. (1990). *PCPFS president's challenge physical fitness program test manual.* Washington, DC: Author.

59. *President's Council on Physical Fitness and Sports.* (2000). Current issues in flexibility fitness. *President's Council on Physical Fitness and Sports Research Digest,* Washington, DC: Author.

60. Schultz, A., Andersson, G., Ortengren, R., Haderspeck, K., & Nachemson, A. (1982). Loads on the lumbar spine: Validation of a biomechanical analysis by measurement of intradiscal pressures and myoelectric signals. *Journal of Bone and Joint Surgery, 64A,* 713–720.

61. Shephard, R. J., Berridge, M., & Montelpare, W. (1990). On the generality of the "sit and reach" test: An analysis of flexibility data for an aging population. *Research Quarterly for Exercise and Sport, 61,* 326–330.

62. Shrier, I. (1999). Stretching before exercise does not reduce the risk of local muscle injury: A critical review of the clinical and basic science literature. *Clinical Journal of Sports Medicine, 9,* 221–227.

63. Sullivan, M. K., Dejulia, J. J., & Worrell, T. W. (1992). Effect of pelvic position and stretching method on hamstring muscle flexibility. *Medicine and Science in Sports and Exercise, 24,* 1383–1389.

64. Wear, C. L. (1963). Relationships of flexibility measurements to length of body segments. *Research Quarterly, 23,* 115–118.

65. Wells, C. L. (1985). *Women, sport, and performance: A physiological perspective.* Champaign, IL: Human Kinetics.

66. Wells, K. F., & Dillon, E. K. (1952). The sit and reach test: A test of back and leg flexibility. *Research Quarterly, 34,* 234–238.

67. Worrell, T., Perrin, D., Gansneder, B., & Gieck, J. (1991). Comparison of isokinetic strength and flexibility measures between injured and noninjured athletes. *Journal of Orthopaedic Sports Physical Therapy, 13,* 118–125.

BODY COMPOSITION

Within the field of kinanthropometry (*kin* = movement; *anthropo* = human; *metry* = measure) there is a subarea called body composition. *Body composition* is a term referring to the components of the human body. Body composition may refer to the amounts of constituents at the submicroscopic level—atoms and molecules—or at the microscopic level—cells—or at the macroscopic level— tissues and whole body.[16] In exercise physiology, body composition often means dividing the body into a two-component model of a fat-free mass and a fat mass.

The purpose of numerous body composition methods is to determine the desirable weight of a person (Table 1). Some of these methods (e.g., stature-weight-age charts) do not indicate the body composition per se but do make an assumption that too much weight for a certain height and age is an indicator of excess fat. Desirable weight can be more validly assessed by examining body composition than by examining standard stature-weight-age charts. For

example, the body masses of lean, muscular athletes may be 30 % greater than the average body mass for stature (height) listed in standard stature-weight-age tables.[17,a] Obviously, these muscular athletes should not be classified as overweight. Thus, a body mass that is above average has a much different meaning if it is due to a preponderance of lean mass, such as muscle, rather than fat mass. Another example can be made of typical major-league baseball coaches who were found to weigh approximately the same as the average major-league baseball player; however, body composition assessments revealed that the coaches averaged 6.4 kg less lean mass than the players. This resulted in a body fat percentage of 20 % in the baseball coach versus 12.6 % in the major league baseball player.[4] Thus, the measurement of body composition is a more valid method of determining desirable weight than is body weight alone.

When studying the various methods of determining body composition, it should be remembered that there is no direct measure of all the fat in the body in living persons— all methods make assumptions.[9] One sure method is to "blenderize" the body and then make a chemical analysis of the constituents, obviously a very traumatic and complicated procedure. Very few human cadavers have

---

[a]All numbered references are found in the References of Chapter 23.

Table 1 **Some Indirect Methods of Determining Body Composition**

Linear-Anthropometry	Densitometry	Spectrometry	Radiology
Stature-weight	Hydrostatic weighing	Potassium	Computer axial tomography (CAT)
		Deuterium	
Body mass index	Buoyancy	Tritiium	X-ray
Ponderal index	Volume displacement	Electrical conductivity	Neutron activation analysis (NAA)
Body surface area	Water	Total body (TOBEC)	Nitrogen
	Air plethysmograph	Bioimpedance	Potassium (^{40}K)
		Bioresistance	Magnetic resonance imaging (MR)
Diameters	Ultrasonic	Metabolic	Nuclear (NMRI)
Girths	A-mode	Urinary creatinine	Photon absorptiometry [1,25]
Skinfolds	B-mode	Plasma creatinine	Dual photon absorptiometry (DPA)
Somatotype	Portable	Urinary 3-methylhistidine	Dual energy X-ray absorptiometry
Somatogram	Hydrometry	N_2 balance	Light wave
Visual inspection	Total body water:	Gas absorption	Infrared
	D^2O-Deuterium and tritium oxide	Xenon; cyclopropane;	Near infrared
	Antipyrine-ethanol	radiokrypton; O_2-labeled water	

been analyzed by chemical extraction of lipids for direct assessment of body composition. All of the body composition methods on living organisms are indirect estimates, ranging greatly in sophistication and expense. A list of many of the indirect methods of determining body composition is presented in Table 1. These methods range in expense from zero dollars, such as visual inspection,[10] to six-figure dollars, such as dual-energy X-ray absorptiometry (DEXA).[24]

The human body can be categorized into component models. Although physiologists usually assign the criterion label of "gold-standard" to the hydrostatic weighing method of predicting percent body fat, the traditional two equations—Brozek[3] and Siri[33]—use the less accurate two-component model. Theoretically, equations based on three-component models and four-component models will provide more accurate predictions of percent body fat.[2] (Table 2)

Table 2 Component Models for Estimating Body Composition

Two Components	Three Components[a]		Four Components
Fat-free	Fat	Fat	Fat
Fat	Water	Mineral	Water
Example: Traditional (Brozek or Siri) equations used with hydrostatic weighing and skinfolds	Solids	Lean soft issues	Mineral
		Example: DEXA	Protein

Note: [a]Researchers provide two subdivisions for the three-component model.

BODY MASS INDEX

The body mass index (BMI), the term proposed by Keys and his colleagues[18] in 1972,[37] also has been referred to as Quetelet's Index,[20] named after its 1869 originator, who is sometimes considered the Father of Anthropometry.[14] The most popular stature-weight index, the Body Mass Index (BMI), has been used to categorize persons with respect to their health-related fitness,[1] their degree of obesity,[6,7] and mortality risk. The U.S. surgeon general recognizes that high body mass indexes relate to various health problems, such as Type II diabetes, hypertension, and heart disease.[36] Using BMI as an indicator of overweight, a progress review by *Healthy People 2000* revealed White and Black American men and women have steadily been increasing their BM indexes over the past few decades.[15] This has led to a 54.9 % prevalence of overweightness in the United States. The United States has the highest mean BMI in the Western world.[31] Based on follow-up home interviews of more than 3000 adults over 65 y of age, it appears that either very low BMI or very high BMI persons are at greater risk of functional impairment.[13] Obviously, BMI plays an important role in establishing standards of overweightness (BMI ≥ 25) and obesity (BMI ≥ 30) from epidemiological studies. Table 23.1 presents the percentages of Americans who are either overweight or obese.

Method

Body weight can be assessed from various stature/weight indexes, thus indicating the degree of obesity. Stature-weight indexes for assessing body weight are probably the simplest and least expensive methods of all, requiring only the measurement of body mass and stature (height). See Box 23.1 for a discussion on the accuracy of BMI.

Procedure

The first two steps in obtaining the BMI are to measure body mass and stature. Both of these were described in Chapter 3. The third and final step in obtaining the BMI requires a simple calculation or the use of a nomogram (Figure 23.1).[35]

Calculation of BMI

As presented in Equation 23.1, BMI is a ratio of the person's body mass (kg) to the height squared (m^2). In other words, BMI (kg/m^2 or $kg \cdot m^{-2}$) is the result of dividing a person's weight by the square of that person's height.[a]

$$BMI = Wt (kg) \div Ht^2 (m) \qquad \text{Eq. 23.1}$$

where:

m = meters; 100 cm = 1 m

For example, if a person weighs 68.0 kg (149.6 lb) and is 174.0 cm tall (1.740 m; 68.5 in.), then Equation 23.1 is used to calculate the BMI as follows:

$$BMI = 68.0 \text{ kg} \div 1.74 \text{ m}^2$$

$$= 68 \text{ kg} \div 3.03$$

$$= 22.44 \text{ (22.4 to closest tenth)}$$

[a]Instead of squaring height, you could divide by height twice. The equation using American units is BMI = (lb ÷ in. ÷ in.) × 703.

Table 23.1 Percentages (%) of U.S. Men (M) and Women (W) Overweight Based on BMI ≥ 25[a]

Years	M and W	Men				Women			
		All	White	Black	Mex-Am	All	White	Black	Mex-Am
1960–1962	43.3	48.2	48.8	43.1		38.7	36.1	57.0	
1971–1974	46.1	52.9	53.7	48.9		39.7	37.6	57.6	
1976–1980	46.0	51.4	52.3	49.0	59.7	40.8	38.4	61.0	60.1
1988–1994	54.9	59.4	61.0	56.5	63.9	50.7	49.2	65.8	65.9
20 y to 29 y of Age									
1988–1994	43.1					33.1			

Adapted from National Heart, Lung, and Blood Institute. (1998). *Clinical guidelines on the identification, evaluation, and treatment of overweight and obesity in adults. The evidence report.* (NIH Publication No. 98-4083). Washington, DC: U.S. Department of Health and Human Services.
Note:[a]Includes those persons classified as obese (BMI ≥ 30).

Calculation of Percent Body Fat from BMI

One reason for including such an error-prone prediction of percent body fat from BMI is to expose its clearly mistaken estimates to students. BMI should not be the single predictor of body fatness. Indeed, some authorities say not to use it to estimate body fatness in a fitness assessment.[21] Percent body fat (% BF) can be estimated in adults up to 83 years of age by using Equation 23.2.[6]

$$\% \text{ BF} = 1.20 \times \text{BMI} + (0.23 \times \text{Age}) \quad \text{Eq. 23.2}$$
$$- (10.8 \text{ sex}) - 5.4$$

where:

sex = 0 for women; 1 for men

For example, if a 30-year-old woman's BMI is 20 $kg \cdot m^{-2}$, then the following calculation predicts her hydrodensitometry (underwater weight) percent fat as 25.5 %.

$$\% \text{ BF} = 1.20 \times 20 \text{ } kg \cdot m^{-2} + (0.23 \times 30 \text{ y}) - (10.8 \times 0) - 5.4$$

$$= 24 + 6.9 - 0 - 5.4$$

$$= 25.5\%$$

If a 30-year-old man's BMI is also 20 $kg \cdot m^{-2}$, then his predicted underwater-determined percent body fat is 14.7 %.

$$\% \text{ BF} = 1.20 \times 20 \text{ } kg \cdot m^{-2} + (0.23 \times 30 \text{ y}) - (10.8 \times 1) - 5.4$$

$$= 24 + 6.9 - 10.8 - 5.4$$

$$= 14.7\%$$

Results and Discussion

Considering the substantial inherent weakness of BMI, it is logical to ask "Why do people use it?" First, it is a better indicator of body composition than traditional stature-body mass tables. Second, population studies of BMI over a long period of time can indicate health problems or trends. For example, Table 23.1 shows the incidence of overweight (BMI ≥ 25) in Americans for the last four decades.[27] The BMI data reveal changes over time and clarify differences among genders, ages, and racial groups.

Cautious interpretation should be made of the BMI value as a direct measurement of the degree of fatness. Norms for BMI may imply that, the higher the BMI value, the greater the fat percentage; this would not be the case in "athletic" persons with high amounts of lean mass. AAHPERD established health fitness standards for 18-year-olds as 18 to 26 $kg \cdot m^{-2}$.[1] The Canadian Standardization Test of Fitness (CSTF) provides percentiles for men and women ages 20 y to 69 y (Table 23.2).[12] The CSTF places percentiles greater than the 84th (low BMI) into the *excellent* category and percentiles less than the 25th (high BMI) into the *poor* category. Consistent with the *poor* criterion, some researchers define obesity as an index higher than 85 % of the population between 18 and 24 years old (or below the 15th %ile in Table 23.2). Overweight has been defined as a BMI between 25.0 and 29.9 $kg \cdot m^{-2}$, whereas obesity's criterion is a BMI ≥ 30.0.[2,11] Using a BMI of 30 as the criterion for obesity, 25 % of American

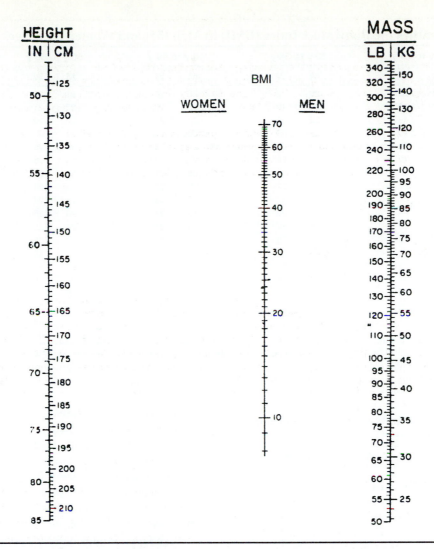

Figure 23.1 A nomogram for assessing body weight. Adapted from Thomas, A. E., McKay, D. A., & Cutlip, M. B. (1976). A nomograph method for assessing body weight. *The American Journal of Clinical Nutrition, 29,* 302–304. Reprinted with permission of American Society for Clinical Nutrition.

women and 20 % of the men are obese according to the Centers of Disease Control's National Center for Health Statistics.[27]

The Canadian norms show that BMI increases in both genders from the 20s through the 40s, then plateaus through the 60s age group. The body mass indexes of a large group (n = 7183) of community-residing, predominantly white, older adults (60 y to 94 y) averaged 25.8 $kg \cdot m^{-2}$ and 26.6 $kg \cdot m^{-2}$ in American men and women, respectively. Their indexes steadily decreased from the 70 y to 74 y age group to the 90 y to 94 y age group in both genders.[29]

Classifications in Table 23.3 relate to the degree of obesity, normality, and underweight for men and women.[27] As of 1980 the average White woman aged 25 y to 34 y of age had a BMI of 23.8 $kg \cdot m^{-2}$, whereas the average Black woman averaged 26.2 $kg \cdot m^{-2}$. The mean BMI for a large

group of 43-year-old men was 25.4 (SD = 3.1 $kg \cdot m^{-2}$), ranging from an extremely lean BMI of 16.96 $kg \cdot m^{-2}$ to a morbidly obese 46.63 $kg \cdot m^{-2}$ BMI.[22] A typical nonobese adult, who has about 25 billion fat cells, is likely to weigh less at a given height, than the obese person, who has about 75 billion fat cells.[34]

BMI in men is directly related to mortality, indicating a greater risk of death the higher the BMI.[2,8,19,23] For women, BMI values over 29 represent a doubling of mortality risk.[23] The increase in mortality is small for overweight persons ($\geq$ 25.0 BMI) but is 50 % to 100 % higher in obese persons ($\geq$ 30 BMI) than in persons with BMI between 20 $kg \cdot m^{-2}$ and 25 $kg \cdot m^{-2}$.[11] For an older adult ($\geq$ 60 y), a BMI greater than 25 $kg \cdot m^{-2}$ indicates a greater risk of losing functional mobility, such as walking, stair climbing, and standing up from the chair or the toilet.[32]

Table 23.2 Percentiles for Body Mass Index (BMI) in Men (M) and Women (W), Ages 20 y to 69 y

%ile	20 y to 29 y		30 y to 39 y		40 y to 49 y		50 y to 59 y		60 y to 69 y	
	M	W	M	W	M	W	M	W	M	W
95	19	18	20	19	21	19	21	20	21	20
90	20	18	21	19	22	20	22	21	22	21
85	21	19	22	20	23	20	23	22	23	22
80	21	19	22	20	23	21	24	22	24	22
75	22	20	23	21	24	21	24	23	25	23
70	22	20	23	21	24	22	24	23	25	23
65	22	20	24	22	25	22	25	23	25	24
60	23	21	24	22	25	23	25	24	26	24
55	23	21	24	22	25	23	25	24	26	25
50	23	21	25	23	26	24	26	25	27	25
45	24	22	25	23	26	24	26	25	27	26
40	24	22	26	23	27	25	27	26	27	26
35	25	22	26	24	27	25	27	26	28	27
30	25	23	27	24	28	26	28	27	28	28
25	26	23	28	25	28	27	28	28	28	28
20	27	24	28	26	29	28	29	29	29	29
15	27	25	29	27	30	29	30	30	30	30
10	28	26	30	29	31	31	31	31	31	32
5	30	28	32	31	32	34	32	34	33	34

Source: Data from Fitness and Amateur Sport Canada, Canadian Standardized Test of Fitness (CSTF) Operations Manual, 3d edition, Appendix I: Table 1, p. 30, 1987 by Canadian Association of Sport Sciences, Ottawa, Ontario.

Table 23.3 Classifications of Body Mass Index (BMI; $kg \cdot m^{-2}$)

Classification	BMI ($kg \cdot m^{-2}$)	Obesity Class
Underweight	< 18.5	
Normal	18.5–24.9	
Overweight	25.0–29.9	
Obesity	30.0–34.9	I
	35.0–39.9	II
Extreme obesity	> 40	III

Adapted from National Heart, Lung, and Blood Institute. (1998). *Clinical guidelines on the identification, evaluation, and treatment of overweight and obesity in adults. The evidence report.* (NIH Publication No. 98-4083). Washington, DC: U.S. Department of Health and Human Services.

References

1. American Alliance for Health, Physical Education, Recreation and Dance. (1988). *Physical best.* Reston, VA: Author.

2. American College of Sports Medicine. (2000). *ACSM's guidelines for exercise testing and prescription.* Philadelphia: Lippincott Williams & Wilkins.

3. Brozek, J., Grande, F., Anderson, J., & Keys, A. (1963). Densitometric analysis of body composition: Revision of some quantitative assumptions. *Annals of New York Academy of Science, 110,* 113–140.

4. Coleman, A. G. (1981). Skinfold estimates of body fat in major league baseball players. *The Physician and Sportsmedicine, 9* (10), 77–82.

5. Cureton, K. J. (1984). A reaction to the manuscript of Jackson. *Medicine and Science in Sports and Exercise, 16,* 621–622.

6. Deurenberg, P., Weststrate, J. A., & Seidell, J. C. (1991). Body mass index as a measure of body fatness: Age- and sex-specific prediction formulas. *Journal of Nutrition, 65,* 105–114.

7. DiGirolamo, M. (1986). Body composition—Roundtable. *The Physician and Sportsmedicine, 14* (3) 144–152, 157, 161, 162.

8. Dorn, J. P., Trevisan, M., & Winkelstein, W. (1996). The long-term relationship between body mass index, coronary heart disease and all-cause mortality. *Medicine and Science in Sports and Exercise, 28* (Suppl.), Abstract #662, p. S111.

9. Dugdale, A. E., & Griffiths, M. (1979). Estimating fat mass from anthropometric data. *American Journal of Clinical Nutrition, 32,* 2400–2403.

10. Eckerson, J. M., Housh, T. J., & Johnson, G. O. (1992). The validity of visual estimations of percent body fat in lean males. *Medicine and Science in Sports and Exercise, 24,* 615–618.

11. Expert Panel. (1998). Executive summary of the clinical guidelines on the identification, evaluation, and treatment of overweight and obesity in adults. *Archives of Internal Medicine, 158,* 1855–1867.

12. Fitness and Amateur Sport Canada. (1987). *Canadian Standardized Test of Fitness (CSTF) operations manual.* Ottawa, Ontario: Canadian Association of Sport Sciences.

13. Galanos, A. N., Pieper, C. F., Cornoni-Huntley, J. C., Bales, C. W., & Fillenbaum, G. G. (1994). Nutrition and function: Is there a relationship between body mass index and the functional capabilities of community-dwelling elderly? *Journal of American Geriatric Society, 42,* 368–373.

Methods for Girth Ratios and Equations

The equipment for measuring girth is very simple. Ideally, a measuring tape made of reinforced fiberglass or metal should be used. Some anthropometric tapes have a calibrated spring at the tip. The purported advantage of anthropometric spring tapes is that the proper tape pressure can be applied repeatedly, although not everyone recommends these.[46] It is helpful to make a "handle" or "tab" from masking tape or adhesive tape attached at the tip of a regular tape. This prevents the technician's thumb and finger from obscuring the zero/index line when reading the circumference. The most practical tapes have an inch scale on one side and a metric scale on the other side. The accuracy of girth measurements is presented in Box 24.1

Because both girth methods for the women and two of the three 2-Girth and 3-Girth Methods for the men require a stature measurement, familiarity with anthropometers or stadiometers is essential. The same is true for weight scales because of the body mass measurements in men for the 1-Girth Method. These instruments and the proper procedures for measuring stature and body mass are described in Chapter 3.

Nomograms are provided in the manual for deriving the percent fat for the men's and women's 1-Girth Method. To determine percent fat from the 2-Girth Method or the 3-Girth Method, a good pocket calculator (or computer-calculator) with "log" function, or estimation tables can be used.

BOX 24.1 Accuracy of Girth Measurements

All measures of fat in living bodies are merely estimates. The first anthropometric prediction of body fat was published in 1951.[12] Since then, more than 100 predictive equations have been developed.

Traditionally, hydrostatic weighing has been the criterion by which other predictive methods are evaluated. The standard error of estimate (SEE) is about 3.5 % for most linear (not hydrostatic) anthropometric predictive tests.[35,37] For example, if an individual was predicted to be 20 % fat by girth, skinfold, and/or diameter measures, then an assumed error of 3.5 % would mean that there is a 67 % chance that the "true" value as predicted by hydrostatic weighing is between 16.5, and 23.5 % (20 % ± 3.5 %).

The 2-Girth and 3-Girth Methods, which were developed from data on large samples of Navy women and men, have moderate to high correlations (r = .85 and .90, respectively) and reasonable standard errors (SEE = 3.7 % and 2.7 % body fat units, respectively) when compared with hydrostatic weighing. In general, the Naval Health Research equations tend to overpredict body fat in lean persons and underestimate it in fat persons.[23,24]

Investigators evaluating the accuracy of three different military equations (Army, Marine, and Navy) concluded that only the Navy equation was not significantly different from hydrostatic weight for group estimations of percent fat in 50-year-old women, but none were a substitute for underwater weighing for individual estimations for middle-aged women.[53]

Test-retest reliabilities of girth measures are .97 or higher.[9]

Procedures for Measuring Girth

1. With the participant standing, the technician measures the body mass and records it to the closest pound or 0.5 kg onto Form 24.1.
2. The technician measures the height of the man or woman and records it to the closest one-fourth in. or 0.5 cm onto Form 24.1.
3. The technician determines the exact anatomical sites of the girth measurements as shown in Figure 24.1. The measurement sites for the 1-Girth[54] and 2- or 3-Girth Methods[23,24] are explained in Table 24.1.
4. The technician measures the girths, careful to avoid any air space between the skin and the tape. On the other hand, the tape should not be pulled so tightly that it indents the skin.[25]
5. The technician holds the tape horizontally, except for neck girth, and reads the tape to the closest one-fourth in. and 0.5 cm. Metric measures are used for the 2-Girth and 3-Girth equations and the Canadian Fitness Test (CSTF); however, either system provides the same ratio value.
6. The technician reads off the values as another technician records them onto the form.

Calculation of Waist (Android; Abdominal) to Hip (Gynoid; Gluteal) Ratio (W:H; A:G)

Although a W:H (A:G) nomogram is available from various sources,[10] the ratio is so simple to calculate that the nomogram is actually less convenient than a pocket calculator. The girth sites (Figure 24.1) and the calculation of the W:H (A:G) ratio are the same for men and women. The ratio is found simply by dividing the waist (upper abdominal; A) girth by the hip (gluteal; G) girth (Eq. 24.1).

$$W:H (A:G) = \text{Upper A} \div \text{G girth} \qquad \text{Eq. 24.1}$$

For example, if a woman's upper waist (upper abdominal) girth is 30 in. ($\approx$ 76 cm) and her hip (gluteal) girth is 40 in. ($\approx$ 101.5 cm), then her W:H (A:G) ratio is calculated as follows:

$$W:H (A:G) = \frac{30 \text{ in.}}{40 \text{ in.}} \quad \text{or} \quad \frac{76 \text{ cm}}{101.5 \text{ cm}} = 0.75$$

Determination of Percent Body Fat from Girth

The following four methods use girth measurements to predict percent body fat: (1) 1-Girth for Men; (2) 1-Girth for Women; (3) 2-Girth for Men; and (4) 3-Girth for Women. The 1-Girth Methods estimate percent body fat by using nomograms, whereas the 2- and 3-Girth Methods use tables or regression equations.

1-Girth for Men

The 1-Girth Method uses the nomogram for men (Figure 24.2). Thus, a straight-edge is placed on the body mass (vertical) axis

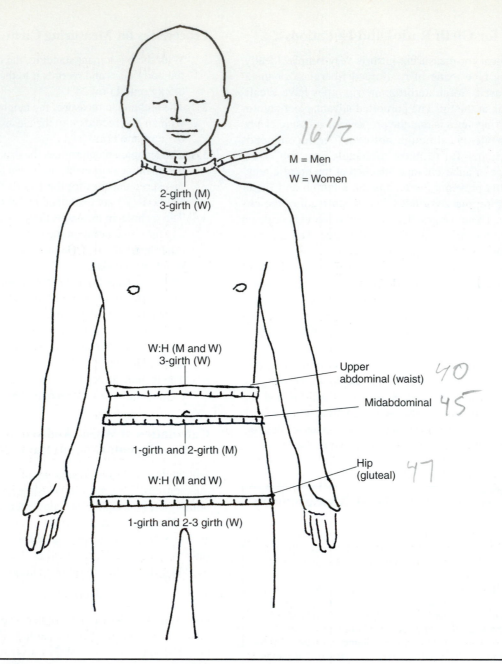

Figure 24.1 Girth sites for the 1-Girth-Method (men: midabdominal; women: hip/gluteal) and 2- or 3-Girth Method (men: neck and midabdominal; women: neck, upper abdominal/waist, hip/gluteal).

Table 24.1 Measurement Sites for the 1-Girth, 2-Girth, and 3-Girth Methods

Men (M)	Women (W)
1-Girth Method	**1-Girth Method**
Weight (closest lb; 0.5 kg)	Height (closest one-fourth in.; 0.5 cm)
Midabdominal girth—level of umbilicus (navel)	Hip girth—widest point
2-Girth Method (Naval Health Research Center)	**3-Girth Method (Naval Health Research Center)**
	Height (closest one-fourth in.; 0.5 cm)
Neck girth—same as women's site	Neck girth—just inferior to the larynx (Adam's apple) with the tape sloping slightly downward to the front
Mid-abdominal girth—level of umbilicus (navel)	Upper abdominal girth (waist)—at the narrowest point above navel; often midway between xiphoid process and navel
	Hip (gluteal)—at the level of symphysis pubis and greatest protrusion of the gluteal muscles
Men's A:G (W:H) Sites	**Women's A:G (W:H) Sites**
Upper abdominal (waist) and hip (gluteal)	Upper abdominal and gluteal

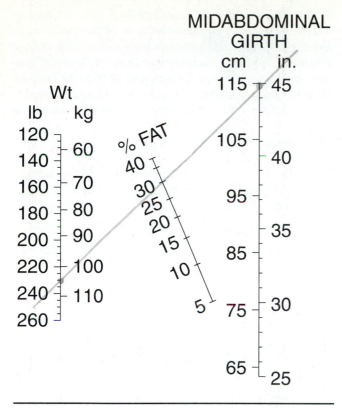

Figure 24.2 Men's nomogram for determination of percent body fat (% fat) from weight and midabdominal girth. From J. H. Wilmore, *Sensible Fitness*, Fig. 13, p. 30, 1988. Copyright © 1988. Human Kinetics Publishers, Champaign, Il.

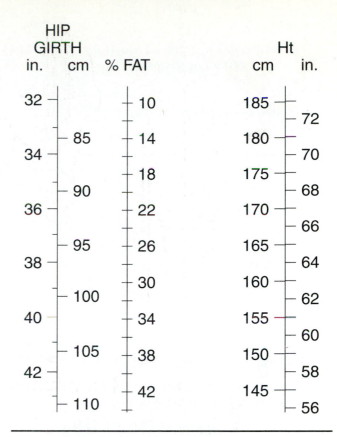

Figure 24.3 Women's nomogram for determination of percent body fat (% fat) from height and hip girth. From J. H. Wilmore, *Sensible Fitness*, Fig. 14, p. 31, 1988. Copyright © 1988. Human Kinetics Publishers, Champaign, IL.

and then pivoted to the midabdominal girth's (vertical) axis; percent fat is then read where the straight-edge intersects the percent fat diagonal axis.

1-Girth for Women

For the women, the percent fat is found by placing the straight-edge on the hip girth on the left vertical axis and then pivoted to the height on the right vertical axis (Figure 24.3). As much as possible, the placements should be at the closest pound or 0.5 kg, and at the closest 0.25 in. or 0.5 cm.

2-Girth and 3-Girth Method (*Naval Health Research*)

The 2- and 3-Girth Methods use tables[1,23,24] or multiple regression equations—Equation 24.2 (men)[23] and Equation 24.3 (women)[24]—to predict body density from circumferences (cm) and stature (cm). The extensive tables (24.2 and 24.3) also require calculations but are not as intimidating as the multiple regression equations. The men's equation uses two girth sites—neck and midabdominal—and stature. The women's equation uses three girth sites—neck, upper abdominal, and hip—and stature. The advantage of the multiple regression equations is that they can be programmed into a calculator or computer quite easily, thus avoiding the search through the tables. The Siri[50] equation (Eq. 24.4) for converting body density to percent fat can also be programmed into the calculator

or computer. Thus, there is an ultimate savings in time and convenience by using the regression equation instead of the tables, especially if testing many people.[a]

Men:

$$D_b = 1.0324 + [0.15456 \times Log_{10}(Ht)] \quad \text{Eq. 24.2}$$
$$- [0.19077 \times Log_{10}(Ab - N)]$$

where:

$$D_b = \text{body density}$$

$$Log_{10}(Ht) = \text{expressed in cm}^b; \text{enter ht, then press "log" on calculator}$$

$$Ab = \text{midabdominal girth (cm)}$$

$$N = \text{neck girth (cm)}$$

---

[a]The body density portion of predicting percent fat (% F) can be bypassed by using the following equations and inches.[25] Men % F = 86.010 × log₁₀ (mid-ab – N) – 70.041 × log₁₀(Ht) + 36.76 (*SEE* = 3.52 % F) Women % F= 163.205 × log₁₀ (up-ab + hip + N) – 97.684 × log₁₀ (Ht) – 78.37 (*SEE* = 3.61 % F)
[b]Logarithm—the exponent expressing the power to which a fixed number (the base) must be raised in order to produce a given number (the antilogarithm): logs are normally computed to the base of 10 and are used for shortening math calculations.

Women:

$$D_b = 1.29579 + [0.22100 \times \mathrm{Log}_{10}(\mathrm{Ht})] \qquad \text{Eq. 24.3}$$
$$- [0.35004 \times \mathrm{Log}_{10}(\text{Up-Ab} + \mathrm{Hip} - \mathrm{N})]$$

where:

Up-Ab = upper abdomen (waist)

For example, if a man, who is 174.0 cm (68.5 in.) tall, has a midabdominal girth of 80.0 cm (31.5 in.), and a neck girth of 41.9 cm (16.5 in.) then the following process would calculate this body density:

$$D_b = 1.0324 + [0.15456 \times \mathrm{Log}_{10}(174)]$$
$$- [0.19077 \times \mathrm{Log}_{10}(80 - 41.9)]$$

$$= 1.0324 + (0.15456 \times 2.2405)$$
$$- [0.19077 \times \mathrm{Log}_{10}(38.1)]$$

$$= 1.0324 + 0.3463 - (0.19077 \times 1.5809)$$

$$= 1.3787 - 0.3016$$

$$= 1.0771$$

$$\% \text{ Fat} = 100 \times [(4.95 \div D_b) - 4.50] \qquad \text{Eq. 24.4}$$

Using the same man as in our prior example, his body density of 1.0771 converts to 9.6 % body fat:

$$\% \text{ Fat} = 100 \times [(4.95 \div 1.0771) - 4.50]$$

$$= 100 \times (4.596 - 4.50)$$

$$= 100 \times 0.096$$

$$= 9.6 \%$$

The rounded-off percentage of 10 % fat is also derived by using Table 24.2 for males (use Table 24.3 for females). For example, the intersecting row (height; 68.0–69.0 in.) and column (circumference; 15.0 in.) meet at 10 % fat.

Calculation of Ideal Weight

After the percent fat is known, a person usually wishes to know how much fat should be lost (occasionally, gained) in order to be ideal or perfect. The criterion for what is perfect is open to speculation and is based on health, aesthetics, and performance or, simply, in the eyes of the beholder. A formerly proposed value of 14 % fat for men and 20 % fat for women[30] may be used as an example for demonstrating the calculation of ideal or desired weight. A range of ideal values, rather than a single ideal percent fat value, for each gender is suitable, and its selection should be left up to the discretion of the counselor and/or investigator and the participant.

The calculation of ideal weight may be performed by using various equations. Equation 24.5 may be referred to as the approximate equation because of its approximation

of ideal weight, whereas Equations 24.6 and 24.7 may be referred to as exact equations because of their more exact and logical approach. Although the examples for the approximated and the exact equations use 14 % as the constant ideal fat percentage for men and 20 % as the constant ideal fat percentage for women, other desired values (or ranges) for percent body fat may be chosen and inserted in their places.

The **approximate** equation is based upon a very simple concept and often can be calculated in one's head. It basically calls for the subtraction of the unwanted fat from the initial body mass (BM) of the man (M) or woman (W).

Approximate Equation:

$$\text{Ideal Wt} = \mathrm{BM} - [(F - 0.14_M \text{ or } 0.20_W) \times \mathrm{BM}] \quad \text{Eq. 24.5}$$

where:

F = percent fat in decimal form for men (M) or women (W)

For example, if a man weighing 70 kg (154 lb) was estimated to be 20 % body fat, then the following calculation would approximate his ideal weight:

$$\text{Ideal Wt (kg)} = 70 \text{ kg} - [(0.20 - 0.14) \times 70 \text{ kg}]$$

$$= 70 \text{ kg} - (0.06 \times 70 \text{ kg})$$

$$= 70 \text{ kg} - 4.2 \text{ kg}$$

$$= 65.8 \text{ kg}$$

The **exact** equations (Eq. 24.6 and 24.7) for calculating ideal body weight are based upon the lean body mass (LBM) of the individual.[7,45] These equations emphasize the importance of maintaining or gaining lean weight while losing fat weight when dieting and/or exercising. Both equations use the ideal (I-% Fat) criteria of 14 % and 20 % fat for men and women, respectively.

Exact Equation (A):

$$\text{Ideal Wt} = \left[\frac{100 - \% \text{ Fat}}{100 - \text{I-}\% \text{ Fat}} \right] \times \mathrm{BM} \qquad \text{Eq. 24.6}$$

where:

% Fat and BM = the measured % Fat and body mass

I-% Fat = the ideal % Fat (e.g., 14 % in men; 20 % in women)

Exact Equation (B):

$$\text{Ideal Wt} = \frac{\mathrm{LBM}}{\text{Ideal LBM Fraction of BM}} \qquad \text{Eq. 24.7}$$

$$= \frac{\mathrm{BM} - \text{Fat wt}}{0.86 \text{ (men) or } 0.80 \text{ (women)}}$$

Table 24.2 Estimation of Percent Body Fat in Males from the Combination of Midabdominal and Neck Girths

Circumference Value (in.) = Midabdominal Girth (in.) − Neck Girth (in.)

Height (in.)	11.0	11.5	12.0	12.5	13.0	13.5	14.0	14.5	15.0	15.5	16.0	16.5	17.0	17.5	18.0	18.5	19.0	19.5
60.0	4	5	6	8	9	10	11	12	14	15	16	17	18	19	20	21	22	23
61.0	3	5	6	7	8	10	11	12	13	14	15	16	17	18	19	20	21	22
62.0	3	4	5	7	8	9	10	12	13	14	15	16	17	18	19	20	21	22
63.0	2	4	5	6	8	9	10	11	12	13	14	15	16	17	18	19	20	21
64.0	2	3	5	6	7	8	10	11	12	13	14	15	16	17	18	19	20	21
65.0	2	3	4	6	7	8	9	10	11	13	14	15	16	17	18	18	19	20
66.0		3	4	5	6	8	9	10	11	12	13	14	15	16	17	18	19	20
67.0		2	3	5	6	7	8	10	11	12	13	14	15	16	17	18	19	19
68.0		2	3	4	6	7	8	9	10	11	12	13	14	15	16	17	18	19
69.0			3	4	5	6	8	9	10	11	12	13	14	15	16	17	18	19
70.0			2	4	5	6	7	8	10	11	12	13	14	15	15	16	17	18
71.0			2	3	5	6	7	8	9	10	11	12	13	14	15	16	17	18
72.0			2	3	4	5	7	8	9	10	11	12	13	14	15	16	17	17
73.0				3	4	5	6	7	8	9	11	12	13	13	14	15	16	17
74.0				2	3	5	6	7	8	9	10	11	12	13	14	15	16	17
75.0				2	3	4	5	7	8	9	10	11	12	13	14	15	15	16
76.0				2	2	4	5	6	7	8	9	10	11	12	13	14	15	16
77.0					2	4	5	6	7	8	9	10	11	12	13	14	15	16
78.0					2	3	4	6	7	8	9	10	11	12	13	14	14	15

Circumference Value (in.) = Midabdominal Girth (in.) − Neck Girth (in.)

Height (in.)	20.0	20.5	21.0	21.5	22.0	22.5	23.0	23.5	24.0	24.5	25.0	25.5	26.0	26.5	27.0	27.5	28.0	28.5
60.0	23	24	25	26	27	28	28	29	30	31	31	32	33	33	34	35	35	36
61.0	23	24	25	25	26	27	28	29	29	30	31	31	32	33	34	34	35	36
62.0	22	23	24	25	26	27	27	28	29	30	30	31	32	32	33	34	34	35
63.0	22	23	24	25	25	26	27	28	28	29	30	31	31	32	33	33	34	35
64.0	22	22	23	24	25	26	26	27	28	29	29	30	31	31	32	33	33	34
65.0	21	22	23	24	24	25	26	27	27	28	29	30	30	31	32	32	33	34
66.0	21	22	22	23	24	25	26	26	27	28	29	29	30	31	31	32	33	33
67.0	20	21	22	23	23	24	25	26	27	27	28	29	29	30	31	31	32	33
68.0	20	21	22	22	23	24	25	25	26	27	28	28	29	30	30	31	32	32
69.0	19	20	21	22	23	23	24	25	26	26	27	28	29	29	30	31	31	32
70.0	19	20	21	22	22	23	24	25	25	26	27	28	28	29	30	30	31	31
71.0	19	20	20	21	22	23	23	24	25	26	26	27	28	28	29	30	30	31
72.0	18	19	20	21	22	22	23	24	25	25	26	27	27	28	29	29	30	31
73.0	18	19	20	21	21	22	23	23	24	25	26	26	27	28	28	29	30	30
74.0	18	18	19	20	21	22	22	23	24	25	25	26	27	27	28	29	29	30
75.0	17	18	19	20	20	21	22	23	23	24	25	26	26	27	28	28	29	29
76.0	17	18	18	19	20	21	22	22	23	24	24	25	26	27	27	28	28	29
77.0	16	17	18	19	20	20	21	22	23	23	24	25	25	26	27	27	28	29
78.0	16	17	18	19	19	20	21	22	22	23	24	24	25	26	26	27	28	28

Original Naval Health Research Center's tables were reduced in number through the courtesy of Dr. W. C. Beam.

Table 24.3 Estimation of Percent Body Fat in Females from the Combination of Upper-Abdominal, Hip, and Neck Girths

Circumference Value (in.) = Upper-Abdominal Girth (in.) + Hip Girth (in.) − Neck Girth (in.)

Height (in.)	37.0	37.5	38.0	38.5	39.0	39.5	40.0	40.5	41.0	41.5	42.0	42.5	43.0	43.5	44.0	44.5	45.0	45.5
58.0	7	8	9	10	10	11	12	13	13	14	15	16	16	17	18	18	19	20
59.0	7	7	8	9	10	11	11	12	13	13	14	15	16	16	17	18	18	19
60.0	6	7	8	8	9	10	11	11	12	13	14	14	15	16	16	17	18	19
61.0	5	6	7	8	8	9	10	11	11	12	13	14	14	15	16	16	17	18
62.0	5	6	6	7	8	9	9	10	11	12	12	13	14	14	15	16	17	17
63.0		5	6	7	7	8	9	10	10	11	12	12	13	14	14	15	16	16
64.0			5	6	7	7	8	9	10	10	11	12	13	13	14	15	15	16
65.0			5	5	6	7	8	8	9	10	11	11	12	13	13	14	15	15
66.0				5	6	6	7	8	9	9	10	11	11	12	13	13	14	15
67.0				5	5	6	6	7	8	9	9	10	11	11	12	13	14	14
68.0						5	6	6	7	8	9	10	10	11	12	12	13	14
69.0						5	5	6	7	8	9	9	10	10	11	12	13	13
70.0							5	6	6	7	8	8	9	10	11	11	12	13
71.0								5	6	6	7	8	9	9	10	11	12	12
72.0								5	5	6	7	7	8	9	9	10	11	11
73.0									5	5	6	7	8	8	9	10	11	11
74.0										5	6	6	7	8	8	9	10	10
75.0											5	6	7	7	8	9	9	10
76.0											5	5	6	7	7	8	9	9

Circumference Value (in.) = Midabdominal Girth (in.) − Neck Girth (in.)

Height (in.)	46.0	46.5	47.0	47.5	48.0	48.5	49.0	49.5	50.0	50.5	51.0	51.5	52.0	52.5	53.0	53.5	54.0	54.5
60.0	19	20	21	21	22	23	23	24	24	25	26	26	27	28	28	29	29	30
61.0	19	19	20	21	21	22	23	23	24	24	25	26	26	27	28	28	29	29
62.0	18	19	19	20	21	21	22	22	23	24	24	25	26	26	27	27	28	29
63.0	17	18	19	19	20	21	21	22	22	23	24	24	25	26	26	27	27	28
64.0	17	17	18	19	19	20	21	21	22	22	23	24	24	25	26	26	27	27
65.0	16	17	17	18	19	19	20	21	21	22	22	23	24	24	25	26	26	27
66.0	15	16	16	17	18	19	19	20	21	21	22	23	23	24	24	25	26	26
67.0	15	15	16	17	17	18	19	19	20	21	21	22	23	23	24	24	25	26
68.0	14	15	16	16	17	18	18	19	19	20	21	21	22	23	23	24	24	25
69.0	14	14	15	16	16	17	18	18	19	20	20	21	21	22	23	23	24	24
70.0	13	14	14	15	16	16	17	18	18	19	20	20	21	22	22	23	24	24
71.0	13	13	14	15	15	16	17	17	18	18	19	20	20	21	22	22	23	24
72.0	12	13	13	14	15	15	16	16	17	18	18	19	20	20	21	21	22	23
73.0	12	12	13	14	14	15	15	16	17	17	18	18	19	20	20	21	21	22
74.0	11	12	12	13	14	14	15	15	16	16	17	18	18	19	19	20	21	22
75.0	11	11	12	12	13	14	15	15	16	16	17	18	18	19	19	20	20	21
76.0	10	11	11	12	13	13	14	15	16	16	17	18	18	19	19	20	20	21
77.0	10	10	11	11	12	13	13	14	15	15	16	16	17	18	18	19	19	20
78.0	9	10	10	11	12	12	13	13	14	15	15	16	17	17	18	18	19	19

Original Naval Health Research Center's tables were reduced in number through the courtesy of Dr. W. C. Beam.

If the exact equation (Eq. 24.6) is used to calculate the ideal or desired weight of the same man in the previous example, then the following calculations would be made:

$$\text{Ideal wt} = \left[\frac{100 - 20 \text{ \% Fat}}{100 - 14 \text{ \% Fat}} \right] \times 70 \text{ kg}$$

$$= (80 / 86) \times 70$$

$$= 0.93 \times 70$$

$$= 65.1 \text{ kg}$$

As can be seen in the two examples, the exact method produces a greater amount of fat mass that must be lost (4.9 kg) than does the approximate method (4.2 kg).

Results and Discussion

Percent Fat Interpretation

Authorities differ as to the recommended body composition for the average person. Average values may not always be recommended values. For example, we do not know if the 16 % body fat of babies born in the United States[21] is healthy even though infant mortality is very low. Also, some feel that elderly persons should carry slightly extra fat in case of severe prolonged illness.

The recommended body composition for athletes also varies; usually, it is dependent upon the sport and/or gender. For example, successful male marathoners are about 7.5 % fat,[14] whereas female marathoners usually are less than 20 % fat. However, some investigators[13] caution that there may be a critical set point of percent body fat for each female amenorrheic (absence of menstruation) runner, although this has not been confirmed by most studies.[47] Successful middle distance and distance swimmers tend to carry more fat than successful sprint swimmers.[42] If high school wrestlers drop below 5 % fat, they are either banned from competition in some conferences[33] or are advised to obtain medical clearance.[3] One authority[52] advises a minimum of 7 % fat for wrestlers under 16 y of age. Thus, it appears that the ideal percent fat is dependent upon the goal of the individual. It may be inappropriate to use a single value as a standard for specific-sport athletes, using instead a suitable range of values.[56] Also, if an indirect method is used, then a person's predicted percent fat should be presented as a value within the range of the standard error; thus, a percent fat of 20 % should be presented as 14 % to 26 % if the standard error is 6 %. Some of the fat categories suggested by various investigators are presented in Tables 24.4 and 24.5.

Although some investigators have reported percent fat values of less than 3 % fat in some persons, these are "generally considered to be underestimates of the true relative body fat."[56] For example, one study of a group of professional football players reported one player at 0 % body fat and eight players at less than 0 % fat![2] Olga Korbut, the girl

Table 24.4 Health and Fitness Standards for Percent Body Fat

Classification	Men	Women
Essential fat	5 %	8 %
Optimal fitness	12 % to 18 %	16 % to 25 %
Optimal health	10 % to 25 %	18 % to 30 %
Overfat	> 25 %	> 30 %

Source: From M. DiGirolamo, "Body Composition: A Roundtable" in The Physician and Sportsmedicine, 14, 144–162, March 1986.

Table 24.5 Percent Fat Categories in College-Age People

Category	Percent Fat (%)	
	Men	Women
Very lean[18]	8	14
Underweight[39]		< 17[a]
Lean[18]	11	20
Average	10.5 ± 5	23 ± 6
	12–16[55]	22–26[55]
	15[18]	25[18]
	15	27
	10–15[16]	15–20[16]
Suitable	10–22[36]	20–32[36]
Optimal health	10–25[47]	18–30[47]
Recommended (goal-dependent)	15–20[29]	22–28[29]
	8–10[41]	
	10–14[31]	
Optimal fitness	12–18[47]	16–25[47]
Adult fitness	15–22[7]	23–28[7]
Navy standard		< 30[53]
Overfat	> 20[39]	> 30[39]
Moderately overfat	> 20[18]	> 31[18]
Obese	> 25[38]	> 34[38]
	> 25[47]	> 30[47]
	> 25[53]	> 35[53]
		> 38[49]
	> 30[18]	> 44[18]
Massively obese	> 55[40]	> 55[40]

Note: [a]Accompanied by < 20th %ile in body mass by stature.

who helped popularize gymnastics, was found to be 1.5 % body fat.[44] The lowest I have ever measured was 4 % fat in a Black wrestler trying out for the U.S. Olympic team. Underfat males and females of less than 5 % and 15 % fat,[47] respectively, may not be healthy. A 70 % body fat is the highest value I have ever seen reported.[51]

The military services use a combination of body mass index (BMI) and girth-prediction of percent fat as their standards.[26] Military men and women with BMI over 25 kg·m^{-2} and percentages of fat between 20 % and 26 % (men), or 30 % and 36 % (women), would be in a "cautionary zone." Persons in this zone would still meet the military standards if they passed the service's physical fitness test.

%ile	15 y to 19 y M	15 y to 19 y W	20 y to 29 y M	20 y to 29 y W	30 y to 39 y M	30 y to 39 y W	40 y to 49 y M	40 y to 49 y W	50 y to 59 y M	50 y to 59 y W	60 y to 69 y M	60 y to 69 y W
95	.73	.65	.76	.65	.80	.66	.81	.66	.82	.67	.84	.71
90	.75	.67	.80	.67	.81	.68	.83	.69	.85	.71	.88	.73
85	.76	.68	.81	.68	.82	.69	.84	.71	.87	.72	.89	.74
80	.77	.69	.81	.69	.83	.71	.86	.72	.89	.73	.90	.75
75	.79	.71	.82	.71	.84	.72	.87	.73	.89	.74	.90	.76
70	.80	.72	.83	.72	.84	.73	.88	.74	.90	.75	.91	.77
65	.81	.73	.83	.73	.85	.74	.89	.75	.91	.76	.92	.78
60	.81	.73	.84	.73	.86	.75	.90	.76	.92	.77	.93	.79
55	.82	.74	.85	.74	.87	.75	.91	.76	.92	.77	.94	.80
50	.83	.75	.85	.75	.88	.76	.92	.77	.93	.78	.94	.81
45	.83	.75	.86	.76	.89	.77	.92	.78	.94	.79	.95	.82
40	.84	.76	.87	.76	.90	.78	.93	.79	.95	.80	.96	.83
35	.85	.77	.87	.77	.91	.78	.94	.79	.95	.81	.97	.84
30	.85	.78	.88	.78	.92	.79	.95	.80	.96	.82	.98	.85
25	.86	.78	.89	.78	.93	.80	.95	.82	.98	.84	.99	.86
20	.87	.79	.91	.79	.94	.81	.97	.84	.99	.85	1.00	.87
15	.87	.80	.93	.80	.95	.83	.99	.86	1.01	.86	1.02	.88
10	.88	.82	.94	.82	.96	.85	1.01	.87	1.02	.88	1.03	.91
5	.92	.86	.96	.85	1.01	.87	1.03	.92	1.04	.92	1.04	.94

Source: Data from Canadian Standardized Test of Fitness (CSTF) Operations Manual, pp. 30–31, 1987. Fitness and Amateur Sport Canada, Ottawa, Ontario, Canada.

Waist: Hip (Abdominal: Gluteal) Ratio Interpretation

W:H (A:G) ratios of a large Canadian sample are presented in Table 24.6.[19] Percentiles above the 84th are in the excellent category; those between the 65th and 84th are better than average; the average includes persons between the 45th and 64th percentiles, and the below average are between the 25th and 44th; the poorest category includes those lower than the 25th percentile.

A waist-hip ratio below 0.80[31] or 0.86[5] for women and 0.95[31] or 1.0[6] for men are the criteria ratios to avoid a greater risk for several diseases. Ratios above 0.94 for young men and above 0.82 for young women produce very high health risks.[10,21] However, the waist circumference alone when over 102 cm (40 in.) in men or over 88 cm (35 in.) in women is an indicator of increased relative risk.[18,26,41]

References

1. Adams, G. M. (1994). *Exercise physiology laboratory manual.* Dubuque, IA: Brown & Benchmark.

2. Adams, J., Mottola, M., Bagnall, K. M., & McFadden, K. D. (1982). Total body fat content in a group of professional football players. *Canadian Journal of Applied Sport Science, 7,* 36–40.

3. American College of Sports Medicine. (1979). Position statement on weight loss in wrestlers. *Sports Medicine Bulletin, 22,* 2–3.

4. American College of Sports Medicine. (1995). *ACSM's guidelines for exercise testing and prescription.* Philadelphia: Williams & Wilkins.

5. American College of Sports Medicine. (2000). *ACSM's guidelines for exercise testing and prescription.* Philadelphia: Lippincott Williams & Wilkins.

6. American Heart Association. (1991). *1992 heart and stroke facts.* Dallas: Author.

7. Baumgartner, T. A., & Jackson, A. S. (1987). *Measurement for evaluation in physical education and exercise science.* Dubuque, IA: Wm. C. Brown.

8. Behnke, A. R., & Wilmore, J. H. (1974). *Evaluation and regulation of body build and composition.* Englewood Cliffs, NJ: Prentice-Hall.

9. Bemben, M. G., Massey, B. H., Bemben, D. A., Boileau, R. A., & Misner, J. E. (1995). Age-related patterns in body composition for men aged 20–79 y. *Medicine and Science in Sports and Exercise, 27,* 264–269.

10. Bray, G. A., & Gray, D. S. (1988). Obesity, Part 1—Pathogenesis. *Western Journal of Medicine, 149,* 429–441.

11. Brooks, G. A., Fahey, T. D., White, T. P., & Baldwin, K. M. (2000). *Exercise physiology: Human bioenergetics and its application* (p. 582). Mountain View, CA: Mayfield.

12. Brozek, J., & Keys, A. (1951). The evaluation of leanness-fatness in man: Norms and intercorrelations. *British Journal of Nutrition, 5,* 194–205.

13. Carlberg, K. A., Buckman, M. T., Peake, G. T., & Riedesel, M. L. (1983). Body composition of oligo/amenorrheic athletes. *Medicine and Science in Sports and Exercise, 15,* 215–217.

14. Costill, D. L., Bowers, R., & Kammer, W. F. (1970). Skinfold estimates of body fat among marathon runners. *Medicine and Science in Sports, 2,* 93–95.

15. Despres, J.-P., Moorjani, S., Lupien, P. J., Tremblay, A., Nadeau, A., & Bouchard, C. (1990). Regional distribution of body fat, plasma lipoproteins, and cardiovascular disease. *Arteriosclerosis, 10,* 497–511.

16. deVries, H. A. (1986). *Physiology of exercise for physical education and athletics.* Dubuque, IA: Wm. C. Brown.

17. DiGirolomo, M. (1986). Body composition: A roundtable. *The Physician and Sports Medicine, 14,* 144–162.

18. Expert Panel. (1998). Executive summary of the clinical guidelines on the identification, evaluation, and treatment of overweight and obesity in adults. *Archives of Internal Medicine, 158,* 1855–1867.

19. Falls, H. B., Baylor, A. M., & Dishman, R. K. (1980). *Essentials of fitness.* Philadelphia: Saunders College Publishing.

20. Fitness and Amateur Sport Canada. (1987). *Canadian Standardized Test of Fitness operations manual* (3rd ed.). Ottawa, Ontario: Minister of Supply and Services Canada.

21. Hager, A., et al. (1977). Body fat and adipose tissue cellularity in infants: A longitudinal study. *Metabolism, 26,* 607–614.

22. Heyward, V. H., & Stolarczyk, L. M. (1996). *Applied body composition assessment.* Champaign, IL: Human Kinetics.

23. Hodgdon, J. A., & Beckett, M. B. (1984). *Prediction of percent body fat for U.S. Navy men from body circumferences and height.* Report No. 84-11. San Diego, CA: Naval Health Research Center.

24. Hodgdon, J. A., & Beckett, M. B. (1984). *Prediction of percent body fat for U.S. Navy women from body circumferences and height.* Report No. 84-29. San Diego, CA: Naval Health Research Center.

25. Hodgdon, J. A., & Beckett, M. B. (1984). *Technique for measuring body circumferences and skinfold thicknesses.* Report No. 84-39. San Diego, CA: Naval Health Research Center.

26. Hodgdon, J. A., & Freidl, K. (1999, September). Development of the DoD body composition estimation equations. Technical Document 99-2B. Washington, DC: Bureau of Medicine and Surgery. Department of Defense.

27. Howley, E. T. (2000). You asked for it. *ACSM's Health & Fitness Journal, 4*(6), 6, 26.

28. Jackson, A. S. (1984). Research design and analysis of data procedures for predicting body density. *Medicine and Science in Sports and Exercise, 16,* 616–620.

29. Jackson, A. S., & Pollock, M. L. (1985). Practical assessment of body composition. *The Physician and Sportsmedicine,* 76–80, 82–90.

30. Johnson, P. B. (1968). Metabolism and weight control. *JOHPER,* 39–40.

31. Johnson, P. B., Updyke, W. F., Schaefer, M., & Stolberg, D. C. (1975). *Sport, exercise, and you.* San Francisco: Holt, Rinehart & Winston.

32. Joint Dietary Guidelines Advisory Committee of the United States, Department of Agriculture, Health, and Human Services. (1990). U.S. Dept of Agriculture.

33. Larsson, B., Svardsudd, K., Welin, L., Wilhelmsen, L., Bjorntorp, P., & Tibblin, G. (1984). Abdominal adipose tissue distribution, obesity, and risk of cardiovascular disease and death: 13-year follow-up of participants in the study of men born in 1913. *British Medical Journal, 288,* 1401–1404.

34. Legwold, G. (1984). When sports medicine groups speak, who listens? *The Physician and Sportsmedicine,* 162–166.

35. Lohman, T. G. (1981). Skinfolds and body density and their relation to body fatness: A review. *Human Biology, 53,* 181–225.

36. Lohman, T. G. (1982). Body composition methodology in sportsmedicine. *The Physician and Sportsmedicine,* 46–58.

37. Lohman, T. G. (1986). Body composition—A round table. *The Physician and Sportsmedicine,* 157, 161, 162.

38. Mayer, J. (1968). *Overweight.* Englewood Cliffs, NJ: Prentice-Hall.

39. McArdle, W. D., Katch, F. I., & Katch, V. L. (1991, 1996). *Exercise physiology: Energy, nutrition, and human performance.* Philadelphia: Lea & Febiger.

40. McArdle, W. D., Katch, F. I., & Katch, V. L. (1994). *Essentials of exercise physiology.* Philadelphia: Lea & Febiger.

41. Myers, C. R., Golding, L. A., & Sinning, W. E. (1973). *The Y's Way to Fitness.* Rodale Press.

42. National Heart, Lung, and Blood Institute. (1998). *Clinical guidelines on the identification, evaluation, and treatment of overweight and obesity in adults.* Washington, DC: U.S. Government Printing Office.

43. Noble, B. J. (1986). *Physiology of exercise and sport.* St. Louis: Times/Mirror.

44. Parizkova, J. (1977). Nutritional practices in athletics abroad. *The Physician and Sportsmedicine,* 32–36, 39–40, 42–44.

45. Pate, R. R., McClenaghan, B., & Rotella, R. (1984). *Foundation of coaching.* Philadelphia: Saunders.

46. Ross, W. D., & Marfell-Jones, M. J. (1991). Kinanthopometry. In J. D. MacDougall, H. A. Wenger, & H. J. Green (Eds.), *Physiological testing of the high performance athlete* (pp. 223–308). Champaign, IL: Human Kinetics.

47. Roundtable. (1986). Body composition methodology in sportsmedicine. *The Physician and Sportsmedicine,* 46–58.

48. Sanborn, C. F., Albrecht, B. H., & Wagner, W. W. (1987). Athletic amenorrhea: Lack of association with body fat. *Medicine and Science in Sports and Exercise, 19,* 207–212.

49. Sharkey, B. J. (1975). *Physiology and physical activity.* San Francisco: Harper & Row.

50. Siri, W. E. (1961). *Body composition from fluid spaces and density: Analysis of methods in techniques for measuring body composition.* Washington, DC: National Academy of Science, National Research Council.

51. Stern, J. S. (1973, May). *Adipose cellularity: Metabolic and chemical significances.* Symposium at ACSM 20th Annual Convention, Seattle, WA.

52. Tipton, C. M. (1987). Commentary: Physicians should advise wrestlers about weight loss. *The Physician and Sportsmedicine,* 160, 163.

53. U.S. Department of the Navy, Navy Military Personnel Command, Code 6H. (1986, August). Office of the Chief of Naval Operations Instruction 6110.1C. Physical Readiness Program.

54. Van Itallie, T. B. (1988). Topography of body fat: Relationship to risk of cardiovascular and other diseases. In T. G. Lohman, A. F. Roche, & R. Martorell (Eds.), *Anthropometric standardization reference manual* (pp. 143–149). Champaign, IL: Human Kinetics.

55. Wells, C. L., & Plowman, S. A. (1983). Sexual differences in athletic performance: Biological or behavioral? *The Physician and Sportsmedicine,* 52–56, 59–63.

56. Wilmore, J. H. (1986). *Sensible fitness.* Champaign, IL: Human Kinetics.

57. Wilmore, J. H., & Behnke, A. R. (1969). An anthropometric estimation of body density and lean body weight in young men. *Journal of Applied Physiology, 27,* 25–31.

Form 24.2

Group Data for Girth-Prediction of % Fat and W:H Ratio

MEN				WOMEN			
Initials (or ID#)	1-Girth % Fat	2-Girth % Fat	W:H (A:G) Ratio	Initials (or ID#)	1-Girth % Fat	3-Girth % Fat	W:H (A:G) Ratio
1.				1.			
2.				2.			
3.				3.			
4.				4.			
5.				5.			
6.				6.			
7.				7.			
8.				8.			
9.				9.			
10.				10.			
11.				11.			
12.				12.			
13.				13.			
14.				14.			
15.				15.			
16.				16.			
17.				17.			
18.				18.			
19.				19.			
20.				20.			
M				M			
Range				Range			

The use of calipers to measure subcutaneous skinfolds for predicting percent body fat is popular not only in laboratories and health clinics but also in commercial fitness centers. Although traditionally the skinfold caliper has been thought of as a laboratory instrument, its portability and recent modification to an inexpensive plastic caliper would qualify it also as a field instrument. In addition, the recommendation of AAHPERD to incorporate skinfold measures in physical education classes,[2,3] characterizes skinfold testing as a field test. Because the location of fat (regional distribution) may be as important clinically and aesthetically as the total amount of fat, skinfolds have an advantage over some other body composition measures.

Physiological Rationale

Fat is not bad. In fact, it is a very economical way to store energy. For instance, one gram of fat contains slightly more than twice the amount of kilocalories (or kilojoules) as do either carbohydrates or proteins. In addition to its economical storage of fuel, fat also provides a storage place for vitamins. Also, fat is important because it serves as an insulator. Because of these important roles, fat is often subdivided into two compartments—storage fat and essential fat.

The **essential** fat necessary to sustain life in the theoretical reference male (ht = 174 cm or 68.5 in.; 70 kg or 154 lb) represents about 2 % to 5 % of total body mass[40] and that of the reference female (ht = 163.8 cm or 64.5 in.; 57 kg or 125 lb) up to 12 % of total body mass (Table 25.1).[8,40] Essential fat may be stored in the bone marrow, heart, intestines, kidneys, liver, spleen, central nervous system (myelination), muscles, and other organs and tissues. In women, an additional, gender-related site for essential fat is the breast area and possibly the pelvis, buttocks, and thighs.[40]

Storage fat is stored subcutaneously between the skin and muscles; it is also between muscles (intermuscularly) and surrounding various organs. The subcutaneous fat represents about half of the fat in the body of a young adult,[44] whereas the other half is internalized. In older adults the visceral (internal) fat becomes proportionally greater.[40]

Regression equations for predicting percent body fat and/or body density are based upon correlations between anthropometric measures (e.g., skinfolds) and hydrostatic measures of body density. Numerous skinfold sites may be measured originally, with the combination of sites best pre-

Table 25.1	**Body Composition of the Reference Man and Woman, 20 y to 30 y of Age**					
	Reference Man[a]			Reference Woman[a]		
	kg	lb	%[b]	kg	lb	%[b]
Total fat wt	11	23	15	16	35	27
Essential fat	2	5	3	7	15	12
Stored fat	9	19	12	9	20	15
Total lean mass	59	131	85	41	91	73
Muscle	31	69	45	20	45	36
Bone	10	23	15	7	15	12
Remainder	18	39	25	14	31	25
Total body mass	70	154	100	57	126	100

Source: Data from Behnke, A. R., & Wilmore, J. H. (1974). *Evaluation and regulation of body build and composition.* Englewood Cliffs, NJ: Prentice-Hall. *Note:* [a]Rounded values. [b]Percent of total body mass.

dicting body density and/or body fat being chosen for the regression equation. In some cases, the regression equation is transformed into a table or nomogram based upon two or more skinfolds (or their sum), which is then used to find the corresponding percent body fat.

Methods of AAHPERD and Jackson-Pollack

A detailed description of skinfold techniques is found in Chapter 5 of *Anthropometric Standardization Reference Manual.*[25] The technique of measuring skinfolds accurately requires practice—the technician must learn to sense (feel) the participant's subcutaneous fold. This feel, however, is not consistent in participants or from one site to another in the same participant. Thus, the ease with which the skinfold, or fatfold, can be separated from the underlying muscle varies between persons and at different sites within the same person. There are also variations in the compressibility of the skin or adipose tissue, which may affect the feel and the measurement. For example, the skinfold is more likely to change its dimension while being grasped in younger persons due to their greater tissue hydration.[25] A description of the accuracy of predicting percent body fat from skinfold dimensions is presented in Box 25.1.

Equipment

The caliper is the basic instrument for skinfold measurements. It simplifies and improves the crude use of a ruler to

BOX 25.1 Accuracy of the Skinfold-Prediction of Body Fat

Of the more than 100 equations for the prediction of body density from anthropometric data (with subsequent conversion to percent body fat), the ones from skinfold measurements are considered the most accurate.[30] The relationship between body density and skinfold fat is nonlinear. Thus, when using a linear equation, accurate predictions would be made for those in the middle values but not at the extremes where the obese person would be underestimated and the lean person overestimated. On the other hand, quadratic equations eliminate this bias.[30]

Validity

Correlation coefficients between skinfolds and hydrostatically determined body fatness have consistently ranged from .70 to .90.[1,4] In general, the inclusion of three skinfold sites in the regression equation produces a better prediction (lower standard error of estimate; *SEE*) of body density than fewer sites. However, neither the feasibility nor accuracy is improved by using more than three sites.[43] The standard error of the estimate for skinfold prediction of hydrodensitometrically determined body fat is about 3.5 % body fat units with the acceptable *SEE* of 1 % to 1.5 % probably impossible to attain via skinfold methods.[9,28,31,48,53] For example, using the sum of three skinfolds, described as the J-P Method in this chapter, resulted in an *SEE* of 2.7 % fat in young adult men.[51] The skinfold *SEE* should be added to the error of hydrodensitometry, making the error of determining true body fat from skinfolds about 4.6 %.[17] The sum of the skinfolds itself may be a more valid indicator of adiposity and better for progressive monitoring of fatness than the prediction of percent fat derived from the skinfolds. The J-P researchers used Lange® calipers, which reportedly overestimate measures from Harpenden® calipers.[24,37] This leads to an underestimation of 1 % to 2 % body fat relative to J-P estimations.[24] Consequently, one group of reviewers recommends that the sum of Harpenden® skinfolds be adjusted upward by multiplying them by 1.10 to account for the 10 % difference.[42]

Reliability

The reliability of skinfold measurements is high. The test-retest correlation was .96 in 28 persons after a one-day waiting period.[a] This is consistent with test-retest reliabilities (*r* = .94 – .98) of other researchers.[10,33]

As with girth estimations, skinfold predictions of body fat are not without controversy. One investigator said that using skinfolds to predict body fat mass "is like trying to find the weight of the peel of an orange by measuring the thickness of the peel, but ignoring the size of the orange."[19] Nevertheless, for the determination of desirable weights, it is logical to conclude that skinfolds are superior to the stature-weight-age tables, girths, and diameters.

[a]Adams, G. M. (1970). Unpublished raw data.

---

measure the pinch of skinfold held by the technician's fingers. Thus, calipers apply a standard pinch pressure and provide an easily read measure of the width (mm) of the pinch. High-quality calipers, such as the Harpenden®, Holtain®, Lafayette®, and Lange®, have scales that can be read within a range of 0.2 mm and 1.0 mm. Lesser-quality calipers, such as McGaw®, Ross®, Fat-O-Meter®, and Slim-Guide®, can usually be read to the nearest 2 mm.[26] These cheaper calipers are apparently acceptable for nonresearch purposes.[37] Descriptions of several calipers are in various sources.[14,41] Comments on the calibration of calipers are in Box 25.2.

A tape measure is used to locate the precise site of some skinfolds (e.g., triceps). It is best to use a metric tape because the midpoint of any measure is often simpler to find using a metric dimension than an inches dimension (e.g., the halfway point of 13.75 in. vs. 34.2 cm). A felt marker (or body marker) or ballpoint pen marks the site of the skinfolds on the participant.

Participant Preparation

Participants should wear loose-fitting shirts and shorts. The males are encouraged to go shirtless, while the females are encouraged to wear a bathing-suit top. Leotards should not be worn. The participant should not be overheated while being measured, due to the increased fluid volume in the skinfold from cutaneous capillary blood flow. On the other hand, the skinfold will be reduced up to 15 % if the participant is hypohydrated.[11]

General Procedures for Measuring Skinfolds

Position of Participant

The participant stands while all skinfold sites are measured. However, the technician measures the calf skinfold at either the sitting or standing position. Although some authorities state that there is little practical difference as to which side of the body to use for girth measures,[39] it appears that most skinfold equations, including those in this manual, are based on right-side measurements. The description of the skinfold sites corresponds mainly with those methods described by AAHPERD,[1,2] Jackson and Pollock (J-P),[29,32] and the *Anthropometric Standardization Reference Manual*.[25,38]

Skinfold Technique

The caliper should be handled very carefully; use the wrist strap, if one is present. While holding it in the right hand, the technician uses the thumb and index finger of the left hand to pinch the skinfold at a distance of about 1 cm above the skinfold site (or mark). This fold represents two layers of skin and fat. The long axis of the fold is a natural, smooth, and untwisted fold. This may be referred to as the natural cleavage of the skin. The axis direction of the cleavage may be different in obese persons than in those of normal weight.

The points of the caliper should be placed perpendicular across the long axis of the skinfold at the designated skinfold site (mark). The 1 cm separation between the technician's fingers and the caliper should prevent the skinfold dimension from being affected by the pressure of the fingers. The depth of caliper placement is about half the distance between the base of the normal skin perimeter and the crest (top) of the skinfold.

Because of the compressibility of the skinfold,[7] the jaws of the caliper should not press longer than 4 s at the skinfold site so they do not force fluid from the tissues and reduce the measurement.[34,44] However, the technician should wait 1 s to 2 s before reading the gauge.[4] Technicians should be consistent in the timing of the reading, not relying on the end of the rapid decrease in the measurement.[25] For example, all technicians should agree that they will record the reading observed at the third or fourth second. While still holding the skinfold, the technician reads the gauge (dial) of the skinfold caliper to the closest 0.5 mm or 1 mm (e.g., Lange® caliper) to 0.1 mm or 0.2 mm (e.g., Harpenden® caliper), depending on what type of caliper is used.

Number of Measurements

Although many technicians repeat two or three measurements at one site before moving onto another skinfold site, some make a complete circuit of the measurement sites, then repeat the circuit. In the case of the AAHPERD skinfold test, this would mean that one of the skinfolds (e.g., triceps) would be measured once and not repeated until the other skinfold (e.g., subscapular) is measured. The measurements should be repeated three times (three circuits) or more if the skinfold thicknesses differ by more than 10 %[55] or 2 mm.[4] If making consecutive measurements at the same site, the technician should give enough time to allow the skin to return to normal texture and thickness.[4] Either the median (middle) or mean value of the two or three trials is used for evaluation, depending on the instructions for the different skinfold equations. There is no need for a third measurement if the first two are the same for equations using median values.

Summary of General Procedures

1. The technician marks the sites to be measured on the right side of the participant's body.
2. The technician pinches the skinfold, at about 1 cm proximal to the marked site, using the thumb and index finger.
3. The jaw points of the caliper are placed on the marked site at a depth of about half the distance between the base of the normal skin perimeter and the crest of the fold.
4. The technician maintains a firm grip on the skinfold while reading the gauge of the skinfold caliper within 4 s to the closest 0.5 mm to 1 mm (e.g., Lange®) or closest 0.1 mm to 0.2 mm (e.g., Harpenden®).
5. The technician makes three circuits of skinfold measurements and records for each site during each circuit.
6. The technician uses the median value for analytical purposes.

Specific Procedures for the AAHPERD and the J-P Methods

Two popular methods of predicting percent fat from skinfold measurements are those using the tables provided by the American Alliance for Health, Physical Education, Recreation and Dance (AAHPERD) and those using the Jackson and Pollock (J-P) multiple-skinfold equations or nomogram[6] for a generalized population of men[29] and women.[32]

AAHPERD Skinfold Measurements

The AAHPERD method derives percent fat from the sum of only two skinfolds—the triceps and subscapular. The calf measurement was substituted later for the subscapular site in younger students partly to circumvent the sensitive situation of lifting the shirt of the participant.[3] The calf value is added to the triceps skinfold, and this sum is compared with accepted standards for students under college age.[3] The procedures for measuring triceps, subscapular, and calf skinfolds are as follows:

Triceps (Figure 25.1a)

1. The participant bends the right arm at a right angle, keeping the elbow close to the side.
2. The technician, standing behind the participant, places the start of the measuring tape at the top lateral portion of the shoulder (acromion process of the scapula) and runs it down the arms (straightest line possible) to the tip of the bent elbow (the olecrenon process of the ulna).
3. The technician marks the arm at the midpoint between the acromion and olecrenon, extending the mark to the most posterior point on the arm.
4. The participant allows the arm to fall to a hanging position.
5. With the thumb and index finger pointed downward, the technician grasps a vertical skinfold at the back of the arm, 1 cm above the mark.
6. The technician applies the points of the caliper to the back of the arm at the marked level.
7. The median value of the three measurements is recorded onto Form 25.1 (males) or 25.2 (females).
8. This value is added to the subscapular value in order to obtain percent fat from Table 25.2 (men) or 25.3 (women).

Subscapular (Figure 25.1b)

1. The technician locates by inspection or palpation the inferior angle of the scapula (lowest point). It helps if the participant places the arm behind the back in an armlock position.
2. The technician marks the skin of the participant just inferior (about 1 cm; 0.5 in.) to the lower tip of the scapula.
3. The technician grasps the skinfold on a diagonal (about 45°) plane directed from the upper medial position to the lower lateral position. This typically follows the natural cleavage of the skin.

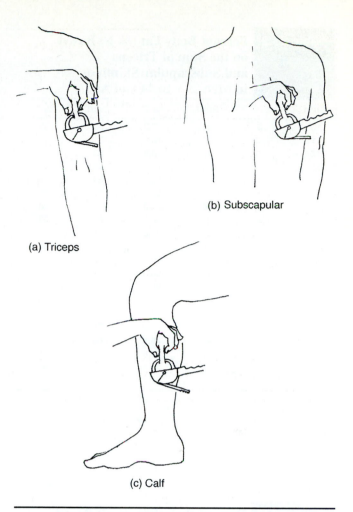

(a) Triceps

(b) Subscapular

(c) Calf

Figure 25.1 The skinfold sites for the AAHPERD method. The sites for college-age population are (a) triceps and (b) subscapular; for students younger than college age: (a) triceps and (c) calf.

4. The technician applies the jaw points of the caliper at the mark about 1 cm distal from the grasp.
5. The median value of the three measurements is recorded onto Form 25.1 (males) or 25.2 (females).
6. To estimate percent body fat for the college-age population, first sum the median values of the triceps and subscapular skinfolds.
7. Second, refer the sum to Table 25.2 (men) or 25.3 (women) for the associated percent body fat. For example, a man with a sum of skinfolds equal to 26 mm has 14 % fat; a woman with a sum of 24 mm has 23 % fat.

Calf (Figure 25.1c) (Not Necessary for Ages 18 y to 35 y)

1. The participant sits or stands with the right knee bent about 90° and the right foot resting comfortably at a right angle. If the participant is standing, the right foot rests upon a bench or the seat of a chair.
2. The technician marks the caliper site at the level of the medial side of the maximum calf circumference.

Table 25.2 Percent Body Fat (% F) Based on the Sum of Triceps and Subscapular Skinfolds in Men 20 y to 44 y of Age

Sum	% F	Sum	% F	Sum	% F
10	2	30	17.3	50	33
11	2	31	18.1	51	34
12	3	32	18.9	52	35
13	4	33	19.6	53	35
14	5	34	20.4	54	36
15	6	35	21.2	55	37
16	6	36	22.0	56	38
17	7	37	22.8	57	38
18	8	38	23.6	58	39
19	9	39	24.3	59	40
20	9	40	25.1	60	41
21	10	41	25.9	61	42
22	11	42	26.7	62	42
23	12	43	27.5	63	43
24	13	44	28.3	64	44
25	13	45	29.0	65	45
26	14	46	29.8	66	45
27	15	47	30.6	67	46
28	16	48	31.4	68	47
29	17	49	32.2	69	48

Sources: Slaughter, M. H., Lohman, T. G., Boileau, R. A., Horswill, C. A., Stillman, R. J., Van Loan, M. D., & Bemben, D. A. (1988). Skinfold equations for estimation of body fatness in children and youth. *Human Biology, 60,* 709–723.
Note: % F = (0.783 Sum) – 6.2.

Table 25.3 Percent Body Fat (% F) Based on the Sum of Triceps and Subscapular Skinfolds in Woman 20 y to 44 y of Age

Sum	% F	Sum	% F	Sum	% F
10	15	30	26	50	37
11	16	31	27	51	38
12	16	32	27	52	38
13	17	33	28	53	39
14	17	34	28	54	39
15	18	35	29	55	40
16	18	36	29	56	40
17	19	37	30	57	41
18	20	38	31	58	42
19	20	39	31	59	42
20	21	40	32	60	43
21	21	41	32	61	43
22	22	42	33	62	44
23	22	43	33	63	44
24	23	44	34	64	45
25	23	45	34	65	45
26	24	46	35	66	46
27	25	47	36	67	46
28	25	48	36	68	47
29	26	49	37	69	48

Sources: Slaughter, M. H., Lohman, T. G., Boileau, R. A., Horswill, C. A., Stillman, R. J., Van Loan, M. D., & Bemben, D. A. (1988). Skinfold equations for estimation of body fatness in children and youth. *Human Biology, 60,* 709–723.
Note: % F = (0.549 Sum) + 9.7.

3. The technician grasps the fold parallel to the long axis of the calf on its medial aspect.
4. The technician applies the jaw points of the caliper at the mark about 1 cm distal from the grasp.
5. The technician records the median value of the three measurements onto Form 25.1 or 25.2.
6. The technician sums the median values for the tricep and calf skinfolds.
7. The technician refers the sum to the AAHPERD Standard box[3] presented in the "Results" section of this chapter.

J-P Skinfold Measurements

The Jackson/Pollock (J-P) Method utilizes a nomogram, equations, or tables in order to determine the percent body fat from the sum of *three* skinfolds for each gender. The three sites for the men are (1) thigh, (2) chest, and (3) abdomen, whereas those for women are (1) thigh, (2) triceps, and (3) suprailium.

Thigh (Male and Female) (Figure 25.2a)

1. The participant flexes the right hip in order to help the technician visualize the location of the inguinal crease at the junction of the hip and the right leg.
2. The technician places the top of the measuring tape at the anterior groin area of the hip (the midpoint of the inguinal ligament, which is halfway between the anterior superior iliac spine and the symphysis pubis).
3. The technician extends the tape to the top (proximal or superior) border of the patella.
4. The technician marks the midpoint on the anterior-most aspect of the thigh.
5. The participant relaxes the thigh muscles of the right leg by standing mainly on the left leg.
6. The technician grasps a vertical skinfold about 1 cm above the mark and then places the caliper's jaw points perpendicularly across the axis of the skinfold at the mark.
7. The technician records the median value of three measurements onto Form 25.1 (males) or 25.2 (females).

Chest (Male) (Figure 25.2b)

1. After visual inspection, the technician makes a mark at half the distance from the anterior axillary fold (the front of the armpit) to the nipple of the participant.
2. The technician grasps the chest skinfold about 1 cm diagonally above the mark—that is, with the long axis of the fold towards the nipple.
3. The technician applies the caliper's jaw points across the fold 1 cm inferior to the grasp.
4. The technician records the median value of the three chest measurements onto Form 25.1 (males).

Abdomen (Male) (Figure 25.2c)

1. The technician marks the site about 2 cm (slightly less than 1 in.) to the right of the umbilicus. (A tape measure is not always necessary for experienced technicians.)

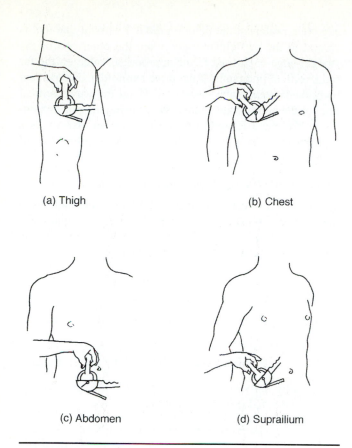

(a) Thigh

(b) Chest

(c) Abdomen

(d) Suprailium

Figure 25.2 Skinfold sites for the J-P Method. Men: (a) thigh, (b) chest, and (c) abdomen. Women: (a) thigh, (d) supraillium and triceps.

2. The technician grasps a vertical skinfold at a point about 1 cm above the marked site.[a]
3. The technician places the points of the caliper at the marked site across the long axis of the skinfold.
4. The technician records the median value onto Form 25.1.

Triceps (Female) (Figure 25.1a)

The technician follows the same procedures as for the AAHPERD method.

Suprailium (Female) (Figure 25.2d)

1. The technician marks the site just above the right iliac crest of the ilium in the anterior axillary line.[b]
2. The technician grasps the skinfold posterior and superior to the marked site; the natural cleavage of the skinfold normally runs diagonally from the crest toward the umbilicus.
3. The technician places the points of the caliper across the long axis of the typically diagonal fold.

---

[a]Some recommend taking horizontal fold, 3 cm to right, and 1 cm inferior, to the center of the umbilicus.[25]

[b]Some recommend taking the measurement 3 cm above the crest[22] or at the midaxillary line.[25]

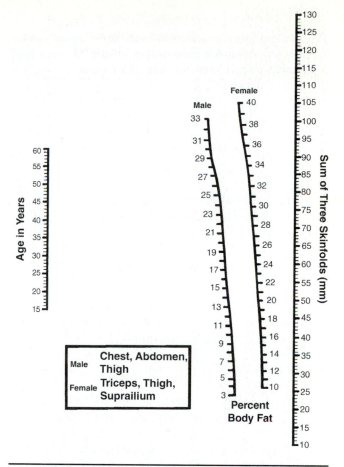

Figure 25.3 The J-P nomogram for the estimate of percent body fat. From W. B. Baun et al., "A nomogram for the estimate of percent body fat from generalized equations," from *Research Quarterly for Exercise and Sport, 52,* 380–384. Permission of Tenneco Health & Fitness Dept., PO Box 2511, Houston, TX 77001; and Copyright © 1981, AAHPERD.

4. The technician records the median value onto Form 25.2.
5. The technician uses any of the following three procedures to derive the percent body fat from the three skinfolds of the J-P Method:
   a. Sum the three skinfolds; then insert the sum into the equations for men and women. Because the skinfolds from Lange® calipers, which J-P investigators used, are about 10 % greater than those from Harpenden® calipers, the 10 % difference in the sum should be added if using Harpenden® calipers.[42]
   b. Refer the sum to a special nomogram[6] derived from the equations (Figure 25.3).
   c. Use tables that are available for the J-P Method but are not presented in this manual.[18,21,30,44,56] You can generate your own tables by inserting the equations into a computer software program (e.g., Microsoft Excel™).

The J-P Equation for Predicting % Fat

The J-P nomogram was derived from the following gender-specific regression equations (Eq. 25.1 and 25.2) for body density (D_b) in combination with the equation (Eq. 25.3) for percent body fat.[49]

Male:

$$D_b = 1.1093800 - 0.0008267\ SSF + 0.0000016\ SSF^2 - 0.0002574\ Age \qquad \text{Eq. 25.1}$$

Female:

$$D_b = 1.0994921 - 0.0009929\ SSF + 0.0000023\ SSF^2 - 0.0001392\ Age \qquad \text{Eq. 25.2}$$

where:

D_b = body density in $g \cdot mL^{-1}$

SSF (male) = sum of chest, abdomen, and thigh skinfolds (mm)

SSF (female) = sum of triceps, thigh, and suprailium (mm)

$$\%\ \text{Body Fat} = \left[\frac{495}{D_b}\right] - 450 \qquad \text{Eq. 25.3}$$

The modified Siri equation eliminates the need to multiply by 100. Obviously, the calculations can be quite cumbersome when done without the aid of a computer.[5] Nevertheless, the solutions are obtained, somewhat tediously (about 5 min), using a pocket calculator. For example, if a 48-year-old man's skinfold sum is 43 mm, then the following calculations reveal his percent body fat as 15 %, the same answer obtained from the nomogram.

$$D_b = 1.1093800 - (0.0008267 \times 43) + (0.0000016 \times 43^2) - (0.0002574 \times 48)$$

$$= 1.1093800 - 0.0355481 + (0.0000016 \times 1849) - 0.0123552$$

$$= 1.0738319 + 0.0029584 - 0.0123552$$

$$= 1.064 \ \text{(rounded off to nearest thousandths)}$$

$$\%\ \text{Fat} = \left[\frac{495}{1.064}\right] - 450$$

$$= 465 - 450$$

$$= 15\ \%$$

The higher body density of African Americans justifies a different percent-fat equation (Eq. 25.4).[15,46,52]

$$\%\ \text{Body Fat} = \left[\frac{437.4}{D_b}\right] - 392.8 \times 100 \qquad \text{Eq. 25.4}$$

The J-P Nomogram for Predicting % Fat

The nomogram in Figure 25.3 is nearly self-explanatory.[6] The percent body fat is determined by placing a straight-edge (e.g., ruler) at the point on the left vertical line that is closest to the participant's age; then the other end of the straight-edge is pivoted to the appropriate value on the far right vertical line (sum of the three skinfolds). The percent body fat is read to the closest 0.5 % on the wavy vertical line for the appropriate gender. When using the same example as for the J-P equation, the nomogram also gives a value of 15 % for a 48-year-old man with a skinfold sum of 43 mm.

Resting Daily Energy Expenditure (RDEE)

An approximate estimate of the RDEE may be made from the fat-free mass (FFM) by a simple regression equation.[16] First, the fat mass is obtained by multiplying the total body mass (TBM) by the percent fat (Eq. 25.5).

$$\text{FM (kg)} = \%\ F \times \text{TBM (kg)} \qquad \text{Eq. 25.5}$$

The fat-free mass (FFM) is calculated by subtracting the fat mass (FM) from the total body mass (TBM), as in Equation 25.6.

$$\text{FFM (kg)} = \text{TBM} - \text{FM} \qquad \text{Eq. 25.6}$$

The resting daily energy expenditure (RDEE) in kilocalories is calculated from Equation 25.7.

$$\text{RDEE (kcal)} = 370 + (21.6 \times \text{FFM}) \qquad \text{Eq. 25.7}$$

For example, if a man's body mass is 70 kg and body fat percentage is 15 %, then his RDEE is estimated as 1655 kcal, or 6919 kJ, according to the following calculations:

$$\text{FM (kg)} = 0.15 \times 70\ \text{kg}$$

$$= 10.5\ \text{kg}$$

$$\text{FFM (kg)} = 70\ \text{kg} - 10.5\ \text{kg}$$

$$= 59.5\ \text{kg}$$

$$\text{RDEE (kcal)} = 370 + (21.6 \times 59.5)$$

$$= 370 + 1285$$

$$= 1655\ \text{kcal}$$

$$\text{RDEE (kJ)} = 1655\ \text{kcal} \times 4.18$$

$$= 6919\ \text{kJ}$$

Results and Discussion

Fat varies from 1 % to 2 % of body mass in a severely starved person to 50 % in a clinically normal, but obese, person.[49] The lowest acceptable percent fat in adult men is about 3 % to 5 %—that is, the amount of essential fat in bone marrow, central nervous system, and internal organs. The lower limit for adult women is about 8 % to 12 % and includes the same amount of essential fat as in the men, but, additionally, the amount of sex-specific fat, such as that in the breasts.

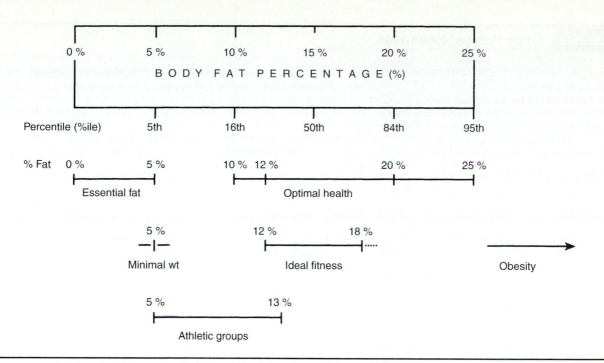

Figure 25.4 Criteria for various categories of percent fat and percentiles in men. Source: Courtesy of Dr. Timothy Lohman.

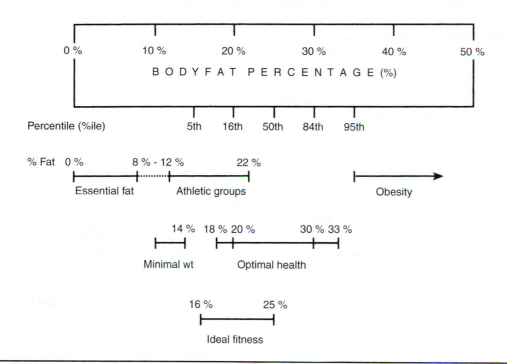

Figure 25.5 Criteria for various categories of percent fat and percentiles for women. Source: Courtesy of Dr. Timothy Lohman.

AAHPERD Interpretation

AAHPERD standards for younger students (under 19 y) simply use the sum (mm) of skinfolds (triceps + calf).[3]

AAHPERD Health Fitness Standards (Ages 5 y to 18 y)	
Boys: 12 mm to 25 mm	Girls: 16 mm to 36 mm

Although various criteria for fatness and leanness are presented in *Exercise Physiology Laboratory Manual,* the criteria presented also in Figures 25.4 and 25.5 emphasize the importance of using ranges, rather than one specific value, for the criteria.[35] The figures should not be interpreted rigidly because not all authorities would have the same criteria. For example, Figure 25.5 shows that a woman with 16 % body fat would be categorized as

Because the AAHPERD and J-P procedures apply mainly to college-age persons and those less than 60 y of age, respectively, the "older adult" equations and procedures are more suitable for persons older than 60 y of age and, perhaps, as young as 35 y.[54,55] These men's and women's equations are derived from a three-component model (fat and two fat-free body components—water and bone) that enhances their validity (*SEE* = 2.9 % and 3.8 % for men and women, respectively) compared with the AAHPERD and J-P two-component models (fat and fat-free weight).

The fourth skinfold for the men is taken vertically at the midaxillary site at the level of the xiphoid-sternal junction.[25] The regression equation for the prediction of percent fat from body density, body water, and bone (PFDWB) of men is presented as Equation 25.8.[54]

Men: (*M* age = 60 y; *SEE* = 2.9 %) $PFDWB = (0.486 \times Sum\ 4\ SF) - (0.0015 \times Sum\ 4\ SF^2) + (0.067 \times Age) - 3.83$ Eq. 25.8

where:

Sum of 4 SF (mm) = Chest + Subscapular + Midaxillary + Thigh; PF = percent fat; D = body density; W = body water; B = bone

For women, an additional skinfold to the AAHPERD's subscapular, triceps, and calf is the abdomen site. Equation 25.9[54] presents the regression for the prediction of percent fat from density of water and bone (PFDWB).

Women:[54] (*M* age = 58 y; *SEE* = 3.8 %) $PFDWB = (0.428 \times Sum\ 4\ SF) - (0.0011 \times Sum\ 4\ SF^2) + (0.127 \times Age) - 3.01$ Eq. 25.9

"ideal," whereas other investigators[40] would suggest that any woman under 17 % fat meets one of the criteria for being classified as "underweight." Also, caution is advised when using only one skinfold as an indicator of obesity.[41] For example, triceps skinfolds of 20 mm and 29 mm are obesity criteria for 25-year-old men and women, respectively,[47] but these criteria might unfairly categorize those persons with a greater tendency to deposit fat in the triceps area. The greater percent body fat in women for any given sum of skinfolds is attributed presumably to a smaller lean body mass and more essential fat.

J-P Interpretation

The J-P generalized method of predicting body density for adult men was based on the data from more than 300 men between the ages of 18 y and 61 y (*M* = 33 y) and who ranged from 1 % to 33 % fat (*M* = 18 %).[29] The J-P Method for women was based on about 250 women between the ages of 18 y and 55 y (*M* = 31 y) and who ranged from 4 % to 44 % fat (*M* = 24 %).[32]

The J-P nomogram illustrates the fact that age is an independent factor in body composition. Thus, the same skinfold total in an old person and a young adult would predict a higher fat percentage in the older person. Aging is associated with an increase in internal (besides subcutaneous) fat and a decrease in bone density. Unless age is factored into the equation an underestimation of percent fat with skinfolds will occur in the older person.[12] Box 25.3 includes age modifications of prior procedures and equations.

References

1. American Alliance for Health, Physical Education, Recreation and Dance (AAHPERD). (1980). *AAHPERD health-related physical fitness test.* Reston, VA: Author.

2. American Alliance for Health, Physical Education, Recreation and Dance (AAHPERD). (1985). *Norms for college students.* Reston, VA: Author.

3. American Alliance for Health, Physical Education, Recreation and Dance (AAHPERD). (1988). *Physical best.* Reston, VA: Author.

4. American College of Sports Medicine. (2000). *ACSM's guidelines for exercise testing and prescription* (pp. 60–66). Philadelphia: Lippincott Williams & Wilkins.

5. Baumgartner, T. A., & Jackson, A. S. (1987). *Measurement for evaluation in physical education and exercise science.* Dubuque, IA: Wm. C. Brown.

6. Baun, W. B., Baun, M. R., & Raven P. B. (1981). A nomogram for the estimate of percent body fat from generalized equations. *Research Quarterly for Exercise and Sport, 52,* 380–384.

7. Becque, B. D., Katch, V. L., & Moffatt, K. J. (1986). Time course of skin-plus-fat compression in males and females. *Human Biology, 58,* 33–42.

8. Behnke, A. R., & Wilmore, J. H. (1974). *Evaluation and regulation of body build and composition.* Englewood Cliffs, NJ: Prentice-Hall.

9. Bouchard, C. (1985). General discussion of sports medicine. In A. F. Roche (Ed.), *Body-composition assessments in youth and adults* (p. 95). Columbus, OH: Ross Laboratories.

10. Bouchard, C. (1985). Reproducibility of body-composition and adipose-tissue measurements in humans. In A. F. Roche (Ed.), *Body-composition assessments in youth and adults* (pp. 9–13). Columbus, OH: Ross Laboratories.

11. Brooks, G. A., Fahey, T. D., & White, T. P. (1996). *Exercise physiology: Human bioenergetics and its application.* Mountain View, CA: Mayfield.

12. Bunt, J. C., Lohman, T. G., Slaughter, M. H., Boileau, R. A., Lussier, L., & Van Loan, M. (1983). Bone mineral content as a source of variation in body density in children and youth. *Medicine and Science in Sports and Exercise, 15* (Abstract), 172.

13. Carlyon, R., Bryant, R., Gore, C., & Walker, R. (1998). Apparatus for precision calibration of skinfold calipers. *American Journal of Human Biology, 10,* 689–697.

14. Cataldo, D., & Heyward, V. H. (2000). Pinch an inch: A comparison of several high-quality and plastic skinfold calipers. *ACSM's Health and Fitness Journal, 4*(3), 12–16.

15. Clark, R. R., Kuta, J. M., & Sullivan, J. C. (1994). Cross-validation of methods to predict body fat in African-American and Caucasian collegiate football players. *Research Quarterly for Exercise and Sport, 65,* 21–30.

16. Cunningham, J. J. (1982). Body composition and resting metabolic rate: The myth of feminine metabolism. *American Journal of Clinical Nutrition, 36,* 721.

17. Cureton, K. J. (1984). A reaction to the manuscript of Jackson. *Medicine and Science in Sports and Exercise, 16,* 621–622.

18. deVries, H. A., & Housh, T. J. (1994). *Physiology of exercise for physical education and athletics.* Dubuque, IA: Wm. C. Brown.

19. Dugdale, A. E., & Griffiths, M. (1979). Estimating fat body mass from anthropometric data. *American Journal of Clinical Nutrition, 32,* 2400–2403.

20. Edwards, D. A. W., Hammond, W. H., Healy, M. J. R., Tanner, J. M., & Whitehouse, R. H. (1955). Design and accuracy of calipers for measuring subcutaneous tissue thickness. *British Journal of Nutrition, 9,* 133–143.

21. Fahey, T. D., Insel, P. M., & Roth, W. T. (1994). *Fit and well.* Mountain View, CA: Mayfield.

22. Fitness and Amateur Sport Canada. (1987). *Canadian Standardized Test of Fitness (CSTF) operations manual.* Ottawa, Ontario, Canada: Author.

23. Gore, C. J., Carlyon, R. G., Franks, S. W., & Woolford, S. M. (2000). Skinfold thickness varies directly with spring coefficient and inversely with jaw pressure. *Medicine and Science in Sports and Exercise, 32,* 540–546.

24. Gruber, J. J., Pollock, M. L., Graves, J. E., Colvin, A. B., & Braith, R. W. (1990). Comparison of Harpenden and Lange calipers in predicting body composition. *Research Quarterly for Exercise and Sport, 61,* 184–190.

25. Harrison, G. G., Buskirk, E. R., Carter, J. E. L., Johnston, F. E., Lohman, T. G., Pollock, M. L., Roche, A. F., & Wilmore, J. H. (1988). Skinfold thicknesses and measurement technique. In T. G. Lohman, A. F. Roche, & R. Martorell (Eds.), *Anthropometric standardization reference manual* (pp. 55–70). Champaign, IL: Human Kinetics.

26. Heyward, V. H. (1991). *Advanced fitness assessment and exercise prescription.* Champaign, IL: Human Kinetics.

27. Ishida, Y., Kanehisa, H., Carroll, J. F., Pollock, M. L., Graves, J. E., & Leggett, S. H. (1995). Body fat and muscle thickness distributions in untrained young females. *Medicine and Science in Sports and Exercise, 27,* 270–274.

28. Israel, R. G., Houmard, J. A., O'Brien, K. F., McCammon, M. R., Zamora, B. S., & Eaton, A. W. (1989). Validity of a near-infrared spectrophotometry device for estimating human body composition. *Research Quarterly for Exercise and Sport, 60,* 379–383.

29. Jackson, A. S., & Pollock, M. L. (1978). Generalized equations for predicting body density of men. *British Journal of Nutrition, 40,* 497–504.

30. Jackson, A. S., & Pollock, M. L. (1985). Practical assessment of body composition. *The Physician and Sportsmedicine, 13*(5), 76–80, 82–90.

31. Jackson, A. S., Pollock, M. L., Graves, J. E., & Mahar, M. T. (1988). Reliability and validity of bioelectrical impedance in determining body composition. *Journal of Applied Physiology, 64,* 529–534.

32. Jackson, A. S., Pollock, M. L., & Ward, A. (1980). Generalized equations for predicting body density of women. *Medicine and Science in Sports and Exercise, 12,* 175–182.

33. Kolkhorst, F. W., & Dolgener, F. A. (1994). Nonexercise model fails to predict aerobic capacity in college students with high VO_2 peak. *Research Quarterly for Exercise and Sport, 65,* 78–83.

34. Lohman, T. G. (1987). *Measuring body fat using skinfolds* [Video]. Champaign, IL: Human Kinetics.

35. Lohman, T. G. (1989, June). *Tutorial on body composition.* Presented at ACSM Convention, Baltimore.

36. Lohman, T. G., Houtkooper, L., & Going, S. B. (1997). Body fat measurement goes high-tech. *ACSM's Health and Fitness Journal, 1*(1), 30–35.

37. Lohman, T. G., Pollock, M. L., Slaughter, M. H., Brandon, L. J., & Boileau, R. A. (1984). Methodological factors and the predicting of body fat in female athletes. *Medicine and Science in Sports and Exercise, 16,* 92–96.

38. Lohman, T. G., Roche, A. F., & Martorell, R. (Eds.). (1988). *Anthropometric standardization reference manual.* Champaign, IL: Human Kinetics.

39. Martorell, R., Mendoza, F., Mueller, W. H., & Pawson, I. G. (1988). Which side to measure: Right or left? In A. F. Roche (Ed.), *Body-composition assessments in youth and adults* (pp. 73–78). Columbus, OH: Ross Laboratories.

40. McArdle, W. D., Katch, F. I., & Katch, V. L. (1996). *Exercise physiology: Energy, nutrition, and human performance.* (4th ed.). Baltimore: Williams & Wilkins.

41. Nieman, D. C. (1999). *Exercise testing and prescription: A health-related approach.* Mountain View, CA: Mayfield.

42. Pollock, M. L., Garzarella, L., & Graves, J. E. (1995). The measurement of body composition. In P. J. Maud & Carl Foster (Eds.), *Physiological assessment of human fitness* (pp. 167–204). Champaign, IL: Human Kinetics.

43. Pollock, M. L., & Jackson, A. S. (1984). Research progress in validation of clinical methods of assessing body composition. *Medicine and Science in Sports and Exercise, 16,* 606–613.

44. Pollock, M. L., Schmidt, D. H., & Jackson, A. S. (1980). Measurement of cardiorespiratory fitness and body composition in the clinical setting. *Comprehensive Therapy, 6,* 12–27.

45. Schmidt, P. K., & Carter, J. E. L. (1990). Static and dynamic differences among five types of skinfold calipers. *Human Biology, 62,* 369–388.

46. Schutte, J. E., Townsend, E. J., Hugg, H., Schoup, R. F., Malina, R. M., & Bloomquist, C. G. (1984). Density of lean body mass is greater in blacks than in whites. *Journal of Applied Physiology, 56,* 1647–1649.

47. Selzer, C. C., & Mayer, J. (1965). A simple criterion of obesity. *Postgraduate Medicine, 38*(2), A-101.

48. Sinning, W. E., Dolny, D. G., Little, K. D., Cunningham, L. N., Racaniello, A., Siconolfi, S. F., & Sholes, J. L. (1985). Validity of "generalized" equations for body composition in male athletes. *Medicine and Science in Sports and Exercise, 17,* 124–130.

49. Siri, W. E. (1961). *Body composition from fluid spaces and density: Analysis of methods in techniques for measuring body composition.* Washington, DC: National Academy of Science, National Research Council.

50. Slaughter, M. H., Lohman, T. G., Boileau, R. A., Horswill, C. A., Stillman, R. J., Van Loan, M. D., & Bemben, D. A. (1988). Skinfold equations for estimation of body fatness in children and youth. *Human Biology, 60,* 709–723.

51. Stout, J. R., Eckerson, J. M., Housh, T. J., Johnson, G. O., & Betts, N. M. (1994). Validity of percent body fat estimations in males. *Medicine and Science in Sports and Exercise, 26,* 632–636.

52. Thorland, W. G., Johnson, G. O., & Housh, T. J. (1993). Estimation of body composition in black adolescent male athletes. *Pediatric Exercise Science, 5,* 116–124.

53. Thorland, W. G., Johnson, G. O., & Tharp, G. D (1984). Validity of anthropometric equations for the estimation of body density in adolescent athletes. *Medicine and Science in Sports and Exercise, 16,* 77–81.

54. Williams, D. P., Going, S. B., Lohman, T. G., Hewitt, M. J., & Haber, A. E. (1992). Estimation of body fat from skinfold thickness in middle-aged and older men and women: A multiple component approach. *American Journal of Human Biology, 4,* 595–605.

55. Williams, D. P., Going, S. B., Milliken, L. A., Hall, M. C., & Lohman, T. G. (1995). Practical techniques for assessing body composition in middle-aged and older adults. *Medicine and Science in Sports and Exercise, 27,* 776–783.

56. Wilmore, J. H., & Costill, D. L. (1988). *Training for sport and activity.* Dubuque, IA: Wm. C. Brown.

Form 25.1

Individual Data for Skinfolds—Males

Name [　　　　　　　　　　　　　] Date [　　　　　] Time [　　] A.M. [　] P.M. [　]

Age [　] y   Gender (M or W) [　]   Ht [　　　] cm   Wt [　　　] kg   Tech. Initials [　]

Meteorological Data

T [　] °C (closest 0.1 °C)   RH % [　] P_B [　] mm Hg × 1.333 = [　] hPa

Caliper Model [　　　　]   Body Mass [　　　] kg

Skinfolds (mm): Circle median value of each site.

SKINFOLD SITE	TRIAL #1	TRIAL #2	TRIAL #3
Triceps			
Subscapular			
Calf (< 19 y)			
Chest			
Abdomen			
Thigh			
Midaxillary (> 44 y)			

AAHPERD (Median Values)

≥ 19 y

Triceps [　　　] mm
+
Subscapular [　　　] mm

Sum [　　　] mm = [　　　] % Fat (Table 25.2)

5 y to 18 y Age

Triceps [　　　] mm
+
Calf [　　　] mm

Sum [　　　] mm

AAHPERD Standard for triceps + calf (12 mm to 25 mm) [　] Yes [　] No

J-P Nomogram (Median Values; mm)

Chest [　　] + Abdomen [　　] + Thigh [　　] = [　　] mm = [　　] % F (Fig. 25.3)

D_b = 1.1093800 − (0.0008267 × SSF [　] mm) + [0.0000016 × (SSF [　] mm)^2] − (0.0002574 × Age [　] y)

= 1.1093800 − [　　] mm + (0.0000016 × [　　] mm) − [　　] y
  　　　　(0.0008267 × SSF)　　　(SSF^2)　　(0.0002574 × Age)

= [　　] + [　　] − [　　] = [　　] g·mL^{-1} (rounded to closest fourth decimal place)

% Fat = (495/ [　　] g·mL^{-1}) − 450 = [　　] − 450 = [　　] % Fat = [　　] %ile (from Fig. 25.4)
　　　　　(D$_b$)　　　　　　　　(495/D$_b$)

Form 25.2

Individual Data for Skinfolds—Females

Name [   ] Date [   ] Time [   ] A.M. [   ] P.M. [   ]

Age [   ] y   Gender (M or W) [   ]   Ht [   ] cm   Wt [   ] kg   Tech. Initials [   ]

Meteorological Data

T [   ] °C (closest 0.1 °C)   RH % [   ] P_B [   ] mm Hg × 1.333 = [   ] hPa

Caliper Model [   ]   Body Mass [   ] kg

Skinfolds (mm): Circle median value of each site.

SKINFOLD SITE	TRIAL #1	TRIAL #2	TRIAL #3
Subscapular			
Calf (< 19 y)			
Triceps			
Thigh			
Suprailium			
Abdominal (> 44 y)			

AAHPERD (Median Values)

≥ 19 y

Triceps [   ] mm
+
Subscapular [   ] mm

Sum [   ] mm = [   ] % Fat (Table 25.3)

5 y to 18 y Age

Triceps [   ] mm
+
Calf [   ] mm

Sum [   ] mm

AAHPERD Standard for triceps + calf (16 mm to 36 mm) [   ] Yes [   ] No

J-P Nomogram (Median Values; mm)

Triceps [   ] + Thigh [   ] + Suprailium [   ] = [   ] mm = [   ] % F (Fig. 25.3)

D_b = 1.10994921 − (0.0009929 × SSF [   ] mm) + [0.0000023 × (SSF [   ] mm)^2] − (0.0001392 × Age [   ] y)

= 1.10994921 − [___] mm + (0.0000023 × [___] mm) − [___]
       (0.0009929 × SSF)   (SSF^2)   (0.0001392 × Age)

= [___] + [___] − [___] = [___] g·mL^{-1} (rounded to closest fourth decimal place)

% Fat = (495/ [___] g·mL^{-1}) − 450 [___] − 450 = [___] % Fat = [___] %ile (from Fig. 25.5)
        (D$_b$)   (495/D$_b$)

Form 25.3

Group Data for Skinfolds

MEN Initials (or ID#)	PERCENT FAT AAHPERD	J-P	OLDER (PFDWB)
1.			
2.			
3.			
4.			
5.			
6.			
7.			
8.			
9.			
10.			
11.			
12.			
13.			
14.			
15.			
16.			
17.			
18.			
19.			
20.			
M			
Range			

WOMEN Initials (or ID#)	PERCENT FAT AAHPERD	J-P	OLDER (PFDWB)
1.			
2.			
3.			
4.			
5.			
6.			
7.			
8.			
9.			
10.			
11.			
12.			
13.			
14.			
15.			
16.			
17.			
18.			
19.			
20.			
M			
Range			

HYDROSTATIC WEIGHING

H ydrostatic weighing is often referred to as underwater weighing because the participant's weight is measured while being submerged in water. Researchers also refer to it as hydrodensitometry because its unit of measure is body density in units of grams per milliliter $(g \cdot mL^{-1})$. A multicomponent model utilizing the combination of dual energy X-ray absorptiometry (DXA), isotope dilution, and hydrodensitometry "is now widely recognized as the 'gold standard' in body composition assessment,"[62] meaning that it is the criterion by which other methods are compared. Despite hydrostatic weighing's prominent position among tests of body composition, it can qualify as a simple field test under certain conditions. For example, hydrostatic weighings can be performed in any body of water, such as jacuzzis, swimming pools, or lakes. By indirectly predicting residual volume, rather than measuring it, the hydrostatic technique is greatly simplified. However, when residual volume is measured directly and the underwater weight is measured under controlled conditions, it truly is a laboratory test, not a field test.

Physical and Anatomical Rationales

The rationales for hydrostatic weighing are based on the interaction between physical and anatomical factors. For example, the buoyancy of the human body during hydrostatic weighing is affected by its anatomical compartments, some being more buoyant or less dense than others.

Fat can be disadvantageous, both mechanically and aesthetically, because its density—that is, weight (mass) for any given volume—is lower than lean tissue. Thus, 1 g of fat occupies more space than 1 g of protein (Figure 26.1). This means that different gains in circumference occur even if identical weight gains are from fat storage or from protein growth (e.g., muscle hypertrophy). Thus, if two people of identical stature and body mass were of different body compositions, the leaner person would occupy less space than the fatter person.

Physical Rationale

Specifically, hydrostatic weighing is a method to determine the density of the body. Once the density of the body is known, equations can be used to convert it to percent body fat. The density (D) of matter is a function of its

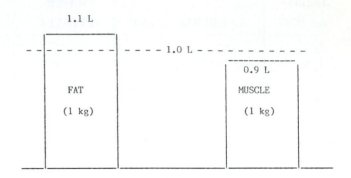

Figure 26.1 Density of 1 kg of fat and muscle produces a smaller volume of muscle than volume of fat.

mass (M) per unit volume (V) and may be calculated from Equation 26.1:

$$D = M / V \text{ or } M \cdot V^{-1} \qquad \text{Eq. 26.1}$$

Thus, the density $(g \cdot mL^{-1})$ of the body can be determined by knowing the mass (or weight in grams) and volume (milliliters) of the body.[7] The mass of the body is referred to as body mass-in-air and often abbreviated as BM_a. The body volume is determined on the basis of Archimedes' principle, whereby the loss of mass of an immersed body is directly proportional to the volume of water displaced by the body. Thus, the principle of deriving body density (D_b) from hydrostatic weighing is conceptualized by Equation 26.2:

$$\text{Body Density } (D_b) = \frac{BM_a}{BM_a - BM_w} \qquad \text{Eq. 26.2}$$

where:

BM_w = body mass in water

$BM_a - BM_w$ = loss of body mass in water

In essence, Archimedes' principle states that an immersed body loses mass equivalent to the mass of the displaced fluid, or, as Archimedes stated, "a body immersed in water is buoyed up with a force equal to the weight of the water displaced."[8,12] The mass of the displaced water converts to an equivalent volume measure. An example of this is the entrance of a person into a jacuzzi filled completely to the top. If all of the water that spills over the brim is collected while the person is completely submerged, then the mass of that collected water is equal to the mass lost by that person at submersion. The loss of mass in gram units of measure converts easily to the milliliter unit of measure for volume. Thus, either the mass of the displaced water (volumetric method) or the mass of the submerged body (hydrostatic method) can be inserted into the proper equations to calculate body density. Usually it is easier to measure the mass of the submerged body rather than the volume of displaced water.[41] The goal of persons wishing to reduce their percent body fat is to increase their body mass in water; this would increase their body density, hence decrease their percent body fat.

$$\uparrow D_b = \downarrow \% \text{ Fat}$$

Anatomical Rationale

In general, the estimation of percent body fat is based upon the two-compartmentalization of total body mass (TBM) into fat mass (FM) and fat-free mass (FFM). The fat mass is stored mainly in fat cells (adipocytes). However, not even this fat is all fat. Dr. Siri, famous for his percent body fat equation, reported that fat cells are about 62 % pure fat, 31 % water, and 7 % protein.[55] The fat-free mass is composed of its two largest components—skeletal (20 % of FFM)[4] and muscle (about 51 % of FFM for a male)—and skin, blood, brain, and organs. The primary constituents of FFM are water, mineral, protein, and glycogen.[6] The fat-free mass is devoid of any fat. Although the terms FFM and lean body mass (LBM) are sometimes used interchangeably, the LBM is a slightly larger mass because it includes essential fat found in internal organs, bone marrow, and the central nervous system.[18,42,58] For example, essential fat is in cell walls and protoplasm of all tissues.[55] The concept of a two-part (FFM and FM) body compartmentalization for total body mass (TBM) is presented in Equation 26.3:

$$\text{TBM} = \text{FFM} + \text{FM} \qquad \text{Eq. 26.3}$$

Thus, fat mass (FM) may be expressed in percentage form as Equation 26.4:

$$\% \text{ Fat} = (\text{FM/TBM}) \times 100 \qquad \text{Eq. 26.4}$$

A person at a given body mass and high relative fat-free mass weighs more in water (BM_w) and, thus, has a higher body density (D_b) and lower percent body fat (% Fat). Hence, the combination of physical and anatomical rationales can be summarized in formula form for a given body mass.

$$\downarrow \% \text{ Fat} = \uparrow \text{FFM} = \uparrow BM_w = \uparrow D_b$$

Interaction of Physical (Density) and Anatomical (Compartmentalization) Rationales

Because fat is less dense than lean body mass, fat weighs less than fat-free tissue when both are placed in water. Thus, greater differences between the person's mass on land (in air) versus the mass in water mean lower densities and, consequently, higher fat percentages.

When the body density is known, that number is inserted into another equation that relates it to the density of lean and fat tissue. Figure 26.1 schematically depicted the fact that the volume of a less dense tissue, such as fat, occupies more space (volume) than that of a more dense tissue, such as muscle, at any given mass.[11] This concept can be stated another way: The mass of a less dense tissue is less than the mass of a more dense tissue for any given volume. Bone is relatively dense and sinkable, having a density of 1.28 g·mL^{-1} [4], compared with 1.100 for lean tissue, ≈ 1.000 for water, and 0.9001 for fat tissue. Fat floats because its density is less than water's density. Fat contains 10 % water in mass, compared with 75 % water in muscle.

Methods of Hydrostatic Weighing

There are at least two methods to determine body density from the submersion of a human in water. One of these methods, the volumetric method, uses a narrow, cylindrical chamber (a volumeter or a spill-over burette) that facilitates the measurement of the displaced water from the submerged human. The conversion of this volume change to a density measure was first proposed in 1942.[8] The hydrostatic weighing method derives body volume by determining body density from the mass of the body when completely submerged in water. Body density is the technique that is the focus of this manual. Box 26.1 contains a discussion of the accuracy of hydrostatic weighing.

Equipment

Scales

For nearly 50 years, most laboratories used the spring-loaded Chatillon autopsy scale to weigh a person underwater. It resembles a supermarket's produce scale and usually has a maximum range of 9 kg to 15 kg (Figure 26.2). In the 9 kg autopsy scale, there are 1 kg, 2 kg, and 3 kg (1000 g, 2000 g, and 3000 g) markers on the main face of the dial; another gauge is on the cycle bar extending from the bottom of the scale, which represents the number of cycles made by the main dial's pointer. For example, if the large-faced dial is at 1500 g (1.5 kg), and the protruding bar is between the 2 and 3, then the actual underwater body mass is 7.5 kg or 7500 g [(2 cycles × 3000 g) + 1500].

Presently, the choice of scale is the strain-gauge, load-cell, or force-transducer scale, which is more precise, is more accurate, and can be interfaced with a recorder and/or a computer.[2,43,50] A regular platform scale may be used to measure the participant's body mass in air (BM_a).

Water Tanks

Water tanks vary in style and weight (e.g., redwood, cedar, plexiglass, stainless steel, fiberglass, tile, etc.), but are usually similar in size—just large enough to allow the participant to sit (usually) totally submerged in the water without touching the bottom or sides of the tank. The water tanks include a water filter and heater. The mass of a body immersed in a fluid varies according to the type of fluid and the temperature of the fluid. For example, the density of gasoline (≈ 0.66 g·mL^{-1}) is much lower than water density (0.99 g·mL^{-1} to 1.0 g·mL^{-1}).[27] Thus, a person's ability to float (buoyancy) in gasoline is more difficult than in water. Consequently, the body mass in gasoline is greater than in water. Also, salt water, which is more dense than fresh water, permits greater buoyancy, thus less body mass during submersion. The temperature of the water can be monitored with a water thermometer, such as a basic pool thermometer. The water density may be monitored with a hydrometer or be derived from an appropriate table for water temperature versus density (Table 26.1). Cool waters are more dense than warm waters. Hence, people are more buoyant in cool water than in warm water.

Tare Mass

The equipment that supports the participant, or attaches to the participant, is called the tare mass equipment. It consists of the supporting device, linkage, and weight belt. The suspension support ("chair") or harness also varies in style and mass (webbing, nylon rope, PVC piping, etc.). Support linkage (chains, rope) attaches the chair to the scale's hook. A weight-belt (e.g., a scuba-type belt) is worn by some participants to aid in submergence and to minimize the oscillations on the scale's dial. Tare mass will usually vary between 3 kg and 6 kg, with overfat persons requiring the higher tare mass.[48]

Lung Volume Equipment

Residual volume (RV) may be measured by nitrogen washout, helium dilution rebreathing, or the simplified method (Chapter 20), requiring only oxygen and carbon dioxide analyzers, not nitrogen or helium ones.[67] RV can be estimated by measuring vital capacity with various spirometers or pneumotachs and then using prediction equations.

BOX 26.1   Accuracy of Hydrostatic Weighing

Although hydrostatic weighing is often considered a gold standard of body composition methods, it does receive some criticism.

Validity

Its validity has been questioned mainly because of the limitations of the cadaver studies that have provided the typical tissue densities. For example, a classic equation for predicting body fat from body density is based upon a sample of only six cadavers.[14] In a study of 12 White cadavers, investigators revealed a much larger variability in muscle and body density than originally supposed.[40] The 1.100 g·mL^{-1} density value for lean tissue used in the equation to predict body fat now is recognized as a varying value within White adults and especially so in various population subgroups. For example, the densities of children (1.085), Blacks (1.113), and the elderly, especially the lower values in postmenopausal women,[24] differ significantly. The greater skeletal densities of Black males[3,61] contribute to their greater lean tissue density. Children have lower densities than adults due to their greater water concentration and lower bone mineral levels in their lean tissue component.[16] Older adults also have a less dense skeleton than younger adults. Thus, unless specific population equations[2,26,53,54] are used, the fat percentage in Blacks will be underestimated and will be overestimated in young and elderly when using such popular equations as the Brozek and the Siri equations.

The variability of the volume component of the density value is a major problem with hydrostatic weighing; consequently, this problem transfers to all of the other anthropometric methods, such as girths and skinfolds, that predict the hydrostatically determined body density. The problem is not with the density of fat but with that of the highly variable density of the fat-free mass.[47] The fallibility of densitometry was apparent in a study of 29 professional football players, 9 of them with 0 % fat or less.[1] The standard error of the estimate by hydrostatic weighing is about 2.5 % body fat,[47] with most of this error attributed to biological variability, not measurement error.[55,56] Ideally, to reduce inherent errors in the two-compartment models or equations (Brozek and Siri), laboratory procedures should measure not only body density but also body water density and bone mineral density. Although equations using the combination of three or four components were once rare,[28] such equations are now available.[2,26]

Errors in body density up to 10 % may result from estimating residual volume.[34] An average error of 0.7 % body fat units occurs for each error of 100 mL in lung volume; the error may accumulate to 3.6 % body fat units.[65] Indirectly measuring residual volume by using the standard 24 % and 28 % vital capacity values for men and women, respectively, may overestimate the residual volume of persons with large vital capacities. Hence, the accuracy of densitometry is improved by directly measuring the residual lung volume (RV) rather than by predicting it from regression equations or from a certain percentage of the vital capacity.[45] The results of various investigators concerning the measurement of residual volume with the participant in air versus in water are conflicting. It appears that it makes little practical difference for training studies as long as the subsequent post-training RV method is performed in the same medium (air or water) as the TLC, FRC, or VC[49] and in the same body position, because RV either decreases or stays the same in water.[10]

Reliability

The reliability of body densitometry is high ($r \geq .95$).[17,63] This obviously can vary with the experience of the investigators, the accuracy of the equipment, and the experience and control of the participant. Correlative statistics, however, are not always the best reflector of the repeatability of a test. Statistics may produce high correlations on a heterogeneous group (e.g., widely varied in fat content). Thus, both the correlation values and the standard error values should be used to interpret the accuracy of a test.

Participant Preparations

The participant takes a towel and skimpy bathing suit (preferably nylon; two-piece for females) to the laboratory if these are not provided. Some persons might bring their own lightweight noseclip or use one provided by the laboratory. These prevent water from entering the nose during submersion. Despite jewelry's negligible weight, it should not be worn because of its high density (for example, gold has a density of 19.3 g·mL^{-1}; that is about 18 times heavier than an equivalent volume of muscle!). The participant

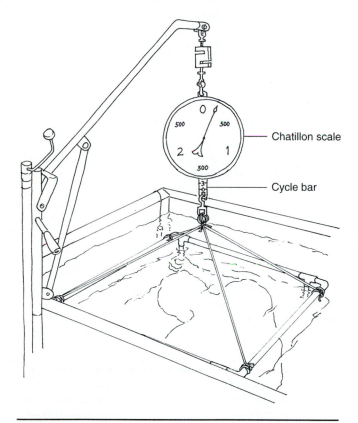

Figure 26.2 A participant's body mass is measured under water in order to determine body density.

should shower just prior to the test in order to remove body oils and lotions. The person should be normally hydrated but should not be tested within 3 h of eating (post-prandial) or more than 12 h after eating. The participant should urinate and defecate before arriving at the laboratory.

Some of the participant preparations are attempts to avoid excess air trapped in the body. Trapped air results in a lower underwater mass, which converts to a higher percent fat. Persons with gastrointestinal (GI) disturbances should be rescheduled.

Anything that is apt to cause hypohydration should be avoided, such as exercise under hot/humid conditions or sauna bathing. Due to higher estimates of percent fat from water retention, it may not be advisable to test females during the bloated period of the menstrual cycle[15] or within seven days on either side of the menstrual cycle.[30] Some investigators think that the fluid retention during normal menstruation may not be enough to affect the body density or percent fat.[19] However, a hydration change equivalent to about 1 kg to 2 kg of body mass may increase the percent body fat estimation by hydrostatic weighing.[25]

Technician Preparations

The water in the tank should be clean, chlorinated, and at the proper temperature. For the comfort of the participants, water temperatures should be at least 33 °C (91 °F), especially for lean persons, but probably no higher than 36 °C (97 °F). The technician should note the temperature of the water and consult Table 26.1 for the water density at that temperature. The ability to float (buoyancy) improves with greater tank-water densities. Water density increases as mineralization (hardness) increases. Densities also increase as water temperature decreases except near and at freezing when water turns into ice at 0 °C and then has the ability to float on water. Because warm water is less dense than cold water, it is found above cold water. The standard density (1.000 g·mL^{-1}) is based on the heaviest density of pure water at 4 °C.[20] In summary, the ability to float will be easier in harder and cooler waters, such as that typical of swimming pools between 25 °C (77 °F) and 27 °C (80 °F), than those typically found in laboratory underwater weighing tanks.

The technician should weigh the tare equipment at the water level likely to be encountered in the actual underwater weighing trials. If an electronic output from a load cell is used, it is likely that the weight (mass) monitor can be zeroed at the tare mass. In the latter case, there will be no need to subtract the tare mass from the underwater mass in Equation 26.7. The position of the participant in the support device, whether it be sitting, semi-prone, or kneeling, should not affect the results of hydrostatic weighing.[29]

Procedures

Besides comforting and positioning the participant, three other concerns in the hydrostatic weighing procedures are

Table 26.1	Relationship between Water Temperature (Tw) and Water Density (Dw)			

Tw		Dw		Tw		Dw
°C	°F	g·mL^{-1}		°C	°F	g·mL^{-1}
0	32	0.999		32	89.5	0.9950
4	39	1.000	Comfort	33	91	0.9947
22	72	0.9978		34	93	0.9944
25	77	0.9971		35	95	0.9941
26	79	0.9968		36	97	0.9937
27	81	0.9965	Range	37	98.6	0.9934
28	82	0.9963		38	100	0.9930
29	84	0.9960		39	102	0.9926
30	86	0.9957		40	104	0.9922
31	88	0.9954				

to account for essential air, to eliminate excess air, and to read the underwater mass accurately.

Nonessential and Essential Air

In addition to fat, only two other parts of the body float: (1) the nonessential air trapped in hair, and (2) the essential air compartments in the lungs and the gastrointestinal (GI) tract.

Nonessential Air

The first thing the participant should do upon entering the water is to dunk under the water and then press the hands against the suit and body hairs in order to push the pockets of nonessential air from these sources. Nylon bathing suits trap air to a lesser extent than most conventional suits.

Essential GI Air

The GI air is a constant value of 100 mL assumed for all persons. Equation 26.8 accounts for this assumed constant value, but gas-producing foods and GI disturbances can increase this value to several hundred milliliters.[55]

Essential Lung Air

The lung volume, which is inserted into Equation 26.10, can be any known volume, such as total lung capacity (TLC), functional residual capacity (FRC), or residual volume (RV). The person does not have to expel air during submersion if using the TLC, FRC, or partial expiration methods. These methods are more comfortable than the RV method but less common.[44] The FRC,[59] TLC,[5,21,60,64] and partial expiration[36] methods appear to be as accurate as the RV method. The TLC or partial exhalation methods may be especially convenient for testing the older adult.[37,57]

The **RV method** of underwater weighing calls for the person to rid the body of all lung air except the residual air by exhaling maximally. Usually, the person is in the seated position and moves the head toward the knees during the effort to expel the air. The technician can observe the formed bubbles of air as they escape from the participant's mouth to the surface of the water. As long as there are noticeable bubbles, the participant still is not down to residual volume. The amount of time that participants can remain under water while exhaling to residual volume is quite variable. Typically, it is 5 s to 10 s, but some persons remain totally submerged for 15 s or more.[60]

Although a true research laboratory test of hydrostatic weighing would include the direct measurement of RV, it is possible to modify the hydrostatic test so that the RV is predicted by equations from either the prior measurement of vital capacity for men (Eq. 26.5) or women (Eq. 26.6).[66] Sometimes the vital capacity is measured with the person submerged to the neck.[57]

Men:

$$RV \ (L) = 24 \ \% \ (\text{or } 0.24) \times VC_{BTPS} \qquad \text{Eq. 26.5}$$

Women:

$$RV = 28 \ \% \ (\text{or } 0.28) \times VC_{BTPS} \qquad \text{Eq. 26.6}$$

Reading the Scale for Underwater Weight

The technician does not have much time to read the oscillating pointer or digital display of the autopsy scale or force transducer, respectively. The time may be dependent upon the participant's breath-holding ability and the degree of oscillation of the scale's indicating pointers or of the display. Force transducers reduce fluctuations, compared with spring autopsy scales but do not eliminate them.[50] The oscillations may be dependent upon the size of the tank, larger tanks requiring greater time. The oscillations should be small enough to be read to the nearest 20 g[31] or 25 g. However, it is not unusual to be able to read it to only the nearest 50 g. The technician reads the midpoint of the oscillations or the consistently highest value. The oscillations can be dampened if the technician loosely grasps the suspension hook of the autopsy scale with the fingers while the participant submerges. Before reading the scale, the technician should check to be sure that all parts of the person's body are submerged and that no air bubbles are visible. When the technician is satisfied with the reading, a prearranged signal (e.g., knocking on the tank) may be given to let the participant know it is time to surface. However, all participants should feel free to ascend according to their own comfort.

The number of trials may vary according to the experience of the participants. Usually, submerged persons will reach their consistently highest expiratory capacities (hence, heaviest weights), within 5 to 12 trials. Some technicians repeat the procedure until 3 trials are within 100 g of each other.[62] Others may exclude the heaviest underwater body mass and use only the mean of the next two highest masses for the body density equations.[32] Other researchers use either the average of the last 2 or 3 trials or the average of the two heaviest weighings. Ideally, none of the readings used to calculate the average should differ by more than 100 g.[9,52]

Summary of Procedures

The following procedures are consistent with the RV method of hydrostatic weighing.

1. The technician measures and records the basic data and water-tank temperature onto Form 26.1.
2. The technician obtains one of the following lung volumes or capacities:
   a. RV—directly measured or predicted from equations 26.5 (men) or 26.6 (women)
   b. TLV (TLC)
   c. FRC
   d. Any partial volume
3. Being of normal hydration and after showering, the participant enters the water tank wearing, ideally, a nylon swimsuit and optional nose clip.
4. The technician records the tare mass and notes the depth of the chair at the participant's expected chin level.

5. The participant briefly submerges and then presses the air out of hair and swimsuit.
6. The participant sits in the chair or platform and, possibly, straps on a weighted belt to avoid floating when submerged.
7. The technician gives instructions for exhalation and demonstrates an exhalation.
8. A signal is clarified by which to alert the participant that the technician is satisfied with the scale reading; the technician reminds participant to ascend if becoming uncomfortable.
9. The participant begins to exhale while lowering head and shoulders under the water.
10. The technician may dampen the scale while observing the bubbles and the oscillations of the scale.
11. Usually near the 10th second, the technician gives the ascent signal and records the underwater body mass (BM_w) to the nearest 20 g to 50 g.
12. The procedure is repeated 5 to 12 times, depending upon the consistency of the values.
13. The average of either the last two or three trials or of the two heaviest weighings is often chosen for the body density equation.

Many modifications of the hydrostatic method have focused on ways to make the participant more comfortable in the water without losing any of the accuracy from the traditional technique. The FRC and TLC methods are two examples. Another example is one that permits the person's head to remain above the water during the procedure.[23] Another modification eliminates the weight scale by having the participant grasp a 5.5 L plastic bottle to achieve neutral buoyancy in the measurement of body volume.[22] In general, it appears that modifications of the hydrodensitometry technique will continue to occur. Until valid electronic see-through techniques become practical and affordable to the exercise physiologist, the hydrostatic technique will continue to be a popular test.

Calculations

The density (D) of matter was shown to be a function of mass (M) per unit volume (V) in Equation 26.1 (D = M/V). This equation was the basis of Equation 26.2, which specifically related to hydrostatic weighing. However, the actual calculation of body density (D_b) from hydrostatic weighing data is slightly more complicated than Equation 26.2. The denominator—volume (V)—is obtained by using Equation 26.7.[68]

$$V = \left[\frac{(BM_a - BM_w)}{D_w} \right] - RV \qquad \text{Eq. 26.7}$$

where:

BM_a = body mass (g) in air

BM_w = body mass in water (minus the tare mass if not zeroed electronically); net mass in water

D_w = density of water at given water temperature

RV = residual volume; other volumes could replace RV in Equation 26.7

When Equations 26.2 and 26.7 are combined and modified from their original form[14] by accounting for the assumed 100 mL of air in the gastrointestinal (V_{GI}) tract, the complete equation (26.8) for body density is formed from the original density equation (D = M/V).

$$D_b = \frac{BM_a}{\left[\dfrac{BM_a - BM_w}{D_w} \right] - (RV + V_{GI})} \qquad \text{Eq. 26.8}$$

Because grams and milliliters are interconvertible, it does not matter which of these units is used in Equation 26.8; the resulting ratio is the same.

The body fat percentage is determined from body density based upon the two-compartment (FW and FFW) models of either the Siri[52] equation (Eq. 26.9) or the Brozek[13] equation (Eq. 26.10), which were developed from the chemical analysis of cadavers. Table 26.2 presents the body densities (1.020 to 1.090) and equivalent body fat percentages (33.8 % to 5.0 %) based on the Brozek equation. The Brozek equation is preferred for elderly persons.[57] Lohman and his colleagues feel that Equation 26.11 is preferable for young adult women.[39] Because indirect or non-vivo measurements have shown that Blacks have denser bones and muscles than Whites, the Schutte equation (Eq. 26.12) is recommended.[53] The Lohman and Schutte equations are multicomponent models based on protein, fat, water, and/or mineral.

$$\text{Siri \% Fat} = (495 / D_b) - 450 \qquad \text{Eq. 26.9}$$

$$\text{Brozek (older) \% Fat} = (457 / D_b) - 414.2 \qquad \text{Eq. 26.10}$$

$$\text{Lohman (young women) \% Fat} \qquad \text{Eq. 26.11}$$
$$= (509 / D_b) - 465$$

$$\text{Schutte (Blacks) \% Fat} = (437.4 / D_b) - 392.8 \qquad \text{Eq. 26.12}$$

Example of Calculating Body Density

A review of the respiratory volumes, such as vital capacity (VC), functional residual capacity (FRC), and residual volume (RV) is helpful in understanding laboratory hydrodensitometry.[1]

Given the following conditions:

Male; Age = 27 y; BM_a = 83.62 kg or 83 620 g

VC_{BTPS} = 6.40 L or 6400 mL

Predicted RV = 1.536 L or 1536 mL (from Eq. 26.5)

Water Temperature (T_w) = 32 °C

Water Density (D_w) = 0.9950 (Table 26.1)

Underwater mass = 6.870 kg or 6870 g

Tare mass = 2500 g

Net BM_w = 6870 g − 2500 g = 4370 g

Table 26.2   Body Densities (D_b) and Body Fat Percentages (% F) Based on the Brozek Equation

D_b (g·mL^{-1})	% F	D_b	% F	D_b	% F	D_b	% F
1.020	33.8	1.038	26.0	1.056	18.5	1.074	11.3
1.021	33.4	1.039	25.6	1.057	18.1	1.075	10.9
1.022	32.9	1.040	25.2	1.058	17.7	1.076	10.5
1.023	32.5	1.041	24.8	1.059	17.3	1.077	10.1
1.024	32.0	1.042	24.3	1.060	16.9	1.078	9.7
1.025	31.6	1.043	23.9	1.061	16.5	1.079	9.3
1.026	31.2	1.044	23.5	1.062	16.1	1.080	8.9
1.027	30.7	1.045	23.1	1.063	15.7	1.081	8.5
1.028	30.3	1.046	22.7	1.064	15.3	1.082	8.1
1.029	29.9	1.047	22.2	1.065	14.9	1.083	7.7
1.030	29.5	1.048	21.8	1.066	14.5	1.084	7.3
1.031	29.0	1.049	21.4	1.067	14.1	1.085	6.9
1.032	28.6	1.050	21.0	1.068	13.7	1.086	6.5
1.033	28.2	1.051	20.6	1.069	13.3	1.087	6.1
1.034	27.8	1.052	20.2	1.070	12.9	1.088	5.7
1.035	27.3	1.053	19.8	1.071	12.5	1.089	5.3
1.036	26.9	1.054	19.4	1.072	12.1	1.090	5.0
1.037	26.5	1.055	19.0	1.073	11.7		

Table derived from Brazek, J., & Keys, A. (1951). The evaluation of leanness-fatness in man: Norms and intercorrelations. *British Journal of Nutrition, 5,* 194–205.

The calculation is performed as follows by using Equation 26.8:

$$D_b = \frac{83\,620\text{ g}}{\left[\dfrac{83\,620\text{ g} - 4370\text{ g}}{0.9950}\right] - (1536 + 100\text{ mL})}$$

$$= \frac{83\,620}{\left[\dfrac{79\,250}{0.9950}\right] - 1636}$$

$$= \frac{83\,620}{79\,648 - 1636}$$

$$= \frac{83\,620}{78\,012}$$

$$= 1.0719\text{ g·mL}^{-1}$$

The percentage of fat from the known body density of the man in our example can be found by using the Brozek equation (Eq. 26.10), Table 26.2, or the Siri equation (Eq. 26.9). The Brozek table gives a percent fat of 12.1 % for a body density of 1.0720 (rounded). If we use the Siri equation (Eq. 26.9), which is not expected to differ by more than 1 % body fat units from the Brozek-derived % Fat,[42] the percent fat is 11.8 % based on the following calculation:

Given: $D_b = 1.0720$

then: % Fat = (495 / D_b) − 450

$\qquad$ = (495 / 1.0720) − 450

$\qquad$ = 461.75 − 450

$\qquad$ = 11.8 % (rounded to closest tenth percent)

If testing young adult women, then the Lohman equation (Eq. 26.11) is preferred. If testing Blacks, then the Schutte equation (Eq. 26.12) is appropriate.

Results and Discussion

Because the prediction of percent fat from body density makes assumptions that are not totally valid, it may be advisable to rely on body density alone for interpretive purposes.[40] Density may range from a low of about 0.93 g·mL^{-1} in a very obese person to 1.10 g·mL^{-1} in a very lean man.[40] Most persons, however, will range from about 1.020 (≈ 34 % fat) to about 1.077 (≈ 10 % fat).

One authority feels that fat percentages between 10 % and 22 % for men and 20 % and 32 % for women are compatible with health.[36] Persons with percent body fats at and above the 85th percentile (26 % fat for men; 31.5 % fat for women) may be considered obese.[44] Persons not satisfied with their body fat percentage will be more successful in altering it by combining diet and exercise rather than by modifying diet alone. It is not unusual for 35 % to 45 % of the total weight loss to be lean body tissue when dieting and not exercising.[49] Many clinicians and researchers suggest a minimal fat percentage for men and women of 3 % to 7 % and 10 % to 20 %, respectively.[36] Persons known to have large muscle masses, such as body builders, power lifters, and Olympic lifters, have body fat percentages typically between 9 % and 11 %.[33]

References

1. Adams, J., Mottola, M., Bagnall, K. M., & McFadden, K. D. (1982). Total body fat content in a group of professional football players. *Canadian Journal of Applied Sport Science, 7,* 36–40.
2. American College of Sports Medicine. (2000). *ACSM's guidelines for exercise testing and prescription* (p. 62). Philadelphia: Lippincott Williams & Wilkins.

3. Baker, P. T., & Angel, J. L. (1965). Old age changes in body density: Sex and race factors in the United States. *Human Biology, 37,* 104–119.

4. Bakker, H. K., & Struikenkamp, R. S. (1977). Biological variability and lean body mass estimates. *Human Biology, 49,* 187–202.

5. Ballard, T. (1984). *Hydrostatic weighing at total lung capacity versus residual volume.* Unpublished master's thesis, California State University, Fullerton.

6. Baumgartner, R. N., Heymsfield, S. B., Lichtman, S., Wang, J., & Pierson, R. N. (1991). Body composition in elderly people: Effect of criterion estimates on predictive equations. *American Journal of Clinical Nutrition, 53,* 1343–1353.

7. Behnke, A. R., Feen, B. G., & Welham, A. C. (1942). The specific gravity of healthy men: Body weight divided by volume as an index of obesity. *JAMA: The Journal of the American Medical Association, 118,* 495–498.

8. Behnke, A. R., & Wilmore, J. H. (1974). *Evaluation and regulation of body build and composition.* Englewood Cliffs, NJ: Prentice-Hall.

9. Bonge, D., & Donnelly, J. E. (1989). Trials to criteria for hydrostatic weighing at residual volume. *Research Quarterly for Exercise and Sport, 60,* 176–179.

10. Bosch, P. R., & Wells, C. L. (1991). Effect of immersion on residual volume of able-bodied and spinal cord injured males. *Medicine and Science in Sports and Exercise, 23,* 384–388.

11. Brobek, J. R. (1968). Energy balance and food intake. In V. B. Mountcastle (Ed.), *Medical physiology* (pp. 498–519). St. Louis: C. V. Mosby.

12. Brooks, G. A., Fahey, T. D., & White, T. P. (1996). *Exercise physiology: Human bioenergetics and its application.* Mountain View, CA: Mayfield.

13. Brozek, J., Grande, F., Anderson, J., & Keys, A. (1963). Densitometric analysis of body composition: Revision of some quantitative assumptions. *Annals of New York Academy of Science, 110,* 113–140.

14. Brozek, J., & Keys, A. (1951). The evaluation of leanness-fatness in man: Norms and intercorrelations. *British Journal of Nutrition, 5,* 194–205.

15. Bunt, J. C., Lohman, T. G., & Boileau, R. A. (1989). Impact of total body water fluctuations on estimation of body fat from body density. *Medicine and Science in Sports and Exercise, 21,* 96–100.

16. Bunt, J. C., Lohman, T. G., Slaughter, M. H., Boileau, R. A., Lussier, L., & Van Loan, M. (1983). Bone mineral content as a source of variation in body density in children and youth. *Medicine and Science in Sports and Exercise, 15* (Abstract), 172.

17. Buskirk, E., & Taylor, H. L. (1957). Maximal oxygen intake and its relation to body composition with special reference to chronic physical activity and obesity. *Journal of Applied Physiology, 11,* 72–78.

18. Buskirk, E. R., & Mendez, J. (1984). Sports science and body composition analysis: Emphasis on cell and muscle mass. *Medicine and Science in Sports and Exercise, 16,* 584–593.

19. Byrd, P. J., & Thomas, T. R. (1983). Hydrostatic weighing during different stages of the menstrual cycle. *Research Quarterly for Exercise and Sport, 54,* 296–298.

20. Clarke, G. L. (1954). *Elements of ecology.* New York: John Wiley & Sons.

21. Coffman, J. L., Timson, B. F., Beneke, W. M., & Paulsen, B. K. (1983). Measurement of body composition by hydrostatic weighing at residual volume and total lung capacity. *Medicine and Science in Sports and Exercise, 15* (Abstract), 172–173.

22. Denahan, T., Hortobagyl, T., & Katch, F. I. (1988). Validation of a new method of hydrostatic weighing. *Medicine and Science in Sports and Exercise, 20* (2 Suppl.), Abstract #44, S8.

23. Donnelly, J. E., Brown, T. E., Israel, R. G., Smith-Sintek, S., O'Brien, K. F., & Caslavka, B. (1988). Hydrostatic weighing without head submersion: Description of a method. *Medicine and Science in Sports and Exercise, 20,* 66–69.

24. Freund, B. J., Wilmore, J. H., Boyden, T. W., Stimi, W. A., & Harrington, R. J. (1984). Relationships of aerobic fitness and body composition measurements to bone density in post-menopausal women. *International Journal of Sports Medicine, 5,* 159.

25. Girandola, R. N., Wiswell, R. A., & Romero, G. T. (1977). Body composition changes resulting from fluid ingestion and dehydration. *Research Quarterly for Exercise and Sport, 48,* 299–303.

26. Heyward, V. H., & Stolarczyk, L. M. (1996). *Applied body composition assessment.* Champaign, IL: Human Kinetics.

27. Hill, J. W. (1992). *Chemistry for changing times.* New York: Macmillan.

28. Houtkooper, L. B., & Going, S. B. (1994). Body composition: How should it be measured? Does it affect sport performance? *Sports Science Exchange, 7*(5), 1–9.

29. Hsieh, S., Kline, G., Porcari, J., & Katch, F. I. (1985). Measurement of residual volume sitting and lying in air and water (and during underwater weighing) and its effects on computed body density. *Medicine and Science in Sports and Exercise, 17*(2) (Abstract), S204.

30. Jackson, A. S., Pollock, M. L., & Ward, A. (1980). Generalized equations for predicting body density of women. *Medicine and Science in Sports and Exercise, 12,* 175–182.

31. Jackson, A. S., & Pollock, M. L. (1985). Practical assessment of body composition. *The Physician and Sportsmedicine, 15*(5), 76–80, 82–90.

32. Johansson, A. G., Forslund, A., Sjödin, A., Mallmin, H., Hambraeus, L., & Ljunghall, S. (1993). Determination of body composition of dual-energy X-ray absorptiometry and hydrodensitometry. *American Journal of Clinical Nutrition, 57,* 323–326.

33. Katch, F. I. (1969). Practice curves and errors of measurement in estimating underwater weight by hydrostatic weighing. *Medicine and Science in Sports, 1,* 212–216.

34. Katch, F. I., & Katch, V. L. (1980). Measurement and prediction errors in body composition assessment and the search for the perfect equation. *Research Quarterly for Exercise and Sport, 51,* 249–260.

35. Katch, V. L., Katch, F. I., Moffatt, R., & Gittleson, M. (1980). Muscular development and lean body weight in body builders and weight lifters. *Medicine and Science in Sports and Exercise, 12,* 340–344.

36. Kohrt, W. M., Malley, M. T., Dalsky, G. P., & Holloszy, J. O. (1992). Body composition of healthy sedentary and trained young and older men and women. *Medicine and Science in Sports and Exercise, 24,* 832–837.

37. Latin, R. W., & Ruhling, R. O. (1986). Total lung capacity, residual volume and predicted residual volume in a densitometric study of older men. *British Journal of Sports Medicine, 20* (2), 66–68.

38. Lohman, T. G. (1982). Body composition methodology in sports medicine. *The Physician and Sportsmedicine, 10*(12), 46–48, 51–53, 56–58.

39. Lohman, T. G., Slaughter, M. H., Boileau, R. A., Bunt, J., & Lussier, L. (1984). Bone mineral measurements and their relation to body density in children, youth, and adults. *Human Biology, 56,* 667.

40. Martin, A. D., Drinkwater, D. T., Clarys, J. P., & Ross, W. D. (1981). Estimation of body fat: A new look at some old assumptions. *The Physician and Sportsmedicine, 9,* 21–22.

41. Mathews, D. K., & Fox, E. L. (1976). *The physiological basis of physical education and athletics.* Philadelphia: W. B. Saunders.

42. McArdle, W. D., Katch, F. I., & Katch, V. L. (1996). *Exercise physiology: Energy, nutrition and human performance.* Baltimore: Williams & Wilkins.

43. McClenaghan, B. A., & Rocchis, L. (1986). Design and validation of an automated hydrostatic weighing system. *Medicine and Science in Sports and Exercise, 18,* 479–484.

44. McGarty, J. M., Butts, N. K., Hall, L. K., & Fletcher, R. A. (1983). Comparison of three hydrostatic weighing methods. *Medicine and Science in Sports and Exercise, 15,* (Abstract), 181.

45. Morrow, J. R., Jackson, A. S., Bradley, P. W., & Hartung, G. H. (1986). Accuracy of measured and predicted residual lung volume on body density measurement. *Medicine and Science in Sports and Exercise, 18,* 647–652.

46. Mullins, N. M., & Sinning, W. E. (1996). Diagnostic utility of the body mass index as a measure of obesity in athletes and non-athletes. *Medicine and Science in Sports and Exercise, 28*(5), Abstract #1148, S193.

47. Nash, H. L. (1985). Body fat measurement: Weighing the pros and cons of electrical impedance. *The Physician and Sportsmedicine, 13*(11), 124–128.

48. Nieman, D. C. (1995). *Fitness and sports medicine: A health-related approach.* Palo Alto, CA: Bull.

49. Noble, B. J. (1986). *Physiology of exercise and sport.* St. Louis: Times/Mirror.

50. Organ, L. W., Eklund, A. D., & Ledbetter, J. D. (1994). An automated real time underwater weighing system. *Medicine and Science in Sports and Exercise, 26,* 383–391.

51. Oscai, L. B. (1973). The role of exercise in weight control. In J. H. Wilmore (Ed.), *Exercise and sport sciences reviews* (pp. 103–123). New York: Academic Press.

52. Quatrochi, J. A., Hicks, V. L., Heyward, V. H., Colville, B. C., Cook, K. L., Jenkins, K. A., & Wilson, W. L. (1992). Relationship of optical density and skinfold measurements: Effects of age and level of body fatness. *Research Quarterly for Exercise and Sport, 63,* 402–409.

53. Schutte, J. E. (1984). Density of lean body mass is greater in blacks than whites. *Journal of Applied Physiology, 56,* 1647.

54. Schutte, J. E., Longhurst, J. C., Gaffney, F. A., Bastian, B. C., & Blomqvist, C. G. (1981). Total plasma creatinine: An accurate measure of total striated muscle mass. *Journal of Applied Physiology, 51,* 762–766.

55. Siri, W. E. (1956). The gross composition of the body. *Advances in Biological Medical Physiology, 4,* 239–280.

56. Siri, W. E. (1961). *Body composition from fluid spaces and density: Analysis of methods in techniques for measuring body composition* (pp. 223–244). Washington, DC: National Academy of Science, National Research Council.

57. Snead, D. B., Birge, S. J., & Kohrt, W. M. (1993). Age-related differences in body composition by hydrodensitometry and dual-energy X-ray absorptiometry. *Journal of Applied Physiology, 74,* 770–775.

58. Tanaka, K., Hijama, T., Watanabe, Y., Asano, K., Takedo, M., Hayakawa, Y., & Nakadomo, F. (1993). Assessment of exercise-induced alterations in body composition of patients with coronary heart disease. *European Journal of Applied Physiology, 66,* 321–327.

59. Thomas, T. R., & Etheridge, G. L. (1980). Hydrostatic weighing at residual volume and functional residual capacity. *Journal of Applied Physiology: Respiratory, Environmental and Exercise Physiology, 49,* 157–159.

60. Timson, B. F., & Coffman, J. L. (1984). Body composition by hydrostatic weighing at total lung capacity and residual volume. *Medicine and Science in Sports and Exercise, 16,* 411–414.

61. Trotter, M., Broman, G. E., & Peterson, R. R. (1959). Density of cervical vertebrae and comparison with densities of other bones. *American Journal of Physical Anthropology, 17,* 19–25.

62. Wagner, D. R., & Heyward, V. H. (1999). Techniques of body composition assessment: A review of laboratory and field methods. *Research Quarterly for Exercise and Sport, 70,* 135–149.

63. Ward, A., Pollock, M. L., Jackson, A. S., Ayres, J. J., & Pape, G. (1978). A comparison of body fat determined by underwater weighing and volume displacement. *American Journal of Physiology, 234,* E94–E96.

64. Weltman, A., & Katch, V. (1981). Comparison of hydrostatic weighing at residual volume and total lung capacity. *Medicine and Science in Sports and Exercise, 13,* 210–213.

65. Williams, L., & Davis, J. A. (1987). Influence of functional residual capacity methodology on body fat determined by hydrostatic weighing. *International Journal of Sports Medicine, 8,* (Abstract), 243.

66. Wilmore, J. H. (1969). The use of actual, predicted, and constant residual volumes in the assessment of body composition by underwater weighing. *Medicine and Science in Sports and Exercise, 1,* 87–90.

67. Wilmore, J. H. (1980). A simplified method for determination of residual volume. *Journal of Applied Physiology, 27,* 96–100.

68. Wilmore, J. H., & Behnke, A. R. (1969). An anthropometric estimation of body density and lean body weight in young men. *Journal of Applied Physiology, 27,* 25–31.

Form 26.1

Individual Data for Hydrostatic Weighing

Name _____ Date _____ Time _____ A.M. ____ P.M. ____

Age ____ y   Gender (M or W) ____   Ht _____ cm   Wt _____ kg   Tech. Initials ____

Meteorological Data

T ____ °C (closest 0.1 °C)   RH % ____ P_B ____ mm Hg × 1.333 = ____ hPa

Lung Volumes

VC (BTPS) _____ L   In water: Yes ____ No ____   RV _____ L   In water: Yes ____ No ____

Estimated RV (L):

Men

$RV = 0.24 \times VC_{BTPS}$ _____ L = _____ L = _____ mL

Women

$RV = 0.28 \times VC_{BTPS}$ _____ L = _____ L = _____ mL

Hydrostatic Weighing

Water T (T_w) _____ °C D_w _____   Tare mass _____ g

Body wt in water (BM_w) to closest 25 g or 50 g

Trial #1 _____ #2 _____ #3 _____ #4 _____ #5 _____ #6 _____

Trial #7 _____ #8 _____ #9 _____ #10 _____ #11 _____ #12 _____

[Circle two highest underwater weight (BM_w) values; average the two. Or use another acceptable method for choosing the BM_w.]

Mean BM_w _____ g – Tare mass _____ g = Net BM_w _____ g

Form 26.2

Hydrostatic Weighing Calculation Form

Body Density (D_b) =

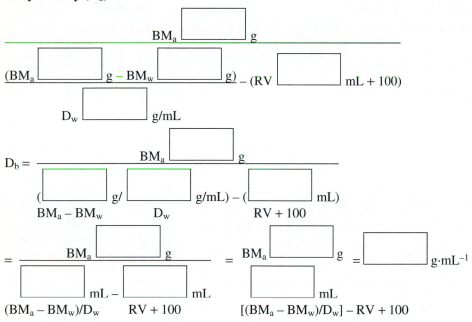

$$D_b = \frac{BM_a \quad \text{g}}{(BM_a \quad \text{g} - BM_w \quad \text{g}) - (RV \quad \text{mL} + 100)}$$
$$D_w \quad \text{g/mL}$$

$D_b =$ ...

D_b = body density		
BM_a = body mass in air		
BM_w = Body mass in water		
RV = residual volume		
D_w = water density		
100 = GI tract air		

Percent Fat (% F):

Siri equation:

% F = (495/D_b [____] g·mL^{-1}) − 450 = [____] − 450 = [____] % F

Lohman equation: (Young Women)

% F = (509/D_b [____] g·mL^{-1}) − 465 = [____] − 465 = [____] % F

Schutte equation: (Blacks)

% F = (437.4/D_b [____] g·mL^{-1}) − 392.8 = [____] − 392.8 = [____] % F

Brozek equation: (Older Men and Women)

% F = (457/D_b) − 414.2 = [____] − 414.2 = [____] % F

Form 26.3

Group Data for Various Body Composition Methods

MEN Initials	PERCENT FAT Girth 1-Girth	2-Girth	Skinfolds AAHPER	J-P	Hydro-Static	WOMEN Initials	PERCENT FAT Girth 1-Girth	3-Girth	Skinfolds AAHPER	J-P	Hydro-Static
1.						1.					
2.						2.					
3.						3.					
4.						4.					
5.						5.					
6.						6.					
7.						7.					
8.						8.					
9.						9.					
10.						10.					
11.						11.					
12.						12.					
13.						13.					
14.						14.					
15.						15.					
16.						16.					
17.						17.					
18.						18.					
19.						19.					
20.						20.					
M						M					

CARDIOPULMONARY RESUSCITATION (CPR)

CPR certification has three general requirements: (1) performing the skills associated with caring for cardiac and pulmonary emergencies; (2) demonstrating appropriate decisions for care; and (3) passing a final written exam.[7] Proper administration of CPR is essential for laboratory personnel who administer exercise stress tests. It appears that, with proper screening, monitoring, and emergency procedures, the incidence of serious problems during exercise testing can be minimal. Successful treatment of a stricken victim often depends upon prompt treatment through basic life support (BLS) methods, followed shortly thereafter by advanced cardiac life support (ACLS) methods.

The following summary of basic life support represents a consensus of experts at the 1985 National Conference on Cardiopulmonary Resuscitation (CPR) and Emergency Cardiac Care (ECC).[10] The goal of BLS is to either (1) prevent circulatory or respiratory arrest or insufficiency or (2) externally support the victim via CPR techniques. The major objective is to promote the oxygenation of brain, heart, and other vital tissues. The key to success is prompt action. Success rates are best when CPR is initiated within 4 min of the time of arrest and when ACLS occurs within 8 min of the start of CPR.[4]

Method

The acronym for remembering CPR techniques is ABC—airway, breathing, and circulation. Each of these has an initial assessment phase to determine (1) unresponsiveness, (2) breathlessness, and (3) pulselessness. The assessment phase should not exceed several seconds. The one-rescuer method is outlined here in more detail than the two-rescuer method.

Airway

(1) Assessment—tap, gently shake, and shout, "Are you OK?"; (2) call for help; (3) position the victim supine on a firm surface; (4) open the airway by the head-tilt/chin-lift maneuver; (5) clear the victim's mouth or throat if obstructed.

Breathing

(1) Assessment—look, feel, and listen for breath; (2) give two breaths, each lasting from 1 s to 1.5 s, which are about two to three times greater (hence, 800 mL to 1200 mL) than a normal breath.

Circulation

(1) Assessment—feel carotid artery; (2) use the heel of the hand to perform 15 external chest (sternum) compressions at a rate of 80 to 100 per min; count 1, 2, etc., to 15; (3) open the airway (tilt) and administer two breaths as before; (4) repeat the 15 chest compressions; (5) perform four complete cycles of 15 compressions and two ventilations.

Reassessment

After the four cycles (15:2 ratio), reevaluate the victim. Check the carotid pulse (5 s); if it is absent, resume the cycle, starting with two breaths. Check breathing (3 s to 5 s). Do not interrupt CPR for more than 7 s.

Two-Rescuer Technique

Personnel should learn both the one-rescuer and the two-rescuer techniques. A compression rate of 80 to 100 per min is used for both the one- and two-rescuer CPR method; however, the compression–ventilation ratio is 5:1, with a 1 s to 1.5 s pause for ventilation in the two-rescuer technique.

Defibrillators

Only medical practitioners, or others specifically authorized by law, can legally use defibrillators.[1] Authorized personnel should be immediately available if maximal exercise testing persons with known heart disease. Having emergency equipment readily available along with the knowledge of how to use a defibrillator would be ideal. Technology has simplified and reduced the size of defibrillators. They are now being used at some public places, such as golf courses and commercial airlines. These automated external defibrillators are no bigger than laptop computers and are less than 10 lb in weight. They restore viable heart rhythms, albeit irregular rhythms, by delivering one or more separate electric shocks. Usually serious cases involve persons with ventricular fibrillation (VF), which consists of erratic rhythm emanating from the two heart ventricles. Because VF causes an asynchronous action of the myocardial fibers, the heart's pumping ability is negligible.

Automated external defibrillators (AED) are most effective if they are used within 3 min of the cardiac event.[16] For example, the survival dropped from a 74 % rate if the shock was delivered in less than 3 min, to a 49 % rate if the shock was delivered after 3 min. Time is critical because there is a 7 % decrease to 10 % decrease in survival for each minute that defibrillation is postponed—this is based upon Emergency Medical Services contacts.[13] A fully automatic AED analyzes the rhythm and then delivers the shock without the operator's input. A semiautomatic AED uses a voice prompt telling the rescuer to press the defibrillator button if the heart rhythm is either in VF or ventricular tachycardia without a pulse.[14] The cost of an AED ranges between $2500 and $3000. Legally, only persons who have been certified in their use can operate AED instruments.

Personnel in exercise testing laboratories, fitness centers, health clubs, or most public places should hold emergency practice drills twice[11] or four[2] times per year.

The Laboratory Emergency Plan

1. All laboratory personnel know the location of the telephone and the emergency equipment (if available).
2. The most experienced person(s) in CPR[a] attend(s) to the victim.
3. Another person calls the emergency number (e.g., paramedics): **911.** The caller gives the following information calmly and clearly:
   a. General location (city, university):

   _____ (fortunately, some systems pinpoint the caller's location).
   Building: _____ Room _____
   b. Telephone number from which the call is made:

   _____
   c. Number of victims: _____
   d. Brief description of trauma (e.g., heart attacks) and present aid and condition of the victim.
4. The caller hangs up **after** the emergency station hangs up.
5. The caller goes to a strategic location to meet the emergency team.

Discussion

Submaximal exercise tests are less risky than maximal tests—the maximal tests having percent death and myocardial infarction (MI) risks of ≤ 0.01 % and 0.04 %, respectively, during or immediately after the test.[1] When exercise testing to 85 % of the performer's predicted maximal heart rate, one group of investigators reported no deaths, cardiac arrests, or ventricular fibrillation in more than five years involving more than 1000 tests.[12]

It appears that exercise testing is less risky in apparently healthy persons having preventive medicine exams than in symptomatic persons having diagnostic exams. In 1981, Dr. Ken Cooper said that his clinic had no deaths and only one resuscitation in more than 41 000 maximal Balke protocol tests in 20 years;[8] in the same preventive medicine clinic, as of 1989 there still had been no deaths in more than 70 000 maximal exercise tests.[5] When considering the noneventful exercise tests administered at fitness clinics, Ys, corporations, safety and emergency facilities, and schools, it is clear that the risk associated with exercise testing is very low in the general population.

Only three fatalities in more than 100 000 exercise tests occurred on steps, cycle ergometers, and treadmills in apparently healthy persons and heart disease patients.[6] Based upon a survey of over 500 000 exercise tests at more than 1000 facilities, only 1.0 deaths occurred per 20 000 tests; about 9 complications (total of MI, serious arrhythmias, and deaths) occurred per 10 000 tests.[15] No deaths were reported in 25 862 tests by Seattle-area physicians testing both symptomatic (63 % with CHD) and asymptomatic persons in a 9-year period.[3]

The complication rates of tests supervised by certified clinical exercise physiologists are similar to physician-supervised rates; the nonphysician-supervised tests having mortality, acute MI, and ventricular fibrillation rates of 0.0, 1.42, and 1.78, respectively, per 10 000 tests.[9] Low rates in a population that includes a high-risk sample is due to the constant monitoring of the exerciser by trained personnel and to the proper application of emergency procedures. Laboratory personnel need to maintain their CPR certifications and participate in periodic rehearsals of emergencies.

References

1. American College of Sports Medicine (ACSM). (2000). *ACSM's guidelines for exercise testing and prescription* (p. 284). Baltimore: Lippincott Williams & Wilkins.
2. American College of Sports Medicine & American Heart Association. (1998). Joint position statement: Recommendations for cardiovascular screening, staffing, and emergency policies at health/fitness facilities. *Medicine & Science in Sports & Exercise, 30*(6), 1009–1018.
3. Bruce, R. A. (1981). Maximal exercise testing: Prognostic value for assessment of coronary heart disease risk. *Postgraduate Medicine, 70,* 161–168.
4. Eisenberg, M. S., Bergner, L., & Hallstrom, A. (1979). Cardiac resuscitation in the community. Importance of rapid provision and implications for program planning *JAMA: The Journal of the American Medical Association 241,* 1905–1907.

---

[a]At least two people in the laboratory should be familiar with cardiopulmonary resuscitation (CPR) techniques; one of these may be familiar with basic life support (BLS) and the other should be familiar with advanced cardiac life support (ACLS).

5. Gibbons, L. W., Blair, S. N., Kohl, H. W., & Cooper, K. H. (1989). The safety of maximal exercise testing. *Circulation, 80,* 846–852.

6. Hornsten, T. R., & Bruce, R. A. (1986). Stress testing, safety precautions, and cardiovascular health. *Journal of Occupational Medicine, 10,* 640–648.

7. Isaacs, L. D., & Pohlman, R. (1998). *Preparing for the health fitness instructor certification examination.* Champaign, IL: Human Kinetics.

8. Jopke, T. (1981). Choosing an exercise testing protocol. *The Physician and Sportsmedicine, 9*(3), 141–146.

9. Knight, J. A., Laubach, C. A., Butcher, R. J., & Menapace, F. J. (1995). Supervision of clinical exercise testing by exercise physiologists. *American Journal of Cardiology, 75,* 390–391.

10. National Conference on Cardiopulmonary Resuscitation (CPR) and Emergency Cardiac Care (ECC). (1986). Standards and guidelines for cardiopulmonary resuscitation (CPR) and emergency cardiac care (ECC). *JAMA: The Journal of the American Medical Association, 255,* 2905–2989.

11. Peterson, J. A., & Tharrett, S. J. (1997). *ACSM's Health/Fitness Facility Standards and Guidelines,* (2nd ed. p. 33). Champaign, IL: Human Kinetics.

12. Sheffield, L. T., Holt, J. H., & Reeves, T. J. (1965). Exercise graded by heart rate in electrocardiographic testing for angina pectoris. *Circulation 32,* 622–628.

13. Starr, L. M. (2000). AED use in your club. *Fitness Management, 16*(13), 40–44.

14. Stoike, P. J. (2001). Automated external defibrillators. *ACSM's Health & Fitness Journal, 5*(4), 20–26.

15. Stuart, R. J., & Ellestad, M. H. 1980. National survey of exercise stress testing facilities. *Chest, 77*(1), 94–97.

16. Valenzuela, T. D., Roe, D. J., Nichol, G. et al. (2000). Outcomes of rapid defibrillation by security officers after cardiac arrest in casinos. *New England Journal of Medicine, 343,* 1206–1209.

REPORTING UNITS AND SYMBOLS

In addition to those presented in Chapter 2, the following units and symbols are noted here along with some general comments. Some symbols, such as approximately (≈), middle dot (·), and equal to or greater than (≥) are not discerned by observing the computer keyboard. In such cases, a diligent search through the symbol tables on the computer's word processor usually uncovers these symbols.

The American Heart Association Task Force on Blood Pressure (1987) has not adopted the SI-approved kilopascals as the unit of measure for blood pressure, thus retaining the mm Hg metric unit.[2] When referring to pressure inside the body, such as for blood pressure or dissolved gases, mm Hg units are acceptable in the United States. When referring to pressures outside the body, such as atmospheric pressures, pascals is the International System's (SI) approved unit of measure.[3]

The symbol for the *micro* unit is not found in some computers; thus, the symbol u is an acceptable replacement (e.g., uV = microvolt).

A number expressed by a negative exponent (e.g., $^{-1}$) is equal to the reciprocal of that number (e.g., 1/10) raised to the respective positive power. The following are examples:

1. $10^{-1} = 1/10$; $10^{-2} = 1/100$
2. $mL \times kg^{-1} = mL \times 1/kg = mL/kg = mL \cdot kg^{-1}$
3. $9.9 \times 10^{-6} = 0.0000099$; decimal moved 6 places to left
4. $1.2 \times 10^{6} = 1\ 200\ 000$; decimal moved 6 places to the right

The International System[3] does not approve the hyphenation of a unit. Thus, scientific writers are discouraged from making such descriptives as "a 54-kg woman" or "a 3-L syringe."

The Exponential law of half-life is defined as the time it takes for half of the substance to disintegrate, deplete, or decay.

Avogadro's (A.D. 1776–A.D. 1856) number is the number of molecules in a mole of any substance: 6.02217×10^{23}. At standard temperature and pressure (STP), one mole of any gas occupies a volume of 22.414 L.

The International Unit (IU) is a measure of biological activity, not mass or volume. IU is sometimes used for vitamins, but it is slowly disappearing in usage.

Although the term *subjects* is acceptable when discussing statistics, scientific writers are encouraged to replace *subjects* with more personal terms, such as *participants, performers,* and *persons.*[1]

The style for the citations in the reference lists of *Exercise Physiology Laboratory Manual* is from the *Publication Manual of the American Psychological Association* (APA).[1] The citations, however, are numbered rather than presented with authors' names. The numbering system is not APA style but is common for various scientific journals (e.g., *Medicine and Science in Sports and Exercise*).

References

1. American Psychological Association. (2001). *Publication manual of the American Psychological Association.* (5th ed.) Washington, DC: Author.
2. Frohlich, E. D., Grim, C., Labarthe, D. R., Maxwell, M. H., Perloff, D., & Weidman, W. H. (1987). *Recommendations for human blood pressure determination by sphygmomanometers: Report of a special task force appointed by the steering committee, American Heart Association.* Dallas: National Center, American Heart Association.
3. Taylor, B. N. (1995). *NIST special publication 811, 1995 edition: Guide for the use of the International System of Units (SI).* Gaithersburg, MD: United States Department of Commerce. National Institute of Standards and Technology.

Most of the problems presented here may be solved in more than one way. These different approaches to the same problem may sometimes produce small differences in the answers. Also, differences may be produced due to differences in rounding off the various conversion factors. These differences are small enough to be of little practical significance in most exercise physiology laboratory classes.

Before starting any calculations, students are encouraged to guess the answer. Guessing will prevent making obvious errors, such as in the placing of the decimal point, and will force metric thinking and visualization.

1. How tall in centimeters and meters is a six-footer?

    6 ft × 12 in. = 72 in.

    2.54 cm = 1 in.

    Therefore: 2.54 cm × 72 in. = 182.88 cm = 182.9 cm

    = 1.83 m

    Optional solutions:

    a. 1 ft = 0.3048 m; 0.3048 m × 6 = 1.83 m (183 cm)
    b. 72 ÷ 0.3937 = 182.9 cm

2. 160 lb = ? kg

    1 kg = 2.2 lb; therefore: 160 ÷ 2.2 = 72.7 kg

    Option: 1 lb = 0.454 kg; thus 0.454 × 160 = 72.6 kg

3. A person loads 200 crates weighing 30 lb each into a truck bed that is 3 ft above the location of the crates. What is the total positive work in N·m and joules?

    + w = F × D; F = 30 lb ÷ 2.2 = 13.6 kg = 136 N

    D in meters = (200 lifts × 3 ft × 0.3048) = 183 m;

    $^+$w = 183 m × 136 N = 24 888 N·m = 24 888 J or

    24.89 kJ

4. Suppose the task in problem 3 takes 20 min. What is the rate of the work (power) in N·m·min^{-1} and watts?

    P = w / t = 24 888 N·m ÷ 20 min

    = 1244 N·m·min^{-1} = 20.7 N·m·s^{-1} = 20.7 W

5. A person with a body mass of 120 lb walks from an elevation of 900 ft to 3400 ft. How much positive work ($^+$w) was accomplished in this ascent?

    $^+$w = F × D; D = 3400 ft – 900 ft = 2500 ft

    1 m = 3.28 ft; thus, 2500 ft ÷ 3.28 = 762 m

    120 lb ÷ 2.2 = 54.5 kg = 545 N

    545 N × 762 m = 415 290 N·m or 415 290 J

    or 415.3 kJ

    Option: 1 ft = 0.3048 m; thus, 0.3048 × 2500 ft

    = 762 m

    Option: 1 lb = 0.454 kg; thus, 0.454 × 120 = 54.5 kg

    = 545 N

6. In problem 5, the return descent resulted in how much negative (eccentric) work?

    [assumes negative work ($^-$w) = 1/3 positive work ($^+$w)]

    $^-$w = 415 290 N·m ÷ 3 = 138 430 N·m = 138 430 J

    = 138.4 kJ

7. During the 1.5 mile run test, a person consumes 35 L of oxygen. How many kcal are burned?

    L $\dot{V}O_2$ = 5 kcal; thus, 35 L × 5 = 175 kcal

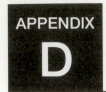

INFORMED CONSENT FOR PARTICIPATING IN EXERCISE PHYSIOLOGY LABORATORY

Explanation of the Graded (Progressive) Exercise Test

You will perform a graded exercise test on a cycle ergometer and/or treadmill. The exercise intensity will increase each 2 to 4 minutes. Depending on your heart rate or other symptoms and variables, you may continue to work harder or the test will end. We may stop the test at any time because of signs of fatigue or discomfort. Also, you may stop the test for any reason at any time.

Explanation of Other Tests

You will also perform several other tests, including evaluations of your muscular strength, anaerobic power, body composition, pulmonary function, blood pressure, and flexibility.

Risks and Discomforts

The possibility does exist that certain changes will occur during the graded exercise test. They include abnormal blood pressure, fainting, disorders of heart beat, and in very rare instances heart attack or death. Every effort will be made to minimize the risk of these changes through preliminary screening and by observation during the testing. Emergency procedures and trained laboratory personnel are available to deal with any unusual situations that may arise. All of the other tests involve minimal risk but could result in muscle strains, respiratory difficulties, and light headedness. Psychological distress is possible when performing these tests in front of your student peers and the instructor. Although informed consents contain statements indicating the confidentiality of test results, this Consent for Participating in Exercise Physiology Laboratory states that not only is it difficult in an instructional setting to keep test data confidential but confidentiality may minimize learning. Discussing freely the individual and group data enhances the visualization, personalization, and retention of information. Therefore, confidentiality cannot be guaranteed in most instances.

Please inform the instructor of your present health status, medications, or former symptoms of concern associated with the tests mentioned within this Informed Consent, Course Syllabus (Outline), or *Exercise Physiology Laboratory Manual*. Symptoms of special importance are those related to your heart, such as pain in the chest, neck, jaw, back, and arms, or shortness of breath. Report symptoms immediately upon their occurrence during the test. The Physical Activity Readiness Questionnaire (PAR-Q) form is a popular questionnaire that can guide you and the laboratory personnel toward a safe test.

Benefits to Be Expected

The results obtained from the graded exercise test and related tests will assist in the assessment of your current level of physical fitness. You will learn how it feels to perform these tests and how to administer them, in addition to learning how to interpret them.

Inquiries

Any questions about the procedures used in the exercise tests are encouraged. If you have any doubts or questions, please ask us for further explanations.

Freedom of Consent

Your permission to perform the tests is voluntary. We will work together toward making an effort to find a substitute assignment for any of the tests in which you do not feel comfortable in performing.

"I have read this form and I understand the test procedures that I will perform. I freely consent to participate voluntarily in all of the described laboratory tests."

_____   _____
(Signature of Participant)   (Date)

_____   _____
(Witness)   (Date)

PAR - Q & YOU

(A Questionnaire for People Aged 15 to 69)

Regular physical activity is fun and healthy, and increasingly more people are starting to become more active every day. Being more active is very safe for most people. However, some people should check with their doctor before they start becoming much more physically active.

If you are planning to become much more physically active than you are now, start by answering the seven questions in the box below. If you are between the ages of 15 and 69, the PAR-Q will tell you if you should check with your doctor before you start. If you are over 69 years of age, and you are not used to being very active, check with your doctor.

Common sense is your best guide when you answer these questions. Please read the questions carefully and answer each one honestly: check YES or NO.

YES	NO		
☐	☐	1.	Has your doctor ever said that you have a heart condition <u>and</u> that you should only do physical activity recommended by a doctor?
☐	☐	2.	Do you feel pain in your chest when you do physical activity?
☐	☐	3.	In the past month, have you had chest pain when you were not doing physical activity?
☐	☐	4.	Do you lose your balance because of dizziness or do you ever lose consciousness?
☐	☐	5.	Do you have a bone or joint problem that could be made worse by a change in your physical activity?
☐	☐	6.	Is your doctor currently prescribing drugs (for example, water pills) for your blood pressure or heart condition?
☐	☐	7.	Do you know of <u>any other reason</u> why you should not do physical activity?

If you answered

YES to one or more questions

Talk with your doctor by phone or in person BEFORE you start becoming much more physically active or BEFORE you have a fitness appraisal. Tell your doctor about the PAR-Q and which questions you answered YES.

- You may be able to do any activity you want — as long as you start slowly and build up gradually. Or, you may need to restrict your activities to those which are safe for you. Talk with your doctor about the kinds of activities you wish to participate in and follow his/her advice.
- Find out which community programs are safe and helpful for you.

NO to all questions

If you answered NO honestly to <u>all</u> PAR-Q questions, you can be reasonably sure that you can:

- start becoming much more physically active — begin slowly and build up gradually. This is the safest and easiest way to go.
- take part in a fitness appraisal — this is an excellent way to determine your basic fitness so that you can plan the best way for you to live actively.

DELAY BECOMING MUCH MORE ACTIVE:

- if you are not feeling well because of a temporary illness such as a cold or a fever — wait until you feel better; or
- if you are or may be pregnant — talk to your doctor before you start becoming more active.

Please note: If your health changes so that you then answer YES to any of the above questions, tell your fitness or health professional. Ask whether you should change your physical activity plan.

<u>Informed Use of the PAR-Q</u>: The Canadian Society for Exercise Physiology, Health Canada, and their agents assume no liability for persons who undertake physical activity, and if in doubt after completing this questionnaire, consult your doctor prior to physical activity.

You are encouraged to copy the PAR-Q but only if you use the entire form

NOTE: If the PAR-Q is being given to a person before he or she participates in a physical activity program or a fitness appraisal, this section may be used for legal or administrative purposes.

I have read, understood and completed this questionnaire. Any questions I had were answered to my full satisfaction.

NAME _____

SIGNATURE _____ DATE _____

SIGNATURE OF PARENT _____ WITNESS _____
or GUARDIAN (for participants under the age of majority)

continued on other side...

© *Canadian Society for Exercise Physiology*
Société canadienne de physiologie de l'exercice

Supported by: Health   Santé
Canada   Canada

PAR-Q form. Reprinted with permission from the Canadian Society for Exercise Physiology, Inc., 1994.

PAR - Q & YOU

We know that being physically active provides benefits for all of us. Not being physically active is recognized by the Heart and Stroke Foundation of Canada as one of the four modifiable primary risk factors for coronary heart disease (along with high blood pressure, high blood cholesterol, and smoking). People are physically active for many reasons — play, work, competition, health, creativity, enjoying the outdoors, being with friends. There are also as many ways of being active as there are reasons. What we choose to do depends on our own abilities and desires. No matter what the reason or type of activity, physical activity can improve our well-being and quality of life. Well-being can also be enhanced by integrating physical activity with enjoyable healthy eating and positive self and body image. Together, all three equal VITALITY. So take a fresh approach to living. Check out the VITALITY tips below!

Active Living:

- accumulate 30 minutes or more of moderate physical activity most days of the week
- take the stairs instead of an elevator
- get off the bus early and walk home
- join friends in a sport activity
- take the dog for a walk with the family
- follow a fitness program

Healthy Eating:

- follow Canada's Food Guide to Healthy Eating
- enjoy a variety of foods
- emphasize cereals, breads, other grain products, vegetables and fruit
- choose lower-fat dairy products, leaner meats and foods prepared with little or no fat
- achieve and maintain a healthy body weight by enjoying regular physical activity and healthy eating
- limit salt, alcohol and caffeine
- don't give up foods you enjoy — aim for moderation and variety

Positive Self and Body Image:

- accept who you are and how you look
- remember, a healthy weight range is one that is realistic for your own body make-up (body fat levels should neither be too high nor too low)
- try a new challenge
- compliment yourself
- reflect positively on your abilities
- laugh a lot

Enjoy eating well, being active and feeling good about yourself. That's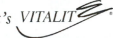

FITNESS AND HEALTH PROFESSIONALS MAY BE INTERESTED IN THE INFORMATION BELOW.

The following companion forms are available for doctors' use by contacting the Canadian Society for Exercise Physiology (address below):

The **Physical Activity Readiness Medical Examination (PARmed-X)** - to be used by doctors with people who answer YES to one or more questions on the PAR-Q.

The **Physical Activity Readiness Medical Examination for Pregnancy (PARmed-X for PREGNANCY)** - to be used by doctors with pregnant patients who wish to become more active.

References:
Arraix, G.A., Wigle, D.T., Mao, Y. (1992). Risk Assessment of Physical Activity and Physical Fitness in the Canada Health Survey Follow-Up Study. **J. Clin. Epidemiol.** 45:4 419-428.
Mottola, M., Wolfe, L.A. (1994). Active Living and Pregnancy, In: A. Quinney, L. Gauvin, T. Wall (eds.), **Toward Active Living: Proceedings of the International Conference on Physical Activity, Fitness and Health**. Champaign, IL: Human Kinetics.
PAR-Q Validation Report, British Columbia Ministry of Health, 1978.
Thomas, S., Reading, J., Shephard, R.J. (1992). Revision of the Physical Activity Readiness Questionnaire (PAR-Q). **Can. J. Spt. Sci.** 17:4 338-345.

To order multiple printed copies of the PAR-Q, please contact the

Canadian Society for Exercise Physiology
1600 James Naismith Dr., Suite 311
Gloucester, Ontario CANADA K1B 5N4
Tel. (613) 748-5768 FAX: (613) 748-5763

The original PAR-Q was developed by the British Columbia Ministry of Health. It has been revised by an Expert Advisory Committee assembled by the Canadian Society for Exercise Physiology and Fitness Canada (1994).

Disponible en français sous le titre «Questionnaire sur l'aptitude à l'activité physique - Q-AAP (revisé 1994)».

© Canadian Society for Exercise Physiology
Société canadienne de physiologie de l'exercice

Supported by: Health   Santé
Canada   Canada

Index

METRIC–AMERICAN CONVERSIONS

Length

1 m = 39.370 in. = 3.281 ft = 1.0936 yd
1 cm = 0.3937 in.
1 mm = 0.03937 in.
1 km = 0.62137 mile
1 in. = 2.54 cm = 25.4 mm = 0.0254 m
1 ft = 0.3048 m
1 yd = 0.914 m = 91.44 cm
1 mile = 1609.35 m = 1.609 km

Mass (M) or Weight (Wt)

1 kg = 2.2046 lb
1 g = 0.0022 lb = 0.0352 oz
1 lb = 453.59 g = 0.454 kg
1 oz = 28.3495 g

Force (F)

1 kg = 9.80665 N
1 N = 0.10197 kg = 0.2248 lb

Volume (V)

1 L = 1.0567 US qt (1 US qt and 1 US gal are > 1 Imperial qt
   and gal)
1 mL = 1 cm^3 (1 cc)^a = 0.03381 fluid oz = 0.061 cu in.
1 US qt = 0.9464 L
1 US gal = 3.785 L
1 cup liquid = 250 mL
1 tablespoon = 15 mL
1 teaspoon = 5 mL

Work (w) and Energy (E)

1 N·m = 1 J = 0.7375 ft·lb
1 kg·m = 9.80665 J = 7.2307 ft–lb
1 ft·lb = 0.1383 kg·m = 1.3559 N·m
1 kJ = 0.239 kcal
1 kcal = 4186 J = 4.186 kJ
1 kcal = 426.85 kg·m at 100 % efficiency
1 J = 1 N·m 0.10197 kg·m
1 L $\dot{V}O_2$ ≈ 21 kJ at R of 1.0

Velocity (v)

1 m·s^{-1} = 2.2371 miles per hour (mph)
1 m·min^{-1} = 0.03728 mph
1 km·h^{-1} = 0.6215 mph
1 mph = 26.822 m·min^{-1} = 1.6093 km·h^{-1} = 0.4470 m·s^{-1}
       = 1.4667 ft·s^{-1}

Radial Velocity

1 rad·s^{-1} = 57.3°·s^{-1}
rad = radian = 57.3°
1° = 0.01745 rad
Π = 3.1416 = ratio of the circumference of a circle to its
    diameter.

Power (P)

1 W = 1 J·s^{-1} = 60 J·min^{-1} = 0.060 kJ·min^{-1} = 60 N·m·min^{-1}
      = 6.12 kg·m·min^{-1} = 0.1019 kg·m·s^{-1}
1 kW = 1000 W = 1.34 horsepower (hp)
1 kg·m·min^{-1} = 0.1635 W = 0.000219 hp
1 hp = 745.7 W = 745.7 J·s^{-1} = 75 kg·m·s^{-1}
      =4562 kg·m·min^{-1} = 10.688 kcal·min^{-1}

Acceleration (a)

a of gravity (g) = 9.81 m·s^{-2} = 32.2 ft·s^{-2}

Temperature (T)

each °C = 1 K = 1.8 °F
each °F = 0.56 °C = 0.56 K

Pressure

1 pascal (Pa) = 1 N·m^{-2}
Barometric Pressure (P$_B$): 1 in. Hg = 25.4 torr = 25.4 mm Hg
29.92 in. Hg = 760 mm Hg = 1 atmosphere (atm)
            = 14.7 lb/in^2 = 101 325 Pa = 1013 hPa
1 mbar = 0.750 mm Hg = 0.750 torr = 1 hPa
1 mm Hg = 1.333 mbar = 1.333 hPa

---

^{a}cc is not an SI-approved unit of measure

Looking for more resources on exercise physiology?

Check out any of these McGraw-Hill textbooks:

- *Exercise Physiology: Human Bioenergetics and Its Applications*, Third Edition
  By George A. Brooks, Thomas D. Fahey, Timothy P. White, and
  Kenneth M. Baldwin
  ISBN 0–7674–1024–6

- *Fox's Physiological Basis for Exercise and Sport* with Study Guide, Dynamic
  Human CD-ROM, and PowerWeb: Health & Human Performance, Sixth Edition
  By Steven J. Keteyian and Merle L. Foss
  ISBN 0–07–250958–2

- *Exercise Physiology: Theory and Application to Fitness and Performance* with
  e-Text and PowerWeb: Health & Human Performance, Fourth Edition
  By Scott K. Powers and Edward T. Howley
  ISBN 0–07–235551–4

- *Fundamental Principles of Exercise Physiology: For Fitness, Performance, and
  Health* with PowerWeb: Health & Human Performance
  By Robert A. Robergs and Scott O. Roberts
  ISBN 0–07–246704–5

To learn more...

For additional resources, check out McGraw-Hill's Health & Human Performance
discipline page at **www.mhhe.com/hhp**

New copies of this book come with a free passcard for PowerWeb, a
comprehensive website that gives you a database of current
articles, sport news, study tips, and other great features. Go to
www.dushkin.com/powerweb to get started now!

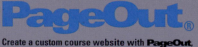

Create a custom course website with **PageOut**,
free to instructors using a McGraw-Hill textbook.

To learn more, contact your McGraw-Hill publisher's
representative or visit www.mhhe.com/solutions.

Create a custom course website with PageOut®,
free to instructors who use a McGraw-Hill
textbook in any of their courses. To learn more,
contact your McGraw-Hill representative or visit
www.mhhe.com/solutions

McGraw-Hill Higher Education
A Division of The *McGraw-Hill* Companies

ISBN 0-07-232903-3

9 780072 329032

www.mhhe.com